THE CASE MANAGER'S SURVIVAL GUIDE

WINNING STRATEGIES IN THE NEW HEALTHCARE ENVIRONMENT

THIRD EDITION

TONI G. CESTA, PhD, RN, FAAN
Partner and Consultant
Case Management Concepts, LLC.
North Bellmore, New York

HUSSEIN M. TAHAN, PhD, RN
System Vice President
Nursing Professional Development and Workforce Planning
MedStar Health
Columbia, Maryland

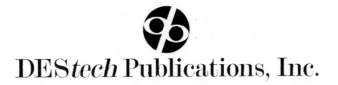

DEStech Publications, Inc.

The Case Manager's Survival Guide

DEStech Publications, Inc.
439 North Duke Street
Lancaster, Pennsylvania 17602 U.S.A.

Printed in the United States of America
10 9 8 7 6 5 4 3 2 1

Main entry under title:
The Case Manager's Survival Guide: Winning Strategies in the New Healthcare Environment, Third Edition

A DEStech Publications book
Bibliography: p.
Includes index p. 503

Library of Congress Control Number: 2016941267
ISBN No. 978-1-60595-288-8

HOW TO ORDER THIS BOOK

BY PHONE: 877-500-4337 or 717-290-1660, 9AM–5PM Eastern Time

BY FAX: 717-509-6100

BY MAIL: Order Department
DEStech Publications, Inc.
439 North Duke Street
Lancaster, PA 17602, U.S.A.

BY CREDIT CARD: American Express, VISA, MasterCard, Discover

BY WWW SITE: http://www.destechpub.com

Table of Contents

v

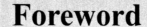

Foreword

As healthcare spending continues to rise, quality of care is questioned, and consumers strive to take a more active role in their health and healthcare, payers and providers have an urgent mission to address. They must find specific ways to control costs, address quality gaps, stem the tide of chronic diseases, and deliver care that meets the needs, but more importantly the goals, of each consumer they serve in an efficient manner.

No one person can tackle these challenges alone, but a fully engaged collaborative team can. Organizations must educate and empower their teams to work together. These collaborative teams work toward a common goal that meets the demands placed on quality, outcomes, and patient satisfaction that will impact their organizational goals and survivability.

The professional case manager is the one objective member of the team who can bring together the various professionals who make up today's interdisciplinary healthcare team to address cost, quality, safety, and access: the four pillars of a successful healthcare organization or system.

The role of the case manager is to identify patients (consumers) who are at increased risk, work to break down barriers that impact their ability to manage their own health and healthcare, and ensure they have the resources to meet their individual needs. To be effective, case managers must always have their "finger on the pulse" and be able to address challenges that come from various stakeholders, including the consumer, in a creative and knowledgeable manner.

Professional case managers must be clinically competent, understand the changing dynamics of the healthcare system, be patient and family centered, and be able to communicate effectively with each member of the healthcare team, especially patients and their caregivers.

The Case Manger's Survival Guide: Winning Strategies in the New Healthcare Environment by Toni G. Cesta and Hussein M. Tahan delivers a resource that each member of the interdisciplinary care team can use to gain insight into what effective case management is and how it should be delivered irrespective of the setting.

The authors share their collective expertise as clinicians but also as leaders in the profession of case management in this comprehensive textbook that should be on every case manager's shelf. They challenge case managers to take their place at the table to ensure the consumer is the central member of the team and has a voice in all aspects of their own care.

Through their writings, the authors provide information that will educate and empower readers with tools and strategies to improve their practice and to achieve the outcomes necessary to remain relevant in today's dynamic and competitive healthcare system.

This textbook is to be used by leaders in healthcare as they redesign systems to meet regulatory, accreditation, and reimbursement challenges that providers and payers face as we move into an accountable care environment where value replaces volume.

This textbook is a valuable resource to those new to the profession of case management as well as those currently in the practice. Healthcare is changing with new care models replacing existing ones to contain cost and improve the quality of care.

This textbook provides essential information that each professional can use to meet the industry's demands. The material will strengthen case management programs and provide organizations with ways to prove their value through the outcomes produced. It serves as an educational tool for academics and professionals involved in continuing education charged with clarifing what case management is and what case management can be.

This textbook also provides a resource that directors and supervisors of case management programs can use to reinforce the fundamentals of the practice to experienced case managers and introduce concepts as new professionals move into the the practice of case management.

As a leader in the practice of case management, I know you will find this textbook a great investment to help you understand and address the challenges you face in the exciting yet disruptive world of today's healthcare system. Use it well!

I would like to thank the authors for asking me to write the Foreword for *The Case Manager's Survival Guide: Winning Strategies in the New Healthcare Environment*. It is an honor for me as a case management leader and someone who has recently experienced first-hand how the healthcare system works or rather does not work.

I thank Toni and Hussein for pouring their passion and expertise into this textbook. It is our hope the information provided on each page improves the care delivered to each patient who enters the complex healthcare system through your practice of case management.

Anne Llewellyn, RN-BC, MS, BHSA, CCM, CRRN
Nurse Advocate

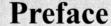

Preface

It has been ten years since we published the last edition of the *"Case Manager's Survival Guide: Winning Strategies for Clinical Practice."* So much has changed in the field of case management, the Medicare and Medicaid benefit programs, and the U.S. healthcare delivery system in general. Terms like coordination and transitions of care and the healthcare continuum have become common parts of the language of healthcare. Bundled payments, accountable care organizations, and the patient experience of care have driven the increased need for case management across the continuum, today and going forward.

It is without a doubt that case management is one of the strategic interventions that is most needed to assist healthcare organizations and providers in balancing the quality of the care they provide to patients and their support systems with the reimbursement they receive. It is also without a doubt that case managers are necessary at every level of care across the continuum. And finally, it is without a doubt that case managers must communicate and transition patients across care settings and providers with a critical eye on quality, safety, care experience, and cost.

It is for these reasons that we have written the third edition of the "Survival Guide." We have heard from

you, our readers, our students and our colleagues, and we have responded with our most comprehensive textbook yet. Building on the first two editions and adding ten years worth of updates have resulted in a textbook that takes you, the reader, from the beginnings of our wonderful specialty profession to the present day and beyond. We feel that it is also time to update the title so that it is consistent with the changing healthcare landscape. We therefore have chosen *"The Case Manager's Survival Guide: Winning Strategies in the New Healthcare Environment."* We believe that this title better reflects the third edition's focus on the new world of healthcare that we live in.

As with our other editions, this one combines practical knowledge with a theoretical framework that allows each reader to take from it the specific components they believe they need to enhance their own work and performance as case managers, interdisciplinary healthcare team members, and colleagues. As always, we hope that you find the "Survival Guide" useful in the ways we designed it; ultimately it is our goal to contribute to the improvement of patient care wherever our patients may seek it.

We hope you enjoy reading this textbook as much as we have enjoyed writing it!

Toni G. Cesta, PhD, RN, FAAN
Hussein M. Tahan, PhD, RN

1

Introduction to Case Management

If you have purchased or borrowed this book, you must be a case manager, or you are thinking of becoming one. If you are *already working* in the field, you are probably beginning to experience many of the conflicts and confusions that come with this role. If you are *thinking of becoming* a case manager, you are probably reading as much as you can about this delivery system and the role you will play in it.

Because case management is relatively new to many nurses and social workers, it may be difficult to find other nurses working with you or colleagues who have been case managers. Although there are tens of thousands of case managers across the country, there may not be many in your organization or your part of the country. This book is written with you in mind. Although the book's overall objective is to provide comprehensive information on the role of the case manager and on case management, its format is designed so that it is a ready reference for the on-the-job questions and issues you may face every day.

The case management process is often an intangible one—a behind-the-scenes process and outcomes role that is, at its worst, very stressful and, at its best, very rewarding. The role is complex and eclectic. Not for the meek or mild, it requires confidence and comprehension of a vast array of topics, many of which are reviewed in this book.

Although case management has become somewhat of a household word in healthcare, there is still a tremendous amount of confusion about what it is, how it applies to various settings, how its success can be measured, and what the role of the case manager is (Box 1.1). As a profession, we have yet to answer all of these questions consistently. There are core components of

---

Box 1.1 Commonly Asked Questions About Case Management

1. What is it?
2. How does it apply to various healthcare settings?
3. How can its success be measured?
4. What is the role of the case manager?

---

the model and of the case manager role that can be taken and applied in a variety of ways. The objective is to find what works best for you and your organization without losing the essence of case management.

1.1. USING THIS GUIDE

The purpose of this book is to provide the hands-on information you will need to be an effective and successful case manager. This book contains a lot of information that can be used in the study of case management and in the implementation of case management models. To be a successful case manager you need to understand the role itself, but you also need to understand how case management fits into the bigger pictures of healthcare delivery, healthcare reform, and the future of healthcare. Pick up this book whenever you have a general or specific question. Use it as a ready reference as you develop your expertise in case management.

Broad topics are addressed, and their specific implementation techniques and strategies follow. It is important to understand both the concepts and their application. We suggest that you review both.

1.2. HEALTHCARE INDUSTRY UNDER HEALTHCARE REFORM

The healthcare industry continues to be in crisis—a chronic crisis of epic proportion, and brought about by many factors (Box 1.2). Both the prospective payment system and managed care infiltration have necessitated a reassessment of the industry's work, how it is organized, and how it is evaluated. Healthcare reform has now added to the need for reassessment of the business of healthcare. The process of getting reform in healthcare was a long one taking over 20 years. Reform was a major issue for the presidency of Bill Clinton. The first program of reform introduced by Hillary Clinton in 1993 was not enacted into law. During the Bush administration, several acts introduced were aimed at reducing the overall growth of healthcare costs. Other programs looked at proposals to guarantee access to coverage in the individual health insurance market and for improving the quality and safety of the U.S. healthcare system. These programs continued to be debated through the 2008 presidential election by candidates McCain and Obama.

The game changer came in 2009 when the Congressional Budget Office (CBO) issued a preliminary analysis for the Patient Protection and Affordable Care Act. The CBO estimated the 10-year cost to the federal government of the major insurance-related provisions of the bill to be approximately $1 trillion (Congressional Budget Office, 2009.) It also provided for a reduction in the number of uninsured by about 16 million people. After President Obama was inaugurated, he announced his intent to work with Congress to construct a plan for healthcare reform. The Senate developed its own proposals while the House of Representatives worked on the Patient Protection and Affordable Care Act. After debate in both the Senate and the House, and after many versions of the bill, it was finally voted into law on March 23, 2010. The amended bill was titled The Health Care and Education Reconciliation Act.

The Health Care and Education Reconciliation Act ensures that all Americans have access to quality, affordable health insurance and puts students ahead of private banks. The CBO has determined that together these two bills are fully paid for and will ensure more than 94% of Americans have access to quality, affordable healthcare, will bend the healthcare cost curve, and will reduce the deficit by $143 billion over 10 years with further deficit reduction in the following decade.

1.3. VALUE-BASED PURCHASING

Value-based purchasing has added another significant change to the business of healthcare. The Centers for Medicare and Medicaid Services (CMS) have instituted linkages between cost and quality through value-based purchasing and other cost-saving measures such as payment penalties for high readmission rates. These changes have created the first links between the cost and quality of healthcare. Many hospitals and health systems are now testing bundled payment methods and accountable care organizational structures which will be discussed in Chapter 2. While the entire act does not directly relate to case management, many of its elements do, whether directly or indirectly. The changing demographics of the patient population have forced us to re-examine our values and our expectations or expected outcomes of the work we perform particularly as they relate to patient care. These changes have come about as a result of an aging patient population with a concomitant increase in chronic illnesses and a more educated patient as the consumer of healthcare. Technology, including medical informatics, has driven up the cost of healthcare. The advent of the electronic medical record has been a positive change for the healthcare industry, but one that has resulted in higher cost. It is hoped that eventually these hardwired electronic processes will reduce errors and associated costs due to these errors in the following ways:

- Improve care quality, safety, efficiency, and reduce health disparities
  —Quality and safety measurement
  —Clinical decision support (automated advice) for providers

---

Box 1.2 Factors Affecting the Healthcare Industry

1. Changes in healthcare reimbursement
2. Increases in auditing by the Centers for Medicare and Medicaid Services
3. Links between cost and quality of care
4. An aging patient population
5. Over-crowded emergency departments
6. Continuosly rising costs
7. Shortages of some types of providers
8. Increasingly complex and chronic illnesses
9. Lack of coordination across the continuum of care
10. Technology, including advances in surgical procedures such as robotics and minimally invasive surgery
11. Information technology such as electronic medical records and physician order entry
12. Educated patients as consumers of healthcare

—Patient registries (e.g., "a directory of patients with diabetes")
■ Improve care coordination
■ Engage patients and families in their care
■ Improve population and public health
—Electronic laboratory reporting for reportable conditions (hospitals)
—Immunization reporting to immunization registries
—Syndromic surveillance (health event awareness)
■ Ensure adequate privacy and security protections (Centers for Medicare and Medicaid Services, 2011)

In 2015 hospitals began to receive financial penalties for not using electronic medical records as required by the Health Information Technology for Economic and Clinical Health (HITECH) Act of 2009.

Complex, high-tech and minimally invasive surgery; expensive, life-prolonging treatments such as kidney dialysis; costly antibiotics; computerization; and the need for more and more durable medical equipment to support the care and recuperation of the elderly and the chronically ill have all contributed to escalating costs as we have never seen before.

In recent years, emergency departments have become overcrowded and congested resulting in patient flow, safety, and quality of care issues. As the CMS have moved to different payment methods, negative issues surrounding coordination of care across the continuum have become more obvious. Lack of coordination across the continuum haved affected readmission rates, cost of care, quality, and patient satisfaction, and have required new analysis and interventions of care coordination. While coordination of care has always been a foundational role of case management, it has only become part of the vernacular of health care in recent years.

The frenzy of activity going on in every healthcare setting across the country is an indicator of the need to bring massive and significant change to the industry. Many of the changes involve cost-cutting efforts that many criticize as compromising the quality of care. Managed care is one change that has been consistently criticized for its cost-cutting approach that has appeared to be less concerned with quality of care (Curtin, 1996; Kongstvedt, 2001). Other changes are intended to control both cost and quality. Case management is one such effort. It is designed to manage care, which results in a monitoring and control of resources and cost regarding management of the resources applied and the cost of the care. It is also de-

signed to be an outcomes model, and it has, as part of its methodology, a close monitoring of the products of the care it manages and their effects on the patient and family. Case management is not equivalent to managed care. They are not interchangeable concepts or phrases. Whereas managed care is a system of cost-containment programs, case management is a process of care delivery sometimes used within the managed care system.

1.4. HISTORY OF CASE MANAGEMENT

Case management is not a new concept. It has been around for more than 90 years (Box 1.3). As a means of providing care, it originated in the 1920s out of the fields of psychiatry and social work and focused on long-term, chronic illnesses that were managed in the outpatient, community-based settings. Case management processes were also used by visiting nurses in the 1930s. The original public health nursing models used community-based case management approaches in their care of patients (Knollmueller, 1989). As a care delivery system, case management is a relatively new concept to the acute care setting, having developed and flourished in the mid-1980s. Between the 1930s and the 1980s the model remained essentially in the community setting. It was not until the introduction of the prospective payment system that the model shifted to the acute care, hospital-based setting.

1.4.1. Definition of Case Management

Whether case management is being applied in the acute care, community, or long-term care setting, its underlying principles and goals are consistent. As a system for providing patient care, case management is designed to ensure that quality care is provided in the most cost-effective manner possible. This is accomplished by improving the processes of care delivery, making these processes more efficient and effective. Other strategies involved include the management of product and personnel resources. By better administration and control over the ways in which care is provided and the resources used, outcomes can be achieved while ensuring that quality is maintained or improved.

There are a variety of definitions of case management, including the following:

■ "A collaborative process of assessment, planning, facilitation and advocacy for options and services to meet an individual's health needs through communication and available resources to promote quality cost-effective outcomes," (CMSA, 2010).

Box 1.3   Coverage, Medicare, Medicaid, and Revenues (Finance Committee Provisions)

Coverage

- Makes plans in the Exchange more affordable by further limiting the cost of premiums and cost-sharing for individuals under 400% of poverty (a family of four with income less than $88,000). Ensures that if costs grow faster than expected, the amount of tax credits will be reduced to more closely track the overall inflation rate.
- Modifies the assessment that individuals who remain uninsured pay by exempting income below the filing threshold. The individual assessment is the greater of a flat dollar payment, which has been lowered, and a percentage of income, which has been raised, as compared to the Patient Protection and Affordable Care Act.
- Improves the employer responsibility provisions.
    - Large employer penalty cap raised from $750 per worker to $2,000 per worker.
    - Strikes the penalty for waiting periods between 60 and 90 days.
    - Counts full-time equivalents toward the threshold for triggering a penalty, but does NOT impose any penalties for part-time workers.
    - Phases in the penalties as employers become larger by discounting 30 full-time workers from the per-worker penalty, eliminating a disincentive to creating new jobs.
    - Eliminates the special rule for construction industry employers.

Medicare

- Provides a $250 rebate for beneficiaries who hit the coverage gap or "donut hole" in 2010 and fills the donut hole for brand and generic drugs by 2020.
- Reduces Medicare Advantage overpayments in a targeted way that reflects the different needs of urban and rural areas. Provides a more refined approach that varies rates by local fee-for-service costs on a sliding scale. Includes 3–7 year phase-in and increases Medicare Advantage benchmarks for high-performance plans. Ensures that Medicare Advantage plans spend at least 85% of revenue on medical costs or activities that improve quality of care.
- Lowers Medicare Disproportionate Share Hospital (DSH) cuts in the Patient Protection and Affordable Care Act from $25.1 billion to $22.1 billion and revises market basket updates to hospitals by $9.9 billion.
- Adjusts the utilization rate changes included in the Patient Protection and Affordable Care Act to take into account the Centers for Medicare and Medicaid Services imaging rule that went into effect on January 1, 2010. Sets the assumed utilization rate at 75% for the practice expense portion of advanced diagnostic imaging services.

Medicaid

- Equalizes and increases funding for the Medicaid expansion by providing 100% federal match in 2014, 2015, and 2016; 95% match in 2017; 94% match in 2018; 93% match in 2019; and 90% thereafter.
- For early expansion states, provides additional federal funding to reduce the cost of covering nonpregnant childless adults beginning in 2014. In 2019 and thereafter, all states will bear the same costs for covering nonpregnant childless adults.
- Increases payments for Medicaid primary care to Medicare rates in 2013 and 2014 and provides full federal support to do so.
- Lowers the reduction in federal Medicaid DSH payments in the Patient Protection and Affordable Care Act from $18.1 billion to $14.1 billion over 10 years.
- Increases funding for the territories by $2 billion and provides territories the option to establish an Exchange.
- Delays Community First Choice Option for one year.
- Narrows the definition of new drug formulations for purposes of applying the Medicaid drug rebate.

Fraud, Waste, and Abuse

- Establishes new requirements for community mental health centers to prevent fraud and abuse.
- Modifies Medicare prepayment medical review limitations.
- Increases funding to fight fraud, waste, and abuse by $250 million.
- Requires a 90-day period of oversight for initial claims of Durable Medical Equipment suppliers.

Revenue

- Delays implementation of the excise tax on high cost health plans until 2018; increases the thresholds for imposing the tax to $10,200 for self-only plans and $27,500 for family coverage. Adds adjustments for age and gender of enrollees.
- Delays the establishment of a $2,500 cap on FSA contributions until 2013.
- For individuals with adjusted gross income above $200,000 for a single taxpayer and $250,000 for a married couple, equalizes the Medicare contribution treatment for earned and unearned income.
- Closes the "black liquor" loophole that allows certain taxpayers to get an unintended tax credit for cellulosic biofuels.
- Establishes, in statute, the "economic substance doctrine" to prevent the use of transactions that generate tax benefits but which otherwise have no business purpose.

Higher Education Provisions Under the Finance Title

- Provides $2 billion for community colleges to develop and improve educational or career training programs.

- "A professional and collaborative process that assesses, plans, implements, coordinates, monitors, and evaluates the options and services required to meet an individual's health needs. It uses communication and available resources to promote health, quality, and cost-effective outcomes in support of the 'Triple Aim' of improving the experience of care, improving the health of populations, and reducing per capita costs of healthcare," (CCMC, 2015).

- A nursing care delivery system that supports cost-effective, patient-outcome-oriented care (Cohen and Cesta, 1997).

- A role and process that focuses on procuring, negotiating, and coordinating the care, services, and resources needed by individuals with complex issues throughout an episode or continuum (Bower and Falk, 1996).

- Case management is a system of healthcare delivery designed to facilitate achievement of expected patient outcomes within an appropriate length of stay. The goals of case management are the provision of quality healthcare along a continuum, decreased fragmentation of care across settings, enhancement of the client's quality of life, efficient utilization of patient care resources, and cost containment (American Nurses Association, 1988).

- A multidisciplinary clinical system that uses registered nurse (RN) case managers to coordinate the care for select patients across the continuum of a healthcare episode (Frink and Strassner, 1996).

- A process of care delivery that aims at managing the clinical services needed by patients ensuring appropriate resource utilization, enhancing the quality of care, and facilitating cost-effective patient care outcomes (Tahan, 1999).

1.4.2. Care Coordination

Care coordination has recently become a popular term, although different, often replacing the use of the term case management. The work of the National Quality Forum (NQF) in the mid-2000s gave rise to care coordination and legitimized its use and value for the effective management of patient care and healthcare services. However, experts argue that coordinating care is one function of case management and is integral to implementation of the case management plan of care. Care coordination is the provision of personalized, quality, and safe care to patients and their families across the continuum of health and human services. A case manager may achieve this through effective integration of services and personnel from various care settings, professional disciplines, and the optimal use of health information technology systems especially for communication and transfer/sharing of important information.

NQF (2010a, 2010b) defined care coordination as a function that helps ensure the patient's needs and preferences for health services and information sharing across people, functions, and sites are met over time. Coordination of care maximizes the value of services delivered to patients by facilitating beneficial, efficient, safe, and high-quality experiences and improved healthcare outcomes. It also identified five key domains of care coordination as follows:

1. *The healthcare "home"*: A setting or provider (e.g., practitioner, a community health center, a hospital outpatient clinic, or a physician practice) committed to organizing and coordinating care based on patients' needs, preferences, and priorities; communicating directly with patients and their families; and integrating care across settings and clinicians/practitioners.

2. *A proactive plan of care and follow-up*: A written plan that anticipates patient's needs and tracks progress toward achieving goals. It serves as a central care coordinating mechanism for all patients, families, and care team members and as a guidepost between clinician-driven care and patient self-management. It also is vital during handoffs and transitions of care, because it can serve as the main communication document between clinicians and care settings and outline elements such as the medication list, follow-up steps, identification of care problems, and resources needed.

3. *Communication*: Open and ongoing dialogue among members of the care team, the patient, and his or her family, primary care provider, and nonclinical resources in the community. This entails the care team, patient, and family agreeing upon and working within the plan of care, sharing important information, making decision, and maintaining privacy.

4. *Health information systems*: Technology systems that support patient care, patient engagement and education, communication, and performance measurement. Specifically, technology should provide a foundation for the healthcare home, such as providing important patient information to members of the care team across various stages of care and settings; support meaningful clinician-patient communication; enable timely and accurate performance measurement and improvement; and improve accessibility of the care team to critical patient health information.

5. *Transitions of care*: Systems that engage patients and families in self-management after being transferred from one care setting or provider to another along the continuum of health and human services. A key strategy here is open, timely, and purposeful communication among the parties involved to enhance patient safety during the transition, and reduce the risk for medical errors or rehospitalizations.

1.4.3. Guiding Principles for Case Management Practice

The practice of case management is based on a number of guiding principles which aim to enhance the value of healthcare delivery and services for all: the clients/support systems, providers, payers, employers, regulators, advocates, and other stakeholders. When designed and implemented in an effective and successful way, case management programs and roles:

- Ensure patient's needs and preferences for health services and information are understood and shared across the involved parties and sites of care at all times and as the patient navigates the healthcare system.
- Result in articulating a proactive plan of care for the individual patient to be used by the patient, family members and caregivers, and healthcare team members.
- Are important for every patient; however, some populations (e.g., children with special healthcare needs, the frail elderly, those with multiple chronic illnesses) are particularly vulnerable to fragmented, uncoordinated care.
- Contribute to organizational or program's strategy for improving quality, safety, and reducing cost.
- Communicate where the responsibility for care lies—the primary care provider (e.g., physician, nurse practitioner, physician assistant, ambulatory clinic) in concert with the rest of the interdisciplinary care team.
- Support the patient centered medical home (PCMH) and other primary care or accountable care programs.
- Ensure the provision of culturally competent and patient-centered, safe care.
- Maximize the value of services delivered to patients and their families.
- Facilitate efficient, safe, cost-conscious, and high-quality patient and family experiences including patient engagement for effective self-management and adherence.
- Improve healthcare outcomes (e.g., clinical, financial, functional, satisfaction).

- Employ innovative information technology systems that ensure removal of barriers and allow for seamless and timely communication across providers, care settings and patients, families, or caregivers.
- Build effective partnerships among healthcare providers across the continuum of care (e.g., hospital and primary care settings), other healthcare organization and community-based resources and leaders.
- Place special emphasis on safe and effective hand-offs and transitions of care.
- Adhere to regulatory and accreditation standards.

1.4.4. Case Management and the Role of Case Manager

It is difficult to separate the model of case management from the role of the case manager. Case management as a model provides the system, but it is the case manager who implements the model and makes it come alive. In other words, the model provides the foundation and organizational structure within which the case manager role is implemented. This may be the reason for the added confusion related to what case management really is and how it works. It is difficult to understand the model without understanding the role, and vice versa. Once the various adaptations of the role and the model are mixed and matched, things really get complicated. The best way to understand the role and the model is to think of them in terms of what the goals of case management are (Box 1.4), and the drivers behind the application of case management over time (Box 1.5).

Regardless of the setting in which case management is implemented, there are goals that can be identified that are consistent across the healthcare continuum (see Box 1.4). Whether it is a hospital, a nursing home, or a community care setting, the model attempts to address both cost and quality issues and to deliver care in ways that result in the most positive patient and organizational outcomes.

The case manager accomplishes these goals by performing a number of complex role functions. These may include but are not limited to care coordination, facilitation, education, advocacy, transitional planning, discharge planning, utilization management, avoidable delay management, resource management, and outcomes management. These functions remain consistent across care settings and levels of care along the continuum.

1.4.5. Case Management as an Outcomes Model

Case management is not only a process model but also an outcomes model in that it provides a prospective

---

Box 1.4 Goals of Case Management and the Case Manager's Role Functions

Overall Goals

1. Manage cost, quality, and safety
2. Achieve positive patient and organizational outcomes
3. Enhance timely access to healthcare services and resources

Role Functions

1. Care coordination
2. Facilitation
3. Avoidable delay management
4. Education
5. Advocacy
6. Brokerage of community services and resources
7. Transitional/discharge planning
8. Resource and utilization management
9. Outcomes management

Goals and Role Function

Goals and role functions are usually driven by the functional areas a case management program consists of. Often case management programs include some or all the following:

1. Clinical care management (facilitation and coordination of care)
2. Utilization review and management (including allocation of resources, certification/authorization for care and services)
3. Transitional/discharge planning and handoffs
4. Access management and patient flow
5. Outcomes evaluation and management
6. Variance management (e.g., delays in care, ommissions or overuse of unnecessary resources)
7. Clinical documentation improvement

Box 1.5 Evolutionary Process of Case Management Application

1. 1920—Psychiatry and social work; outpatient settings
2. 1930—Public health nursing
3. 1950—Behavioral health across the continuum
4. 1985—Acute care
5. 1990—All healthcare settings
6. 2010—Healthcare reform increasing the role of community-based care (patient centered medical home and accountable care organizations)

---

cause most healthcare reimbursement was based on a fee-for-service (FFS) structure, there were no financial incentives to reduce costs. In fact, because the use of resources was financially rewarded by the system, overuse abounded. This overuse and misuse of healthcare resources, particularly those in the acute care setting, resulted in spiraling costs for the consumers of care (Box 1.6). Concurrently, the costs of pharmaceuticals, radiology, and supplies continued to escalate with minimal management of those costs. In the 1990s and beyond, healthcare in the United States is a trillion-dollar business.

It is therefore no great surprise that the healthcare system eventually broke down. Consumers and third-party payers were no longer willing to pay these high costs when the quality of the services they were receiving was barely keeping pace. In fact, it appeared to most consumers of healthcare that the quality of the services they were receiving was diminishing and that the value of the care was reduced. The costs were rising while the value was subsiding.

The mid-1980s were witness to a flurry of activities all designed to figure out how to improve the quality of healthcare while reducing the cost. The expected result was an increase in value. On the payer side, we first saw the introduction of the prospective payment sys-

---

Box 1.6 Forces Driving the Move Toward Case Management

1. 1970s—Escalating healthcare costs
2. 1980s—Prospective payment system in acute care settings
3. 1990s—Managed care infiltration
4. 2000s—Prospective payment system in home care, outpatient care, rehabilitation services, and long-term care
5. 2010s—Healthcare reform and value-based purchasing

---

approach for planning the ways in which care will be provided, the steps in the care process, and the desired outcomes of care. In other words, for each step in the process, there is also an expected outcome that can be predetermined and managed. All steps in the process are designed to move the patient toward the desired outcome.

1.5. CHANGES IN REIMBURSEMENT: THE DRIVING FORCE BEHIND CASE MANAGEMENT

It was not until the 1980s that case management truly came into its own. Before 1983, healthcare costs were not of major concern to the healthcare provider. Betem with the diagnosis-related groups (DRGs) as the reimbursement scheme. Shortly after that, the western United States saw an increase in the use of managed care and health maintenance organizations (HMOs). DRGs and managed care are discussed in Chapter 2. Employers saw the use of HMOs as a way to reduce the cost of providing healthcare insurance to their employees. Several states, including Minnesota, California, Arizona, and Tennessee, have since adopted broad-based managed care programs. By the turn of the twenty-first century, managed care reimbursement systems had permeated throughout the United States.

Unfortunately, many of the efforts resulting in changes in reimbursement and the introduction of managed care were perceived solely as cost cutting. Although much lip service was given to the notion of quality, effective and consistent outcome measures, as well as measures of quality of care, were lacking. What did exist were financial parameters that guided outcomes evaluation, such as length of stay and cost per case. Within 3–5 years organizations began to recognize the need to incorporate quality into the agenda. Much of this came out of healthcare organizations themselves. Two major quality improvement models drove the quality initiatives. The first was total quality management and the use of continuous quality improvement (CQI) methods. The second was case management. Ultimately, both of these concepts became the framework for redesign efforts and patient-focused care.

1.6. THE COST/QUALITY RATIO

CQI has been linked in philosophy and practice to case management. CQI methods are used to drive case management processes and to monitor outcomes (Cesta, 1993). Other methods used to improve quality of care now include Six Sigma™ as a commonly used framework for quality improvement (Pande, Neuman, & Cavanaugh, 2000). Case management is now recognized as a system for delivering care that coordinates interdisciplinary care services, plans care, identifies expected outcomes, and helps facilitate the patient and family toward those expected outcomes. The case manager is responsible for ensuring that the patient's needs are being met and that care is being provided in the most cost-effective setting or level of care.

CQI and/or Six Sigma can address both system and practice issues, looking for opportunities for improvement that will result in reduced cost and improved quality of care. Without addressing and improving these processes, case management as a delivery system will not be effective. When implemented, case management affects the patient population served as well

as every part of the organization, every discipline, and every department. Therefore it is sometimes necessary to correct existing systems or interdisciplinary problems before the model can be successfully implemented. CQI can then be applied to measure and continuously monitor the progress and outcomes of the model.

1.7. NURSING CASE MANAGEMENT

Nursing case management evolved as a hospital-based care delivery system in 1985. Before that time there had been a number of other nursing care delivery systems, including functional, team, and primary nursing. It has been said that nursing case management incorporates elements of both team and primary nursing. In team nursing, a nurse team leader directs the care being provided by all the members of the nursing team, including RNs, licensed practical nurses, and nurse aides. The team leader generally does not provide direct patient care but directs the care being provided by the members of the team.

1.7.1. Move from Team to Primary Nursing

In the 1970s team nursing evolved to primary nursing. In primary nursing, the RN is responsible for providing all aspects of care to an assigned group of patients. With the assistance of a nurse aide, the RN carries out all direct and indirect nursing functions for the patient. One of the goals of primary nursing is the reduction in fragmentation of nursing care. The primary nurse provides all facets of care to the patient but works independently. It was anticipated that primary nursing would enhance the professionalism of nursing by upgrading the level of autonomy and independent practice.

1.7.2. Breakdown of Primary Nursing

With the advent of the prospective payment system in 1983, primary nursing became increasingly difficult to implement. Although it provided a structure for the RN to function autonomously and independently, it did not address the cost/quality issues affecting the healthcare delivery system in the 1980s. As lengths of stay began to shorten, care activities had to be accelerated. At the same time the nursing profession began to experience a nursing shortage, and various strategies were put into place to recruit and retain nurses. One of these was flexible (flex) time, including 12-hour shifts. Twelve-hour shifts provided the RN with more flexibility in terms of the work schedule. This might mean more time to spend raising a family, or it might mean time to return to school. In any case, nurses working three days a week, combined with accelerated hospital stays, resulted in increasing difficulty in maintaining a primary nursing model. Continuity of patient care was all but destroyed as nurses worked only three days a week. With shortened lengths of stay, it was possible that the nurse who began caring for the patient on admission might not be the same nurse caring for the patient on discharge. It was very expensive to staff nursing units to the extent necessary to maintain as much continuity as possible. In addition to the cost of personnel, primary nursing was not designed to manage care in shorter timeframes or place an emphasis on the management of resources. Care was not outcome focused, and the healthcare providers were fragmented.

1.7.3. Early Hospital-Based Case Management

Two hospitals attempted to respond to the changing times by addressing the changes in healthcare reimbursement, shortened lengths of stay, and dwindling hospital resources. Carondelet St. Mary's Hospital in Tucson, Arizona, and New England Medical Center in Boston, Massachusetts, were the first to recognize the need to redesign their nursing departments. Each introduced nursing case management models that incorporated elements of both team and primary nursing within a context of controlled resources and shortened lengths of stay. The early case management models were structured on using hospital-based nurse case managers to monitor the patient's progress toward discharge.

Carondelet's model was initially designed as an acute care case management model. The job title "Professional Nurse Case Manager" described an RN with the minimum educational preparation of a bachelor's degree. The case manager assumed responsibility for managing patients toward expected outcomes along a continuum of care. Carondelet collected data for the first 4 years after implementation of the model and found that quality and cost were both improved. Job satisfaction improved for nurses, and their job stress decreased. In addition, patient satisfaction increased (Ethridge, 1991).

Perhaps the most compelling finding was that some patients with chronic illnesses were not hospitalized at all (Ethridge & Lamb, 1989). Those who were admitted had lower acuity levels. They were immediately linked to the healthcare system so that the length of stay at the beginning of the hospitalization was decreased. This resulted in lower costs for the hospital (Ethridge, 1991).

These findings resulted in the development of the first nursing HMO. The initial program, began in 1989, focused on case-managing patients from a senior-care HMO. The nurse case manager screened all patients admitted under the Senior Plan contract. The assessment included determining the necessary nursing services before discharge, monitoring of any community services being provided, and ensuring a continuation of care in the community if necessary. Because the fees were capitated, the case manager could match the patient's needs with the appropriate services.

New England Medical Center Hospitals (NEMCH) in Boston, Massachusetts, used RNs in positions of senior staff nurses to pilot the case manager role. The case managers carried a core group of patients for whom they provided direct patient care. They worked closely with physicians, social workers, utilization managers, and discharge planners. The core of the care delivery system was that outcomes should drive the care process. Several versions of critical pathways were developed for planning, managing, documenting, and evaluating patient care. During those early years the "tools of the trade" moved more and more toward care management tools that structured the care process and outcomes and were more interdisciplinary (Zander, 1996).

Both models were deemed successes by their organizations. Across the country other hospitals began turning to these two role models for ideas, direction, and support. This was a watershed moment in healthcare delivery. Unprecedented numbers of healthcare organizations began to think about or implement case management. Its position in the healthcare arena was secured.

Although case management initially addressed the changes necessary for organizations to survive prospective payment, it was even more effective in its management of cases under a managed care system. In both reimbursement systems, patient care must be managed and controlled, with a tight rein on the use of resources, the length of stay, and continuing care needs.

The majority of the models of the 1980s did little in terms of changing the role functions of the other members of the healthcare team. Whereas nursing provided the driving force for the movement toward hospital-based case management, the other disciplines were slower in recognizing the value of such a system. Additionally, serious downsizing was only just beginning in the industry. Corporate America had already begun its massive layoffs and downsizing initiatives. Thousands of people lost their jobs. Healthcare had not yet begun to feel the economic pinch as it was being felt in other businesses; therefore the incentive for merging and downsizing departments was not yet there.

Shortly after these early models, case management began to mature as more and more hospitals began to implement case management models. One could see a direct correlation between the degree of managed care infiltration and the use of case management. In nursing case management, the nurse essentially functions as the leader of the team, similar to the team nursing approach. The difference was that the team did not consist of nurses only. Now the team was an interdisciplinary one, and each healthcare provider had a say in terms of how a patient's care would be delivered and monitored.

Shortly after this popularity of the nursing case management models, other disciplines caught on and began to pursue the design and implementation of case management systems. This increased buy-in from other disciplines resulted in an outbreak of these models throughout the country, leading to the birth of interdisciplinary approaches in the design; hence dropping "nursing" from the label to better reflect the models because they no longer were nursing in nature. Today, case management departments most commonly report to the chief operations or medical officers of an organization rather than to nursing services. This shift in reporting structure has resulted in giving case management departments more credence and power in an organization.

1.8. EARLY COMMUNITY-BASED CASE MANAGEMENT

Case management, although more commonly thought of as an acute or hospital-based model, has its roots in the community. Long before hospitals were considered the center of the healthcare universe, case management was being used for a variety of purposes and to meet the needs of diverse populations of patients.

Case management finds its roots in public health nursing, social work, and behavioral health. We can find evidence of case management in the 1860s, where case management techniques were used in the settlement houses occupied by immigrants and the poor. "Patient care records" consisted of cards that catalogued the individual's and family's needs and/or follow-up needs, all aimed at ensuring that the patient/family received the services that they needed and that additional services would be provided as necessary (Tahan, 1998).

Another example of a case management application, also in the 1860s, was the first Board of Charities established in Massachusetts. Aimed toward the sick and the poor, public human services were coordinated with a primary goal of conserving public funds (Tahan,

1998). Even in the 1860s, cost containment was a concern as it related to the distribution of public funds to the poor. Social workers were the health professionals responsible for managing these processes.

In the early 1900s case management strategies were implemented by public health nurses at the Yale University School of Nursing. A collaborative effort was established between a clergyman and the superintendent of the school. The clergyman described the nurse's role and the requirements he sought in the following ways:

1. Knowledge and expertise
2. Communication skills
3. Cost containment
4. Collaboration with physicians
5. Appropriate allocation of resources
6. Responsibility for overall care of the patient and family
7. Provision of emotional and psychosocial support and the assurance of a dignified and peaceful death
8. Coordination and management of care
9. Facilitation of the delivery of patient care activities
10. Obtaining funds for special programs (Tahan, 1998)

Review a contemporary case manager's job description and you are likely to find the superintendent's expected role functions and requirements there.

Around the same time that public health nursing was embracing case management concepts and techniques, the field of social work was using care coordination techniques with a focus on linking patients and families to available resources. Social work began to emerge as the discipline focused on linking or brokering healthcare services for individuals. Conversely, the early nursing case management models included both coordination and care delivery functions. In many ways these differences remain in the approaches taken by both disciplines in the delivery of contemporary case management.

The 1950s was the decade in which behavioral health workers began to use case management tools and strategies. Targeted were World War II veterans who presented mental and emotional problems in addition to physical disabilities. *Continuum of care* was labeled for the first time, and in this context it related to the myriad of community health services these individuals required and accessed. Behavioral health case managers accessed, coordinated, and ensured that service needs were met on a continuous basis. These strategies can still be found today in many behavioral health models of care delivery.

1.8.1. The 1970s and 1980s

During the 1970s and 1980s the federal government provided funding to support the development of several demonstration projects focused on long-term care. Legislation was enacted at the state and federal levels to incorporate these projects into strategic planning policies. Reimbursement was established through Medicare and Medicaid waivers. Some of the better known projects included the Triage Program in Connecticut, the Wisconsin Community Care Organization, the On Look Project in San Francisco, the New York City Home Care Project, and the Long-Term Care Channeling Demonstration Project in San Francisco (Cohen & Cesta, 1994).

By the late 1980s, community-based case management programs were emerging in many parts of the country as a mechanism for managing patients and resources in capitated environments. One important example is the Carondelet Saint Mary's Model in Tucson, Arizona (Cohen & Cesta, 2001). These emerging and contemporary models returned case managed to its original roots, the community. Case management had now completed a circle that took over 100 years to circumnavigate.

1.8.2. The 1990s

As a result of the re-emergence of community-based case management, the CMS, formerly the Health Care Financing Administration (HCFA), funded five demonstration projects that used registered professional nurses in the role of community case managers to coordinate care for the Medicare beneficiaries. These projects were called *community nursing centers*, and they are as follows:

1. The Carle Clinic at the Carle Organization in Urbana, Illinois (Schraeder & Britt, 1997)
2. A School-Based Health Center at The University of Rochester in Rochester, New York (Walker & Chiverton, 1997)
3. The Silver Spring Community Nursing Center at the University of Wisconsin, Milwaukee (Lundeen, 1997)
4. The University Community Health Services Group Practice at Vanderbilt University in Nashville, Tennessee (Spitzer, 1997)
5. The Carondelet Health Care Corporation at Carondelet St. Mary's Hospital in Tucson, Arizona (Ethridge, 1997)

A special feature of these centers is that they relied on nurses as the main providers of care with physicians in consultative roles. These centers demonstrated the ability to affect both the process and outcomes of care. Examples of the services provided or arranged for and coordinated by the nurse case managers were health risk assessments; authorization, coordination, evaluation, and payment of services; services such as home care, transportation, respite care, and home-delivered meals; preventive and psychiatric mental health; health promotion activities such as exercise, nutrition, and lifestyle changes; durable medical equipment; and medical or minor surgical care.

1.9. HISTORY OF EVIDENCE-BASED GUIDELINES

It has been almost two decades since the introduction of case management plans as a method of controlling cost and quality in healthcare. First known as critical pathways, these tools have grown in scope and sophistication over the years (Box 1.7). Critical pathways were originally designed and implemented by nursing departments as a paper-and-pencil system for outlining the course of events for treating patients in a particular DRG for each day of hospitalization (Zander, 1991; Nelson, 1994; Cohen & Cesta, 1997).

In a broader fashion, critical pathways outlined the key or critical steps in the treatment of the DRG in a one-page summary. Because DRGs are broad groupings or classifications of similar types of patients, the critical pathway also had to be broad and nonspecific in nature (Edelstein & Cesta, 1993). The original critical pathways were mainly focused on nursing interventions and tasks. The daily interventions such as blood work or other diagnostics and therapeutics were outlined generically and were applicable to a host of different patient types. Because of the generic nature of the plans, they did little to control the use of resources, types of medications, route of administration, or other factors related to cost and quality. Although they did suggest the appropriate number of hospital days to allocate to the DRG, they did little beyond that to control the kinds of product resources applied to the particular broad grouping of patients.

Box 1.7   Elements of an Effective Case Management Plan

1. Interdisciplinary in nature
2. Outcomes based
3. Clinically specific
4. Care provider documentation included
5. Flexible enough to meet individual patient's care needs

1.10. CASE MANAGEMENT PLANS TODAY

Critical pathways were a good first attempt at providing a framework for controlling cost and quality within the prospective payment system of the acute care setting. Subsequent adaptations of the critical pathway concept began to use more specific and direct clinical content in a multidisciplinary format and multiple settings or levels of care. These more sophisticated case management plans are called multidisciplinary action plans (MAPs), clinical guidelines, practice guidelines, practice parameters, care maps, and so on. Today's case management plans are clinically specific, incorporate other disciplines, are outcome oriented, and may include care provider documentation. In addition to being more clinically specific, these plans are focused around specific clinical case types rather than DRGs. Thus the content applies to the clinical issue being planned out. This may be a medical problem, surgical procedure, or workup plan (Hampton, 1993; Tahan & Cesta, 1994; Cohen & Cesta, 1997). Chapter 12 contains more detailed information on the various adaptations of the current "tools of the trade" in case management. Appendices 1 and 2 present examples of several different types of case management plans.

1.10.1. Benchmarking

Evolutionary changes involved much more specificity in terms of the content of the case management plan. Benchmarking is used as a strategy for understanding internal processes and performance levels; it provides a basis for understanding where the performance gaps are. It brings the best ideas that identify opportunities and helps the organization to rally around a consensus. In addition, it results in the implementation of better-quality products and services (Czarnecki, 1994).

The clinical content for the case management plans should be based on benchmarks such as those established by the following:

- Professional societies
- Professional journals
- Health systems and hospital corporations
- Texts and manuals
- National databases

One or more of these benchmarks can be used to develop any one plan. In this way much of the subjectivity is taken out of the plan of care and instead the care is based on sound judgment, expert opinion, and research outcomes. With this step in the evolutionary process, the plans became much more clinically directive and began to provide a framework for controlling resource application for specific case types.

1.11. MULTIDISCIPLINARY CARE PLANNING

The next step in the evolutionary process was the introduction of plans that had a more multi-disciplinary focus and that incorporated the plan of care for all disciplines represented (Goode & Blegan, 1993; Adler, Bryk, & Cesta, 1995). The final step was the addition of expected outcomes of care that applied to the specific interventions on the plan. In other words, for each intervention there was an expected outcome for the patient to achieve before the patient could move on to the next phase of care (Sperry & Birdsall, 1994). Box 1.8 presents an example of expected outcomes.

1.12. CHOOSING A CASE MANAGEMENT TOOL

A variety of case management tools are available today. The tool chosen by any organization should be based on that organization's needs and goals. Some issues to be addressed during the design and implementation process are summarized in Case Manager's Tip 1.1 and are described in more detail in the following paragraphs.

1.12.1. Format: Critical Pathway Versus Multidisciplinary Action Plan

A critical pathway is generally formatted as a one-

Box 1.8   Expected Outcomes as They Might Appear on a Multidisciplinary Action Plan for Community-Acquired Pneumonia

Intermediate Outcomes (Also Known as Milestones or Trigger Points)

Convert from intravenous to oral antibiotics when the patient:

1. Has two consecutive oral temperatures of less than 100.4°F obtained at least 8 hours apart in the absence of antipyretics
2. Shows a decrease in leukocytosis to less than 12,000
3. Exhibits improved pulmonary signs/symptoms
4. Is able to tolerate oral medications

Discharge Outcomes

In less severe pneumonia, discharging the patient from the hospital may occur simultaneously or up to 24 hours after switch to oral antibiotics, providing there is no deterioration or other reason for continued hospitalization.

CASE MANAGER'S TIP 1.1

Choosing a Case Management Tool

When choosing a case management tool, be sure to address the following issues during the design and implementation process:

1. Format: critical pathway versus MAP
2. Utility as a documentation system
3. Inclusion as a permanent part of the medical record
4. Interdisciplinary nature
5. Legal issues related to care providers' use of the tool
6. Fulfillment of the standards and requirements of accreditation (e.g., The Joint Commission [TJC]) and regulatory agencies (CMS)

---

page summary of the tasks to be accomplished for a specific diagnosis or DRG. It does not include outcomes and is usually not used as a documentation tool. In addition, it is customarily not a part of the patient's medical record. MAPs, however, are more comprehensive in nature, are usually a part of the patient's permanent record, include outcomes, and are interdisciplinary.

1.12.2. Utility as a Documentation System for Nurses and Other Healthcare Providers

The MAP is intended to be used as a documentation tool. This is most often accomplished by using the MAP in conjunction with a documentation-by-exception system, whereby the expected patient outcomes are prospectively identified and then charted against the timeframes established. To date the majority of such documentation systems incorporate only nursing documentation. Some organizations have successfully included other disciplines such as social work, nutrition, and physical and occupational therapy. The format can be adjusted to include other disciplines such as physicians by including more narrative note space within the document and medical orders as a preprinted order set.

1.12.3. Inclusion as a Permanent Part of the Medical Record

If the MAP is to be used as a documentation tool, then it clearly must be included as part of the permanent medical record. Some organizations, out of fear of legal liability, opt not to include the MAP as a part of the record. It is believed that this reduces their liabil-

ity. In reality, if the plan is the standard of care for the organization, then the organization is responsible for producing the standard should a legal issue arise (Hirshfeld, 1993); therefore it is discoverable and admissible in court regardless of whether it is a part of the medical record. If the MAP is used to guide the clinical care of a particular patient the hospital is being sued for, the court may demand that the MAP be made available. If the physician did indeed follow the MAP, then it will afford legal protection to the physician and the organization.

In any case, some organizations may choose to test the MAP outside the medical record first before sanctioning it. In situations such as this in which the MAP has not been approved by the hospital, patient consent may be necessary. Otherwise the use of two different standards of care cannot be justified.

Including the MAP as part of the medical record lends the medical record more weight and credibility than not including it. Including the MAP clearly gives the message that the organization stands behind it as the standard of care and believes that the MAP represents state-of-the-art care.

1.12.4. Interdisciplinary Nature, Incorporating All Disciplines in the Care Process, and Expected Outcomes

Early case management plans did not include all disciplines but had a heavy nursing focus and emphasis. As case management has evolved and matured, case management plans have become more multidisciplinary. Although it may be more difficult to include the documentation of all care providers, it should be easier to include all disciplines in the actual plan itself. Expected outcomes for each discipline can be prospectively identified and incorporated. The biggest advantage to creating an interdisciplinary plan is that it reduces duplication and fragmentation and provides proof of an integrated plan of care for accrediting and regulatory agencies. Opportunities to reduce redundancy become more obvious when the plans for each discipline can be reviewed and compared. This approach also enhances the use of existing personnel by ensuring that all are carrying out the care activities most appropriate to their disciplines. Areas in which this becomes obvious include patient education and discharge planning, where there is greater likelihood that duplication of effort may take place.

Because quality and length of stay are affected by the efforts of each and every member of the healthcare team, it only makes sense to include all of them in the planning process.

1.12.5. Legal Issues for Physicians, Nurses, and Other Providers

Many healthcare providers may feel anxiety related to the use of MAPs and other case management plans. This may be due to a lack of understanding related to the legal issues concerning these kinds of tools. Legal issues should be carefully discussed with the organization's risk management department after a thorough review of the literature is completed. Each organization must weigh the legal pros and cons and draw its own conclusions as to whether this is a concept that the physicians can adopt and embrace. Another strategy to reduce legal risk and curtail providers' hesitancy to using the MAPs is to review the stance taken by the various professional societies and associations, such as the American Medical Association and the American Nurses Association. Almost all professional societies are in favor of using MAPs in some form or another.

1.12.6. Fulfillment of The Joint Commission Requirements for Care Planning, Patient Teaching, and Discharge Planning

The standards for TJCs focus on the incorporation of all disciplines into the plan of care for those tasks that are interdisciplinary in nature (www.jointcommission.org). The MAP, by nature of its format and philosophy, is designed to ensure that all disciplines are represented and integrated in the plan.

1.13. PHYSICIAN SUPPORT

Physician support is a key component in the success or failure of any case management plan, no matter what format it takes. Although these plans were once feared as legally dangerous, physicians are beginning to realize some of their legal benefits. Conceptually, case management plans can meet physician, hospital, and patient needs in a number of ways.

1.13.1. Aid to Shortening Length of Stay

To maintain financial viability, acute care settings must shorten the number of inpatient hospital days. Whether the reimbursement system is negotiated managed care or the prospective payment system, length of stay can translate to financial success or failure for any hospital in today's healthcare environment.

1.13.2. Selling Tool for Managed Care/HMOs

An ability to demonstrate systems that control cost and

quality is essential to any forward-thinking healthcare organization in the 2000s and beyond. Case management plans that are prospective and outcome oriented and outline both the appropriate length of stay and expected outcomes and the appropriate use of resources for a particular case type provide a structure for controlling cost and quality. These plans can be shared with managed care organizations before admission to demonstrate how the hospital manages a particular case type, or they can be used as a concurrent review tool to justify the length of stay and resource allocation.

1.13.3. Means of Legal Protection

Practice guidelines and case management plans can protect physicians from a risk liability perspective in that they outline what is appropriate to do, as well as what is not appropriate to do. They provide for a plan of care that is supported by the organization in which they work (West, 1994).

1.13.4. Aid to Regulatory Agency Compliance

For TJC or other regulatory bodies, case management plans are recognized as an excellent vehicle for integration of care and maintaining and improving quality. By outlining the expected clinical outcomes and documenting deviations from those outcomes, the organization can identify opportunities for clinical process improvements (www.jointcommission.org).

1.13.5. Means of Providing a Competitive Edge

Clearly the organizations that maintain market-share advantage will be the ones that will remain competitive in the managed care environment. If "covered lives" is the name of the game, a competitive edge will lie with those organizations that have captured the greatest market share. This means that they will have negotiated managed care contracts that provide for maximum reimbursement and that have large patient populations.

1.13.6. Source of Practice Parameters

A variety of respected organizations have developed practice guidelines (see Section 1.10.1). Physicians, nurses, and other providers can refer to their own specialty organizations regarding state-of-the-art guidelines (Holzer, 1990).

1.14. BENEFITS OF CASE MANAGEMENT

Internally there are many reasons why case manage-

CASE MANAGER'S TIP 1.2

Benefits of Case Management Plans

When soliciting support for case management plans, focus on the ways in which they can help to ensure the healthcare organization's success. Case management plans help do the following:

1. Simplify and integrate care
2. Improve reimbursement
3. Objectify decision making
4. Contain cost
5. Prioritize resources
6. Ensure quality outcomes

ment plans spell success or failure (see Case Manager's Tip 1.2).

1.14.1. Simplify Care

Case management plans provide a systematic format for all disciplines to use in the treatment of specific case types. All disciplines involved in the care of the specific group of patients represented are included in one interdisciplinary plan of care. In some cases, documentation is also included so that the entire course of events is seen in one documentation tool (Adler et al., 1995).

1.14.2. Improve Reimbursement

Because documentation is enhanced, there is greater opportunity for the medical record to be coded properly and for managed care organizations to authorize needed services. Proper coding and authorizations mean maximization of reimbursement.

1.14.3. Objectify Decision Making

Although a tremendous amount of subjectivity and judgment goes into the art of practicing medicine, there still remains a core of safe and appropriate clinical practice that is based on research and state-of-the-art recommendations. Case management plans provide a vehicle for communicating these clinical recommendations in an objective manner.

1.14.4. Contain Cost

Because case management plans provide a foundation for reducing variability in medical treatment, they serve

as a tool for controlling cost. Care needs, both product and personnel, are prospectively determined so that the organization can predict its resource needs and reduce the need for a variety of different brands and types of the same product. This ultimately has an effect on cost. The plans outline the expected length of stay, thereby controlling the number of hospital days and resulting in cost savings to the hospital. Daily resource application is also outlined, which will translate to saved dollars for the organization (Edelstein & Cesta, 1993; Jijon & Jijon-Letort, 1995).

1.14.5. Prioritize Resources

Resource use is closely tied to cost containment. By properly using resources, costs are reduced. Other issues involve the appropriate use of existing resources, both product and personnel. Case management plans can provide a framework for identifying which members of the healthcare team will provide which services. So much of the misutilization and/or overutilization of healthcare resources occurs because of lack of communication between departments and disciplines. Through case management, the work to be done can be allocated to the most appropriate member of the team. Responsibilities are outlined prospectively rather than on a case-by-case basis. This reduces the opportunity for redundancy or for things to fall through the cracks and not be done at all. For example, discharge planning functions can be allocated to the most appropriate care provider, thereby using personnel most appropriately and as early in the process as possible (Tahan & Cesta, 1994).

1.15. INTERDISCIPLINARY TEAM

Case management has provided a structure for healthcare providers to develop teams that are truly interdisciplinary and collaborative. In the past, either various disciplines have controlled the team or the team was composed of only one discipline. For example, "patient care rounds" were generally physician dominated and focused on the medical plan. In team nursing, the team was composed of only nurses. The team leader was a nurse, members of the team were nurses, and so on. Discharge planning rounds were often interdisciplinary but were focused on the patient's discharge plan and social services.

1.16. CHANGE PROCESS

Case management as a delivery model crosses all boundaries within the organization. Therefore it is critical that the members involved in the development of the team represent all those affected. The roles most closely affiliated with that of the case manager are utilization management, transitional/discharge planning, and home care. During the design process, an interdisciplinary team representing these departments should be brought together to examine current practice and to look for opportunities to redefine role functions within the organization.

Logically the membership should consist of those individuals who have the power and authority to make the necessary changes in the role functions of these departments. During the analysis phase, some disciplines may feel threatened or defensive about their current functions within the organization and may interpret the need to change as a criticism of their current job performance rather than as identifying opportunities to make the organization more productive and efficient.

This period while current processes are analyzed and critiqued may cause some anxiety. How well this group works through the process will greatly depend on the members' interpersonal relationships, their vision, and their ability to collaborate.

Using the techniques of CQI, Six Sigma, and other methods for performance improvement will help to facilitate this process (Cesta, 1993).Quality improvement helps to place everyone on an equal playing field as processes are analyzed and changed (see Chapter 13). The team should first examine current practice by looking at what the various departments and disciplines are currently doing, where there may be overlap or redundancy, and where things may be falling through the cracks. Only then can opportunities for improvement be initiated. One useful tool for this technique is the flow diagram. The flow diagram provides the team with a visual representation of their current practice, where quality barriers may be, and where opportunities for improvement may lie (Figure 1.1).

The social worker and the case manager may be duplicating some discharge planning functions. There may be confusion between them in terms of who is doing what; specific tasks must then be negotiated as they arise. This results in confusion and delays because each episode requires an analysis, a discussion, and a resolution.

This executive-level team essentially designs the case management model after a thorough analysis has taken place. The role functions of each member of the team are clearly outlined and delineated prospectively before going further with the implementation process.

Once these role functions have been determined,

the members of the interdisciplinary case management team can be assembled to carry out a number of important functions. The team members are those clinicians and others who are directly involved in the care process. The team first prospectively develops the case management plan. The plan, as discussed in Chapter 12, is collaboratively developed by the team to manage the case as efficiently and cost-effectively as possible. The team also individualizes the plan to the specific patient. Finally, the team implements the plan. The case manager serves as the thread that binds the interdisciplinary team together. The case manager does not lead the team but essentially guides the team and the patient/family toward the achievement of the expected outcomes as identified in the plan.

The members of the team are fluid and depend on the patient's location, clinical problem, and expected long-term needs. Core members of the team should always include the physician, nurse, case manager, social worker, discharge planner, and patient/family. Additional members depend on the picture presented. For example, orthopedic problems warrant the physical therapist's membership on the team; pulmonary problems necessitate the respiratory therapist. For the diabetic or other patient with metabolic problems, the nutritionist should be a member of the team. Clearly, members should be those healthcare providers who have some relevance to the case and who have something to contribute to the interdisciplinary plan of care.

In a time when containing costs has never been more important, a collaborative, interdisciplinary approach is critical to the success of any case management model. Without it, true case management can never take place.

1.17. MANAGED CARE

It has not been uncommon for the terms *case management* and *managed care* to sometimes be used interchangeably. However, there are specific differences between the terms. Although linked philosophically, managed care is a broader term that refers to an organized delivery of services by a select panel of providers (Rehberg, 1996; Kongstvedt, 2001). These services are managed under a prepayment arrangement between a provider of services and a managed care organization. Managed care is a system that provides the generalized structure and focus when managing the use, cost, quality, and effectiveness of healthcare services. HMOs and preferred provider organizations (PPOs) are the two most common types of managed care arrangements. They are essentially health insurance plans that link the

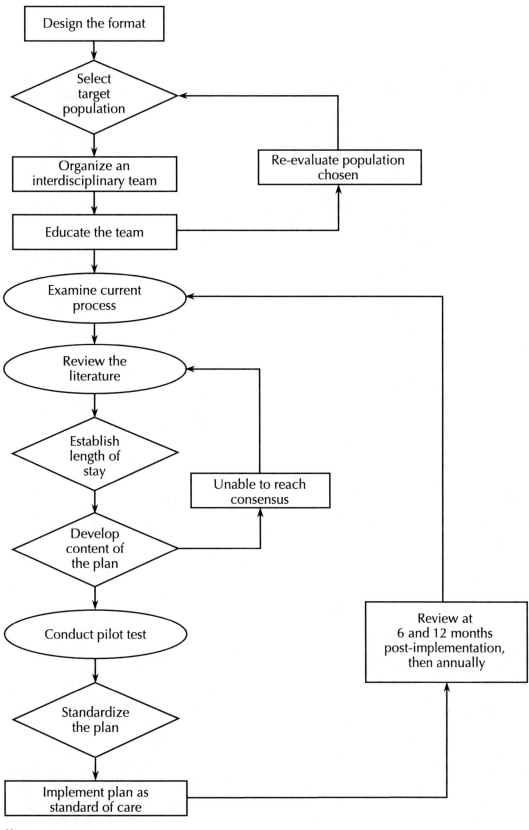

Key:
Box = Activities
Circle = Inputs to/outputs from
Diamond = Decision to be made
Arrow = Direction of flow of activities

Figure 1.1 Flow diagram: Developing a case management plan.

patient to provider services, and their purpose is to improve the efficiency of the healthcare delivery system (Mullahy, 1995, 1998; Kongstvedt, 2001).

Because some physicians' only exposure to case managers has been through a managed care organization, they may see the two as synonymous. They may believe that case managers and case management means managed care. In reality, although case managers can be found in managed care organizations, they are also found in a wide variety of other practice settings (see Chapters 3 and 4).

Case management is a patient care delivery system. Perhaps the most profound difference between case management and managed care is the fact that managed care is a function of a healthcare reimbursement system, whereas case management is a structure for providing care within a managed care reimbursement system. Case management also applies to provider areas that are not reimbursed under managed care. *Managed care* is defined as a means of providing healthcare services within a defined network of providers. These providers are responsible for managing the care in a quality, cost-effective manner (Baldor, 1996).

The initial driving force for case management in the hospital setting was the prospective payment system because of the dwindling reimbursement associated with the DRGs. As managed care continues to proliferate, it has become an even greater force in the movement toward case management. Under full capitation, the incentive is greatest (see Chapter 2). In between full capitation and FFS we now find a wide variety of combinations of insurers, reimbursement systems, and service settings. It may be many more years or more before the dust settles nationally, systems are in place and integrated, and the continuum of care has been defined.

1.18. KEY POINTS

1. Case management originated as a community-based model in the late 1800s and early 1900s.

2. In the 1950s case management emerged in the field of behavioral health, in which the term "continuum of care" was first applied.

3. Case management applications in the 1980s evolved out of changes in the healthcare reimbursement system, specifically the prospective payment system.

4. Healthcare reform has had an effect on the business of case management.

5. Case management can be defined in a number of ways but is essentially a process and out-

comes model designed to manage resources and maintain quality of care.

6. Case management tools such as pathways and guidelines can help facilitate the case manager role.

7. It is important for physicians to be part of the design, implementation, and evaluation processes related to case management.

8. Case management uses a team approach and incorporates elements of quality improvement.

1.19. REFERENCES

Adler S.L., Bryk, E., Cesta, T.G., & McEachen, I. (1995). Collaboration: The solution to multidisciplinary care planning, *Orthop Nurs 14*(2):21–29.

American Nurses Association. (1988). *Task force on case management*, Kansas City, Mo.

Baldor, R.A. (1996). *Managed care made simple*, Cambridge, Mass, Blackwell Science.

Bower, K. & Falk, C. (1996). Case management as a response to quality, cost, and access imperatives. In Cohen E, Ed.: *Nurse case management in the 21st century*, Mosby, St Louis,.

Case Management Society of America (CMSA). (2010). *CMSA's Standards of practice for case manangement*. Little Rock, AR.

Centers for Medicare & Medicaid Services. (2011). CMS EHR meaningful use overview, EHR incentive programs, October 12.

Cesta, T.G. (1993). The link between continuous quality improvement and case management, *J Nurse Adm 24*(12):49–58.

Cohen, E.L. & Cesta, T.G. (1994). Case management in the acute care setting: a model for health care reform, *J Case Manag 3*(3):110–116.

Cohen, E.L. & Cesta, T.G. (1997). *Nursing case management: From concept to evaluation*, ed 2, Mosby, St Louis,.

Cohen, E.L. & Cesta, T.G. (2001). *Nursing case management: From essentials to advanced practice applications*, Mosby, St Louis.

Commission for Case Manager Certification (CCMC). (2015). *Code of professional conduct for case managers with standards, rules, procedures and penalties*. Mount Laurel, NJ.

Congressional Budget Office. (2009). Preliminary analysis of major provisions related to health insurance coverage under the affordable health choices act, Washington, D.C., June 15.

Curtin, L. (1996). The ethics of managed care—Part 1: proposing a new ethos? *Nurs Manage 27*(8):18–19.

Czarnecki, M.T. (1994). *Benchmarking strategies for health care management*, Aspen, Gaithersburg, Md.

Edelstein, E.L. & Cesta, T.G. (1993). Nursing case management: an innovative model of care for hospitalized patients with diabetes, *Diabetes Educ 19*(6):517–521.

Ethridge, P. (1991). A nursing HMO: Carondelet St Mary's experience, *Nurs Manage 22*(7):22–27.

Ethridge, P. (1997). The Carondelet experience, *Nurs Manage 28*(3):26–28.

Ethridge, P. & Lamb, G.S. (1989). Professional nursing case management improves quality, access and costs, *Nurs Manage* 20(3):30–35.

Frink, B.B. & Strassner, L. (1996). Variance analysis. In Flarey DL, Blancett SS, editors: *Handbook of nursing case management,* Aspen, Gaithersburg, Md.

Goode, C.J. & Blegan, M.A. (1993). Developing a CareMap for patients with a cesarean birth: A multidisciplinary approach, *J Perinat Neonat Nurse* 7(2):40–49.

Hampton, D.C. (1993). Implementing a managed care framework through care maps, *J Nurs Adm* 23(5):21–27.

Hirshfeld, E. (1993). Use of practice parameters as standards of care and in health care reform: A view from the American Medical Association, *J Qual Improve* 19(8):322–329.

Holzer, J.F. (1990). The advent of clinical standards for professional liability, *Qual Rev Bull* 16(2):71–79.

Jijon, C.R. & Jijon-Letort, F.X. (1995). Perinatal predictors of duration and cost of hospitalization for premature infants, *Clin Pediatr* 34(2): 79–85.

Knollmueller, RN. (1989). Case management: what's in a name? *Nurs Manage* 20(10):38–42.

Kongstvedt, P. (2001). *Essentials of managed health care*, 4th ed., Aspen, Gaithersburg, Md.

Lundeen, S. (1997). Community Nursing Center: issues for managed care, *Nurs Manage* 28(3):35–37.

Mullahy, C.M. (1995). *The case manager's handbook*, Aspen, Gaithersburg, Md.

Mullahy, C.M. (1989). *The case manager's handbook*, 2nd ed., Aspen, Gaithersburg, Md,.

National Quality Forum (NQF). October, (2010a). Care Coordination. NQF Quality Connections, pp: 1–12.

National Quality Forum (NQF). October, (2010b). Preferred practices and performance measures for measuring and reporting care coordination: A consensus report. Washington, DC.

Nelson, M.S. (1994). Critical pathways in the emergency department, *J Emerg Nurs* 19(2):110–114.

Pande, P.S., Neuman, R.P., & Cavanaugh, R.R. (2000). The Six Sigma Way, McGraw Hill, New York.

Rehberg, C.A. (1996). Managed care contracts: a guide for clinical case managers, *Nurs Case Manag* 1(1):11–17.

Schraeder, C. & Britt, T. (1997). The Carle Clinic, *Nurs Manage* 28(3):32–34.

Sperry, S. & Birdsall, C. (1994). Outcomes of a pneumonia critical path, *Nurs Econ* 12(6):332–345.

Spitzer, R. (1997). The Vanderbilt University experience, *Nurs Manage* 28(3):38–40.

Tahan, H.A. (1998). Case management: a heritage more than a century old, *Nurs Case Manag* 3(2):55–60.

Tahan, H.A. (1999). Clarifying case management: what is in a label? *Nurs Case Manag* 4(6):268–278.

Tahan, H.A & Cesta, T.G. (1994). Developing case management plans using a quality improvement model, *J Nurs Adm* 24(12):49–58.

The Joint Commission. (2015). www.jointcommission.org

Walker, H. & Chiverton, P. (1997). The University of Rochester experience, *Nurse Manage* 28(3):29–31.

West, J.C.C. (1994). The legal implications of medical practice guidelines, *J Health Hosp Law* 27(4):97–103.

Zander, K. (1991). CareMaps: the core of cost and quality care, *New Definition* 6(3):3.

Zander, K. (1996). The early years: the evolution of nursing case management. In Flarey DL, Blancett SS, editors: *Handbook of nursing case management*, Aspen, Gaithersburg, Md,.

2

Financial Reimbursement Systems

2.1. ORIGINS OF THE PROSPECTIVE PAYMENT SYSTEM: AN OVERVIEW

The prospective payment system (PPS) and DRGs *Diagnosis related group* were probably the strongest catalysts for the movement of case management from the community to the acute care setting. Under FFS plans there were no financial incentives for hospitals to reduce cost and length of stay. In the 1960s and 1970s public policy was focused on improving access to services. Medicare, Medicaid, and other entitlement programs were designed to make services available to the poor, the disabled, and the elderly.

By the early 1980s cost containment had become the driving issue. Healthcare policy had begun to shift from the issues of access and entitlements to quality, cost, and fiscal monitoring. The PPS was initiated to control hospital costs by providing a price-per-case reimbursement. The onus of responsibility was shifted to the provider to manage resource utilization as a set reimbursement would be allotted. The tool designed to determine the amount of reimbursement was the DRG. It was believed that the DRG would encourage physicians, nurses, ancillary departments, and administrators to work together to provide the most efficient care and to manage the patient through the system as efficiently as possible. It was also believed that the PPS would help to standardize care and improve the efficiency of the care process. In reality, although the DRG controlled the payment rate the hospital was to receive, it did not control the cost of care. Therefore despite these rather dramatic and strict reimbursement schemes, hospital costs continued to escalate. This resulted in the resurgence of the managed care reimbursement systems in the 1990s, especially capitation.

2.2. USE OF DOCUMENTATION

Under the PPS, it was believed that proper documentation could ensure that the DRG assignment would be timely and accurate and that the hospital would be reimbursed as quickly as possible. Therefore it became clear that much of the financial success of the hospital would depend on accurate and appropriate documentation. Some hospitals introduced a new position known as DRG manager, DRG coordinator, or documentation specialist. The DRG coordinator/manager was responsible for disseminating information related to the DRGs, particularly data regarding how the hospital was doing in terms of length of stay, cost of care, and case mix. The coordinator, based on analytical findings, could make recommendations regarding areas for improvement in length of stay or cost, where the hospital might be able to maximize revenues or work with the healthcare providers to help them enhance coding through improvements in their documentation.

In 1982 the Tax Equity and Fiscal Responsibility Act (TEFRA) enacted the DRGs (Richards, 1996). They were initially designed to set limits on Medicare reimbursement. The development of the methodology that would determine the reimbursement rates was intricate, complex, and laborious. The first generation of DRGs was based on the International Classification of Diseases, Adapted, Eighth Revision (ICDA-8) and Hospital Adaptation of ICDA, Second Revision (HICDA-2) diagnostic coding schemes. The second generation was based on the International Classification of

21

Diseases, Ninth Revision, Clinical Modification (ICD-9-CM) codes. The "I-8" was a four-digit scheme used to measure the incidence of disease, injury, or illness (Commission on Professional and Hospital Activities, 1975). The "I-9," introduced in 1979, is a five-digit scheme and adds more specificity in terms of location and precision in the reporting of clinical conditions. For example, the I-8 described all fractures (e.g., fracture of the femur), whereas the I-9 added the actual location of the fracture (top or bottom). Tumors of the large intestine could be identified, as well as whether there was an associated obstruction.

In October 2015, ICD-10-CM went into effect and the CMS expects claims submitted must include a valid ICD-10 code. ICD-9 codes are no longer accepted. ICD-10-CM is composed of codes with three, four, five, six, or seven characters, indicating more specificity of illness and treatment compared to codes used previously in ICD-9-CM. Codes with three characters reflect the heading of a category of codes that may be further subdivided by the use of fourth, fifth, sixth, or seventh characters to provide greater specificity of a patient's condition and services provided. Codes within a category are clinically related and provide differences in capturing specific information on the type of condition. For example, category H25 (age-related cataract) contains a number of specific codes that capture information on the type of cataract as well as information on the eye involved. A three-character code alone is used only if the category of an illness is not further subdivided. For example, using the C81 code (i.e., Hodgkin's lymphoma) by itself is considered inappropriate or not valid because this category contains five characters, such as C81.00 (nodular lymphocyte predominant Hodgkin's lymphoma, unspecified site), C81.03 (nodular lymphocyte predominant Hodgkin's lymphoma, intra-abdominal lymph nodes), C81.10 (nodular sclerosis classical Hodgkin's lymphoma, unspecified site), and C81.90 (Hodgkin's lymphoma, unspecified, unspecified site).

2.2.1. Diagnosis-Related Groups

The DRGs are a patient classification scheme that provides a means of relating the type of patient a hospital treats (also known as its case mix) to the costs incurred by the hospital. The DRGs lump "like" patients together. Patients are considered alike if they demonstrate similar resource utilization and length of stay. Resource utilization is defined by the product or personnel resources used to care for that type of patient. Product resources refer to diagnostic and therapeutic interventions such as use of medications, laboratory tests, radiology, and so on. Personnel costs refer to the use of nursing hours per case or other personnel. Length of stay refers to the number of days that the patient remains in the hospital (also known as bed days).

2.2.2. Major Diagnostic Categories

The DRGs are categorized into major diagnostic categories (MDCs). The number of DRGs in each MDC varies from one to twenty or more. The MDCs are consistent with anatomical or pathophysiological groupings and/or the ways in which patients would be clinically managed. Examples include diseases of the central nervous system, diseases of bone and cartilage, and diseases and disorders of the kidney and urinary tract. The major diagnostic categories are broken down into either medical or surgical, meaning the presence or absence of a surgical procedure.

2.2.3. Relative Weights and Case Mix Index

Each DRG is assigned a relative weight. Weights are based on length of stay and cost. The assigned weight is relative to the number 1.00, meaning that the number 1.00 represents a DRG class using an average amount of resources. The assigned weight is intended to reflect the relative resource consumption associated with each DRG. The higher the relative weight, the greater the payment to the hospital. DRGs with relative weights above 1.00 represent those of greater case mix complexity and the use of greater amounts of resources. Those with a relative weight that falls below 1.00 represent lower resource use and lesser complexity.

The weight assigned to the DRG for the hospital is based on the case mix index (CMI). The CMI is the sum of all DRG-relative weights divided by the number of cases (patients) cared for over a period, usually one calendar year. The higher the CMI, the higher the assumed case mix complexity of the hospital. Case mix is affected by the following:

- Severity of illness
- Prognosis
- Treatment difficulty
- Need for intervention
- Resource intensity
- Presence of complications and comorbidities

Hospital payment is calculated by multiplying the CMI with the hospital's assigned base rate. Each hospital is assigned a base rate for reimbursement by the federal government, that is, the CMS. The base rate is determined by the specific hospital (teaching, academic, community), geographical location, population

TABLE 2.1. Examples of the Components of the Early Medicare DRG (HCFA, 1995).

DRG	Description	Relative Weight	Mean LOS	Outlier
001	Craniotomy age >17 except for trauma	3.1565	13.5 days	32 days
90	Simpole pneumonia and pleurisy age >17 without CC	0.6924	5.7 days	15 days

CC: Complication and comorbidity; LOS: length of stay.

served, cost of living in that area, and types of services provided. CMI and base rates are reviewed periodically by the CMS and adjustments made as needed based on actuarial data.

2.2.4. Measuring the Elements in Case Mix

Severity of illness and prognosis reflect the complexity of services or the types of services provided. Severity of illness is made up of objective, clinical indicators of the patient's illness that reflect the need for hospitalization (Box 2.1). Prognosis indicates the patient's likelihood of recovering and to what extent. Treatment difficulty, need for intervention, and resource intensity comprise the intensity of service or the number of services per patient day or hospital stay (Box 2.2). The case mix influences hospital costs. It is not the number of patients that affects the costs incurred by the hospital but rather the types of patients and their use of resources. Table 2.1 presents some examples of the components of a Medicare DRG.

2.2.5. Assigning the DRG

Assignment of a DRG is made based on the documentation in the medical record. For the proper information to be obtained the record must be comprehensive and complete. The documentation must be timely, legible, thorough, and proper.

The DRG assignment is made after discharge. Once that assignment has been made, the hospital receives one lump-sum payment based on the relative weight (Case Manager's Tip 2.1). Some DRGs are given a higher relative weight based on existing complications or comorbidities. Complications are defined as conditions occurring during the hospitalization that prolong the length of stay at least 1 day in 75% of the cases. Comorbidities are pre-existing conditions that increase the length of stay about 1 day in 75% of the cases.

2.2.6. Outliers

Patients with atypically long or short lengths of stay are referred to as outliers. All other patients are considered to be inliers. The placement of a patient as an outlier depends on the trim points for the DRG. Each DRG has a high length-of-stay trim. Some DRGs also have a short length-of-stay trim. Trim points are based on medical and statistical criteria and represent the lowest and highest average lengths of stay for the DRG (see components of a DRG, Table 2.1). Patients may also fall into a cost outlier category. These are patients who have fallen within the appropriate length of stay

 CASE MANAGER'S TIP 2.1

Elements of Diagnosis-Related Groups

When choosing a case management tool, be sure to address the following issues during the design and implementation process:

1. The DRG is assigned after discharge.
2. Payment to the hospital is made once the DRG has been assigned.
3. One lump-sum payment is made for:
   - DRGs with complications or comorbidities.
   - Cost outlier payments.

but who have used an exceptional amount of resources. This may be determined by a flat amount (such as $500) or by determining that the charges exceed the rate by at least 50%.

2.2.7. Managing the DRGs

In 1985 the PPS was advanced to allow some states to designate reimbursement rates for Medicaid and all other third-party payers. Based on hospitals' experiences with the Medicare DRGs and the advent of the system at the state level, strong incentives appeared for the control of hospital resources. Regardless of the cost incurred for caring for a particular case type, the hospital would still be reimbursed a fixed amount of money based on the coded DRG.

It was recognized rather quickly that the RN could play a vital role in managing these dwindling healthcare dollars. The RN's role became increasingly important in terms of the following:

- Coordination of tests, treatments, and procedures
- Confirmation of physician orders
- Accurate documentation
- Timely admissions
- Necessary patient and family teaching
- Timely discharges

In the past, much of the care process had a life of its own, running its course to completion. There were few financial incentives to control the healthcare process; in fact, there were disincentives. In an FFS environment, longer lengths of stay and greater use of product resources translated into greater revenue and financial success for the hospital. The PPS changed all that. It became important to maximize the patient's hospital stay by coordinating the flow of patient care activities. This meant coordination of the patient's tests, treatments, and procedures so that delays could be avoided. Additional strategies included the confirmation of physician orders and/or questioning of their appropriateness when necessary. Getting the patient into the hospital on time and out of the hospital on time were other strategies for maximization.

Finally, documentation in the medical record, although always important, carried even greater weight under this system. Because reimbursement is contingent on the diagnoses and surgical procedures, charting must be complete and accurate. In some hospitals the utilization manager monitors the medical record documentation to ensure that it is accurate, timely, and reflective of what is currently happening in the case. Under case management this is often a role assigned to the case manager.

2.2.8. Diagnosis-Related Groups Assignment

After discharge, the medical record coders review the patient's record. The DRG assignment requires a thorough accounting of the following:

- Principal diagnosis
- Secondary diagnosis
- Operating room procedures
- Complications
- Comorbidities
- Age
- Discharge status

The principal diagnosis (or primary diagnosis) is the condition determined to have been chiefly responsible for the admission to the hospital. The major diagnosis is that which consumed the most hospital resources. The principal diagnosis and the major diagnosis are not necessarily the same. The secondary diagnosis is the next priority in terms of resource consumption. Principal procedures are those performed to treat the chief complaint or complication rather than those performed for diagnostic purposes. If more than one procedure is performed, then the one most closely related to the principal diagnosis will become the principal procedure. Any other surgical procedures are considered as secondary. Operating room procedures other than those performed for diagnostic purposes are also considered as principal procedures. Complications and comorbidities, as defined previously, are also considered. Age is a determining factor for about one-fifth of the DRGs. Age 65 is a demarcation line for some. For a small number of DRGs, the patient's discharge status is considered. Discharge status refers to the final patient destination after discharge, such as nursing home, home, or home with services.

In some cases the DRG is used for per diem rate setting. States with these rate-setting programs use the DRGs to adjust per diem rates. In addition, there are some DRG-exempt categories in some states. These may include the following:

- HIV/AIDS
- Psychiatry
- Pediatrics (if children's hospital)
- Other specialty hospitals (such as cancer hospitals)

Payments are calculated by multiplying the relative weight by the current reimbursement rate. The relative weight is determined by the final DRG coding. Short stays, or patients discharged below the short trim point, are paid at 150% of the daily rate. Outliers, those above the high trim point, are paid 60% of the daily rate for each day above (Box 2.3).

Box 2.3 Severity of Illness Criteria

Example 1: Average Relative Weight

Payment = Relative weight × Current inlier rate
Payment = 1.0 × $1,000.00
Payment = $1,000.00

Example 2: Light Relative Weight

Payment = Relative weight × Current inlier rate
Payment = 0.5 × $1,000.00
Payment = $500.00

Example 3: Heavy Relative Weight

Payment = Relative weight × Current inlier rate
Payment = 22 × $1,000.00
Payment = $22,000.00

Example 4: Short-Stay Payments Before the Short-Trim Point

Short-trim point = 2 Days
Average length of stay = 5 Days
Relative weight = 1.0
Current inlier payment = $1,000.00
Each day's payment = 1.0 × 1,000.00/5 Days
Each day = $200.00
Patient stays in hospital 1 day
Payment = $200.00 × 150%
Payment = $300.00
Revenue loss = $700.00

Example 5: Outlier Payments Above the High-Trim Point

Outlier point = Day 20
Average length of stay = 10 Days
Relative weight = 2.0
Current inlier payment = $1,000.00
Payment = $2,000.00
Each day = $200.00
Patient stays 2 days
Payment = DRG payment + $200.00 = 60%
Payment = $2,000.00 + $120.00
Final payment = $2,120.00

---

*Figures are for example only; they do not reflect actual hospital reimbursements. $1,000.00 is used arbitrarily as the current inlier rate for the purpose of this illustration.

2.3. IMPACT OF DRGs ON THE HEALTHCARE INDUSTRY

In addition to the move toward case management after the institution of the DRG system, other changes have occurred in response to this reimbursement system.

2.3.1. Increased Number of Outpatient Procedures

For some low relative weight DRGs it is more financially lucrative for the hospital to treat patients on an outpatient basis. Generally, the adjusted per diem rate will reimburse less than the DRG reimbursement but more than the short trim outlier payment. This financial incentive led many hospitals to open ambulatory or day surgery facilities, outpatient dialysis, and same-day surgery programs.

2.3.2. Reduced Length of Stay via Preoperative Testing, Home Healthcare, and Discharge Planning

The industry quickly realized that the management of the length of stay on the preadmission and postdischarge sides was extremely important. No longer could the focus be on the inpatient days only. Preoperative or preadmission testing departments were created to respond to these changes. The expense to the hospital and the reimbursement were greater if the hospital did as many tests before admission as possible. Conversely, the better the discharge planning process, as well as the availability of community-based programs, the sooner the patient could be discharged to a less costly care setting.

2.4. USE OF DIAGNOSIS-RELATED GROUPS TODAY

2.4.1. Medicare Severity Diagnosis-Related Groups

The latest version (version 25) of the DRGs was created in 2007. Known as the MS-DRGs (Medicare Severity) at that time, the CMS DRGs were further refined to replace the previous pairing of DRGs to a trifurcated or three-tiered system (Table 2.2). In this new design three tiers were created for some DRGs which included no complication or comorbidity (CC), the presence of a CC, or the presence of a major CC. As a result of this change, the historical list of diagnoses that qualified for membership on the CC list was substantially redefined and replaced with a new standard CC list and a new Major CC list (Mays, 2007).

Another refinement included the elimination of the use of a strict numerical sequencing as was done in prior versions. In the past, newly created DRG classifications would be added to the end of the list. In version 25, there are gaps within the numbering system that will allow modifications over time, and also allow for

TABLE 2.2. Example of a Three-Tiered Diagnosis-Related Group.

DRG	Major Diagnostic Category	Type	Description	Relative Weight	Geometric Mean LOS	Arithmetic Mean LOS
190	04	Medical	Chronic Obstructive Pulmonary Disease W MCC	1.1684	4.4	5.3
191	04	Medical	Chronic Obstructive Pulmonary Disease W CC	0.9628	3.7	4.5
192	04	Medical	Chronic Obstructive Pulmonary Disease W/O CC/MCC	0.7081	3.0	3.5

new MS-DRGs in the same body system to be located more closely together in the numerical sequence.

The sequencing looks like this:

- Major complication/comorbidity (MCC)
- Complication/comorbidity (CC)
- Noncomplication/comorbidity (Non-CC)

These levels are calculated based on clinical factors—principally the patient's secondary diagnosis codes (such as pneumonia or sepsis) in addition to the primary diagnosis (hip fracture). DRG systems focused more on the resources and length of stay of the DRG rather than on the diseases or specifics associated with the patients. It was believed that this would provide more clinical relevance to the DRG system by aligning the diagnoses and patients with the DRG rather than resource consumption of length of stay (Mays, 2007).

In Table 2.2 we can see the relative weights, and therefore reimbursement, drop as the level of patient complications and/or co-morbidities drops. We can also see the expected lengths of stay drop as well. These tiers demonstrate the clinical severity associated with the care of these patients and allows for differences in complexity of care in the amount of reimbursement.

2.5. OBSERVATION STATUS

The Medicare program has had a reimbursement structure for observation status for decades. Some hospitals chose to utilize this level of payment while others did not. The notion of observation has always been to allow providers the additional time they may need in order to make a decision as to whether to admit a patient to the inpatient setting. This decision was to be made based on the patient's condition and the provider's clinical judgement as to what the further needs of that patient might be.

The CMS defines observation status in this way:

"A well-defined set of specific, clinically appropriate services, which include treatment, assessment, and reassessment before a decision can be made regarding whether patients will require further treatment as hospital inpatients or if they are able to be discharged

from the hospital and in the majority of cases the decision can be made in less than 48 hours, usually in less than 24 hours. In only rare and exceptional cases do outpatient observation services span more than 48 hours," (CMS Publication 100-02, 2014).

Observation is considered an outpatient level of care and is billed as such under Medicare Part B. If patients are billed as observation level patients, then they may have to pay a deductible (if not already met) as well as a 20% co-pay. If large amounts of pharmaceuticals are used during the period of observation, the the co-pay can be highly variable and place a great financial burden on the patient.

2.6. THE TWO-MIDNIGHT RULE

A predictable, yet perhaps unwanted, change went into effect on October 1, 2013. Despite protests and a concerted effort on the part of the healthcare industry to keep it away, CMS enacted this new rule as part of the 2014 Hospital Inpatient Prospective Payment System (IPPS) Final Rules. CMS had been scrutinizing one- and two-day hospital stays for years, but no one saw this rather drastic change coming. It is a game changer for case management, but also for all hospitals reimbursed under the IPPS. The rule impacts many things including length of stay, the definition of medical necessity and hospital inpatient status, the use of observation status, and physician documentation. It requires that case managers apply due diligence at the hospital's routes of entry, particularly the emergency department.

2.6.1. A Time-Based System

In the past CMS had defined 24 hours as the amount of time the patient might have *needed hospital care*. With the two-midnight rule new logic is being applied. Known as the Medicare Utilization Day (MUD), CMS has applied language and logic in a new way as it redefines a 24-hour benchmark process. It is defined as the 24 hours (that begin at midnight) of the first calendar day that a patient is in a bed and continues until the following midnight. While CMS states that this is still a 24-hour benchmark, it goes on to say that "the relevant 24 hours are those encompassed by two midnights." This leaves the potential for the MUD to last up to 48 hours when patients are admitted just after the first midnight benchmark.

The rule requires that when a physician expects that a patient's hospital stay will encompass at least two midnights that the patient be admitted to the hospital as an inpatient. The time that the patient spends in the emergency department receiving treatment, and/or the time that that patient spends in surgery, is counted as part of this time period. Therefore the patient's time of presentation will affect whether or not they get admitted, rather than their medical condition in some instances. It also requires that physicians be able to anticipate and project the expected treatment duration, something that can often be quite difficult. The physician must have a reasonable expectation that the patient's stay will cross two midnights and admit the patient based on that expectation.

2.6.2. Outpatient and Observation Status

In addition to delineating what an admission requires, the rule also clarifies what is inappropriate for an inpatient hospital stay. It stipulates that surgical procedures, diagnostic tests, and other treatments that require that the patient be in the hospital for a more limited time period, and do not cross two midnights, are generally not appropriate for admission to the inpatient setting.

Our view of observation status, as providers, also changes with this new rule. Observation had been used as a "time-extender," allowing the physician additional time following care in the emergency department to determine if the patient needed to be admitted to the hospital. Now CMS is directing hospitals to place any patient whose stay will not span two midnights into observation status. It goes on to say that once the physician has additional information, the status may be changed to inpatient or the patient may be discharged.

This distinction between the previous use of observation and the 2014 use of observation warrants further explanation. In the 2014 use of observation status, the physician's selection of inpatient versus observation status is strictly based on his anticipated duration of care and not on the patient's level of illness or needed services. CMS further explains that even a patient requiring care in a critical care bed or telemetry, but whose stay will not span at least two midnights, should be placed in observation status. CMS explains that the majority of patient stays under two midnights will gen-

erally not be appropriate for an inpatient admission, with the following exceptions: death, transfer, patients leaving against medical advice, unforeseen recovery, and election of hospice care. Should patients fall under any of these categories, the hospital will be able to bill the stay as an inpatient admission. It is important that your hospital checks its policies regarding the use of certain specialty hospital beds, such as critical care beds, to ensure that observation patients placed in these beds are not outside the hospital's own policies about use of these beds.

Under very limited circumstances the physician may admit the patient to the inpatient setting even though the expectation is that that stay will not span at least two midnights. These include: medically necessary procedures on the inpatient only list, new onset mechanical ventilation (not including intubations expected as part of a surgical procedure), and others approved by CMS and outlined in sub regulatory guidance.

2.6.3. Physician Documentation

In addition to changes in the use of observation status, there are changes in the final rules as they apply to physician documentation expectations. The new rule requires that every inpatient admission is certified by the physician of record, that is, the physician who is most familiar with the patient's needs and reason for hospitalization. Certification is fulfilled when there is a valid order for admission that is authenticated prior to discharge and is in compliance with the two midnight rule. In addition the medical record must also include a history and physical outlining the diagnosis and treatment plans for the patient, and a documented discharge plan at the time of discharge. The physician must also be sure to document other complex medical factors such as comorbidities, the severity of the signs and symptoms, current medical needs, and the risk of adverse events. The physician does not need to include a separate attestation for the expected length of stay. Rather this information is inferred from the physician's standard medical documentation. Examples of this include the plan of care, treatments orders, and physician's notes.

Case managers must be sure that they discuss the discharge plan with the physician of record and the agreement with the discharge plan is clearly documented in the medical record by the physician of record. CMS does not require that the physician complete a "certification form," although some hospitals have chosen to use a form or template in their electronic medical record. Whether a form is used or the hospital depends solely on the presence of the physician's documentation in the medical record is a choice that each hospital must make.

2.6.4. The Use of Screening Criteria—A Change for Case Managers

The CMS, in the final rules, explains their take on the use of inpatient level utilization review screening criteria. While the hospital may continue to use existing utilization review criteria, these criteria are not binding on the hospital, CMS, or outside review contractors. When a Medicare external review contractor reviews the medical record they assess for the following:

- The reasonableness of the physician's expectation of the need for and duration of care based on complex medical factors such as history and comorbidities
- The severity of the signs and symptoms
- Current medical needs
- Risk of an adverse event

This is a change from the traditional use of utilization review criteria to determine the medical necessity of admission. In the past, case managers in the emergency department (ED) have used commercial screening criteria to determine whether or not the patient should be admitted to the hospital. When the patient did not meet these criteria, the case manager would have a conversation with the admitting physician to see if an alternative plan could be created, thereby preventing the admission to the hospital. While CMS does not direct hospitals to stop doing this, clearly the decision to admit will now be based on the expected duration of the stay and not on whether or not the patient meets the medical necessity criteria for admission. This is a significant change in the approach of utilization review in the emergency department. ED case managers will now need to review the patient's expected length of stay and guide the physician in determining whether or not the patient should be admitted to the hospital.

2.6.5. Care Following Surgical Procedures

The CMS explains how to manage patients who may need additional recovery time following a minor surgical procedure. When the determination is made that the patient needs additional recovery time, the physician should reassess the expected length of stay. Generally speaking, if the expected length of stay is unclear, and/or the physician can determine that the patient's expected length of stay will not span two midnights, then the physician should continue to treat the patient as an outpatient. If additional information is obtained during

that time that suggests that the patient's stay will span greater than two midnights, then the physician may admit the patient to the hospital as an inpatient.

2.6.6. Other Roles for the Hospital Case Manager

When the patient is placed in observation status, the patient should be notified in writing of this decision. It is prudent to have the patient sign the written notice and the case manager should place a copy of the signed document in the medical record.

The case manager should explain the differences between inpatient admission and observation status to the patient in a manner that they can understand. The implications of the increase in out-of-pocket expenses that may be incurred by the patient if they remain in observation status throughout the stay should also be explained. These expenses may include a co-pay as well as a deductible. In some instances, the patient may also be billed for medications that are not related to the reason for the period of observation such as diabetic or antihypertensive medications.

One point of clarification is important to note: While the total time in the hospital will be taken into consideration when the physician is making an admission decision (expectation of hospital care for two or more midnights), the inpatient admission does not begin until the inpatient order and formal admission occur.

Today we find a mixture of reimbursement systems and schemes. Although more and more patients are being reimbursed under managed care contracts, which is the subject of the next section, others remain under either state or federal reimbursement systems. These systems continue to use the DRG as a measuring stick for either flat rates of reimbursement for the hospital stay or in negotiating discounted rates.

2.7. AMBULATORY PAYMENT CLASSIFICATIONS: MEDICARE'S OUTPATIENT PROSPECTIVE PAYMENT SYSTEM

Years after the implementation of the inpatient PPS, the CMS, formerly the HCFA, turned its attention to other care delivery settings across the continuum. It was only logical that great attention would be paid to ambulatory and outpatient settings, including ambulatory surgery, EDs, and clinics. As healthcare delivery shifted away from the acute care setting, more and more complex (and therefore more expensive) services were being provided in outpatient settings.

The Balanced Budget Act of 1997 (see page 39) instructed CMS to develop and implement a PPS for hospital outpatient services. The September 1998 Federal

Register published, in review form, the proposed form for the outpatient prospective payment system (OPPS), including the implementation regulations. Finally, in 1999, the Balanced Budget Refinement Act (BBRA) was passed and the OPPS was a go.

As a follow-up to the previous publication in the Federal Register, the final regulations were published in the April 2000 edition, including an expected implementation date of July 1, 2000. With such an ambitious implementation date, it was no surprise when CMS extended the deadline by 1 month to August 1, 2000.

2.7.1. Ambulatory Payment Classification

The ambulatory payment classification (APC) system is an encounter-based patient classification system. The system approaches outpatient reimbursement from the same philosophical vantage point as the inpatient PPS. Similar groupings of patients are identified, and predetermined reimbursement amounts are allotted (Case Manager's Tip 2.2). The system attempts to predict the amount and type of resources used for a variety of types of ambulatory visits.

The initial program identified 451 ambulatory payment classification groups. Table 2.3 outlines the categories of APCs and the number of APCs in each category. The groups and payment rates are based on categories of services that are similar in cost and resource utilization. Current Procedural Terminology (CPT)-4 or Health Care Financing Administrators Common Procedure Coding System (HCPCS) codes are mapped, or identified with, an APC (see page 30 for more detail on CPT codes). Each APC has an associated status indicator. The status indicator defines if and how a service will be paid. Some status indicators are paid under an APC, whereas others are not. In total, 936 new codes have been added; 645 of these are codes for billing pass-through and new technology items.

CMS has also identified certain procedures as "in-

TABLE 2.3. Ambulatory Payment Classification Groupings.

Category	Number of APCs
Significant procedures	240
Medical visits	7
Ancillary	39
New technology	15
Transitional pass through	132
Extensive pharmaceuticals	17
Partial hospitalization	1
Total	**451**

patient only." These are mainly surgeries that CMS has identified as requiring more services than can be provided in an outpatient setting. Hospitals must be very careful to ensure that patients are placed in the appropriate setting so that revenue is not lost (see Chapter 5).

Procedure APCs include surgical and nonsurgical procedures (see Table 2.3). Included under nonsurgical procedures are nuclear medicine, magnetic resonance imaging (MRI), radiation therapy, and psychotherapy.

Pass-through items include drugs, biologicals, and devices that can be claimed for reimbursement in addition to the APC payment if they meet certain criteria as set by CMS. Examples of these items would be pacemaker devices, cataract lenses, and cardiac catheterization lead wires.

In addition, certain services are packaged. Packaged services include the following:

- Operating room
- Recovery and treatment rooms
- Anesthesia
- Observation services
- Medical/surgical supplies
- Drugs and pharmaceuticals (with exceptions)
- Donor tissue
- Implantable devices

Exceptions to packaged services include the following:

- Drugs, pharmaceuticals, biologicals, and/or devices that are eligible for transitional pass-through payments
- Other specific services defined by CMS:
  —Corneal tissue acquisition
  —Casting, splinting, and strapping
  —Blood and blood products
  —Certain other high-cost drugs

 CASE MANAGER'S TIP 2.2

Comparing Ambulatory Payment Classifications and Diagnosis-Related Groups

1. APCs follow the same methodology as DRGs.
2. Similar groupings of patient types are prospectively identified with corresponding reimbursement amounts.
3. Unlike DRGs, a single outpatient encounter can result in the payment of one or more APCs.

It is important to note that, unlike the inpatient PPS in which only one DRG can be assigned to a hospital stay, under an OPPS, an outpatient visit may consist of multiple APCs. The total reimbursement equals the sum of the individual payments for each service. Therefore a single outpatient visit might include APC as well as non-APC-related payments. The total of all of these will determine the final reimbursement.

2.7.2. The Scope of the Outpatient Prospective Payment System

OPPS applies to acute care hospitals and includes hospitals that are currently exempt from an inpatient PPS. Also included are partial hospitalization services provided by community mental health centers (CMHCs). Cancer centers that are exempted from the inpatient PPS are not exempt from OPPS, but they are held permanently harmless for payment reductions. Simply stated, this means that they must implement the same infrastructure for mapping and billing under the OPPS, but should their reimbursement be negatively affected, the reimbursement will be supplemented. Similarly, small rural hospitals of less than 100 beds will be held harmless, but only through 2003.

Box 2.4 lists the services included in the OPPS. Additionally, there are services that are excluded from OPPS (Box 2.5).

2.7.3. Clinics, Emergency Departments, and Critical Care Services

Clinic visits, ED visits, and critical care are assigned to one of seven Medical APC groups. Assignment into the APC is based on 31 Evaluation and Management (E & M) CPT-4 codes. Hospital-based clinics have three APCs, identified as low, medium, and high. Assignment into one of these would be based on the CPT-4 code identified. The ED also has three categories, identified as low, medium, and high, and these would also be identified based on the CPT-4 code. Critical care has one CPT (CPT 99291).

Box 2.4   Included Services

- Emergency department visits
- Clinic visits
- Surgical procedures
- Radiology
- Chemotherapy
- Most ancillary services
- Partial hospitalization program services

Box 2.5   Excluded Services

- Ambulance services
- Rehabilitation therapy services
- Laboratory services paid under a fee schedule
- End-stage renal disease (routine dialysis services) and Epoetin (EPO)
- Services provided by critical access hospitals
- Durable medical equipment
- Orthotic/prosthetic devices
- Screening mammography

2.7.4. Observation Services

Under the new system, observation is no longer reimbursed separately but would be included as part of the APC payment, either ED or ambulatory surgery. Exceptions to this are congestive heart failure, asthma, and chest pain. Patients admitted to observation with one of these diagnoses are mapped to their own APC.

2.7.5. Mapping

Hospitals are required to develop their own internal system for "mapping" provided services to the different levels of resource utilization represented by the APC groupings. The process includes each hospital's own identification of which CPT-4 codes they would map into either the low, medium, or high APC groupings and then to derive computerized systems for linking the coding to the APC and, finally, to the billing.

2.8. HOME CARE PROSPECTIVE PAYMENT SYSTEM

On October 1, 2000, CMS implemented prospective payment for home care visits. Unlike inpatient PPS, home care's system would be based on a prospective nursing assessment completed at the time the patient was entered for home care services. Home care, like acute care before it, was no longer paid based on a visit. Care would be reimbursed for an episode of care or 60 days. The dollar amount reimbursed would be fixed regardless of the number of visits the patient received. The final dollar amount reimbursed is based on the Outcome and Assessment Information Set (OASIS) (Case Manager's Tip 2.3).

2.8.1. Outcome and Assessment Information Set

Scores in the OASIS are based on three categories. The first category is clinical and consists of four items;

CASE MANAGER'S TIP 2.3

Understanding Home Care Prospective Payment System

1. Home Care PPS is the only PPS that relies on a nursing assessment as the driver for reimbursement.
2. The OASIS data must be accurate because this is what drives reimbursement.
3. HHRGs are similar to DRGs and APCs.

the second category is functional and consists of five items; and the third category includes service utilization and consists of four items. The final score results in the assignment of 1 of 80 resource groups called home health resource groups (HHRGs). Like the DRGs, each HHRG has a dollar amount attached to it.

2.8.2. Initial Claims

Home care agencies can make an initial claim for payment known as an advance request for payment (ARP) at the time the initial OASIS assessment is completed. This initial payment equals 60% of the designated HHRG. One of home care's first challenges following the implementation of this new system was to be sure that claims were processed as quickly as possible after the first assessment (no greater than 48 hours). A rapid turnaround time would better ensure that cash flow problems did not occur.

The dollar amount reimbursed for the HHRG is calculated based on several factors. The payment rate corresponds to the level of home health services for that HHRG. The national payment rate for a 60-day episode of home healthcare services is standard and is then adjusted based on several factors. The standard amount is for all home health services, excluding durable medical equipment, and osteoporosis drugs will continue to be paid by a fee schedule. It is inclusive of the per-visit amounts for all disciplines, as well as nonroutine medical supplies and the cost of managing the OASIS process. The national payment rate is proportioned at 77.668% for labor and 22.332% for nonlabor. It is expected that the national rate ($2,037.04) will be adjusted at predetermined times to allow for changes in the cost of goods and services necessary to provide home health services. Adjustments will be made to this rate on a periodic basis.

2.8.3. Final Payment

The final claim is paid at the end of the episode and must include all line-item visit information that was rendered during the 60-day period.

2.8.4. Adjustments

The national payment rate is adjusted for the case mix and the wage index area of the patient. The case mix payment rate is based on the level of home health services for the particular HHRG. Finally, an adjustment is made for the wage index for the area in which the patient lives. This is split by labor and nonlabor in the percentages previously mentioned (see the following example).

Example

Standard Prospective Payment Rate	$2,037.04
Case Mix Payment Rate for C0F050	× 0.5265%
Case Mix Adjusted PPS Payment Amount	$1,072.50

Wage Index Adjustments	
Case Mix Adjusted PPS Payment Amount	$1,072.50
Labor Percentage of PPS Payment Rate	× 0.77668%
Labor Portion	$832.99

The labor portion is then multiplied by the Wage Index Factor:	$832.99
Wage Index Factor	× 1.1 (example)
Adjusted Labor Portion	$916.29

Nonlabor Portion	
Case Mix Adjusted Amount	$1,072.50
Nonlabor Percentage	× 0.2233%
Adjusted Nonlabor Portion	$239.49

Labor Portion	$916.29
Nonlabor Portion	+ 239.49
Total Case Mix and Wage Adjusted PPS Rate	$1,155.78

2.8.5. Partial Episode Payments

Similar to a short-trim point in the DRG system, CMS has allowed for situations in which the 60 days for home care services are interrupted. These Partial Episode Payments (PEPs) occur under only two circumstances. The first would be when a patient elects to transfer from one home health agency to another. The second would be when a patient is discharged and then returns to the same agency within the 60-day period. The PEP would only apply if the transfer or discharge/return was not related to a significant change in the patient's condition. The reimbursable amount is prorated based on the number of days the patient was seen. For example, if the patient was seen for 15 of the 60 days, the PEP would be calculated as 15/60 multiplied by the full original payment amount.

2.8.6. Significant Change in Condition Payment

For circumstances in which the patient's condition results in a new OASIS, a new HHRG, and a new set of physician orders, CMS has established a special payment rate. The change must not have been originally expected and must signify an interruption in the 60-day episode and the plan of care. As in the PEP, a prorated amount would be determined. Of the 60 days, a partial amount would be paid at the original HHRG level, and an additional payment would be made at the significant change in condition payment (SCIC) level (see the following example).

Example

Original HHRG 20 days of 60 days	$1,155.78
	× 0.33
	$381.40
SCIC HHRG 40 days of 60 days	$2,200.00
	× 0.66
	$1,452.00
	$381.40
	$1,452.00
(new HHRG reimbursement)	$1,833.40
Total Reimbursement	

2.8.7. Low-Utilization Payment

A low-utilization payment adjustment (LUPA) would be made for patients who require minimal visits during their 60-day episode. For patients who receive four or fewer visits during their 60-day encounter period, the home health agency will be paid based on the national standard per visit amount by discipline. These amounts are adjusted based on wage area index but not on case mix.

2.8.8. Outlier Payments

Finally, when unusual variations occur in the amount of medically necessary home health services, an outlier payment may be considered. These unusual variations are determined based on two principles: (1) that the cost of services should exceed the payment and (2)

that the outlier payment should cover less than the total amount of cost above the outlier threshold.

The amount of the outlier payment is limited to 5% of the total PPS payment. The fixed dollar loss amount is now 1.13 times the standard episode amount (see the following example).

Example

Standard Prospective	$2,037.04 Payment Rate
Fixed Dollar Loss Amount	$2,037.04
	× 1.13
	$2,301.86
Case Mix Adjusted PPS	+ 1,072.50
Payment Amount	
Outlier Threshold Total Amount	$3,374.36

2.8.9. Important Points to Consider

Under the home care PPS, the old paradigm of more visits, more incurred cost, more Medicare reimbursement is now extinct. Under PPS it is essential to coordinate the clinical and financial aspects of the agency. In other words, it is imperative that the patient receives the appropriate number of visits by the appropriate clinicians but that those visits not be in excess of the patient's true clinical needs.

In addition, the OASIS data must be accurate and timely because this is what drives reimbursement. Going forward, home care agencies, like hospitals before them, will need to identify their costs on an HHRG basis. This data will serve as the benchmark for identifying areas of profit and loss for the agency and lead to new product lines, elimination of old ones, or improvement in resource utilization for existing patient groups.

Home health agencies need to implement strategies similar to those applied in the acute care setting. For example, implementation of clinical practice guidelines will help to prospectively identify the expected resources to be applied to various case types and to standardize the care for that group of patients. Strategies such as this will better ensure that patients receive just the right amount of resources: not too much and not too little. Case managers will be deployed to manage high-risk populations who have a greater likelihood of falling outside the norms of the clinical practice guidelines. Because of the variation in these high-risk groups, it can be assumed that they will have a greater likelihood of using excess resources if not proactively managed.

Identification of these high-risk groups will have to be made based on high-risk assessment strategies so that patients can be immediately identified and the case manager can be deployed as quickly as possible. The OASIS data may provide the foundation for much of the data that will be necessary to identify patients at greater risk for poor outcomes or greater resource utilization.

2.9. INPATIENT REHABILITATION FACILITY PROSPECTIVE PAYMENT SYSTEM

Among its other mandates, the Balanced Budget Act of 1997 mandated prospective payment for inpatient or acute rehabilitation effective January 1, 2002. This new reimbursement scheme replaces the prior reimbursement structure as directed by TEFRA in 1982. TEFRA mandated the CMS regulations for Medicare reimbursement, Medicare HMOs, and risk contracts.

Reimbursement is based on patient assessment forms completed on admission to and discharge from the acute rehabilitation unit (Case Manager's Tip 2.4). The assessment form, the Inpatient Rehabilitation Facilities Patient Assessment Instrument (IRF-PAI), contains 54 data items and takes approximately 45 minutes to complete.

The admission assessment reference date is calendar day three of stay. Completion date is calendar day four. The discharge assessment reference date is day of discharge or death. Completion date is calendar day four after discharge/death.

2.9.1. The Inpatient Rehabilitation Facilities Patient Assessment Instrument

The PAI is used to classify patients into distinct groups based on clinical characteristics and expected resource needs. Patients are classified as follows:

- First, patients are assigned to 1 of 21 rehabilitation impairment categories (RICs).
- Second, patients are classified into 1 of 100 distinct case mix groups (CMGs).

Completion of the PAI requires a skilled assessor. It cannot be completed by clerical staff but must be

 CASE MANAGER'S TIP 2.4

Elements of the Acute Inpatient Rehabilitation Prospective Payment System

1. Acute rehabilitation uses CMGs that function just like the DRGs and APCs.
2. This classification is based on the data in the IRF-PAI.

completed by a qualified clinician such as a physician, RN, or physical or occupational therapist. Therefore many organizations use RN case managers to complete the PAI, which contains physician, nursing therapy, and other care elements. In this way the case manager can complete the PAI and perform other case management functions so critical to financial survival under this system, such as monitoring of resource utilization, cost per case, and length of stay.

Each CMG has a relative weight that determines the base payment rate the IRF will receive. Included in the payment rates are the operating costs and capital costs of furnishing covered inpatient rehabilitation hospital services, including routine, ancillary, and capital costs. Not included are the costs of bad debts or approved educational activities.

2.9.2. Payment Adjustments

Payment may be adjusted for the following reasons:

- Labor share percentage, area wage index, disproportionate share, and rural factors
- Comorbidities present during the patient's stay

Although the admission assessment will be used to place a patient into a CMG, the discharge assessment is used to determine the relevant weighting factors associated with any existing comorbidities.

The short-stay category contains only one CMG. For patients who have expired there are the following four CMGs:

- Orthopedic, short-stay
- Orthopedic, regular stay
- Nonorthopedic, short-stay
- Nonorthopedic, regular stay

2.9.3. Method of Payment

A standardized amount per discharge is adjusted based on case mix, DSH, and a rural hospital add-on of 15.89%. Other adjustments include high-cost outlier payments. Transfer cases are reimbursed at a per diem rate. Interrupted stays, defined as cases in which the beneficiary returns to the inpatient rehabilitation facility by midnight of the third day after a discharge, are reimbursed as a single discharge. Payment is based on the CMG classification determined from the initial PAI assessment.

2.9.4. Three-Step Process

Calculating the reimbursement encompasses a three-

Example: CMG Relative Weights for RIC 03: Nontraumatic Brain Injury

CMG	Description	CMG Weight	Payment	Comorbidity Add-On	Payment with Comorbidity Add-On
0301	M = 33–0 and C = 22–35	0.6399	$3,855	12.6%	$4,342
0302	M = 33–0 and C = 5–21	0.8393	$5,056	12.6%	$5,695
0303	M = 46–34	0.9467	$5,703	12.6%	$6,424
0304	M = 56–47	1.2605	$7,593	12.6%	$8,553
0305	M = 78–57	1.7517	$10,552	12.6%	$11,886

C: Cognitive; M: motor.

step process. First the patient is assigned to a RIC. Within the RIC, the patient is assigned to a CMG. Within the CMG, the patient is designated as either having or not having a relevant comorbidity. Relevant comorbidities are represented by codes.

The 21 RICs represent the primary cause of the rehabilitation stay. The RICs are clinically homogeneous (see the example above).

2.9.5. Conversion Factor

As in the inpatient DRG system, each CMG is assigned a relative weight. Weights represent the variance in the cost per discharge and resource utilization among payment groups. Basic payment in 2001 was $6,024, and from that each CMG payment was based on the relative weight multiplied by the payment amount.

2.9.6. Short-Stay Cases

There is one relative weight for short-stay cases. Short-stay cases are defined as patients with a length of stay of less than or equal to 3 days who do not meet the definition of a transfer case; for example, patients who leave against medical advice or patients who are unable to tolerate intensive rehabilitation services (see the example below).

2.9.7. Expired Patients

Relative weights have also been identified for patients who have expired.

2.9.8. Wage Index

The hospital location will determine the classified wage index. The rate excludes 100% of wages for teaching physicians, interns and residents, and nonphysician anesthesiologists. The wage adjustment is to the labor-related portion of the payment only. The labor portion is 71.301%, and the nonlabor portion is 28.699% of the rate.

The disproportionate patient percentage (DPP) is calculated as Medicare supplemental security income (SSI) days (as a percentage of total Medicare days) plus Medicaid days (as a percentage of total days).

2.9.9. Outlier Cases

Additional payments are made for high-cost patients. These are calculated based on 80% of the case loss exceeding a deductible. Loss is determined by charges multiplied by the overall facility-specific ratio of cost-to-charges (RCC) minus the IRF PPS payment. The deductible, also known as the threshold, is $7,066 multiplied by the wage index, multiplied by the DSH adjustment. Outlier payments can be attributed to 3–5% of total program payments.

2.9.10. Transfer Cases

Transfer cases are those with a length of stay less than the arithmetic mean length of stay for the relevant CMG. Transfer cases would include those that were discharged to another inpatient site of care, such as an

Example: CMG Relative Weight for Short-Stay Cases

CMG	Description	CMG Weight	Payment	Comorbidity Add-On	Payment with Comorbidity Add-On
5001	Short-stay	0.1908	$1.149	0.0%	$1,149

(LOS ≤ 3 days)

inpatient hospital, long-term care hospital, rehabilitation facility, or nursing home that accepts Medicare and/or Medicaid. Discharges to home health, outpatient therapy, or day programs are not considered as transfer cases.

Payment is based on a per diem inlier payment, which is divided by the mean length of stay for the CMG, multiplied by the number of actual days, plus an outlier payment. Unlike inpatient prospective payment systems, the first day is reimbursed only one per diem.

2.10. LONG-TERM CARE REIMBURSEMENT (SKILLED NURSING FACILITY)

Under the Balanced Budget Act of 1997, CMS implemented a PPS for services provided to nursing home residents during a Medicare Part A–covered stay. Implemented on July 1, 1998, PPS rates reimburse for routine, ancillary, and capital-related costs.

Residents of the nursing home are assessed on a schedule at certain points during their stay (on the fifth, fourteenth, thirtieth, sixtieth, and ninetieth days after admission to the skilled nursing facility [SNF]). Unlike inpatient rehabilitation, SNFs have a window in which to perform each assessment. As an example, a Day 14 assessment can have a reference date of Days 6, 7, 8, 9, 10, 11, 12, 13, or 14. Additional assessments would be required when a resident experiences a significant change in status or care needs.

The Minimum Data Set (MDS) is the assessment tool used in the SNF setting. The MDS collects comprehensive information, which includes the patient di-

CASE MANAGER'S TIP 2.5

Long-Term Care Reimbursement
1. The RUG III determines the reimbursement amount.
2. The RUG is selected based on the data in the MDS.

agnosis, activities of daily living (ADLs) capabilities, cognition, and minutes per day of rehabilitation services received. The exception to this is the Day five assessment, which requests information regarding estimated rehabilitation minutes.

Based on the data captured in the MDS, the patient is placed into one of 44 Resource Utilization Group III (RUG-III) categories (Case Manager's Tip 2.5). Each MDS assigned is "locked-in" within 7 days of completion of the MDS and cannot be changed. Each RUG is assigned a case mix weight, which is used to adjust the federal portion of the SNF's reimbursement for that resident.

The RUG-III system (Table 2.4) classifies patients into seven major clinical hierarchies and 44 groups. The RUG-III grouper, a computer software program, will classify the patient into the group with the highest payment. The seven major hierarchies are rehabilitation, extensive services, special care, clinically complex, impaired cognition, behavioral problems, and reduced physical function. A patient who classifies into a lower category may be covered if the coverage guidelines of the SNF are met.

TABLE 2.4. The RUG III System.

Clinical Heirarchy	Activities of Daily Living	Problem/Service Split	Number of RUG Groups
Automatically Deemed Medicare Covered			
Rehabilitation	14 Levels	Not used	14 RUGs
Ultra-high			
Very high			
High			
Medium			
Low			
Extensive Services	Not used	Various types of services	3 RUGs
Special Care	3 Levels	Not used	3 RUGs
Clinically Complex	3 Levels	Signs of Depression	6 RUGs
Medicare Covered Based on Skilled Nursing Facility Guidelines			
Impaired Cognition	2 Levels	Nursing rehabilitation	4 RUGs
Behavioral Problems	2 Levels	Nursing rehabilitation	4 RUGs
Reduced Physical Function	5 Levels	Nursing rehabilitation	3.5

2.11. GOVERNMENT PROGRAMS

2.11.1. Medicare

In 1966 the federal government enacted Title XVIII of the Social Security Act. Known as the Medicare program, it was designed to finance medical care for persons age 65 years and older and disabled persons who are entitled to Social Security benefits (Case Manager's Tip 2.6). Medicare also covers individuals with end-stage renal disease. Disabled individuals and those under age 65 with end-stage renal disease make up approximately 12% of Medicare beneficiaries.

The Medicare program is a federal program under the administrative oversight of CMS. CMS is a branch of the United States Department of Health and Human Services (DHHS).

2.11.2. Medicare's Dual Structure

Medicare consists of two parts. Part A is a hospital or acute care insurance program. Included in Part A are the following:

- Inpatient hospital
- Skilled nursing
- Home health
- Hospice
- Administrative expenses

Part A is financed by special payroll taxes collected under the Social Security program. Employer and employee share equally in financing this portion of the Social Security income known as the hospital insurance trust fund. The amount an individual contributes to this fund is distinctly identified on an employee's pay stub. This mandatory tax is paid by all working individuals, including those who are self-employed.

2.11.3. The Omnibus Budget Reconciliation Act of 1993

The Omnibus Budget Reconciliation Act of 1993 (OBRA-93) eliminated the maximum taxable earnings base so that as of 1993, all earnings are now subject to Medicare tax. Despite OBRA, there still remains concern that the Hospital Insurance Trust Fund may eventually run out of money. Debates continue to focus on precisely when this may happen and as to whether the fund should be financially supplemented in some other way. Some politicians have suggested that the minimum age to receive Medicare be increased to age 70.

 CASE MANAGER'S TIP 2.6

Government Programs—Medicare

1. Medicare finances healthcare for the following:
   a. Persons over 65
   b. Disabled persons
2. Part A covers hospitalization.
3. Part B is a voluntary program covering physician services and emergency visits, among others.

2.11.4. Overview of Services

A maximum of 90 days of inpatient hospital care is allowed per benefit period. Once the 90 days are exhausted, there is a lifetime reserve of 60 hospital inpatient days. A benefit period is a spell of illness beginning with hospitalization and ending when a beneficiary has not been an inpatient in a hospital or SNF for 60 consecutive days. There is no limit to the number of benefit periods.

The beneficiary pays a deductible for each benefit period and co-payments based on the duration of services.

Medicare pays for up to 100 days of care in a Medicare-certified SNF, provided that the beneficiary has been hospitalized for at least 3 consecutive days, not including the day of discharge. Admission to the SNF must occur within 30 days of hospital discharge.

Medicare pays for home healthcare when a person is homebound and requires intermittent or part-time skilled nursing care or rehabilitation care. There are no time or visit limits. For terminally ill patients, Medicare pays for care provided by a Medicare-certified hospice.

2.11.5. Supplementary Medical Insurance Part B

The Supplementary Medical Insurance (SMI) program is a voluntary program financed partly by general tax revenues and partly by required premium contributions. The main services covered by SMI include the following:

- Physician services
- Hospital outpatient services such as outpatient surgery, diagnostic tests, and radiology and pathology services
- ED visits
- Outpatient rehabilitation services
- Renal dialysis

- Prosthetics
- Medical equipment and supplies

Services not covered by SMI include the following:

- Vision care and eyeglasses
- Outpatient prescription drugs
- Routine physical examinations
- Preventive services

Exceptions for Part B Enrollees are as follows:

- Screening Pap smears
- Mammography
- Flu shots and vaccinations against pneumonia

2.11.6. Managed Medicare

In September of 1982, the laws treating Medicare HMOs were passed as part of TEFRA. The regulations became effective in 1985. In 1982 CMS funded several demonstration contracts to test the concepts of risk HMOs. These were known as the Medicare competition demonstration projects. These operated under a variety of waivers as part of the Social Security Act. By 1985 there were about 300,000 members enrolled out of a total of about 30 million Medicare beneficiaries. By 1995 nearly 3 million Medicare members had enrolled in TEFRA-risk HMOs.

TEFRA also modified the HMO contracting rules to permit CMS to contract with a new type of entity known as the comprehensive medical plan (CMP). A CMP is defined as an entity that is state licensed, provides healthcare on a prepaid capitated basis, provides care through physicians who are employees or partners of the entity, assumes full financial risk on a prospective basis, and meets the Public Health Service Act requirements against insolvency. Today these differences between HMOs and CMPs no longer exist.

2.11.7. Requirements to Obtain a TEFRA Contract

A nonrural plan must have a minimum of 5,000 prepaid members, and rural plans a minimum of 1,500 members. At all times during the contract, membership cannot exceed 50% combined Medicare and Medicaid.

The entity must be able to render (or contract for) all Medicare services available in the service area. In addition, it must use certified Medicare providers and be able to provide 24-hour emergency services. Other requirements include provisions for emergency claims both within and out of network. All services must be accessible within reasonable promptness.

 CASE MANAGER'S TIP 2.7

Government Programs—Managed Medicare

1. Managed Medicare is an option afforded to Medicare enrollees.
2. The HMO must provide all the Medicare Part A and Part B services that a recipient would normally receive in his or her area.

The HMO must provide all of the Medicare Part A and Part B services that a recipient would receive as available in his or her area. The HMO may provide additional services not traditionally covered under Medicare as additional and covered services or as optional supplemental services that the patient may choose to subscribe to (Case Manager's Tip 2.7). In some instances, additional benefits must be purchased as a condition of enrollment. For example, preventive care, not traditionally covered under Medicare but covered by HMOs, would be financed by mandatory premiums. Some HMOs opt to provide additional services beyond the traditional scope of Medicare at no cost to the patient.

2.11.8. Benefits to Enrollees

Medicare beneficiary enrollment in HMOs has been slow. Portions of the country see greater enrollment than others. Correlations can be found between highly managed care penetrated areas and the percent of Medicare enrollees who have opted for HMO plans. It should also be noted that not all areas offer HMO products to Medicare recipients. Some of the attractions of enrolling include lower out-of-pocket expenses. Some waive the plan premium, which includes the Medicare coinsurance and deductible payments. Most provide additional non-Medicare benefits such as prescription drugs (to a capped amount per year), eyeglasses, and hearing aids.

Resistance to enrollment often has to do with an older person's longstanding relationship with his or her physician. In general, managed care concepts are not familiar to the senior population and therefore some may not realize that the HMO may offer higher coverage at a lower cost.

2.11.9. Medicaid

The Medicaid program is referred to as Title XIX of the Social Security Act and finances healthcare for the indigent. Started in 1966, the program is jointly

CASE MANAGER'S TIP 2.8

Government Programs—Medicaid

Medicaid finances healthcare for the indigent and is funded through the tax structure.

financed by the federal and state governments (Case Manager's Tip 2.8). The federal government provides matching funds to the states based on the per-capita income in each state. Federal matching, known as the Federal Medical Assistance Percentage (FMAP), cannot be less than 50% or greater than 83% of total state Medicaid costs. Wealthier states have a smaller share of their costs reimbursed by the federal government, and federal outlays have no set limit. The federal government must match whatever the individual state provides.

The federal government also shares in the state's expenditures for administration of the program. Most administrative costs are matched at 50%. Each state administers its own Medicaid program. Eligibility criteria, covered services, and payments to providers vary from state to state.

Federal law mandates that every state provide some specific healthcare services. The mandated services include the following:

- Hospital inpatient care
- Hospital outpatient services
- Physician's services
- Laboratory and x-ray services
- SNF care

Home health services for those eligible for SNF services include:

- Prenatal care
- Family planning services and supplies
  —Rural health clinic services
- Medical services for dependent children under age 21
- Nurse-midwife services
- Certain federally qualified ambulatory and health center services

In addition to the mandated services, each state has the option of providing the following additional services:

- Prescription drugs
- Optometrist services
- Eyeglasses
- Dental care

States may impose nominal deductibles and co-payments on some Medicaid recipients for certain services. Some services are exempt from co-payment. These include emergency services, family planning services and supplies, and hospice care.

2.11.10. Eligibility Criteria

Eligibility criteria are based on income and assets. These criteria vary from state to state. Certain individuals are automatically covered if they are already receiving SSI, which includes many of the elderly, the blind and disabled, and families with children receiving support under an "aid to families with dependent children" program.

From the inception of the Medicaid program, there have been problems. The population of Medicaid recipients is composed of mainly women and children under age 18. This population of individuals requires a narrow range of healthcare services, mainly including obstetrical, prenatal, and well-child care. Members of this population have specific problems unique to their social situation, such as transportation issues, and they are more likely to be vulnerable to impoverished lifestyles, especially in urban areas. This type of lifestyle exposes them to violence, inferior living conditions, substance abuse, and other social problems related to poverty and inadequate living situations.

In addition, many healthcare providers have been reticent to care for the Medicaid population because of the low payment rates. This results in additional access issues. Many Medicaid recipients continue to use emergency rooms as their major source of primary care. This is referred to as the Medicaid syndrome and further results in additional expenditures in the ambulatory and inpatient settings (Hurley, Freund, & Paul, 1993).

2.11.11. Managed Medicaid

Traditionally, managed care organizations (MCOs) have not embraced Medicaid. HMOs that moved into this arena in the 1980s tended to provide services to select and small populations to have some greater amount of assurance that they might not experience excessive financial losses. Nevertheless, in recent years many states have turned their attention to managed care for their Medicaid populations (Case Manager's Tip 2.9). For example, Arizona enacted legislation that would provide healthcare to the poor using what were described as alternative healthcare systems that used strategies such as cost containment, improved patient access, and quality care in managed care settings. Arizona was the first state to implement such a statewide program. Other states, such as New York and Virginia, used an incremental approach to enrolling Medicaid beneficiaries.

It was expected that organized services using modalities such as managed care would serve to address some of the inherent problems associated with the Medicaid program, such as overutilization of emergency rooms and issues of access. Focus was placed on primary care as a mechanism for managing cost and resource utilization. Inherent problems occurred as a result of the population itself. Medicaid participants can be transitory, entering and leaving the program as their income eligibility changes over time. The population generally cannot afford the traditional co-payments and penalties for using out-of-network services associated with participation in managed care, thus raising the overall cost for the MCO. An inability to control resource utilization through economic incentives provided unusual challenges to MCOs.

It is unknown whether provider satisfaction is improved through participation in managed care. In addition, it has appeared that overall reductions in ED use have not been achieved. On a positive note, there tends to be more use of primary care physicians as opposed to specialists. This comes more as a result of changes in physicians' practice patterns and less as a result of changes in the behavior of the patients themselves.

In the future, HMOs will need to adjust their administration of these plans to the Medicaid population, who presents with challenges unique and different from the commercial populations. These individuals, with complex medical and social needs, require different approaches to those traditionally employed from healthy populations in commercial products.

2.11.12. Balanced Budget Act of 1997

The Balanced Budget Act of 1997 (BBA) was signed into law in August of 1997 by President Clinton. Titled Public Law 105-33, it enacted the most extensive changes to the Medicare and Medicaid programs since their inception in the 1960s. These changes did the following:

- Extended the life of the Medicare Trust Fund and reduced Medicare spending
- Increased healthcare options available to seniors
- Improved benefits for staying healthy (prevention)
- Fought Medicare fraud and abuse
- Looked at ways to help Medicare work well in the future

In addition to the significant changes the Act made to the government healthcare programs, it also enacted changes to the Child Health Insurance Program (CHIP) (Title XXI). CHIP expands block grants to states, increasing their Medicaid eligibility for low-income and uninsured children. Through CHIP, states are given the autonomy to set up their own programs. States must match the federal grant monies for each 3-year period that they are awarded. The success of CHIP will depend to a great extent on the ability of the states to identify and enroll eligible children. Therefore primary care and outreach become critical to its success. It is predicted that states that do not provide for adequate outreach and therefore do not enroll adequate numbers of children into CHIP may be at risk for some of the grant funding to be rescinded.

2.11.13. The Balanced Budget Act and the Case Manager

Case managers should stay current in all issues related to not only the BBA but all changes in healthcare legislation. Chapter 2 reviews many of the most important changes in the Act as they relate to the new reimbursement structures implemented in the new prospective payment systems. Additional information on the BBA, as well as any of the payment structures discussed in Chapter 2, can be obtained through the Centers for Medicare and Medicaid Services website: http://www.hcfa.gov/rregs/bbaupdat.htm . The most current information available can always be found at this and similar sites (Case Manager's Tip 2.10).

2.11.14. Current Procedure Terminology Codes and International Classification of Diseases-9-CM Codes

Case managers need to be familiar with both the ICD-9-CM and the CPT code systems. ICD-9-CM (American Medical Association, 1996), is used for coding inpatient medical records. In addition, CPT is also used. CPT is a listing of descriptive terms and identifying codes for reporting medical services and procedures performed by physicians. The terminology provides a uniform language that accurately describes medical,

CASE MANAGER'S TIP 2.10

Balanced Budget Act

Case managers can stay current on the BBA and other CMS updates by logging on to https://www.cms.gov/ to access current information related to reimbursement.

surgical, and diagnostic services. By using this coding system, there is a reliable nationwide communication system among physicians, patients, and third-party payers. CPT codes define medical, surgical, and diagnostic procedures. ICD-9-CM codes are used for medical interventions.

2.12. THIRD-PARTY PAYERS/MANAGED CARE ORGANIZATIONS

Like it or not, the healthcare system has taken on a brand new shape. Most healthcare institutions are scurrying to learn how to reduce their costs without reducing their quality.

Managed care has taken on many meanings over the past several years. It has grown to mean different things to different people. Business executives, financial controllers, healthcare providers, and payers are viewing managed care as a means of reducing skyrocketing healthcare costs (Case Manager's Tip 2.11). Healthcare institutions may view it as the mechanism for negotiating better discounted rates for the care of their patients, but only if they can attract a larger volume of patients to their institution. To the physician base it probably seems like an external control over their previously unstandardized methods and treatment modalities. It is probably the patient who views managed care as a protective mechanism that helps keep healthcare costs down while maintaining quality ser-

CASE MANAGER'S TIP 2.11

Diversity of Managed Care Plans and Services

Managed care is both a type of health insurance and a type of healthcare delivery system; that is, it focuses on both delivery and reimbursement of healthcare services. The intensity of the managed care services provided varies widely based on the type of health plan and the type of reimbursement method applied. The involvement of case management also differs based on the degree and complexity of the managed services offered to the consumers or demanded by the payers.

CASE MANAGER'S TIP 2.12

Understanding Types of Health Insurance and Terminology

It is important for a case manager to understand the basic types of health insurance plans and the related terminology to better serve the patient and to help provide the appropriate healthcare services in accordance with a patient's insurance benefits.

vices. However, this may not be as such, considering consumers' concerns about the occurring denials of services by MCOs.

Before a discussion can take place about managed care, it is important to understand and be well versed in health insurance in general (Case Manager's Tip 2.12). Health insurance is the protection one seeks to provide benefits for an illness or injury. A person, group, or employer pays a price (called a premium in managed care terminology) for protection from the potential expenses that could be incurred during an illness or injury. Lack of insurance coverage can mean going without needed healthcare, having to settle for lower-quality healthcare, or having to pay out of pocket—your own pocket—for healthcare. The insurance company gambles that it will take in much more in the way of premiums than it will pay out to the insured as a result of illnesses. The contract a person negotiates states the nature of the benefits or the coverage that is available. It also lists the conditions under which the insurer will cover expenses, either in part or, less commonly, in full. Deductibles and co-payments are those expenses the insured will be responsible for before and after the insurance carrier pays its portion of any medical bills.

The prominent types of health insurance are group and individual coverage. Group insurance is usually provided by an employer or professional organization to which one belongs. Employee group coverage is usually offered to spouses and dependents in addition to the employee. These policies vary from place to place and from one insurance company to another. Commercial or for-profit insurance companies dominate the group type of coverage. Individual health insurance is sometimes referred to as personal insurance. These policies also vary from provider to provider, and their premiums are often more expensive than group policies. Individuals may purchase individual insurance to supplement their group policy in areas that they identify as gaps in benefits (Enteen, 1992).

Currently the fastest-growing coverage option in the healthcare industry is the prepaid health plan—commonly known as HMOs and PPOs. In addition, government-paid coverage (i.e., Medicare, Medicaid, and veteran coverage) has recently undergone much scrutiny regarding its continued financial viability. These policies usually offer coverage for hospital expenses, surgical expenses, physician's expenses, and major medical (major illness or injury expenses). A person can also elect to pay larger premiums to supplement the basic plan for items not covered, such as home care benefits or durable medical equipment (Enteen, 1992).

It is important to discuss each type of insurance plan in more detail before moving on to an explanation of managed care. Each type of insurance plan has its advantages and disadvantages, and each is in such a state of flux that it is difficult to keep current and accurate on the various benefits. Definitions of each type of insurance as it is currently offered follow, but it is important to remember that managed care reform can affect these definitions at any time.

2.12.1. Health Maintenance Organizations Versus Preferred Provider Organizations

Because HMOs and PPOs are the most commonly confused managed care products, it is helpful to detail them more fully. An HMO is a state licensed entity that agrees by contract to provide medical services on a prepaid, capitated basis. It is an indemnity plan that delivers comprehensive, coordinated medical services to an enrolled membership in a defined geographical location on a prepaid basis. There are four main models of HMOs: group model, individual practice association (IPA), network model (health plan), and staff model. Different variations of these models are also available in certain locations of the country. Today there are more HMO models than the four traditional types just mentioned. Examples are open access, closed access, or mixed-type models.

2.12.2. Group Model Health Maintenance Organizations

A group model HMO contracts with multispecialty physicians organized in a partnership, corporation, or association. The physicians are not employed directly by the HMO but are employed directly by the group practice. The plan compensates the medical group for services they have contracted at a negotiated rate, and the group is then responsible for compensating its physicians and for contracting with healthcare providers for their patients. The HMO and the group thus share in the risk. Physicians in the group practice may be allowed to see HMO and non-HMO patients, although

they are primarily available to provide services to the HMO patients.

There are two types of group model HMOs: captive group and independent group. The captive group exists solely to provide services to the HMO's beneficiaries. In most cases the HMO creates the group for that purpose and provides it with administrative services and oversight. An example of this HMO type is the Permanente Medical Group of the Kaiser Foundation Health Plan (Kongstvedt, 2001). In the independent group model HMO, the group is already in existence, and the HMO contracts with it to provide physician services to its members. The group is responsible for all administrative functions and the operations of the group practice. An example of this type is the Geisinger Health Plan in Danville, Pennsylvania (Kongstvedt, 2001).

2.12.3. Individual/Independent Practice Association

An HMO can also contract with an IPA to provide healthcare services for a negotiated fee. The IPA then contracts with physicians who practice in their individual or group practices. These physicians usually care for HMO and non-HMO patients and keep control and responsibility over the way their offices are run. The IPA compensates the physicians on a fee schedule or an FFS basis. Generally, IPAs recruit physicians of different specialties to participate in their plans. This makes their services more desirable and cost-efficient because they are able to provide a wide array of services within the IPA. In turn, this diversity in services makes the IPA more attractive to an HMO. IPA model HMOs are either exclusive or nonexclusive. They are exclusive in providing services to the HMO's beneficiaries if they were created by the HMO. If they were already in existence and contracted with the HMO, they often are not limited in their clients to the HMO's beneficiaries.

2.12.4. Network Model Health Maintenance Organizations

If the HMO contracts with more than one physician group practice, it is referred to as a network health plan. In this arrangement the physicians do not necessarily provide care exclusively to the HMO. The network model HMO, similar to the group practice, consists of physicians from a multitude of specialties. An example of this type is Health Insurance Plan of Greater New York. If an HMO contracts with groups of primary care providers, this forms a primary care network HMO. Other variations of the network model HMO are closed and open panels. A closed network panel is usually limited to contracts with a small group of already existing group practices, whereas in an open network panel, participation in the group practice is open to interested physicians who meet the HMO credentialing criteria (Kongstvedt, 2001).

2.12.5. Staff Model Health Maintenance Organizations

The last HMO model is the staff model. In this type the physicians are employed by the HMO to provide healthcare services to its beneficiaries. The physicians are paid a salary and are offered various incentive programs based on their performance and productivity. Physicians in this model are also of different specialties so that the HMO is able to meet the needs of its beneficiaries. Administrative functions of this model are the responsibility of the HMO. For rare services or specialties, the HMO may contract with independent specialty groups available in the community. The staff model HMO is also known as a closed model because participation of physicians is limited to those employed by the HMO. An interesting feature of the staff model HMO is that the HMO exerts a great degree of control over the physicians' practice.

HMOs in general are a good example of the gatekeeper model, in which a primary care provider is responsible for authorizing all specialist referrals. This serves to control costs and resource consumption.

2.12.6. Preferred Provider Organizations

PPOs are generally neither state licensed nor federally qualified. They function as brokers by offering discounted healthcare services either directly to employers or to third-party payers. Under a PPO agreement, a limited number of providers are contracted as part of the network. The PPO provides this limitation in the size of the panel of providers, almost similar to an incentive, in return for the agreement of participating providers/physicians to abide by its utilization and resource management practices. Typically, capitation and other risk-bearing payment arrangements with

providers are not used in PPOs compared with HMOs, where such payment structures are usually the norm.

Members of PPOs are encouraged to use the physicians and services of the PPO; however, they are permitted to go outside the network for their healthcare if necessary. In this case, members are held responsible for a co-payment or higher levels of cost sharing compared with staying within the network. Those members who do elect to use out-of-network services may be reimbursed at a lower rate than those who remain within the network. Therefore there is incentive for subscribers to remain in the network because those providers will be offering their services at a discounted rate as part of the PPO. Those cost savings are passed on to the consumer. There is a further incentive to employers to contract with a PPO as a means of reducing overall healthcare costs for their employees. PPOs have become more popular than HMOs because their enrollees are less restricted regarding their choice of providers. Table 2.5 summarizes important differences between the two types of healthcare plans: HMOs and PPOs.

2.13. MANAGED CARE AND ITS STAGES OF DEVELOPMENT/MATURATION

There has been an evolution of the healthcare market as it matured into the managed care environment. Managed care can be defined as a system of healthcare delivery aimed at managing and balancing the cost, risk, and quality of access to healthcare. It is both an industry and a process. Ultimately, managed care is nothing more than a range or spectrum of activities designed to control the means by which healthcare is delivered. It is used by HMOs and PPOs to improve the delivery of services and contain costs (Mullahy, 1998; Kongstvedt, 2001). This so-called evolution has been mapped out and studied by many economists, consulting firms, and healthcare experts and futurists. For example, the University Hospital Consortium and American Practice Management, Incorporated Management Consultants (1992) categorized the healthcare market and its evolution to managed care into four stages of development. Today, this categorization has expanded to

TABLE 2.5. Summary of HMO and PPO Characteristics.

Types	Flexibility	Premiums	Reimbursement	Rates	Provider Risks
HMO	Must remain in network Less choice of providers	Prepaid Capitated	Not reimbursed out of network	Usually capitated For-Profit or Not-For-Profit	High incentive to control costs High financial risk sharing
PPO	Less restrictive More choice of providers	Fee-for-Service Not prepaid	Covers services out of network	Not usually capitated	Low incentive to contain costs Less financial risk sharing

---

Box 2.6   Stages of Evolution of the Health Care Market

Stage I: Unstructured

- Independent hospitals
- Independent physicians
- Independent purchases, not price sensitive

Stage II: Loose Framework

- HMO/PPO enrollment rise
- Excess inpatient capacity
- Hospitals/physicians under pressure
- Provider networks form

Stage III: Consolidation

- A few large HMOs/PPOs emerge
- Provider margins erode
- Hospitals form systems
- Hospital systems align with physicians to form integrated systems

Stage IV: Managed Competition

- Employer coalitions purchase health services
- Integrated systems manage patient populations
- Continued consolidation of provider systems and health plans

Stage V: Integrated Delivery Partnerships

- Fully capitated market
- Partnerships between providers, purchasers, and payers
- Providers assume risk for the full continuum of care
- Population health management

(Modified from University Hospital Consortium and American Practice Management, Incorporated Management Consultants, 1992)

---

include a fifth stage. Box 2.6 summarizes the various stages of evolution.

Stage I of this market refers to the "now historical" perspective of healthcare when hospitals, physicians, employers, and HMOs were operating under a more unstructured FFS payment system. At this stage, more options were available to the client and more flexibility within this framework was permissible. The penetration of the HMO market was barely noticeable during this stage—about 5–10%. An example of an HMO at this point of development was the Health Insurance Plan (HIP) of New York, or the oldest HMO, Kaiser Permanente, in California.

Characteristics of the environment of care in this stage were duplication and fragmentation of services and less pressure on hospitals to discharge their patients early or reduce length of stay. Competition was based on technology. Case managers' roles in this stage were

just beginning in the acute care settings, particularly with nurses assuming the role.

Stage II of this market is referred to as the loose framework/alliance. Many areas of the country are currently in this stage and struggling with it. HMOs and PPOs are beginning to emerge in greater numbers (10–30% of the market), and enrollment has skyrocketed. They are no longer unnoticeable in the healthcare market of today. As a result of their large enrollments, they now have the leverage to negotiate pricing and the ability to contract at lower reimbursement rates. During Stage II, the motivation is to lower the cost of providing healthcare so that the value of the money received is not eroded. Several types of HMOs are developing. In the past, HMOs were organized to employ their own staff physicians and service providers and pay them a salary. Soon after, groups began to emerge in which a number of physicians and other providers established partnerships and shared their profits. These groups usually practiced out of a common facility or location. Next came the independent practitioners who formed associations and contracted to be part of a group endeavor while still practicing out of their own offices. The last type of HMO to emerge was the network, in which large areas are covered, perhaps crossing various states or regions or even the entire United States. Networks are most popular among large conglomerates who want to obtain the benefits of HMOs for their employees with the same consistency at any of their sites.

This stage of development witnessed increased focus on eliminating delays, duplication, and unnecessary use of resources, as well as other activities to streamline the delivery of care processes. As the interest in cost effectiveness increased, the use of case managers also arose with a focus on care coordination across the continuum of care. Healthcare executives began to integrate utilization and case management practices with a major focus on transitional planning and expediting the patient's journey across the different levels of care settings.

After these states of development, the market moves into Stage III, consolidation. While HMOs are forming networks, hospitals are simultaneously forming systems and networks themselves. Managed care penetration increases to 30–50% of the market. This now sets up the beginnings of a competitive market in which hospitals are aggressively recruiting physicians and practitioners. These groups of physicians and providers are more commonly becoming known as PPOs. The payment system is based on a per case, per diem, capitation through the PPO. A contract is developed that outlines the cost per covered life in the plan. PPOs are now outgrowing the HMO market primarily as a result of their ability to offer greater savings for employers at a time when employers are extremely concerned about the cost of their employees' health benefits.

Case management programs in this stage became more popular and available in the majority of healthcare organizations and in different settings. These programs were necessary to curtail the rising cost of healthcare and increased risk on the part of the provider. Case management was viewed as the most desired strategy for cost-effectiveness and efficient service delivery. However, these programs took a new and improved structure: an initial integrative approach to case management with merged utilization management, clinical management, and transitional planning functions. In addition, case managers in the payer-based system (i.e., MCOs) assumed the gatekeeper and utilization management role.

Many parts of the country, primarily the West Coast, have lived through Stage III and have now embarked on Stage IV, managed competition. This is the phase in which capitation prevails (50–80%). In this market, purchasers contract with hospital/physician networks to provide a comprehensive healthcare package to their clients. These integrated systems contract with the purchasers to accept the financial risk for managing their utilization of services (utilization management). In other words, they bear the burden of controlling their costs to deliver healthcare. The next level of this system is capitation, where a set fee is given to provide comprehensive care to a given population. This puts an even greater burden on the ability to provide quality care while controlling cost. The managed organization is no longer taking the risk with its premiums; the risk has now shifted to the provider of the healthcare services within the network or physician care group.

This phase of managed care is the most uncomfortable of all because this is where survival of the fittest comes into play. Competition is at its peak during this phase because MCOs are searching for membership from the most frugal yet quality-driven establishments. Report cards are now the judgment mechanism of any MCO and can be the demise of any physician or hospital not meeting the standards of cost containment as set up by the MCOs. An example of capitation is as follows: 1,000 HMO members sign up for a healthcare network as part of a full-risk contract. The network will reimburse approximately $400 per member per month to cover all of their healthcare needs regardless of how much or how little they access the healthcare system. It is the burden of the healthcare network to provide adequate resources to cover their healthcare needs at low cost.

The integrative approaches to case management services in this stage become the norm. Department consolidation also occurs. In Stage III it was possible for healthcare organizations, particularly hospitals, to still have either discharge planning, utilization management, or quality management as separate from case management. However, in Stage IV this lack of integration becomes no longer viable and is seen as a cost-ineffective practice. Because of the development of integrated delivery systems (IDSs), collaborative strategies in case management across the continuum of care and across different sites and settings are developed, strengthening the role of the case manager and its importance. Moreover, case management takes a new focus here to meet the demands of the managed care environment: population risk assessment, categorization, and management with special interest in disease prevention and health maintenance and promotion.

Stage V, integrated delivery partnerships, occurs when the market of managed care expands to include most of the population in such an arrangement of health insurance (> 80%). IDSs (discussed in Section 2.14) mature in size, focus, and method of operation. They also become more popular in almost every geographical location, even though not every market may have reached this stage of development. The environment of healthcare in this stage is characterized by full capitation as the reimbursement method; partnerships between providers, purchasers, and payers; and population health management. Another important characteristic is that the providers assume risk for the full continuum of care.

These characteristics and advanced developments impact the practice of case management in a way that new strategies and innovations are developed, such as telephonic or Internet-based case management services. These approaches tend to also focus on the population served and its needs rather than just the individual patient or person. Therefore proactive programs in demand management and risk reduction are more evident in this stage compared with Stage IV. Furthermore, both the provider and payer groups adopt these strategies and use them in their marketing efforts.

2.14. INTEGRATED DELIVERY SYSTEMS AS A RESPONSE TO MANAGED CARE

IDSs became more popular in the mid-1990s as a response to the mature managed care environment. Today they are present mostly in heavily penetrated managed care markets. The driving forces behind the development of IDSs are as follows:

- The healthcare reform climate
- Managed care contracts and the need to increase competitiveness and negotiating power
- Need to expand market share
- Desire to increase efficiency, productivity, and profitability
- Shift in reimbursement methods away from FFS to capitation
- Increasing activism of employers in seeking control over healthcare costs and spending
- Managed care technology advances
- Sophistication of the utilization management practices of MCOs
- Risk-sharing contracts between the payer and provider
- Shift to a managed health rather than managed illness approach to care
- Employers' desire to be owners and voting participants in the healthcare delivery system rather than only vendors and providers (Hastings, Luce, & Wynstra, 1995)

There is little agreement in the literature and among healthcare providers on how to define IDSs. However, according to Kongstvedt, an IDS can be defined as one or more "type of provider coming together in some type of legal structure to manage healthcare and, in most cases, to contract with payer organizations," (2001). The main goal of an IDS is to improve efficiency in the delivery of healthcare services. Reflecting back on the past decade, we can see that some IDSs have succeeded, but others have failed and completely vanished.

There are no standard rules for the size or type of an IDS. Some are large and others are small; however, larger IDSs are known to gain increased leverage in negotiating contracts with an MCO. Successful IDSs are noted to include an acute care hospital, physician group practices, long-term care facilities, a home care agency, and managed care contracts with major payers. As for the type of an IDS, there are not formal structures. IDSs can be one of the following:

- Systems in which only physicians are integrated: physician practice integration
- Systems in which physicians are integrated with healthcare facilities: physician-hospital integration
- Systems that include insurance agencies (i.e., a payer structure: provider-payer integration) (Kongstvedt, 2001)

Regardless of the type of integration a healthcare institution may be involved in, case management services and departments play an important role in the integration of services to meet the primary goal for the formed IDS: efficiency of service delivery.

In today's healthcare market and after the enactment of the Patient Protection and Affordable Care Act of 2010, a new wave of integrated healthcare delivery networks and systems are emerging. Often these are driven by academic medical centers creating full merger acquisition, sponsorships, or strategic affiliations with other organizations. The main focus of these activities is maintaining or expanding marketshare, leverging contractual agreements with health insurance plans, and increasing revenue while minimizing financial risks. Examples of the organizations these academic medical centers are partnering with include community hospitals, community medical centers, and agencies and facilities from across the care continuum and settings (e.g., skilled care, home care, and physician practice groups). With the Value-based Purchasing Program, Hospital Readmissions Reduction Programs, nontraditional reimbursement methods such as bundled payments, integrated delivery systems, and networks have created competitive advantage among major healthcare providers in specific regions while enhancing opportunities for revenue, reduction in financial risk due to CMS imposed penalties related to performance expectations, and increased access in rural and suburban areas to academic medicine.

2.14.1. Physician Integration

Managed care and healthcare reform resulted in increased reliance on primary care physicians as providers of healthcare services. This shift left specialty care physicians in a bind and worried about the survival of their practice because they were no longer in demand. As a result, specialists and primary care providers pursued integrated group practices that witnessed the creation of IPAs with multispecialty providers. IPAs and physician networks discussed in the previous section are examples of IDSs that are built around physician integration. Other types of physician-integrated IDSs are primary care groups, specialist provider groups, and management service organizations (MSOs). These types of groups function similar to IPAs; however, MSOs are different. The main focus of MSOs is managed care contract negotiation for IPAs and physician networks.

2.14.2. Physician-Hospital Integration

Specialty hospitals experienced the same concerns as specialist physicians. They were afraid that their referral source and base would dwindle; therefore they began to establish relationships with primary care

IPA = Individual/Independent practice association

physicians and expanded their scope of services and providers. As a result, hospitals were found to develop new collaborative or partnership agreements with other physician groups, such as those listed in the Physician Integration section. Other types of integration are physician-hospital organizations (PHOs), particularly for the purpose of managed care contracting power; MSOs, in which hospitals sponsored the physician practices; and physician-hospital integration through direct employment of physicians. The MSOs were a natural development or growth of PHOs. Both PHOs and MSOs are similar in their focus on managed care contracting; however, MSOs include additional hospital administrative services.

Managed care contracts negotiation was the main incentive behind physician-hospital integration efforts. In these ventures, hospitals assisted physicians in the management of their practices (i.e., provided practice management services) and assumed the administrative responsibilities for billing and collections, utilization review and management, and quality assurance activities. In these structures the hospital received a fee as a compensation for the services provided. The fee had to be at market value; otherwise, the MSO could incur legal problems.

2.14.3. Provider-Payer Integration

Provider-payer integration is different from the other two types of integration. Physician and physician-hospital modes of integration are unidimensional (i.e., provider-based). However, provider-payer integration is bidimensional because it merges the provider (physician and hospital) and payer sides of healthcare delivery. This type of integration is the most complex and challenging to manage. Picking the right partner is a leading success factor of this venture. Issues of concern in the provider-payer integration venture are as follows:

- *Governance structure*: Would the party with more capital assume ownership and control?
- *Allocation of risk and profit.*
- *Acquisition versus start-up*: Should a provider partner with an already existing payer or establish a new one? If a new one is established, one should be aware of its cost implications.
- *Management*: Who will run the new entity on a day-to-day basis?
- *Exclusivity that is too expensive and complicated*: Would the parties agree to only deal with each other on all managed care projects?
- *Government regulations*: The new entity must

comply with all the related laws and governmental review.

2.14.4. Government-Related Insurance Structures

Government provision of medical insurance is the final source when reviewing the options for the population at large. Both federal and state governments provide medical insurance benefits. The Medicare program under the federal government provides mandatory basic hospitalization benefits for most U.S. citizens over the age of 65 years and some other special classes of individuals, such as the disabled. This coverage is referred to as Medicare Part A, and it can be supplemented by Medicare Part B, which provides for payment of doctor bills. These plans are not all-inclusive enough for most senior citizens. Recently there have been growing cutbacks to Medicare; therefore it is prudent for any citizen over 65 years of age to supplement Medicare with another insurance plan. Many HMOs/PPOs are now expanding their plans to offer managed care Medicare and managed care Medicaid components.

At the state level, insurance benefits are also offered. These are commonly referred to as the Medicaid program of benefits for the indigent. They are no longer associated with the stigma of the term welfare because more and more citizens must apply for public assistance to cover their medical bills after they have exhausted their income and assets. Medicaid is a pool of funds used to provide insurance benefits for those who cannot afford health insurance. The amount of funds set aside for this purpose is most often a direct result of the economic status of a particular state. The amount of funding is undergoing a great deal of turmoil as many states are tightening their pocketbooks in anticipation of the full impact of managed care in a capitated environment.

A few examples of differing reimbursements for physician services are outlined in dollars in Table 2.6. This is only a representative partial listing of potential physician fees and does not represent all practices or the many varieties of reimbursement schedules.

2.15. OTHER HEALTH BENEFIT PLANS

2.15.1. Workers' Compensation

An additional type of government provision that can vary from state to state is the workers' compensation guidelines. Workers' compensation cases are different from group medical insurance in that the insurers and employers are mandated by legislature guidelines to reimburse for both medical costs and lost wages. It is

TABLE 2.6. Differing Reimbursements for Physician Services.

Service	Fee	Medicare	Medicaid	HMO
Outpatient services	$45	$25	$19	$35
Hospital care	$42	$27	$26	$30
Flexible sigmoidscopy	$335	$86	–	$144
Obstetrical care/Vaginal delivery	$2,250	$1,750	$1,125	$1,850
Appendectomy	$1,000	$525	$375	$875
Cholecystectomy	$1,875	$875	$750	$1,125

imperative that a case manager working with workers' compensation claims be familiar with the state's laws, especially as they reflect the claimant's return to work.

2.15.2. Case Manager's Role in Workers' Compensation Cases

The case manager must be aware that there is a two-pronged effort in workers' compensation cases. That is, the insurance carrier is not only interested in the timely results of medical care but also wants to minimize the outlay of lost wages. Therefore getting the employee back to work as soon as possible, even with a modified work schedule and duties, becomes an additional motivational pressure on the case manager. At times the case manager may have difficulty balancing medical health and the timely return to the workforce. The case manager may be faced with the dilemma of a tight timeframe to return someone to work if the salary losses are a greater expense to the insurer than the medical care expenses.

Case managers specializing in the field of workers' compensation must be well versed in orthopedic injuries because these injuries dominate compensation cases. They must also be knowledgeable enough in rehabilitative medicine to recommend the resources necessary to assist a patient in increasing functionality. It is the goal of the case manager to return an employee to the previous state of well-being or the optimum level of improvement obtainable. The case manager achieves this by ensuring that the appropriate treatment plan is in effect and progressing, along with verifying compliance by the employee. It is also important for the case manager to know the employee/claimant well enough to prevent the person from engaging in any untoward activities that would hinder or sabotage the progress or ultimate recovery.

2.15.3. Automobile Insurance

As with workers' compensation guidelines, automobile policies and/or no-fault policies vary from state to state. Many rules depend on the location of the acci-

dent, where the person resides, or where the person's employment headquarters is located.

Case management usually becomes involved in motor vehicle accident cases when catastrophic injury has occurred. Case managers become very involved in the discharge planning and coordination, such as transfer from acute level of care to rehabilitative settings or decisions involving a chronic injury requiring adaptive equipment, home care, or home modifications.

2.15.4. Disability Insurance

Disability plans are usually referred to as short-term, long-term, or total disability. Each type of plan varies in its amounts of salary replacement and length of time covered. Disability plans will require a case management review. Usually a case manager will become involved as the length of time for disability coverage is winding down. It will be the creativity of a case manager's skills that will determine if the financial plan and the medical plan will balance to the benefit of the insured and the employer.

2.15.5. Long-Term Care

This is a relatively new type of insurance offered. The policy holder has a variety of possibilities for nursing care coverage. Such care as skilled nursing, subacute care, custodial nursing care, extended home care, respite care, or nursing home provisions can be covered. The insurance company usually case manages a claim to confirm the need for services and approves benefit coverage accordingly.

2.16. PROACTIVE TACTICS TO COUNTERACT THE EFFECTS OF MANAGED CARE

Most strategies are incorporating a two-pronged approach to tackle all of the major areas that the MCOs seem to be concentrating on. One approach could fall under the overall operational management. This is the area in which efforts are initiated to control costs and

CASE MANAGER'S TIP 2.13

Case Management Caveat

Case management must not be the catchall for fixing all that ails a facility.

to become more accountable for costs. Work redesigns and changes in the work delivery systems are becoming commonplace in organizations that are taking a more proactive approach. A more active performance and reward system is becoming evident and attempts are being made to integrate physician best practice with a functional integration system so that quality standards of care can be maintained at the lowest cost possible.

The second approach, and the area in which case management has the most direct impact on its overall success, is clinical management. Nursing case management was the first tool used to oversee the patient's journey through the healthcare system. Without a clear system of managing the patient services and resources in the least costly way, particularly in an environment of increased capitation, funds will quickly be wiped out. Capitation clearly requires control over resources, utilization management, length-of-stay reduction, disease management, and clinical process improvement. All of these listed areas can be incorporated into the case management role (see Chapters 4 through 7).

The emergence of the case manager using the clinical pathway was a major step toward a more cost-effective, efficient method of delivering care. By identifying variances to care, the case manager began to identify ways to continuously improve the delivery of care while not compromising quality. The use of clinical paths was the beginning initiative to control and reduce length of stay. An effective case management program can make a significant difference in managing and coordinating the clinical resources available for the patient (Case Manager's Tip 2.13) (Flarey and Blancett, 1996).

Integrating case management into managing a patient group or a specific disease entity is the next level of resource and clinical management. This strategy uses a multidisciplinary approach to care and requires input from the medical, clinical, ancillary, financial, and

CASE MANAGER'S TIP 2.14

Case Management's Focus

The focus must always go beyond illness to include wellness, maintenance, and preventive case management.

administrative teams. Many facilities have developed multidisciplinary teams to meet frequently on units and review the care of the patients to ensure that quality is being maintained while utilization of services is appropriate and cost-efficient. Similarly, length-of-stay committees have been launched to discuss problem cases, high-cost patients or certain areas of overutilization, and more efficient methods of providing services at lower cost. Future strategies must expand efforts beyond the hospital walls to include community services and community-based initiatives of case management (Case Manager's Tip 2.14).

Differentiating between case management and managed care can be somewhat confusing at times because the terms are used interchangeably in many arenas.

2.17. VALUE-BASED PURCHASING

The CMS has implemented two programs that link quality of care to hospital payments under the Medicare program. The first, implemented beginning with fiscal year 2013 (began October 1, 2012), is titled the Hospital Value-Based Purchasing Program (VBP). This program was established under the Affordable Care Act as a pay-for-performance program for hospitals. Under this program, Medicare is adjusting a portion of payments to hospitals on either:

- How well they perform on each measure as compared to all hospitals, or
- How much they improve their own performance on each measure as compared to their performance during a prior baseline period.

The program is considered a demand-side strategy used to measure, report, and reward excellence in healthcare delivery. By reporting quality outcomes and linking them to payment, it is anticipated that patients will begin to demand better quality of care. In this way it becomes an external motivator for providers to lead re-engineering of healthcare delivery efforts. The current system of healthcare is fragmented, inefficient, with wide variation in both cost and quality. Its orientation has always been toward the treatment of illness rather than population health management or management toward desired outcomes of care. The system has incentivized providers to overuse resources and has contributed to the problem. CMS' incentives through the VBP program are geared toward reductions in cost and unnecessary hospital admissions. It is a value-driven system in which ever-increasing quality of care is achieved at the lowest possible cost. It moves CMS away from being an passive purchaser to an active and discriminating one.

The other CMS program is the Hospital Readmissions Reduction Program. This program, which began on October 1, 2012 as part of the Affordable Care Act, authorizes Medicare to reduce payments to acute care hospitals with excess readmissions that are paid under CMS's inpatient prospective payment system. The program initially focused on acute myocardial infarction (AMI), heart failure (HF) and pneumonia (PN). If hospitals rank above the national average for 30 day readmissions, a percentage reduction is made to all Medicare payments to that hospital, as per the tables below. The program continues to expand, both in diagnoses penalized and the percentage of the penalty. These percentages are taken from the total of all Medicare billing and so can add up to a lot of revenue lost to the hospital.

Other meaures of note include the Medicare Spending per Beneficiary measure in which hospitals are rated based on their performance in length of stay and cost per case and the mortality measure. The Spending per Beneficiary Measure (also known as the Efficiceny Measure) provides hospitals with a score. A score greater than one means that the hospital spends more than the average and a score below one means the hospital spends less than the average hosptial. By 2016 there will be financial penalties associated with scores below one.

The Mortality measure determines a hospital's rating on deaths 30 days following an admission to the hospital, regardless of the location of the death. As with other measures, this one ranks hospitals against other Medicare hospitals and follows with a financial penalty for poor performers (Box 2.7).

Box 2.7 Financial Penalty for Poor Performance

Payment Penalty Cap 1%

Initial set for FFY 2013
- Heart attack
- Heart failure
- Pneumonia

Expanded set for FFY 2014
- Heart attack
- Heart failure
- Pneumonia

Expanded set for FFY 2015 and possibly beyond
- Total hip and knee replacements
- Heart attack
- Heart failure
- Pneumonia

2.17.1. Elements of Value Based Purchasing

Listed below are the key elements to consider for a successful approach to value-based purchasing. These elements should not be considered linear. Instead they should be approached as interrelated concepts that depend on each other for success.

Element One: Standardized Performance Measurement—Measurement is based on the ability to access and aggregate data from multiple sources. It should be conducted on multiple levels, including health plans, hospitals, physician groups, and individual healthcare providers. Measurement should be used to answer questions such as, *is care safe, timely, efficient, effective, equitable*, and *patient-centered*? The data should also provide actionable information on cost, quality, and appropriateness of care. Utlimately, the data should move organizations toward outcomes measures, as these will drive performance improvement.

Element Two: Transparency and Public Reporting—Regular and timely public reporting can be a significant external motivator for perfomance improvement. Data to be reported should include both quality outcomes and cost of care.

Element Three: Payment Innovation—Innovations in payment must include ways in which providers will be reimbursed based on demonstrated performance. Pay-for-performance is based on the notion of paying for something based on its quality. It is moving the healthcare industry toward payment for keeping individuals well, rather than treating them only after they are sick.

Element Four: Informed Consumer Choice—A core element of value-based purchasing is the notion of individual consumer choice of selection. As in other competitive industries, the desired goal is for consumers to make choices in health and healthcare on the basis of value.

2.17.2. Bundled Payments

On January 31, 2013, the CMS, began a program for healthcare organizations. The program, called the Bundled Payments for Care Improvement (BPCI), an innovative new payment model. It lasted for 3 years and the outcomes were used by CMS to determine whether the various models being tested resulted in improved patient care and lower costs. If selected to participate, organizations entered into payment arrangements that included both financial and performance accountability for episodes of care. Unlike the prospective payment model of reimbursement, where each provider at each level of care is paid separately, in these models, certain payments are combined, or bundled for providers across the continuum for a specific episode of care. In prospective payment, providers are rewarded for quantity. In bundled payment methodology, providers have aligned incentives which allow them to work closely together across all specialties and settings.

There are four models, or ways, by which the payments for multiple providers can be linked under this program. Organizations who choose to participate, can select one of these. In the first model the organizations agree to provide a standard discount to Medicare from the usual Part A hospital payments. In the second and third models, a retrospecitive bundled payment arrangement is used. In these models, actual expenses are reconciled against a target, or set price, for an episode of care. In model four, a lump sum payment is made to a provider for the entire episode of care.

2.17.2.1. Details of Each Model

Model one: Retrospective acute-care hospital stay only. The episode of care is defined as the inpatient stay in the acute care setting. Based on the IPPS, Medicare will pay the hospital a discounted amount based on what the IPPS payment would have been. Physicians continue to receive separate payments, but in some instances may share gains, arising from redesign efforts, with the hospital.

Model two: Retrospective acute care hospital stay plus post-acute care. The episode of care includes the inpatient stay in the acute care hospital and all related services for that episode. The episode will end either 30, 60, or 90 days after the hospital discharge. Providers who participate can select up to 48 different clinical condition episodes. An example might be a total knee replacement which would include the surgical procedure, hospital stay, and post-acute rehabilitation in any setting or at home.

Model three: Retrospective post-acute care only. Episodes are triggered by an acute care admission and begin at initiation of post-acute care services with either a skilled nursing facility, inpatient rehabilitation facility, long-term care hospital, or home care agency. The post-acute services must begin within 30 days of the acute care discharge, and end either at 30, 60 or 90 days after inititation of the episode. As in model two, participants can select up to forty-eight different clinical condition episodes.

Model four: Acute care hospital stay only. A single bundled payment, prospectively determined that encompassess all services furnished during the inpatient stay. This would include hospital, physician, and other provider payments. The physicians and other providers would be paid by the hospital out of the bundled payment. Related readmission are included in the bundled amount. Hospitals participating can pick from among 48 different clinical condition codes.

2.17.3. Accountable Care Organizations

Accountable care organizations (ACOs), also known as shared savings programs, are groups of doctors, hospitals, and other healthcare providers, who organize to voluntarily provide coordinated high quality care to Medicare patients. The ACO is expected to function as a true patient-centered organization where providers and patients work together in making healthcare decisions. Each ACO must agree to accept responsibility for a minimum of 5,000 Medicare fee-for-service patients. If accepted to participate, they must agree to do so for a period of three years. Implemented as part of the Affordable Care Act, hospitals receive bonuses for achieving predetermined outcomes and penalties for not achieving them. ACOs can participate in one of two tracks. The first track provides for a shared-savings only track. The second track allows for the ACO to share in savings and losses, in return for a higher share of the savings achieved.

The outcomes include measures of improved health and the patient experience of care, improvements for the health of populations of patients and for reducing the rate of growth of healthcare spending. All of this is achieved through the use of evidence-based healthcare and coordination of care. By coordinating care across the continuum, the ACO structure helps to ensure that patient care is provided at the right amount and at the right time. ACOs are particularly focused on patients with chronic conditions as these patients can consume a disproportionately high amount of healthcare resources and therefore dollars. Coordinated care is aimed at also reducing unnecessary duplication of services and reducing medical errors. If an ACO is able to reduce cost while providing high quality care, they share in the savings with the Medicare program. Eleven of the first 23 pioneer ACOs received bonuses from Medicare that totaled $68 million. As of 2012, nearly 350 hospitals and health systems had signed on as ACOs. At the heart of any ACO is care coordination. Case management plays an important role in coordinating care for patients across the continuum. The Medicare patient who is a patient within an ACO can still choose among healthcare providers as they do in the traditional Medicare program. Patients must be notified by their provider that they are participating in an ACO and that they are eligible for receiving payments from Medicare if their provider improves quality and coordination of care. The Medicare beneficiary can then choose to stay with that provider or switch to a non-ACO provider (The Shared Savings Program final rule: http://www.gpo.gov/fdsys/pkg/FR-2011-11-02/pdf/2011-27461.pdf).

In general terms, managed care is the umbrella for several initiatives of cost containment that include case management. Case management is a variation of the components that comprise managed care (i.e., managing cost, quality, and effectiveness of services) (Cohen & Cesta, 1997). Case management is a process that incorporates the components of managed care when attending to the needs of patient care. It can be used in any form of patient delivery system, such as team, functional, primary, or alternative nursing care. Continuous monitoring of care rendered to a patient is maintained through interdisciplinary team meetings and analysis of variances from the outlined plan. Case management is effective because it coordinates, integrates, and evaluates the outcomes of the processes of care (Cohen & Cesta, 1997).

To have an effect on managed care, and the Medicare program, case managers must take an active role in watching for quality outcomes. Benchmarking research used by managed care companies will be an important tool that a case manager must incorporate into the role because it will become clear that adequacy of care will be measured by outcomes. Case managers must demonstrate that they have the flexibility to ensure that care is delivered in a high-quality and cost-effective manner. They will undoubtedly play a vital role in the future of our healthcare industry and the survival of quality healthcare provided to its people.

2.18. KEY POINTS

1. The prospective payment system was one of the forces leading acute care settings toward the adoption of case management models.

2. Case mix helps hospitals to determine their costs, as well as their types of patients and use of resources.

3. In addition to acute care settings, prospective payment methodologies can now be found in ambulatory care, home care, and long-term care.

4. Medicare and managed Medicare are government programs providing healthcare to those age 65 years and over and the disabled.

5. Medicaid and managed Medicaid are state-run healthcare programs for the indigent.

6. Regardless of the reimbursement system under which the patient is eligible, the length of stay will continue to need to remain short, and the use of resources will need to be monitored and controlled.

7. Health insurance is the protection one seeks to provide benefits for an illness or injury.

8. The insurance contract states the nature of the benefits or the coverage available to the insured.

9. The HMO delivers comprehensive medical services to an enrolled membership on a prepaid basis.

10. The PPO offers a more limited number of providers and encourages the use of physicians and services within the network, but patients are permitted to go outside the network for decreased reimbursement.

11. The evolution of the healthcare market has four stages of development in the managed care environment.

12. Work redesigns are becoming commonplace in organizations taking a proactive approach to managed care.

13. Managing patient services and resources in the least costly way while maintaining quality will be the primary goal of case management as it relates to managed care.

14. Managed care is the umbrella for several cost-containment initiatives that include but are not limited to case management.

2.19. REFERENCES

American Medical Association. (1996). *CPT '97*, St. Anthony's Press, Reston, VA.

Blancett, S.S. & Flarey, D.L. (1996). *Case studies in nursing case management: health care delivery in a world of managed care*, Aspen, Gaithersburg, MD.

Centers for Medicare and Medicaid Services. (2014). *Medicare Benefit Policy Manual*. Chapter 6: Hospital Services Covered under Part B. CMS Publication 100-02. Rev. 182. March 21.

Cohen, E.L. & Cesta, T.G. (1997). *Nursing case management: From concept to evaluation*, 2nd Ed., Mosby, St. Louis.

Commission on Professional and Hospital Activities. (1975). *The international classification of diseases*, rev 8, 2 vols, Ann Arbor, MI (adapted for use in the United States).

Enteen, R. (1992). *Health insurance: how to get it, keep it, or improve what you've got*, Paragon House, New York.

Flarey, D.L. & Blancett, S.S. (1996) *Handbook of nursing case management*, Aspen, Gaithersburg, MD.

Hastings, D.A., Luce, G.M., & Wynstra, N.A. (1995). *Fundamentals of health law*, National Health Lawyers Association, Washington, DC.

Hurley, R., Freund, D., & Paul, J. (1993). *Medicaid managed care:*

lessons for policy and program design, Health Administration Press, Ann Arbor, MI.

Kongstvedt, P. (2001). *Essentials of managed health care*, Gaithersburg, MD, Aspen.

Mayes, R. (2007). The Origins, Development, and Passage of Medicare's Revolutionary Prospective Payment System," *Journal of the History of Medicine and Allied Sciences* Volume 62, Number 1, pp. 21–55.

Mullahy, C.M.. (1998). *The case management handbook*, 2nd ed., Aspen, Gaithersburg, MD.

Richards, S. (1996). A closer look at case management, *J Health Qual 18*(4): 8–11.

University *Hospital Consortium and American Practice Management*, Incorporated Management Consultants. (1992). Stages of market evolution, University Hospital Consortium, Chicago, IL.

3

Case Management Models

Case management is a malleable and easily adapted model of care that applies to a variety of healthcare delivery locations, settings, organizations, and systems. It is because of this flexibility that the model has been designed and implemented in various ways that respond to and meet the needs of the individual organization or setting applying it. Although case management has been used in the community practice settings for the longest period, it is now commonly seen as an integrated care delivery model in the acute care setting and other sites along the continuum of care (e.g., home care, skilled nursing facilities, and long-term care facilities). More and more organizations are recognizing the model's ability to manage resources while maintaining or improving patient care quality and safety and enhancing adherence to regulatory and accreditation standards. Most recently, case management has been identified as a strategic tool to be used in accountable care organizations, patient centered medical homes, federally qualified healthcare centers, healthcare systems, and other care delivery models that coordinate patient care across the continuum of care and health and human services.

3.1. SYSTEMNESS AND CASE MANAGEMENT

System models are designed to provide case management services along the continuum. A continuum of care is defined as an integrated, client-oriented system of care composed of both services and integrating mechanisms that guides and tracks clients over time through a comprehensive array of health, mental health, and social services spanning all levels of intensity of care. The continuum contains seven access points to healthcare, as described in Box 3.1.

The case manager works on a client's case at one of the seven access points, depending on where the patient enters the healthcare system. In most cases the case manager is responsible for the patient no matter where the patient is along the healthcare continuum. This may mean that the primary case manager communicates with the case manager in the setting in which the patient currently is. In this case the current setting is considered the transient or episodic setting wheras the primary care setting is the one the patient consistently accesses for ongoing care and is known to be the setting with the primary responsibility, accountability, and ownership for the management of the patient's healthcare condition and needs over time. For example, if a community-based case manager is following the patient, the responsibility for the case may be relinquished to the hospital-based case manager on a temporary basis should the patient be admitted, and for the duration of the hospital stay. The community-based case manager would share relevant information with the hospital-based case manager and might visit the patient. The ultimate responsibility for the management of the case while the patient is in the hospital would be the hospital-based case manager's.

In organizations in which the service line crosses the continuum and there are multiple service programs, patient referrals and continuity of care are not necessarily automatic. In fact, the more complex the organization, the greater the need for client referral, follow-up, and tracking mechanisms. Continuity can be maintained by the case manager for clients at any point along the continuum (Case Manager's Tip 3.1).

What is a model of care? A model is a systematic description used to help visualize something that is ab-

Box 3.1 Healthcare Access Points and Types of Care Offered

1. Primary Care
   a. Clinics
   b. Health fairs
   c. Risk screening programs
   d. Health education programs
   e. Demand management programs

2. Ambulatory Care
   a. Physician offices
   b. Clinics
   c. Diagnostic centers
   d. Day surgery
   e. Patient-Centered Medical Home (PCMH)
   f. Federally qualified health centers (FQHCs)

3. Acute Care
   a. Hospitals
   b. Medical centers
   c. Emergency departments
   d. Critical access hospitals (CHAs)

4. Tertiary Care
   a. Teaching hospitals
   b. Academic medical centers
   c. Acute rehabilitation
   d. Specialty physicians

5. Home Care
   a. Visiting nursing services
   b. Home medical equipment, including IV therapy
   c. Community care programs

6. Long-Term Care
   a. Nursing homes
   b. Subacute care facilities
   c. Long-term rehabilitation centers
   d. Adult homes
   e. Skilled nursing facilities

7. Palliative and Hospice Care
   a. Home hospice programs
   b. Hospital-based programs
   c. End-stage group homes
   d. Ambulatory care programs

Note: The above list is not mutually exclusive. Some access points may be applicable in more than one designation; for example, primary care and ambulatory care can be of same or similar designation as primary care has recently become increasingly popular as a model of care in ambulatory care settings. Another example, tertiary care, is also acute care.

 CASE MANAGER'S TIP 3.1

System Model of Case Management

System models of case management are structured across the continuum of care and/or health and human services. They usually involve multiple care settings and providers. Some models have the same case manager follow a spcific number of patients across the continuum or have a tightly linked and strategically positioned workflow which allows the hand-off of accountability of patient care to the case manager in the setting the patient needs to access.

For organizations in which the service line crosses the continuum and there are multiple service programs, the case manager can help maintain continuity for clients at any point along the continuum by providing referral, follow-up, transitions of care communication, and tracking services.

stract and may not be feasible to directly observe. It is a representation of an object or phenomenon that shares important characteristics of the object or phenomenon. Models can be material, visual, mathematical, or computational. Because care delivery models such as case management models are not easy to imagine or see, we use descriptors to provide a picture of the model in terms of its structure, key elements, differentiating or distinguishing factors, and processes. Chapter 3 discusses the structures and key characteristics of various case management models from different care settings.

Roles of case managers and the set of key categories of accountabilities they perform as they care for patients and their families. Roles are driven from titles we assume in the social structure of our practice and provide the context in which we work and can be applied differently in different settings. Within each role are a set of functions. Functions are the series of activities or tasks that are conducted within each role. They are the specific actions taken by a case manager in the performance of the specific role and are needed to complete each role. Functions may vary from model to model and from one care delivery setting to the next. In Chapter 4 we discuss the roles and processes that are used to bring each model to life in the practice of case managers.

Clearly the most effective models are those that provide a mechanism for managing patients across the continuum of care, thereby providing a seamless, integrated care process. In a managed care environment this is most easily done because of the integrated services inherent in a managed care system. However, due to the many changes in healthcare reimbursement methods, case management is now being applied more readily in medical homes and health homes, discussed later in this chapter. The notion of managing patients in a variety of care settings is more difficult in payer systems in which there are no incentives for the various settings to communicate and/or share resources. With the advent of the medical home and health home concepts, as well as accountable care organizations, Medicare has provided new incentives that reach beyond commercial payers and deeply into the government payer arena. While managed care has traditionally been viewed as the system that provided the generalized structure and focus when managing the use, cost, quality, and effectiveness of healthcare services, it is no longer the only payer interested in managing costs of care.

Many healthcare organizations have opted to first implement case management in the acute care setting. This accomplishes a number of things. First, it allows the organization to design, implement, and perfect its case management system in a more easily controlled environment; the hospital for example. Although it provides greater challenges in terms of the clinical management of patients in the acute care setting, it is still a place where healthcare team members are part of a team that is "within-the-walls." In fact, the term within-the-walls has been used to aggregate those case management models that manage patients' care during the acute care portion of the illness. Among the many applications of the within-the-walls models are a host of types using members of the interdisciplinary healthcare team in various role functions. In most cases the RN is used as the case manager. It is the placement of the RN in the organizational structure and the associated role functions that differentiate the various models.

Case management is difficult to encapsulate because it describes many different approaches, including a patient care delivery system, a professional practice model, a defined group of activities performed by healthcare providers in a particular setting, and services provided by private practitioners.

3.2. TYPES OF CASE MANAGEMENT

Case management can be provided in a variety of model structures. It has become an imbedded feature in many care delivery systems. The mechanisms for describing these applications relies on the level of care in which the model is implemented. These would include the pre-acute, the acute, and the post-acute care models. Box 3.2 summarizes the levels of care and the types of models.

Box 3.2   Case Management Models and Sites in Which They are Used

1. Pre-Acute Care Models
   a. Community-based
   b. Medical homes
   c. Primary care
   d. Chronic care
   e. Managed care
   f. Wellness, screening, and prevention
2. Acute Care Models
   a. Emergency department
   b. Hospital–based
3. Post-Acute Care Models
   a. Long-term care
   b. Acute rehabilitation
   c. Sub-acute services
   d. Palliative care
   e. Hospice care

3.3. PRE-ACUTE CARE MODELS

3.3.1. Community-Based

Community-based case management encompasses any of the case management functions that are performed outside the acute care setting. Community-based case management, whether in the home care arena, the clinic setting (patient centered medical home and federally qualified health centers), or the chronic care setting, is designed to support patients and families in achieving the optimal level of wellness by accessing and using community services. Community-based case management incorporates a focus on the continuum of care (Case Manager's tip 3.2).

In some instances the community-based case manager provides episodic case management. For example, the home care case manager manages the care of a patient through a specific episode of illness, after which

 CASE MANAGER'S TIP 3.2

Community-Based Case Management

By providing ongoing education and support to patients, the case manager can help ensure that the goal of community-based case management is met: to support and empower individuals to reach their optimal level of wellness health and through the use of community resources.

his or her span of responsibility concludes. The community-based case manager, working out of a clinic setting for a patient in a capitated, at-risk contract, may follow this patient from enrollment to disenrollment, passing the case management "baton" to the episodic case manager (e.g., the acute care or home care case manager, see Box 3.3).

Community-based case management models are focused on primary care and primary prevention. They are therefore predominantly focused on healthy individuals in the community who are at risk or who have the potential for needing healthcare services. These models can provide integrated healthcare services found nowhere else. Comprehensive, coordinated, community-based programs can interrelate the client's health, social, physiological, functional, educational, employment, and recreational needs.

Community-based social workers may perform a variety of functions. Generally, a social work model is predicated on some form of referral process whereby the nurse case manager or other members of the interdisciplinary healthcare team refers to the social worker patients that are deemed to be at high risk. High-risk criteria for a community-based social work referral might include such things as the need for psychosocial counseling, emotional support, family counseling, financial counseling, and stress management. Social workers in the community may be referred patients through a physician, a clinic, or through self-referral.

In some high-risk cases, a patient may be case managed by both a nurse case manager and a social worker in the community. The need for both disciplines is determined based on the patient's high-risk needs. Those with both psychosocial and clinical needs may therefore be case managed by both a nurse and a social worker. In this way, the neediest patients receive the care and support of the disciplines best able to meet those needs.

Social workers in the community may provide short-term psychosocial interventions or long-term support, depending on the needs of the patient and family. For example, a family with a child who has cystic fibrosis may need years of psychosocial intervention and support. The social worker may maintain a therapeutic relationship with that child and family for a very long time.

3.3.2. Medical Homes

Medical homes, also known as patient-centered medical homes (PCMH), are a philosophy or model of primary care that is designed to provide "patient centered, comprehensive, team-based, coordinated, accessible care that is focused on quality and safety," (Patient Centered Primary Care Collaborative, 2000). Widely accepted in the primary care arena, medical homes have fast become the gold standard in organizing primary care services. In March 2007, the American Academy of Family Physicians, American Academy of Pediatrics, American College of Physicians, and American Osteopathic Association, the largest primary care physician organizations in the United States, released the *Joint Principles of the Patient-Centered Medical Home* (Box 3.4).

At the center of the medical home philosophy is care coordination. Medical homes use a care coordination model framework to achieve their goals. While there are many definitions of care coordination, the one embraced by the medical home community focuses on the following four elements:

1. Facilitate the provision of comprehensive health promotion and chronic condition care
2. Ensure a focus on ongoing, proactive, planned care activities
3. Build and use effective communication strategies among family, the medical home, schools, specialists, and community professionals and community connections
4. Help improve, measure, monitor, and sustain quality outcomes including clinical, functional, well-being, satisfaction, experience, and cost) (McAllister, Cooley, VanCleave, Boudreau, & Kuhlthau, 2007).

The ultimate aim of the medical home is to provide an infrastructure in which, through responsiveness and collaboration, high quality and high value holistic care is provided. Tools used to support the model include information systems and data bases that interface across the continuum of care. These allow for communication among providers, resulting in reduction of duplication of resources and better coordination among providers. The connecting link among all providers is the case manager who interacts with the patient at all

---

Box 3.4   Joint Principles of the Patient Centered Medical Home

- *Personal physician*: "Each patient has an ongoing relationship with a personal physician trained to provide first contact, continuous, and comprehensive care."
- *Physician directed medical practice*: "The personal physician leads a team of individuals at the practice level who collectively take responsibility for the ongoing care of patients."
- *Whole person orientation*: "The personal physician is responsible for providing for all the patient's healthcare needs or taking responsibility for appropriately arranging care with other qualified professionals."
- *Care:* Care is coordinated and/or integrated between complex healthcare systems, for example across specialists, hospitals, home health agencies, and nursing homes, and also includes the patient's loved ones and community-based services. This goal can be attained though the utilization of registries, health information technology and exchanges, ensuring patients receive culturally and linguistically appropriate care.
- *Quality and safety*:
  —Partnerships between the patient, physicians, and their family are an integral part of the medical home. Practices are encouraged to advocate for their patients and provide compassionate quality, patient-centered care.
  —Guide decision making based on evidence based medicine and with the use of decision-support tools.
  —Physician's voluntary engagement in performance measurements to continuously gauge quality improvement.
  —Patients are involved in decision making and provide feedback to determine if their expectations are met.
  —Utilization of informational technology to ensure optimum patient care, performance measurement, patient education, and enhanced communication.
  —At the practice level, patients and their families participate in quality improvement activities.
- *Enhanced access to care*: Services are available through open scheduling and extended hours.
- *Reimbursement*: Payment must "appropriately recognize the added value provided to patients who have a patient-centered medical home."
  —Payment should reflect the time physician and nonphysician staff spend doing patient-centered care management work outside the face-to-face visit.
  —Services involved with coordination of care should be paid for.
  —It should support measurement of quality and efficiency with the use and adoption of health information technology.
  —Enhanced communication should be supported.
  —It should value the time physicians spend using technology for the monitoring of clinical data.
  —Payments for care management services should not result in deduction in payments for face-to-face service.
  —Payment "should recognize case mix differences in the patient population being treated within the practice."
  —It should allow physicians to share in the savings from reduced hospitalizations.
  —It should allow for additional compensation for achieving measurable and continuous quality improvements.

---

points within the medical home continuum and sometimes beyond. For example, the case manager might interact with a hospital-based case manager should the patient be admitted to the hospital. These interfaces result in reduced fragmentation and the elimination of "care silos" where episodes of care are treated as individual events and not as episodes in the life cycle of the patient and family. PCMHs are most commonly seen in hospital-affiliated clinics and ACOs.

3.4. HEALTH HOMES

3.4.1. The Medicaid Health Home

The Medicaid Health Home State Plan Option, authorized under the Patient Protection and Affordable Care Act of 2010 (Section 2703), allows states to design health homes to provide comprehensive care coordination for Medicaid beneficiaries with chronic conditions. States receive enhanced federal funding during the first eight quarters of implementation to support the roll out of this new integrated model of care.

Not to be confused with patient-centered medical homes, health homes are specifically developed for Medicaid beneficiaries with chronic illnesses. In contrast to the physician-led primary care focus of the medical home, health homes offer person-centered, team-based care coordination with a strong focus on behavioral healthcare and social supports and services. Some states (e.g., New York State) are building health home models based on a medical home framework by expanding links to providers and increasing the breadth of available support services.

The health home (also medical home) concept uses risk stratification as a method for identifying those patients at highest risk who will require more intensive case management services. The identification of the high risk patient can happen in one of two ways:

1. Proactively by identifying these patients while they are still in the community.
2. Once the patient has had multiple encounters with the healthcare system, particularly emergency department visits or acute hospital admissions or readmissions.

From a practical point of view, it is likely that both approaches will need to be used. Even if a patient scored low risk in the community, and then was admitted to the hospital, something in their clinical condition or social situation may have changed or deteriorated, resulting in the visit to the hospital.

Conversely, as patients enter the community system, either the clinic or physician's office, an assessment can be performed there that will categorize the patient as low, moderate, or high risk. Risk level criteria can vary and there are a variety of schools of thought as to what places some patients at higher risk than others. One starting point can be to select the diagnoses that are resulting in the most readmissions to the hospital. One may also decide to focus on the diagnoses that CMS has been focusing on for the hospital readmission penalties. These, for example, include heart failure, acute myocardial infarction, pneumonia and hip and knee replacements. CMS, however, has been adding more to the list of diagnoses of focus each year.

Using this approach, a case management program and leader can then track patients with these diagnoses and also add additional risk factors to the equation (Box 3.5).

A combination of risk factors and chronic diagnoses ensures the identification and selection of the highest risk patients for special care coordination and case management. No single element alone can place a patient at high risk, but rather some combination of the elements shared as seen in Box 3.5. If a patient has

heart failure but is adherent to diet and medication regimen, the patient may need to be classified as high risk. If another patient has heart failure, but routinely winds up in the hospital because he/she does not take the medications as prescribed or goes off diet restrictions, then this patient may need to be classified as high risk. Both patients have heart failure, but one needs much closer case management supervision and support than the other (Figure 3.1).

If approximately 5–10% of the patients one sees fall into the high risk category the case management program for the health home patients is likely on the right track, especially in terms of use of the risk indicators. If the percentage turns out to be higher than that, then revisiting the criteria is necessary. For example, no need to tighten up the criteria unless there are enough program resources (e.g., case managers) available to manage larger numbers of patients.

Another 20% of the patients should fall into the moderate risk category. This is sometimes also referred to as the "rising risk" category as it represents patients who may be on the cusp of becoming high risk if an intervention does not take place. These patients typically do not need professional case management in the form of a registered nurse or social work case manager. They can be managed via telephonic reminders, electronic monitoring of their blood work and appointments, and occasional check-ins if appointments are missed.

These patients should be reassessed for risk level if they have a hospitalization, a visit to the emergency department, miss multiple appointments, or experience worsening of medical conditions. Additional factors may include new comorbidities, a change in socioeconomic status, or an acute illness.

Case management staff in the emergency department or hospital can play an important role helping to identify patients whose risk level has changed. This

---

Box 3.5 Additional Risk Factors For Consideration in Health Home Risk Stratification of Patients

- Number of hospital admissions in the prior months
- Number of hospital readmissions in the prior months
- Number of emergency department visits in past months
- Number of comorbidities
- Number of prescribed medications
- Age
- Gender
- Socioeconomic status
- Health literacy
- Ability and willingness to adhere to health regimen

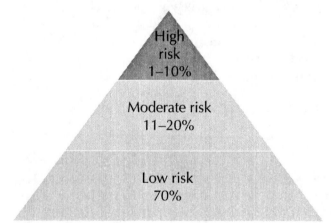

Figure 3.1 Risk level and patient distribution in the health home model.

identification can take place when the patient is initially assessed. At that point, a contact should be made with the community case management department so that they can determine what additional case management services the patient might require.

Risk levels are fluid. Patients may increase or decrease in risk level at any point. For example, if a high risk patient has not been hospitalized or been in the emergency department for a 6-month period and whose clinical status is improving, this patient may be appropriate for a down-grade to moderate risk. Conversely, the patient who is moderate risk and has been frequently to the emergency department or experienced multiple hospitalizations may need to be up-graded to high risk. According to the Advisory Board Company, approximately 18% of the rising risk or moderate risk patient population will become high-risk in any given year (Playbook for Population Health, www.advisory.com/pophealthplaybook).

The remaining 70% of patients fall into the low risk category. These are patients who have none of the risk factors as described above and who are generally stable and self-managing well. They may be completely healthy individuals. They may have chronic conditions that are well-maintained. These patients are as important as the moderate to high risk patients in terms of keeping them healthy and stable and prevent them from progressing to a higher risk category. They need to be connected to the healthcare system as should all patients. The goal of care for these patients would include providing a level of care and involvement with these patients that keeps them loyal to the healthcare system or medical home setting. Another goal is keeping them as healthy as possible by ensuring that annual routine check-ups take place and that these patients do not fall through the cracks. By maintaining a database on the low risk patient population, the healthcare system or medical home is in a better position to treat them should care be needed at any point.

The best way for these patients to interact with the health system is through a patient portal where they can participate in the management of their care and interface with the healthcare system or medical home.

3.4.1.1. Patient Registries

Patient registries (Case Manager's Tip 3.3) are another important tool for managing the high and moderate risk patients. These are clinical information systems that provide a foundation for actively following large numbers of patients with specific health conditions such as diabetes, heart failure, asthma, and end-stage renal failure. Registries provide a technology solution

CASE MANAGER'S TIP 3.3

Use of Patient Registries and the Case Manager

Patient registries are important tools in medical and health homes and any type of chronic care management program. They can be used to track and manage patients suffering a particular chronic illness such as diabetes, heart failure, and asthma. They are for patients of all age groups and assist the interdisciplinary healthcare team and case managers in the effective management of patients and for the improvement of clinical outcomes to ultimately improve the health of a total population of patients.

to managing large populations of patients. For low risk patient groups, they can be used to trigger patient appointment scheduling, routine blood work, or annual health risk assessment tests such as mammograms or colonoscopies.

For moderate risk patients, the registry can be used to trigger the above, plus additional clinical management issues that may be specific to the moderate risk patients. These may include more frequent appointments with the primary care provider. Beyond these issues, the moderate risk patient may need monthly telephonic or face-to-face meetings with the case manager and/or the social worker, depending on the patients' issues.

High risk patients may need to have their blood work monitored closely as well as any other frequent tests or procedures that need to be performed. The risk stratification, electronic documentation and medical records, and electronic tracking software applications can alert the case manager when blood work results are abnormal or when a patient does not keep a scheduled appointment. Expected outcomes can be entered into the patient's database so that all care providers know the patient status and can review while all looking at the same information in the system. In addition, the social worker and case manager will need to keep a close and diligent eye on their status and progress.

Finally, registries can be used to assess populations of patients to determine how an organization is doing in terms of any and all of the issues listed above. This data can be used to identify areas for improvement, gaps in care, or other issues requiring intervention or improvement.

Because health homes are focused on the Medicaid population, they require that they are set up in a way that integrates the medical and behavioral needs of patients. The medical and behavioral health needs of patients are interconnected and if only one is addressed, both will suffer. Unless a single case manager can address both, it is likely that one or the other will suffer. By risk-stratifying the patient, the social worker or the nurse case manager can be deployed according to the needs of the patient. If a behavioral health case manager and a medical case manager are both involved with a health home patient, it is critical that they function as a dyad team, and use an integrated approach to the care of that specific patient. In this way, the psychosocial needs which may be affecting the patient's clinical status and outcomes are addressed in concert with the medical needs. Conversely, medical care planning is coordinated with the psychosocial needs in mind.

3.4.2. Private Case Management

Private case management is used for patients who fall outside the traditional patient care programs. In this type of case management an RN will either be self-employed, an independent practitioner, or work on a case-by-case basis for a MCO or other third-party payer/commercial health insurance plans. The private case manager is contracted for services as needed. The case manager coordinates and manages the care for the patient regardless of the setting.

Because the case manager is independent of the organization, some believe that private case managers can provide the greatest level of completely unbiased services to the patient and family. The case manager functioning under this model is not advocating for anyone but the patient. This case management specialty and practice model has become more popular in the disability management and/or workers' compensation arenas where patients who are severely injured works. Many of the private case managers hired in the 1980s were masters prepared RNs or social workers. In the 1990s this trend continued with case managers who were usually clinical nurse specialists (CNSs) or social workers. Often they were paid privately by the client or subcontracted by a third-party payer. The private case manager may coordinate services for the client, advocate on behalf of the client, and/or provide counseling (Clark, 1996) and manage the patient's benefits based on the insurance/health plan.

3.4.3. Primary Care Case Management

In primary care case management the physician functions as the case manager. The physician is responsible for coordinating and managing patient care services. Some health insurance plans and MCOs are using nurse practitioners as primary care case managers. Nurse practitioners are able to take on this role because

of their ability to function independently or under a collaborative agreement with a physician. The primary care case manager is the gatekeeper who plans, approves, manages, and negotiates care for the patient.

In payer-based organizations such as MCOs, the case manager triages patients and determines their future needs and resource allocation. For example, the primary care case manager evaluating a newly diagnosed asthmatic patient will determine whether the patient needs to be seen by a specialist, in an ED setting, or in a doctor's office. This particular managed care function serves to control expenses by limiting the use of more expensive interventions and ensuring that they are provided in the most appropriate level of care/setting.

In today's primary care case management programs, the role of the nurse case manager has become popular. One case manager works with about three to five primary care physicians. Such case managers focus on the group of patients with the highest risk with the primary goal of improving their health and quality of life, enhancing their self-management skills and abilities, and increasing their engagement. Ultimately the case manager, in collaboration with the primary care provider, is able to reduce costs and unnecessary or unplanned access to healthcare services (e.g., acute and emergency care) by this high risk patient population.

3.5. MANAGED CARE MODELS AND CASE MANAGEMENT

Managed care is a broad, expansive term covering a wide variety of services. Its main objective is to contain costs by controlling utilization of resources and coordinating care. It is used as the generic term for commercial health insurance plans offering managed healthcare services to an enrolled population on a prepaid basis such as capitation (per-member-per-month fixed rate). Access, cost, and quality are controlled by care gatekeepers. The gatekeeper is usually a physician in primary care setting. This physician, after assessing the patient, determines whether the patient needs additional services such as a specialty physician or other service controlled by the MCO. There are many types of MCOs, but the most common is the HMO. The four basic models are the group model HMO, the staff model HMO, the IPA model HMO, and the network model HMO (see Chapter 2 for more details).

In the various managed care models case managers are employed to carry out a variety of functions. Broadly speaking, the case management functions can be classified as either financial case management or clinical case management. The financial functions is what might traditionally be classified as utilization management. The MCO case manager is in communication with the hospital-based case manager or utilization manager determining the patient's admission eligibility; continued stay; or discharge disposition, including eligibility of post-discharge services. The case manager in this role advocates on behalf of the MCO and may have a caseload of several hundred patients. Therefore this role is based on a 'lower intensity—higher volume' approach.

Some MCOs supplement the patients being followed by a financial case manager with a more clinically focused case manager. These case managers tend to have a somewhat smaller caseload. Their focus is more high intensity-low volume in nature. They may be assigned by degree of risk stratification (i.e., low, moderate, or high-risk patient population) as identified by the MCO and through predictive modeling processes or automated systems. These may include such things as catastrophic illness or injury, high-user or high-volume members, chronic or disabling conditions, or cases with high annual cost projections ($25,000–$50,000). It is hoped that assisting in the management of these patients will prevent unnecessary admissions to the hospital and minimize misutilization of healthcare resources (Case Manager's Tip 3.4).

MCOs vary in how they employ the services of case managers. Some have developed case management departments and hired salaried case managers to assume both of the financial and clinical roles. Others have contracted with independent case management entities for these services (i.e., outsourced this function). Still others have a hybrid arrangement in which most case management activities are performed by the MCO while workers' compensation and long-term disability cases are subcontracted to an independent disability manager or private case management provider. However, it is unlikely for a large MCO to outsource this important function. Regardless of the arrangement, the role of the case manager remains basically the same.

Some MCOs are focusing on the management of their older members. The elderly are at greater risk in terms of cost, chronicity, and frequency of care needs. It is hoped that case managing this population will enhance the health status of older adults while containing their use of healthcare resources. MCOs have employed special strategies for managing the care of this population, such as telephonic case management and triage services.

3.5.1. Telephonic Case Management

Member services in MCOs (HMOs and PPOs alike) take place mostly via telephone communication. However, other methods of communication such as paper mailings still exist to some degree, and new ones such as the use of the Internet for electronic mailings are being developed and implemented (Case Manager's Tip 3.5). Regardless of the method employed, communication between the payer, the provider, and the members is an important subject in managed care and case management. The focus on the continuum of care in case management and disease management practices and in demand management programs sponsored by MCOs has led to an expansion in the role of the case manager. New additions include responsibility for interventions or functions that are based on the telecommunication advances such as telephone triage and telephonic case management.

Telephonic case management is defined as the delivery of healthcare services to patients and/or their families or caregivers over the telephone or through correspondence, fax, e-mail, text messaging, or other forms of electronic transfer. It is a patient and family encounter with a healthcare provider, in this case a case manager, applying the case management process (see Chapter 4) to appropriately meet the patient's needs. It

 CASE MANAGER'S TIP 3.5

Communication Between MCOs and the Members

The greatest volume of interactions between MCOs and their members occurs in the form of telephone communications. However, other forms of communication do occur, such as routine paper mailings of the insurance identification cards, member newsletters, and other individualized forms of communication such as claims-related information. It is becoming more popular today for MCOs and their members to use electronic media such as e-mail, online discussion groups, and list serves for certain types of general communications that do not jeopardize an individual's right to privacy and confidentiality.

 CASE MANAGER'S TIP 3.4

Payer-Based and Managed Care Case Management

Payer-based and managed care case managers usually function either as financial case managers (utilization managers) who may have a caseload of hundreds or even thousands, or as more clinically focused case managers who have fewer cases but of higher intensity.

also is considered a cost-effective and proactive strategy for preventing catastrophic health outcomes and high expenses associated with major illness events. Box 3.6 contains additional benefits to telephonic case management.

Telephonic case management services exist across the continuum of care, particularly in the following settings:

- Health insurance plans and MCOs
- Physician offices, primary care, and group practices
- Patient centered medical homes, health homes, and federally qualified health centers
- Major medical centers, especially in pediatric services
- Emergency departments
- Advice or call centers
- Community agencies

Although health advice lines have been in existence for quite some time, they did not become popular for the delivery of case management services until recently. This newer form of case management, known as telephonic case management, is the result of the pressures on managed care for cost containment and improved and timely access to healthcare services. However, MCOs incorporated telephonic case management services as an additional benefit to their members in the form of telephone triage. This service, when provided by the payer, focuses on the financial management (utilization management and resource allocation) aspect of

case management. Today, the clinical aspect of case management is as popular as financial management. However, this is generally a focus of the provider rather than the payer.

Case managers provide telephonic case management services in a variety of forms and around the clock. The managed care case manager focuses on triage services and utilization management. The clinical case manager focuses on the coordination and integration of clinical services as they are needed by patients. Both types of case managers use algorithms, guidelines, or protocols for the delivery of case management services. These guidelines provide the case manager with prospectively developed plans of care that incorporate decision-making steps in the form of decision trees. For example, a mother may call the telephone triage line for an advice regarding her 3-year-old child, who is suffering from a high fever.

The case manager engaged in this telephone conversation will bring up the pediatric fever algorithm on his or her personal computer. The case manager will use this algorithm to guide the assessment and evaluation of the child's signs and symptoms so that he or she can determine the urgency of the child's medical/health condition and the type of advice or intervention he or she will be providing. Depending on how urgent the situation is, the case manager will advise the mother to (1) give the child a dose of Tylenol, (2) continue to observe the child and bring the child to the pediatrician's office, or (3) bring the child to the nearest ED.

In this example, the case manager would provide clinical case management advice and triage the patient to access the appropriate level of care/setting for further healthcare services. Other types of interventions are based on the type of call received. Telephone calls made to the MCO case manager are mostly related to problems with claims, clarifications of benefits, authorizations of services, or triage. Those made to clinical case management programs usually focus on the provision of advice, patient and family education, counseling, health risk management, self-care management skills building, and in some instances triage or brokerage of services. In both types of interventions, case managers apply a process of assessment of the situation/need, analysis of the situation using a related algorithm/protocol, prioritizing/determining the urgency of the situation and planning care, implementing care strategies, and evaluation of the outcomes.

In telephone triage, case managers use their findings of the assessment they complete for each caller to categorize the call (i.e., the patient's condition) into one of three triage categories: emergent, urgent, or nonurgent (Rutenberg, 2000; Van Dinter, 2000).

Box 3.6   Benefits of Telephonic Case Management

- Patient's risk identification, stratification, and management
- Cost reduction
- Empowerment and engagement of patients and families for assuming responsibility for self-care and health management
- Provision of timely interventions and real-time information
- Enhancement and ease of access to healthcare services, providers, and payers
- Patients are more likely to adhere to medical regimen
- One case manager could manage greater numbers of patients/enrollees
- Timely referral of patient/family to other providers, case managers, or community resources
- Provision of timely counseling and support for patient/family in troubleshooting problems
- Enhanced working relationships with patients, providers, and payers

1. *Emergent*: Patients must be seen immediately. Examples are conditions of airway compromise, cardiovascular collapse, wounds or lacerations, strokes, and sensory changes. The case manager refers patients with these conditions to the ED or may call emergency medical services for that purpose.
2. *Urgent*: Patients may be seen within 8–24 hours. Examples are vomiting after minor head injury, signs of infection, soft tissue injury, and increasing edema. The case manager suggests to these patients to see their primary care physician within 8 hours.
3. *Nonurgent*: Patients may be seen routinely or treated at home with appropriate follow-up. Examples are minor bruises or abrasions, persistent cough, and cold symptoms. The case manager may provide such callers with advice and recommend that if symptoms do not improve within 2–3 days that they see their primary care providers.

In deciding on the triage category, the case manager considers the patient's age, gender, past medical history, medication intake, and access to care (Rutenberg, 2000). When uncertain of a caller's situation, case managers may consult with a physician or nurse practitioner or may refer the patient/caller to them (Van Dinter, 2000).

3.5.2. Independent/Private Case Management

Independent/private case management entails the provision of case management services by case managers who are either self-employed or are salaried employees in a privately owned case management firm. They are known as "external" case management services. The terms independent and private refer to the absence of oversight by an MCO or a healthcare organization such as a home care agency or an acute care hospital (Case Manager's Tip 3.6). An insurance company or a healthcare facility usually subcontracts with independent case managers for the provision of case management services, particularly for long- and short-term disability cases. However, a patient or a family member may subcontract case management services from a private case manager for assistance in the coordination of cost-effective and appropriate care, for example, to the chronically ill elderly member of the family (Case Manager's Tip 3.7). Because the structure and services are almost the same in both independent and private case management, their descriptions in this section will be combined.

Independent/private case management focuses on

 CASE MANAGER'S TIP 3.6

Independent and Private Case Management

Although they provide similar services, the terms *independent case management* and *private case management* are not the same and should not be used interchangeably.

Independent case management refers to firms that are not a formal part of an insurance company or a healthcare facility. They exist solely for the provision of case management services based on a contractual agreement between the independent case management firm and the healthcare organization.

Private case management refers to the services provided by an independent case manager privately contracted or hired by a patient or a family member.

enabling the patient to make the necessary transitions along the healthcare continuum and to successfully navigate the healthcare delivery system. It also focuses on monitoring resource utilization, managing costs and health benefits, and ensuring the provision of quality care and services.

Healthcare organizations and MCOs are more likely to subcontract with an independent/private case management firm in the areas of rehabilitation and disability case management than for other clinical services. Subcontracting of such services is considered more cost-effective and is thought to increase patient and family satisfaction. In these arrangements, case managers manage the care of their patients as representatives of the insurance company or healthcare facility unless they are hired directly by the patient or family, in which case they represent the patient.

The goals of independent/private case management are similar to other case management programs/models, particularly the insurance-based models. They include the coordination and facilitation of complex medical services; ensuring the provision of timely, quality, and appropriate services; cost-effectiveness;

 CASE MANAGER'S TIP 3.7

Dual Advocacy Role

Independent/private case managers function in a dual advocacy role that sometimes generates conflict. They are expected to deliver care that is efficient and cost-effective in a manner that is satisfactory for both the patient and the hiring insurance company or healthcare facility.

reduction of fragmentation or duplication of services; and providing the patient/family with a one-to-one personalized relationship with a case manager.

Independent/private case managers may not always receive referrals for their patients at an early stage of illness, trauma, or disability. On the contrary, most often they receive a referral after a patient has been ill or disabled for an extended period, which causes the illness to be considered chronic rather than acute and the focus of care to be rehabilitation and restoration of function rather than curative.

Although in independent case management the insurance company or healthcare facility hires the case managers, they are required to obtain certifications for services from the MCO before they are provided to the patient. Therefore independent case managers are usually seen interacting with the managed care–based case manager on an ongoing basis. They even provide concurrent and periodic review of the patient's condition, progress, and treatment plan to the managed care–based case manager. Usually these reviews are set to occur at a predefined time interval and are discussed. Ongoing authorizations of services are also required every 30 days regardless of whether new services are implemented. The same expectations apply for private case management unless the patient/family who made the arrangement for care is paying privately (self-paying) for the services.

3.5.3. Workers' Compensation

Case management approaches to workers' compensation have been implemented to curtail the increased cost of caring for patients with work-related injuries and reduce the potential for legal litigation. They are even more important today because of the shift in workers' compensation insurance to a managed care structure in the form of HMOs and PPOs and their related utilization management practices. The application of case management in workers' compensation provides another example of the value of case management services and evidence that such models exist across the continuum of care.

Workers' compensation, also known as "workers' comp," is a type of insurance employers are mandated by law to offer to their employees in the event of an on-the-job injury (Case Manager's Tip 3.8). It is a no-fault system of benefits for employees who sustain occupational injury or illness (DiBenedetto, 2001). According to DiBenedetto (2001), a person must sustain the injury or illness while on the job and must incur medical costs, rehabilitation costs, lost wages, or disfigurement to qualify for workers' compensation ben-

 CASE MANAGER'S TIP 3.8

Worker's Compensation Law

It is mandatory that employers provide their employees with a worker's compensation insurance benefit that covers on-the-job injury. This is in accordance with state law, and the mandates vary from state to state. There are some exclusions to this mandate depending on employer size and types of workers.

efits. Employers are mandated by law to provide their employees with three types of benefits: indemnity cash benefits in lieu of lost wages, reimbursement for necessary medical expenses, and survivors' death benefits (Powell, 2000).

Workers' compensation claims are the result of trauma or job-related illness. Case management is an effective strategy used to expedite the return of injured employees to work. Case management services must be directed toward bringing the injured employee to maximal medical improvement and physical functioning and eventually back to work. Case managers are essential for meeting these goals. They assume the responsibility for coordinating medical care and rehabilitation services. They also facilitate the resolution of legal issues by acting as liaisons between the injured employee, legal representatives (lawyers), occupational health department, claims adjusters, and employer. Case managers achieve these goals by following the injured employee from the time the injury occurs until a safe, maximal, modified, or optimal return to work takes place. During this time they collaborate with rehabilitation professionals in the development, implementation, monitoring, and evaluation of the employee's plan of care and return-to-work plan.

The main focus of case management services in the field of workers' compensation is return to work. The case manager develops and achieves the return-to-work plan through the application of the case management process and in collaboration with the injured employee, the employer, and the physician(s) and other healthcare providers involved in the employee's care. Return-to-work plans are of three types (Case Manager's Tip 3.9): full, modified, or temporary. Full plans aim at returning the injured employee to a full work assignment and schedule similar to that which existed before the injury. Modified plans are those adjusted to meet the injured employee's abilities and physical limitations resulting from the injury. Case managers implement these plans to expedite the employee's return to work (Box 3.7). Temporary plans are those that

CASE MANAGER'S TIP 3.9

Return to Work Plans

Case managers involved in the design and implementation of return to work plans must ensure compliance with relevant laws and regulations such as the Americans with Disabilities Act, Family Medical Leave Act, and Occupational Safety and Health Administration.

are adjusted for a limited period during the time the injured employee is still undergoing rehabilitation. These plans include limitations in job functions based on the medical and functional condition of the employee. Before the employee returns to work with this temporary plan, human resources or occupational health services must approve the work schedule and assignment.

Case managers are effective in achieving these plans if they build trusting and humanistic relationships with the injured employee. They must treat their patients with courtesy, dignity, and respect. These relationships are important particularly because injured employees tend to disengage themselves from the work environment. This act of disengagement presents case managers with a greater challenge when facilitating an employee's timely return to work. The process may be delayed if the case manager is not successful in re-engaging the injured employee with the work environment, and this cannot be achieved unless the case manager is able to build an effective relationship with the employee.

3.6. WELLNESS, SCREENING, AND PREVENTION

Wellness and screening for early identification of risks for illness, new health conditions, or exacerbation of existing conditions can be applied to most of the pre-acute models described earlier in Chapter 3. These screenings should be an integral part of any pre-acute case management model.

Box 3.7   Sample Modifications of Return to Work Plans

- Decreased work hours
- Temporary job sharing
- Job modifications (temporary or permanent)
- Reducing responsibilities and tasks
- Acquisition and use of assistive equipment, tools, or other devices
- Work environment modification
- Technology modifications

Typically, screening is focused on the patient's age, sex, and presence or absence of chronic conditions, illnesses, or post-operative states. Examples of elements to be included in a screening analysis include:

- Blood pressure
- Cholesterol
- Mammograms
- Colonoscopies
- Osteoporosis screening
- Obesity
- Lifestyle behaviors such as smoking and alcohol consumption
- Blood test monitoring such as Hemoglobin A1c for diabetes and PSA for prostate cancer
- Annual physical examinations
- Other tests based on existing conditions such as blood urea nitrogen and creatinine levels for patients diagnosed with kidney disease.

By providing a patient-centered approach to care as described in the above models, health and wellness screening becomes a part of the patient's plan of care. Patient care registries are a good way to provide automated reminders to healthcare providers when any of the above tests need to be completed, whether that be monthly, annually, or less frequently. Results can be shared with the entire healthcare team in order to ensure that all elements of the patient's condition are taken into consideration when treating the patient.

3.7. ACUTE CARE CASE MANAGEMENT MODELS

Acute care or hospital-based case management models are also referred to as episodic case management. These models are applied to patients during an episode of illness that is short term and involves care delivery at the acute or critical care level. Case managers in the acute care setting are available at the access points, inpatient units, and at discharge points.

3.7.1. Access Point Case Management

Early acute care case management models did not give great attention to the two fundamental routes of entry to the hospital: the ED and the admitting department. Acute care settings now recognize the importance of gatekeeping these hospital admission points to manage and control the types of patients approved for admission. Before managed care, the need for putting such controls in place was much less obvious and clearly less important. In addition to the imperatives fostered by managed care including notification of emergency admissions and precertification of planned admissions, the CMS has increased the need for access point case management with the implementation of the two-midnight rule and observation status. Never before has gatekeeping of the primary routes of entry to the hospital been more critical than they are now.

Case management in the admitting department provides for a gatekeeping function at one of the two primary routes of entry to the hospital nonemergency admissions including planned and urgent, and direct admissions. Patients are screened through the use of clinical indicators. Through this process, the patient's severity of illness and the intensity of service requirements are compared with the services being requested by the admitting physician. When the patient's needs do not meet the admission criteria (see Chapters 5 and 6), the case manager contacts the physician to discuss care alternatives to the acute care setting.

The case manager may suggest to the physician the use of an alternative level of care/setting such as ambulatory surgery or observation status. It is important that the case manager never deny an admission without providing the physician with alternative settings along the continuum that would more appropriately meet the patient's clinical needs and ensure reimbursement.

The case manager also screens all admissions for which the admitting physician is requesting preoperative days. Using established criteria, the case manager will either approve or disapprove the request. If approval cannot be granted because reimbursement cannot be obtained, the case manager will communicate this to the admitting physician. If the case manager and the physician feel that a patient cannot adequately prepare himself or herself for surgery, such as completing a bowel prep, then despite the lack of reimbursement, the approval will be granted. The patient's intensity of service should be the primary indicator determining whether a preoperative day is necessary.

The admitting department case manager also screens all patients being transferred into the hospital to ensure that the transfer is appropriate and meets all Medicare guidelines. The basic rule of thumb for acute to acute transfers is that the receiving hospital should have the capacity to provide the higher level of service that the patient requires, and that cannot be provided in the transferring hospital. An example of this would be cardiac surgery. The patient may have been admitted to the sending hospital for a cardiac catheterization or on an emergency basis (e.g., acute chest pain). The sending hospital may not have open heart surgery services available, and therefore the patient must be transferred to receive this higher level of service.

Once admission to the hospital has been agreed to,

the admitting case manager is responsible for communicating his or her approval to the admitting department. Generally the clerical staff in the admitting department then obtains a preauthorization or precertification from the insurance company. When the insurance company is requesting clinical information before giving its precertification, the case manager is often the appropriate person to provide that link between the clinicians, the admitting department, and the insurance company.

The admitting case manager reviews all same-day admissions before the scheduled day of surgery to ensure that preauthorization has been obtained. Additionally, the admitting case manager may be responsible for reviewing all "short-stay" medical records. These would be the medical records of patients who have been in the hospital for 24 hours or less and who were not placed in an observation status. The case manager would review the record to assess whether the care rendered and documented met acute care criteria. If the record does not support an inpatient level of reimbursement, the case manager has the authority to revert the hospital bill to the ED services only. In this way an insurance denial is avoided and the hospital is at least assured that it will receive the ED level of reimbursement in a timely manner (Case Manager's Tip 3.10).

3.7.2. Emergency Department Case Management

As a commonly used route of entry to the hospital, acute care case management models should not neglect to staff this important hospital department. As does the admitting department case manager, the ED case manager provides an important gatekeeping function for the hospital. The ED case manager is responsible for facilitating the patient's hospitalization from preadmission through discharge from the ED. The case manager interfaces with physicians, nurses, social workers, and other members of the team to expedite medically appropriate, cost-effective care.

 CASE MANAGER'S TIP 3.10

Admitting Department and Emergency Department Case Management

Admitting department and emergency department case management models are key to any case management program design because they represent routes of entry to the hospital; a location where case managers are able to reduce financial risk (e.g., avoidance of reimbursemenrt denials) by assuring admitted patients meet acute care medical necessity criteria.

The ED case manager manages different groupings of patients. These include the treat-and-release patients, patients admitted to the hospital, patients who can be discharged from the hospital but will require follow-up services such as home care in the community, observation patients, and inappropriate admissions such as social admissions.

3.7.3. Treat-and-Release Patients

This group of ED patients will receive all necessary services during their short-term treatment time in the ED and will be discharged without the need for follow-up home care or other community services beyond the routine follow-up physician or clinic appointment. The ED case manager can assist these patients to receive the care they require in the most expeditious way possible. Patients who typically fall into this category include asthmatics or those with other chronic illnesses and patients with injuries or viruses, colds, and the like. Because of the common misuse of EDs in the United States, many of the treat-and-release patients could have received the care they needed in their primary care physician's office or an urgent center.

The case manager facilitates the initiation of diagnostic services, treatment plans, and therapeutic treatments while the patient is in the ED. The case manager identifies any delays in service and either expedites the process by eliminating barriers or collaborates with other members of the interdisciplinary team to resolve the problem.

3.7.4. Patients Admitted from the Emergency Department

The case manager works with the interdisciplinary team to facilitate diagnostic testing in the ED and to ensure that the treatment plan is initiated immediately once a diagnosis has been rendered. For example, a pneumonia patient who is being admitted to the hospital should have his or her antibiotic therapy initiated while still in the ED once the diagnosis has been established. By initiating the treatment in the ED, hours can be shaved off the length of stay and quality of care is enhanced.

The case manager also works with the team to ensure that the patient is transferred to the inpatient bed as quickly as possible. Patients who are out of their managed care network may choose to be transferred to a hospital within their network. The case manager plays an important role in identifying these patients and discussing their options with them. Patients can only be transferred by their own request and if stable.

So as to not violate any Emergency Medical Treatment and Active Labor Act (EMTALA) regulations, the case manager should only inform the patient that, if they are admitted, they may risk some financial responsibility for the hospital bill. The case manager should make it very clear to the patient that they have every right to remain and that they will receive appropriate care, but that there may be some financial risk associated with this decision.

Case managers working in EDs must have a working knowledge of EMTALA and its requirements. EMTALA (also known as COBRA, Section 1867, or the Federal Antidumping Act), governs the delivery of all hospital-based emergency medical care in the United States. It is an antidiscrimination statute.

Two sections in EMTALA relate directly to the initial interactions of EDs with managed care patients, or the "Appropriate Medical Screening Examination (MSE)" requirement, and the "No Delay on Account of Insurance" provision.

The Appropriate Medical Screening Examination provision states the following:

> If any individual comes to the emergency department and a request is made on the individual's behalf for examination and treatment, the hospital must provide an appropriate medical screening exam within the capability of the hospital's emergency department, including ancillary services routinely available to the emergency department, to determine whether or not an emergency medical condition exists (42 USC 1395dd[a]).

For the case manager in the ED, this simply means that all patients who come to the ED must be given an appropriate medical screening. Patients cannot be turned away for any reason. Case managers should be sensitive to this provision and should never be pressured to transfer a patient to another facility unless by the patient's request and only after an appropriate medical screening.

The No Delay on Account of Insurance provision states the following:

> A hospital may not delay provision of an appropriate medical screening examination or necessary stabilizing treatment . . . in order to inquire about the individual's method of payment or insurance status (42 USC 1395dd[h]).

It should never be the policy of an ED to demand that a patient receive authorization from his or her managed care company before screening takes place. The ED case manager should never interfere in this process. In any event, a managed care company cannot deny authorization for an ED visit under any circumstances unless once triaged it is determined that the presenting condition is not an emergency condition. Under those circumstances, the patient's care may be delayed while authorization is being obtained. The patient may be referred to his or her urgent care center for further treatment of the nonemergent complaint.

If the patient requires hospitalization and is out of network, the ED should have a written procedure for informing the patient of the potential "financial risk" of being admitted to the out-of-network hospital. The patient should be clearly told that he or she may certainly stay at the out-of-network hospital if he or she so chooses and that the patient will receive all needed services if that is his or her decision. At the same time, the patient should know that this decision may result in his or her suffering some financial burden such as a deductible or a co-payment, depending on the patient's coverage. If the patient chooses to transfer to an in-network hospital, the patient must sign a release indicating that he or she is transferring at his or her own request. The patient's plan should be billed for the transportation to the in-network hospital. Under no circumstances can a patient be transferred unless he or she is medically stable. Transfer would also be appropriate under circumstances in which the patient needed transfer to receive a higher level of service than was available in the first hospital.

3.7.5. Emergency Medical Conditions

Under EMTALA, the definition of an emergency medical condition (EMC) is much broader than typical medical usage. An EMC is any condition that is a danger to the health and safety of the patient or unborn fetus, or may result in a risk or impairment or dysfunction to the smallest bodily organ or part if not treated in the foreseeable future, and includes the following range of conditions:

- Undiagnosed, acute pain, sufficient to impair normal functioning
- Pregnancy with contractions present (legally defined as unstable)
- Symptoms of substance abuse such as alcohol ingestion
- Psychiatric disturbances such as severe depression, insomnia, suicide attempt or ideation, dissociative state, and inability to comprehend danger or to care for oneself

The ED case manager plays an important educational role for the hospital and an advocacy role for the patient and should remain cognizant and up-to-date on EMTALA at all times.

The ED case manager performs an intake assessment on admitted patients and communicates this assessment to the inpatient case manager. The assessment should include a discharge planning assessment and referral to the social worker if necessary. The case manager should provide any clinical information needed by the third-party payer during the admission process.

3.7.6. Discharged Patients with Services

The case manager in the ED is responsible for coordinating any needed follow-up services for patients returning to the community. In some instances, this intervention may prevent an unnecessary or nonreimbursable admission. The case manager will coordinate the discharge plan with the team and ensure that the services are covered by the patient's third-party payer. Once this has been completed, the case manager will facilitate and coordinate those services with the community agency. Typically, patients who fall into this category will need home care services. On occasion a patient may be transferred to a long-term care facility directly from the ED. In all instances the case manager should follow established criteria to ensure that the patient is receiving the appropriate level of service.

3.7.7. Observation Patients

Under Medicare, observation is an outpatient category in which the patient needs observation of a condition or following a procedure for less than 24 hours. Patients may be observed in a specific observation unit or scattered within the hospital. If the patient is placed in an inpatient bed, the patient's status remains outpatient and the bill should reflect that this level of care was provided. The hospital may bill the third party for the ED visit and for up to 24 hours after the time of transfer from the ED.

The ED case manager should work directly with the attending medical staff in the ED and assist them in the identification of patients appropriate for observation. The InterQual and Milliman criteria both provide the clinical parameters of the observation status.

3.7.8. Inappropriate Admissions

When it is clear that a patient does not require admission, the case manager should assist the care team in identifying an alternative care regimen appropriate to the needs of the patient. For example, a patient may require admission to a long-term care or subacute setting or may require home care services. Working with the patient, the family and the care team, the case manager can facilitate the movement of the patient to the appropriate level of service and prevent a hospital denial of payment.

3.7.9. Preadmission Testing Case Management

In some organizations the admitting case management functions may be integrated with the preadmission testing process. During the preadmission process the case manager assures that the patient's health insurance plan has been notified of the admission as necessary and authorizations for the inpatient stay and surgical procedure has been obtained; if not, the case manager proceeds with completing these important activities. The case manager also may interview and and complete an "intake" for the preoperative patients. During this interview process the case manager evaluates the patient for any preadmission issues that might affect the hospitalization or post-hospitalization process. Part of this assessment includes exploring discharge planning options and post-discharge services with the patient/family. When appropriate, the patient is referred to the social worker (if psychosocial or financial issues were identified) who is responsible for the patient after admission and the inpatient case manager. The case manager may also collaborate with the attending physician when post-discharge needs can be clearly anticipated. For example, an elderly patient who is scheduled for a hip replacement will most likely need either subacute or home care rehabilitation after surgery. The preadmission case manager can begin to discuss options with the patient, family/caregiver, and physician and can also explore these options with the insurance company. All intake information should be communicated to the inpatient case manager so that a smooth transition can take place for the patient. The case manager should document a "preadmit" note in the patient's record that would include postdischarge needs and options.

3.7.10. Perioperative Services Case Management

Perioperative case management is designed to provide case management services to surgical patients. The process begins at the preadmission phase, continues post-surgery, includes surgery and post-anesthesia recovery, and terminates at the post-operative period. The perioperative case manager provides an important link between the members of the surgical team and the patient. During the preoperative phase the case manager assesses the patient to be sure that the patient is

ready for surgery. Readiness may be defined by the following checklist:

- Preoperative tests completed
- Medical clearance obtained, including any necessary consults from specialty care providers such as cardiology or nephrology
- Informed consent obtained
- Patient scheduled for surgery
- Authorization for surgery obtained from the payer

If any elements on the checklist are not completed and/or are problematic, the case manager can adjust the operating room (OR) schedule so that the patient is not left on the schedule, cancelled, and then another patient placed in that slot. For example, before surgery the patient may refuse to sign consent or may become unstable and unable to go to surgery the next day.

Perioperative case managers can also review same-day surgical admissions to ensure that the minimal requirements for surgery have been completed. They use the American Surgical Association (ASA) classification system (Box 3.8) as the review criteria in addition to any other utilization management criteria as indicated by the organization or the managed care companies. For example, for ASA I and II categories a history and physical must be completed, as well as a complete blood cell count (CBC), ECG, chest x-ray examination, and PT/PTT when indicated. For ASA III and IV, all of these must be completed, the patient must be assessed by an anesthesiologist, and any additional tests as indicated by the patient's primary care

---

Box 3.8 American Surgical Association Classifications

- *ASA Class I*: Patient with no systemic disease; takes no prescription or illicit drugs; pathology limited to surgical site, with no systemic implications.
- *ASA Class II*: Patient with mild systemic disease (e.g., diabetes controlled by diet or oral medications; controlled hypertension; smoker without respiratory symptoms).
- *ASA Class III*: Patient with severe systemic disease that limits activity but is not incapacitating (e.g., diabetic patient on daily insulin; poorly controlled hypertension).
- *ASA Class IV*: Patient with an incapacitating systemic disease that is a constant threat to life (e.g., diabetic patient with history of repeated episodes of ketoacidosis and/or hypoglycemia; patient with severe uncontrolled hypertension; patient with coronary artery disease and frequent episodes of chest pain).

physician must be completed. For example, a patient with hypertension may need additional testing before the medical clearance will be approved.

The perioperative case manager maintains a vital link between the patient, the surgeon, and the OR schedule. Potential delays or cancellations are identified earlier, and adjustments are made to the OR schedule so that OR time can be optimized every day. By identifying potential problems early, the patient can be reassessed and possibly go for the surgery later on the day scheduled rather than the surgery being cancelled, resulting in a potential denial of payment by a third-party payer.

3.7.11. Social Work Case Management

Social workers have used the title case manager for many years. In fact, after the RN, social workers are the other professionals most often seen in the role of case manager (Rantz and Bopp, 1996). The social worker, if functioning as the case manager, can focus on the patient's social, financial, and discharge planning needs. The social worker as case manager is effective in the outpatient setting, where many of the patient's needs are related more to financial or social issues and less to clinical ones. In the hospital setting, a dyad of RN case manager and social worker can be an effective way to manage cases based on needs. If the prevailing issues are clinical or educational in nature, the RN may be more appropriate for case management. If the patient's needs are more social or financial, the social worker may be more appropriate to provide the necessary services.

In the dyad model (Box 3.9) the RN and social worker case managers assess the patient on admission to the hospital; based on that assessment, it is determined which practitioner may be more appropriate to manage the case. In some cases it may be necessary for both disciplines to case manage the same patient.

The case manager's initial assessment would be a clinical or biological review of systems, reason for hospitalization, relevant previous medical history, clinical issues that may affect discharge, and educational needs. The social worker would be focused on the social support and psychological segments of the patient's overall clinical picture. A social assessment includes an evaluation of the patient's lifestyle, activities, interests, and support system. Family support, living environment, and the patient's ability to return to the preadmission environment would be assessed by the social worker. The psychological assessment would consist of an evaluation of the patient's mental

---

Box 3.9   Neonatal Case Management Team Role Responsibilities

Social Work

1. Psychosocial assessment, including evaluation of family situation/home/financial support, other high-risk social factors. Clarify medical coverage. Advocate; refer for such coverage. Refer for appropriate entitlements. Advocate for patients with various systems.
2. Evaluation of coping with illness/hospitalization; evaluation of family support systems; provision of emotional support.
3. Referral to community support agencies/mental health services as indicated.
4. Coordination of child abuse/neglect cases, including substance abuse cases.
5. Act as part of the neonatal intensive care unit (NICU) team in providing coordinated services to families with children in the NICU.

Shareable Skills/Tasks with the Interdisciplinary Healthcare Team

1. Attend regular interdisciplinary NICU rounds to share information.
2. Share in decision making with family.
3. Identify system barriers and solutions.
4. Provide patient/team continuity.
5. Collaborate with utilization management.
6. Optimize patient's adjustment to NICU.

Case Manager

1. Case management plan of care; length of stay.
2. Track data.
3. Follow clinical status.
4. Coordinate/facilitate plan of care.
5. Provide consultation regarding clinical issues.
6. Monitor outcomes.
7. Track clinical resource utilization with team.
8. Provide discharge teaching (e.g., CPR, medications).
9. Provide discharge planning, including equipment and home care referrals.
10. Posthospital follow-up.
11. Make transportation arrangements.

---

status; use of alcohol, tobacco, and drugs; and previous history of mental disorders.

When implementing this model, it is extremely valuable for both disciplines to sit down together and outline what their case management inclusion or selection criteria will be. Through techniques such as case conferencing, an ongoing evaluation can be made as to the patient's progress toward the expected outcomes and as to whether additional providers may need to be added to the case.

This type of model, although extremely patient focused and beneficial to the patient and family, may be too costly for the organization to support. If so, the RN case manager can call the social worker on a referral basis for cases needing more comprehensive social work-type interventions (Case Manager's Tip 3.11).

In an RN/social worker dyad model, another effective strategy can be the use of specific referral criteria adapted to various clinical settings. Working as a team, the nurse and social worker can meet the needs of high-risk patients identified through the use of prospectively determined criteria that reflect the specific issues identified in discreet clinical settings. If you work in a hospital or out-patient setting in which a variety of types of patients are treated, it may be helpful to outline the referral criteria by clinical specialty. The examples in Box 3.10 and Box 3.11 serve as guides only. Each organization must develop its own unique set of criteria to meet its clinical needs, as well as remain appropriate to the specific case management departmental design.

For example, the criteria for referring a social worker to a patient in the ED will vary significantly from the needs of a patient on a maternal/child unit. By using this type of criteria, both disciplines can be deployed to specific patients as needed, and in a timely fashion. In all instances, the division of responsibilities should address the unique skill sets and knowledge base of each discipline. Clinical needs should be addressed by the RN case manager, whereas social/financial needs are best addressed by the social worker. In this way each discipline's knowledge and time are optimized.

3.7.12. Inpatient Registered Nurse Case Manager

The case manager in the acute care/hospital setting performs multiple roles including coordination of patient flow, utilization and resource management, reimbursement denials management, tracking and management of care variances, transitional planning, quality management, and psychosocial assessment and counseling.

 CASE MANAGER'S TIP 3.11

Social Work Case Management

Social work case management is beneficial to patients and families yet may be too costly for the organization to support. One solution is for the nurse case manager to call the social worker on a referral basis for cases that need more comprehensive interventions.

Box 3.10   Guidelines for RN Case Managers and Social Workers: Example in Medical/ Surgical Inpatient Adult Services

RN Case Manager

- Performs admission and concurrent utilization management, including insurance calls
- Coordinates/facilitates plans of care
- Facilitates daily rounds and team meetings
- Assesses all patients for psychosocial needs
- Completes discharge plans, including durable medical equipment, home care, rehabilitation, and long-term care facilities
- Orders transportation
- Completes discharge forms
- Oversees clinical guidelines
- Tracks data (e.g., variances in patient care and systems standards)
- Provides alternate level of care notification
- Issues HINN letters

Social Worker

- Patient/family difficulty coping with new diagnosis (e.g., cancer, ventilator dependency, difficulty understanding/accepting decision making with long-term discharge planning options)
- Psychiatric, cognitive, or behavioral factors that may impede delivery of care and discharge planning process
- Inadequate supports that may impact on compliance with continuing care needs (*Note*: Social workers can provide case managers with information to give to patients and families regarding entitlements)
- Ethical or legal concerns (e.g., patient, family, team conflicts related to medical plan of care, guardianship cases, or end-of-life issues around Advance Directives, DNR order)
- Suspicion or evidence of domestic violence, elder abuse or neglect, child abuse or neglect, rape, sexual assault; known to PSA
- Substance abuse counseling referrals when patient requests or is viewed as amenable to intervention
- Unidentified patient(s) is seriously ill, and there is difficulty locating significant others
- Patients signing out against medical advice
- Homelessness (e.g., new onset, patient is unable to return to prior living situation)
- Long-term nursing facility placements for patients with complex family or financial situations

DNR: Do not resuscitate; HINN: hospital-issued notice of noncoverage; PSA: Protective Services for Adults.

Box 3.11   Guidelines for Referrals: Example in Inpatient Case Management Model for AIDS Patients; Special Focus on Shared Responsibilities

RN Case Manager

- Completes discharge planning forms
- Performs admissions and concurrent utilization management, including insurance calls
- Tracks data (e.g., variances in patient care and systems standards)
- Facilitates daily rounds and team meetings
- Makes referrals to home health services
- Orders transportation, equipment, supplies
- Provides alternate level of care notifications
- Issues HINN letters

Social Worker

- Participates in case conferences
- Collaborates with community agencies, CBO's IDC providers round on complex psychosocial problems
- Initiates referrals to AIDS community services and immigration advocacy groups
- Provides crisis intervention; advocacy; counseling around impact of illness on the patient/significant other, bereavement, and sexual assault; child protection; substance abuse patient education
- Facilitates discussion around healthcare proxies, guardianship, DNR orders
- Provides financial assessments and referrals to entitlement programs
- Maintains contact with each patient through patient's first follow-up medical provider appointment postdischarge
- Refers patients to long-term and subacute placement
- Coordinates Medicaid application as needed and charitable services

RN Case Manager/Social Worker–Shared Responsibilities

- Assesses each patient
- Identifies and communicates with prior and future providers of medical and psychosocial services
- Assists physicians in completing discharge forms
- Participates in interdisciplinary patient care management rounds

CBO: Community-based organization; IDC: infectious disease clinic.

3.7.12.1. Patient Flow Coordination and Facilitation of Care

In the role of patient flow the case manager ensures that all patient care processes that support patients as they move through the acute care continuum are opti-

mized. These processes may include tests, treatments, procedures, consults, any other care interventions, and inpatient bed assignment. The purpose of patient flow is to optimize each day the patient is in the acute care setting, including evenings and weekends. The case manager arranges care interventions so that patient care occurs in the proper sequence and level, and optimizes patients' recovery and discharge back to home and the community setting.

The case manager also facilitates the care interventions to ensure that they occur in a timely manner and without delay. In order to adequately perform this role, the case manager assesses every patient on admission and daily thereafter. The case manager also leads and/or attends interdisciplinary patient care management rounds daily. In addition, the case manager coordinates the key interventions among and between the members of the interdisciplinary care team, and with the patient and/or family caregiver. Finally, the case manager identifies delays in patient care processes and intervenes to correct them.

The goals of patient flow are to correct or expedite efficient through-put. This ensures that care is provided in a timley manner and that the patient moves smoothly through the acute care continuum. Through this process each hospital day is optimized.

Patient flow is critical to the role of the case manager. It is the principle and most important role that the hospital case manager performs. All the other roles stem from this role.

3.7.12.2. Utilization and Resource Management

Utilization review was the first role assumed by hospital case managers. It is the process that is still used by case managers today to communicate with third party payers/commercial health insurance plans including managed care organizations. Sometimes this communication is verbal, sometimes via fax, and sometimes the clinical information is transferred electronically via e-mail. Now called utilization management, this process is used to ensure that the care provided is medically necessary and appropriate and provided in the most relevant setting or level of care. Added to this role today in successful case management models is resource management.

Resource management is a review of patient care services ordered for the patient to ensure that they are not under the amount needed or over the amount needed to diagnose and treat the patient. This assessment is based on nationally recognized care guidelines. Resources include pharmaceuticals, radiology services, laboratory sevices, and others. In the utilization review case management function, it is easy for the case manager to become overloaded. Keeping some of these tasks part of a centralized core utilization management department can help prevent the true case management focus from being lost.

The goals of utilization and resource management are to ensure that resources used are appropriate, are used timely and without unnessary delay, and that reimbursement is ensured (see Chapter 5 for more details).

3.7.12.3. Denial Management

Denial management is the process of monitoring and managing third-party payer reimbursement from pre-admission to post-discharge. The process includes notification, preauthorization, billing, and appeals management. The key functions of denial management include several actions. The first is to ensure that the payer/health insurance plan has been notified about the patient's admission to the acute care setting. Next, verify that the clinical information is available in the medical record, is accurate, and reflects the care rendered to the patient. Third, ensure that this information is provided, when necessary, to the third party payer in a timely manner and is based on nationally established guidelines and the payer's utilization management procedures. Finally, it is to ensure that the patient is transitioned to the next level of care as quickly as possible once the patient no longer meets the clinical criteria for the current level of care.

The case manager works closely with the precertification staff at the front end and the billing staff at the back end. Appeals are managed either internally or outsourced externally. An appeal is the process applied to manage a denial received from the payer. In this case the process aims to rebuttle the denial and counteract its effects to ultimately minimize the hospital's financial risk (see Chapter 5 for more details).

3.7.12.4. Variance Tracking

Also known as avoidable delay or avoidable delay management, this role is used as a mechanism for the identification and correction of patient care delays in through-put, care delivery, or discharge. These delays may or may not result in an increase in the hospital's length of stay, but may affect the quality of care provided due to the service delays. In this role, the case manager identifies delays in services and seeks to correct them as they are identified. The case manager is also responsible for discussing these delays with the interdisciplinary healthcare team during patient care management rounds each day and for cataloging the

delays into the case management or other databases. The purpose of this role is to identify single delays as well as patterns of delays that can be corrected both concurrently but also over the long term. The data is typically aggregated into groupings identifying the category that the variance falls into. These include internal hospital systems, systems outside the hospital, patient issues, family issues, provider issues, and payer issues (see Chapter 11 for more details).

3.7.12.5. Transitional and Discharge Planning

Both transitional and discharge planning focus on the movement of the patients through the acute care continuum and beyond. Transitional planning is the process the case manager applies to ensure that appropriate resources and services are provided in the most relevant setting or level of care based on the patient's condition and care needs. It is also used to identify the point at which the patient is clinically ready to move to the next level of care and to coordinate this process/transition. Transitional planning occurs within the acute care continuum. For example, it encompasses the movement of the patient from the emergency department to a regular floor, out of the intensive care unit (ICU) to a regular floor bed, into a stepdown from the post-anesthesia care unit (PACU), and so on.

Conversely, discharge planning, while following the same principles as transitional planning, applies to the movement of the patient beyond the acute care setting. It includes the assessment of the needs that the patient may have after the hospital environment. The case manager is responsible for ensuring that the patient's discharge is timely, appropriate, and safe, incorporating the best use of resources that the patient may need in the community or at home (see Chapter 6 for more details).

3.7.12.6. Quality Management

The goal of quality management is to ensure that the care that is rendered to the patient and family is at or above quality, regulatory, and accreditation standards. As such, case managers play a supportive role in quality management. They assist in identifying and documenting adverse events and readmissions. Some case managers may also identify the root cause of hospital readmissions. Some may also perform or participate in concurrent core measure (i.e., value-based purchasing program indicators) review. While all case managers may not have a formal responsibility in this process, they have a professional obligation to bring forward any issues that they identify (see Chapters 11 and 12 for more details).

3.7.12.7. Psychosocial Assessment and Counseling

Psychosocial assessment and counsleing are typically performed by the social worker. The purpose of this process is to identify any issues that may impact the patient's recovery and/or transition out of the hospital. This may include crisis intervention, emotional support, behavior management problems, end stage of life support, inadequate social or financial supports, issues of noncompliance, psychiatric and/or substance abuse issues affecting the current hospitalization or discharge plan, homelessness affecting the current hospitalization or discharge plan, and any other barriers associated with psychosocial issues.

3.8. STATE-OF THE-ART ACUTE CARE CASE MANAGEMENT MODELS

Contemporary case management models appl eit r an integrated or collaborative approach to e c e manager's role and functions. Either type of role requires appropriate staff to patient ratios. Effective models also employ other nonpersonnel resources to assure success and to remain cutting edge. These include some or all of the following:

- Dedicated case management software application for use in electronic documentation and as case management tool(s)
- Laptops or other mobile devices case managers carry with them wherever they are seeing patients to allow them easy access to the case management software application and other key systems
- Cell phones or zone phones
- Dedicated locations on the patient care units or departments to be able to privately meet with patients or their families and communicate with payers and other parties
- Use of support personnel who function in associate roles to case managers; for example, to call vendors of durable medical equipment and transportation services

3.8.1. The Integrated Case Management Model

In the integrated model all roles are performed by a single nurse case manager. This model integrates previoulsy disconnected roles and functions. Included in the integrated model are the seven roles listed above. The nurse case manager integrates the roles of patient flow, utilization management, and discharge planning into one role that applies to all patients in her/his casel-

oad. The nurse case manager is also in this case responsible for referring any psychosocially complex patients to the social worker as they are identified.

The integrated model requires that all patients are seen by a nurse case manager. For some patients that are considered "high risk" they may also be followed by a social worker at the same time with the nurse case manager. Table 3.1 and Table 3.2 describe the recommended staffing ratios (nurse case manager and social worker) that are considered and are based on the design and the roles of the RN case manager and the social worker as described above.

3.8.2. Differences in Staffing

To further c rify the differences between the nurse case manager an the social worker ratios and caseloads, the following are the descriptions of each role.

- *Nurse Case Manager*: Assigned 15 fixed beds that are consistent daily. Patients may be discharged from these beds and new admissions received into these beds over the course of a day of work.
- *Social Worker*: Assigned up to 17 patients based on high-risk referral criteria. These 17 patients may be located across more than one unit, depending on the size of the units.

Approximately 30% of all inpatients match with the high-risk social work referral criteria, and of these, 17 are assigned to each social worker. In total, only 30% of all inpatients may require follow up by both a social worker and a nurse case manager.

3.8.3. The Collaborative Case Management Model

In this model, a third team member is added. The

TABLE 3.1. Ratio of Nurse Case Manager to Patients.

Unit Type	Case Manager to Patient
Medical—including sub-specialties such as oncology, cardiology	1:15
Neurology	1:15
Surgical—including sub-specialties such as neurosurgery, orthopedics	1:15
Intensive Care	1:20
Step-down (intermediate)	1:15
Pediatric	1:20
Obstetrics/gynecology	1:20
Acute rehab	1:15

TABLE 3.2. Ratio of Social Worker to Patients.

Unit Type	Social Worker to Patient (Active Cases)
Medical—including sub-specialties such as oncology, cardiology	1:17
Neurology	1:17
Surgical—including subspecialties such as neurosurgery, orthopedics	1:17
Intensive care	1:17
Step-down (intermediate)	1:17
Pediatric	1:17
Obstetrics/gynecology	1:17
Acute rehab	1:17

third member, called the utilization or DRG manager or business associate and is responsible for the "business" aspects of case management such as conducting clinical reviews for the purpose of transferring information to a third party payer. This person in some hospitals may also be responsible for clinical documentation improvement. As such, the staffing ratios are different in the collaborative compared to the integrated model (Box 3.12). The case manager is responsible for assess-

Box 3.12   Staffing Ratios in Collaborative Acute Care Case Management Model

Case Manager: 15–23 patients

Business Associate: 20–40 patients

Social Worker: 1–17 active patients/cases

ing, planning, coordinating care, and outcomes management.

Each of the integrated and collaborative models brings certain advantages and disadvantages (Table 3.3). The key differences between the two models are the integration of utilization management into the role of the case manager versus the separation of the role through the addition of a dedicated third team member.

3.8.4. How are the Integrated and Collaborative Models Alike?

Both the integrated and collaborative models build on the interrelationships of the nursing and social work disciplines to achieve the expected case management outcomes. They both require strong social work sup-

TABLE 3.3. Advantages and Disadvantages of the Integrated and Collaborative Acute Care Case Management Models.

	Integrated Model	Collaborative Model
Advantages	Everything under one umbrella	Consolidates the business functions of case management into one role—builds expertise
	Reduces duplication, fragmentation, and redundancy	Case managers are not consumed with routine payer functions
	Data collected once for multiple purposes	Case managers have time to focus on more leveraged functions
	Case manager in direct communication with third party payers and vendors—they know the case	Expands focus on clinical documentation improvement
	One stop shopping—may be more cost-effective by requiring less hand-offs and less staff	Separates two time-dependent functions
	Physician and other staff only have to communicate with one person for all issues	Creates holistic jobs that optimize skills and talents of different staff
Disadvantages	Bundles highly time-dependent functions of discharge planning and utilization management—can be frustrating for staff to manage	Requires intensive communication between the three team members
	If not done well, can morph into task-oriented approach	Creates some duplication such as chart reviews and assessments
	Detailed work of utilization management may appeal to some staff more than others	Works best if all disciplines report to the same administrator
	Will not work if staffing is not adequate	May be more costly and require more staff. Will not work if staffing is not adequate.

port and will not work if they are adequately staffed. Caseloads and workloads must be balanced.

3.9. POST-ACUTE CARE MODELS

3.9.1. Home Care Case Management

Case management in the home setting is designed with the same goals in mind as case management in the acute care setting. The role of home care in the success of case management is critical, especially because of the ability to care for increasingly complex and chronically ill patients and to prevent avoidable readmissions to the acute care setting. The implementation of chronic care management and disease management programs have provided a unique opportunity for home care case management to reduce the need for acute care services, therefore allowing healthcare providers and executives to curtail cost and reduce the hospital's length of stay and financial risk imposed by the value-based purchasing program and others. The continuum approach to case management programs and managed care have also spurred alternative approaches to the provision of healthcare services, such as subacute care, transitional living centers, infusion centers, day treatment centers, and especially sophisticated home care services that handle individuals requiring higher and alternative levels of care and acuity (Case Manager's Tip 3.12). The goals of home care case management are as follows:

- Optimizing the delivery of care across the continuum
- Keeping patients in less costly care settings
- Facilitating a proactive approach to patient care delivery and management
- Preventing deterioration in patients' conditions
- Reducing patients' risk and the need for acute care services

The demand for case managers to coordinate and integrate healthcare services in the home setting has increased exponentially over the past decade. This has resulted from the growth of managed care, increasing capitation, implementation of the home care prospec-

 CASE MANAGER'S TIP 3.12

Home Care Case Management

Home care case management targets patients with chronic illness and seriously complex medical and psychosocial conditions and those who need immediate postacute care services.

tive payment system by the federal government for Medicare and Medicaid beneficiaries, demand management programs, integrated delivery systems, and the payers' expectations that the providers do more for less. The case manager in the home environment directs the members of the interdisciplinary healthcare team (Box 3.13) toward the achievement of the best-quality care at the lowest possible cost (Case Manager's Tip 3.13). The home care case manager also makes visits to patients in their homes to ensure that they are receiving the appropriate services and that the expected outcomes are being met. During the home visit the case manager may decide to refer the patient to the physician or other healthcare providers as deemed necessary.

The home care case manager receives referrals from the hospital-based case manager. The home care case manager can obtain important information on the patient's condition and related care by visiting the patient in the hospital and/or attending the hospital patient planning or discharge planning rounds. If a face-to-face exchange of information is not practical or possible, then the home care and hospital case managers must develop good systems for the sharing and exchange of information. Information to be shared should include the patient's medical history, physical symptoms and functional abilities or other findings, financial information including entitlements, and relevant psychosocial issues including family support mechanisms.

Patients receiving home care services are not acute enough for hospitalization and are not ambulatory

Box 3.13   Members of the Home Care Case Management Team

Core Members
- Physician
- Nurses
- Case manager
- Physical therapist
- Occupational therapist
- Speech therapist
- Social worker
- Home health aide
- Home companion/homemaker
- Administrator

Ad Hoc Members
- Acute care case manager/discharge planner
- Health education specialist
- Clinical nurse specialist
- Home care intake coordinator
- Consulting/specialty physicians
- Community health worker

CASE MANAGER'S TIP 3.13

Home Care Case Management Services

Case managers in the home care setting are responsible for coordinating and integrating care for patients with complex therapeutic modalities and treatment plans such as the following:

- Nonhealing wounds and wound care management
- Infusion therapy
- Speech therapy
- Physical and occupational therapy; ADLs
- Mechanical ventilation and oxygen therapy
- Polypharmacy management
- Tube feedings
- Psychosocial counseling and social services for the patient and family
- Pain management and palliative care

enough for daily visits to a clinic setting or physician's office. In most cases the cost of home care is a fraction of what a hospital stay would cost. In addition to monitoring the patient's progress during this phase of illness, the case manager will also ensure that the necessary services are being delivered in the home setting and that the patient's optimal level of wellness is being met. Under FFS reimbursement, there was no financial incentive for the home care agency to control the number of home visits. Just as hospital visits were relatively unlimited before the prospective payment system, the home care agencies are only now beginning to face reductions in resources and reimbursement for visits. Under capitated managed care and the prospective payment structure, the number of home visits are the most strictly controlled.

The criteria for selecting patients for the provision of home care case management services are similar to those of traditional home care services and are defined by the conditions of participation in Medicare and/or Medicaid programs. In order for the patients to receive home care case management services, they must meet the following criteria:

- Homebound (Box 3.14)
- In need of skilled services (e.g., care provided by a licensed professional such as a registered nurse, social worker, or physical therapist)
- Under the supervision of a physician
- Show the medical necessity of services
- In need of intermittent or part-time services

Case managers may use some criteria to identify high-risk seniors enrolled in a managed care health

Box 3.14 Definition of Homebound Status: CMS Pub 100-02

For a patient to be eligible to receive covered home health services, the law according to CMS requires that a physician certify in all cases that the patient is confined to his/her home. For purposes of the statute, an individual shall be considered "confined to the home" (homebound) if the following two criteria are met:

Criteria-One:

The patient must either:
   a. Because of illness or injury, need the aid of supportive devices such as crutches, canes, wheelchairs, and walkers; the use of special transportation; or the assistance of another person in order to leave their place of residence.

   OR

   b. Have a condition such that leaving his or her home is medically contraindicated.

If the patient meets one of the criteria-one conditions, then the patient must ALSO meet two additional requirements defined in criteria-two below.

Criteria-Two:

   a. There must exist a normal inability to leave home.

   AND

   b. Leaving home must require a considerable and taxing effort.

For the complete definition of homebound and the law, refer to CMS at www.cms.gov/Regulations-and-Guidance/Guidance/Transmittals/Downloads/R192BP.pdf

plan who would benefit from home care case management services. Case managers use a screening questionnaire for this purpose or receive referrals from other healthcare providers, including physicians, based on the criteria. The criteria are broad in focus, which makes them applicable to any patient population and payer type. Examples of these criteria are as follows:

- *Diagnosis-specific indications (i.e., medical condition)*: such as spinal cord injury, traumatic brain injury, AIDS, chronic obstructive pulmonary disease, premature neonate, high-risk pregnancy, and heart failure
- *Behavioral and functional indicators*: such as nonadherence to medical regimen, impairment in ADLs (e.g., bathing, dressing, toileting), lack of medical follow-up
- *Healthcare resource utilization indicators*: such as frequent readmissions to acute care settings, high clinic encounters, polypharmacy, complex wound

care management, presence of multiple tubes (e.g., gastrostomy tube, Foley catheter, and drains), and frequent use of ED services

■ *Cost indicators*: such as managed care health plans, capitation, benefits still available

Research has shown that a variety of factors may influence home care nurses' decisions regarding management of their clients, including the appropriate number of visits or the necessity for referrals to social service or other agencies. Home care agencies have developed home care protocols similar to those previously developed for hospital care (e.g., pathways and interdisciplinary action plans [IDAPs]). These prospectively developed tools become the case manager's frame of reference as they outline the appropriate number of visits for a particular disease entity or surgical procedure. Expected outcomes for each discipline are predetermined so that the number of patient care visits correlates with the expected outcomes. As a result, allotted visits are not arbitrary but can be validated, and the patient's progress toward these expected outcomes can be benchmarked. The termination point for the case is also clearly defined, and the expectations of the staff in terms of when to close the case are delineated. Cases kept open beyond the appropriate length of time become very costly to the home care agency. By prospectively identifying the criteria for case closure based on outcomes, the care provider no longer has to make a subjective decision regarding when to close the case. Closing cases in a timely fashion allows resources to be appropriated to those cases that truly need extended services beyond the norm.

Home care case managers can be assigned by disease entity or broader clinical specialty. Chronic illnesses, such as diabetes, asthma, HIV and AIDS, or congestive heart failure, may require case management services in the home after an episode of acute exacerbation of the disease. Rehabilitation after joint replacement is another clinical grouping for which case management may work well. These patients will require the services of more than one discipline, such as nursing and physical therapy. By coordinating these services and monitoring the patient's progress closely, the case manager can ensure that the patient is moving toward those outcomes as efficiently as possible without duplication or redundant utilization of resources (Case Manager's Tip 3.14).

3.10. LONG-TERM CARE CASE MANAGEMENT

Long-term care settings such as the nursing home, rehabilitation facility, or skilled nursing facility are set-

 CASE MANAGER'S TIP 3.14

Home Care Case Management

Home care case managers can help ensure that patients achieve expected outcomes without duplication or redundant use of resources by coordinating services and monitoring the patient's progress closely.

tings in which case management can serve the purpose of slowing the deterioration process and improving the functional status of the resident. In long-term care settings, care has been task oriented, with different practitioners providing different services to the resident. Today's typical nursing home patient is sicker, requires more complex medical and nursing care, and will live longer.

Patients with any diagnosis can be admitted to a skilled nursing facility level of service. Care is considered to be either chronic or supportive. The average length of stay is approximately 1.5 years. Physician visits are about once a month, and patients receive about 1.5–3 hours of nursing care per patient day. Rehabilitation services provided to the nursing home resident are limited in scope and when provided are usually less than 30 minutes per day. Patients leave this level of service either when admitted to a hospital or at the time of their death.

As in the subacute setting, the long-term care case manager can provide a vital link between the members of the interdisciplinary team. Increasing focus today is being placed on other subacute care settings as managed care drives the need for less expensive care settings appropriate to the needs of the patient. Conditions that usually are considered subacute are listed in Box 3.15.

Short-term complex medical problems would include problems such as wound care, respiratory management, total parenteral nutrition, dialysis, intravenous therapies, and postsurgical recovery. The goal in case managing this group of patients is recuperative.

Box 3.15 Conditions Typically Considered Sub-Acute

Emphasis on subacute care as a cost-saving mechanism is increasing. The conditions that typically are included in this category include the following:

1. Short-term complex medical problems
2. Short-term rehabilitative conditions
3. Long-term (chronic) conditions

The expected outcome is to bring the patient to the optimal level of wellness.

Short-term rehabilitative subacute care focuses on clinical issues such as stroke, amputation, total hip/knee replacement, and brain injury. The case management goal for this clinical group is restorative, to bring the patient as close to the preinjury condition as possible.

Long-term (chronic) case management is preventive maintenance, assisting the patient to maintain the level of functioning without deterioration for as long as possible. Long-term chronic conditions include coma, ventilator dependence, and head injury.

In response to these changes, nursing homes are adapting and undergoing modifications to the way they provided care in the past. Case management has been used as a mechanism not only for improving patient outcomes in long-term care settings but also for improving job satisfaction of care providers in these settings. With the introduction of a case management model, a healthcare provider can coordinate the services provided by nursing assistants, RNs, physical and occupational therapists, and nutritionists. Integrating these services and identifying interdisciplinary expected outcomes allow the resident's functional status to be closely monitored and managed. Care is managed using an interdisciplinary approach, and therefore goals can be more specific, realistic, and measurable. Furthermore, the move away from a task-oriented approach means that goals are patient-focused instead of staff-focused.

The case manager in the long-term care setting may not be an RN if there is a lack of RN staff in the facility. In some cases it may be necessary to use the licensed practical or licensed vocational nurse in the role of case manager. The case manager provides for ongoing monitoring and evaluation of the resident's progress. Progress is measured against an assessment of the patient's medical problems, functional capabilities, social supports, and psychosocial well-being.

Case management plans (see Chapter 10) can be used to manage the care and expected outcomes. Plans should focus on such things as nursing needs, therapies, ADLs, and personal care (Case Manager's Tip

 CASE MANAGER'S TIP 3.15

Long-Term Care Case Management

To manage the care and expected outcomes of long-term care clients, focus the case management plan on nursing needs, therapies, ADLs, and personal care.

3.15). The chronicity of the residents may mean that the case management plans are reviewed at a maximum of every 3 months or whenever the resident's condition or change in progress warrants a review. The case manager provides an ongoing evaluation process and liaisons between the resident, the physician, the family, and other members of the healthcare team.

3.11. SUB-ACUTE CARE CASE MANAGEMENT

The subacute setting is among the fastest growing care delivery settings within the continuum of care. The reasons for this growth are obvious. Just 10 years ago it was not uncommon to find patients recovering in acute care beds for weeks on end while receiving nothing more than an intravenous (IV) antibiotic, wound care, or ventilator weaning. Because of the high cost of managing these types of patients in acute care beds, MCOs began to expect that patients meeting the clinical criteria of subacute would be transferred to subacute units, whether in hospitals, nursing homes, or freestanding facilities.

Subacute care is considered restorative, meaning that it is expected that the patient's condition will improve as a result of the care rendered. The level of care is somewhere between acute care and traditional nursing home care. Care rendered may be less invasive and less diagnostically oriented as compared with acute care. In comparison with traditional nursing home care it is more intensive and of shorter duration. The average length of stay is generally between 7 and 30 days. Admission criteria would be specific to the program of care, such as neurologic, rehabilitation, or orthopedic, and the patient would have to demonstrate clear outcome potential.

In the subacute setting the physician would visit 1–3 times per week. Average nursing care is 4.5–8 hours of direct nursing care per patient day, with a high use of nurse aides. To qualify for subacute rehabilitation, typically a patient must be able to tolerate a minimum of 1–1.5 hours of therapy per day. Patients are expected to be discharged home after the course of treatment.

Case managers who discharge patients to subacute settings must be familiar with the criteria for the levels of service in the subacute setting. The three categories include (1) short-term rehabilitative or restorative, (2) short-term complex medical or recuperative, and (3) long-term, chronic, or preventive maintenance (Table 3.4). The hospital-based case manager should always consider transferring a patient to a subacute level of care/setting when the acute care outcomes have been met and the patient's care can be rendered in a less intensive setting.

TABLE 3.4. Conditions Typically Considered Subacute.

Short-Term Complex Medical	Short-Term Rehabilitative	Long-Term (Chronic)
Postsurgical recovery	Cerebrovascular accident	Coma
Respiratory management	Stroke	Multiple trauma
Pulmonary management	Brain injury	Ventilator dependency
Oncology	Spinal injury	Head injury
AIDS care	Amputation	
Wound care	Arthritis	
Tracheostomy/suctioning	Total hip/knee replacement	
Total parenteral nutrition	Other neurologic/orthopedic conditions	
Intravenous therapies		
Terminal care		
Dialysis		
Complication as a result of prematurity		

The case manager in the subacute setting coordinates the services of the interdisciplinary team that would include physicians, therapists, nurses, and other professionals such as nutritionists. The case manager is responsible for ensuring that the patient is moving toward expected outcomes of care, whether restorative, recuperative, or end of life. In some instances the patient may be discharged home to continue with home care services, or the patient may need to be moved to a skilled nursing facility level of service. By closely monitoring the patient's progress toward expected outcomes, the case manager can assess that the patient is receiving the appropriate level of service, and if not, the case manager should work with the interdisciplinary team to transition the patient to the appropriate level or to home if outcomes have been met.

3.12. ACUTE REHABILITATION

Patients are admitted to acute rehabilitation units and facilities that have a traumatic injury, debilitating disease, or following certain types of surgery. Acute rehabilitation is appropriate for patients who will benefit from an intensive, multidisciplinary rehabilitation program. Patients receive physical, occupational, and speech therapy as needed and are medically managed by specially trained physicians. There is an attending physician onsite 24 hours a day to manage the medical aspects of each patient's care. Acute rehabilitation is an interdisciplinary process comprised of a team of clinicians that maximize the recovery process for patients that have functional deficits. The goal of inpatient rehabilitation is to gain independent function, promote safe home living, improve quality of life, and establish community reintegration. Acute rehabilitation programs are designed to help patients return home at their highest level of independence (Stam et al., 2012).

The rehabilitation process is different for every patient. Each patient has his/her own unique needs and goals for recovery. As such, an individualized plan of care is developed jointly by the patient, his/her family and care givers, and an interdisciplinary team of rehabilitation professionals. The treatment team incorporates treatment methods and technology to achieve the desired goals.

For patients with neurological diagnoses, a neuropsychologist may be on staff to determine if they are in need of additional psychological or psychiatric treatment. In an acute rehabilitation hospital, the patient is expected to make significant functional gains and medical improvement within a reasonable time frame. Patients receive a minimum of three hours of therapy per day, up to six days a week. Therapy is provided on both a one-to-one and group basis, depending on the needs of the individual patient. Additional services such as respiratory therapy and therapeutic recreation programs are also available for patients during their rehabilitation.

In the acute rehabilitation setting, the case manager's role is to ensure that the patient's needs are being coordinated. Since care in these settings is multidisciplinary, it is important that all members of the team are in constant communication and that care planning includes the patient's clinical, rehabilitative, and psychosocial needs. Once patients have completed their episode of acute rehabilitation, they may go home, go home with home care, or continue with rehabilitation in a less intensive setting such as a subacute unit or facility. The case manager must assess and reassess the patient's progress toward expected goals. The transition may take place when the patient has improved enough to move to a less intensive plan of care, or when no further improvements can be gained from continuing with the rehabilitation at the acute level.

3.13. PALLIATIVE CARE

Palliative care is defined as multidisciplinary approach to specialized medical care for people with serious illnesses (Watson *et al.*, 2009). It focuses on providing patients with relief from the symptoms, pain, and physical and mental stress of a serious illness. It is not dependent on the patient's diagnosis but rather on their symptoms and need for relief from those symptoms. Although the concept of palliative care is not new, most physicians have traditionally concentrated on trying to cure patients. The goal of palliative care therapy is to improve the quality of life of both the patient and the family or family caregivers. Palliative care is provided by a team of physicians, nurses, and other health professionals who work together with the primary care physician and referred specialists to provide an extra layer of support. It is appropriate at any age and at any stage in a serious illness and can be provided along with curative treatment. Palliative care can be used along with curative or aggressive therapies.

Starting in 2006 in the United States, palliative medicine is now a board certified subspecialty of internal medicine with specialized fellowships for physicians who are interested in the field. Palliative care utilizes a multidisciplinary approach to patient care, relying on input from pharmacists, nurses, chaplains, social workers, psychologists, and other allied health professionals in formulating a plan of care to relieve suffering in all areas of a patient's life. This multidisciplinary approach allows the palliative care team to address physical, emotional, spiritual, and social concerns that arise with advanced illness.

The focus on a person's quality of life has increased greatly since the 1990s. In the United States today, 55% of hospitals with more than 100 beds offer a palliative-care program (Buckley, 2008), and nearly one-fifth of community hospitals have palliative-care programs. A relatively recent development is the palliative-care team, a dedicated healthcare team that is entirely geared toward palliative treatment. In some instances, the palliative care team is led by a physician. In other models it is led by a case manager who ensures that care is integrated among all members of the interdisciplinary care team.

Case managers who are involved in care coordination should always consider the benefits of palliative care for their patients. Patients who are in emotional or physical distress will respond poorly to interventions both in the hospital as well as in community settings if these problems are not addressed adequately. The case manager should discuss the benefits of palliative care with the physician while planning for inpatient care as well as during the discharge planning process. In some acute care hospitals, case managers can make direct referrals to the palliative care program.

3.14. HOSPICE CARE

Unlike palliative care, hospice care is end-of-life care. Hospice is a type of care involving palliation without curative intent. A team of healthcare professionals and volunteers provide hospice services which also include medical services and psychological and spiritual support. The goal of hospice care is to help people who are dying have peace, comfort, and dignity. The interdisciplinary care team's goal is to try to control pain and other symptoms so a person can remain as alert and comfortable as possible (Matzo and Sherman, 2014). Hospice programs also provide services to support a patient's family.

Usually, a hospice patient is expected to live 6 months or less. Hospice care can take place:

- At home
- At a hospice center
- In a hospital

Hospice has become an important alternative to patients dying in hospitals, particularly in critical care beds. As with palliative care, case managers should collaborate with the patient's physician and interdisciplinary care team when the patient's prognosis is less than 6 months. As above, hospice is provided in a number of different settings and levels of care. When working with the patient and family, realistic goals should be set so that the patient's needs and the family's needs are met. While some families may want to take a patient home on home hospice, this plan may not be realistic or practical. The social worker should work with the patient, family, and family caregivers as they navigate through this decision-making process. As case managers assess their patient's on admission and daily, they should always remain aware of the potential need for hospice services and plan accordingly.

3.15. CHRONIC CARE CASE MANAGEMENT

Chronic conditions are conditions that patients are expected to have for years or possibly for the rest of their lives. These patients may access and use a variety of healthcare services, providers, and resources in a multitude of care settings during the course of illness. It is the use of these various services and care settings for the chronically ill that places them at risk for receiving less than adequate, duplicative, fragmented, or delayed healthcare services. Typical target populations for

CASE MANAGER'S TIP 3.16

Chronic Care Case Management

The case manager can coordinate the wide range of services needed by chronically ill patients so that care, financing, and information are integrated. This provides a foundation for planning and managing care across settings.

chronic care case management include the frail elderly, survivors of strokes, accident victims, the mentally ill, and children and infants with congenital abnormalities.

Patients with chronic illnesses may access a wide variety of services and specialty providers from the acute care setting to social services, mental illness, home care, or subacute care. It is during these transitions that the greatest opportunity for problems may arise. Case management integrates these wide-ranging services so that care delivery, financing, and information are integrated. It provides a foundation for planning and managing care across settings (Case Manager's Tip 3.16). The focus is more than just providing the patient with access to the various services; it is also geared toward integrating these systems to provide a coordinated, continuing care approach.

The patient population at greatest risk for chronic care needs is the elderly, particularly the frail elderly. This group is at high risk for complex health needs, potential for physical or social complications, and continued use of costly healthcare resources. A multidisciplinary approach such as that provided by a case management model has been documented to reduce cost and improve outcomes for this population. The application of case management to this population may mean providing adult day care programs with transportation. The children of aging parents may be able to maintain their parents in the community if they have access to an adult day care program that provides a flexible structure so that they can drop parents off on their way to work and pick them up in the evening. Other necessary services may be meal preparation, delivery services, housekeeping, or shopping services.

3.15.1. Disability and Rehabilitation Case Management

The application of case management models for disability and rehabilitation management resulted from escalating costs of medical care, rising premiums, and other costs related to lost time from work and litigation of workers' compensation cases. It also became of greater demand because of the use of managed care insurance health plans by employers and the increased number of patients with complex, traumatic, and catastrophic injuries that required intensive short- or long-term disability and rehabilitation services. Employers usually refer their workers' compensation cases for comprehensive case management services because of their desire to control cost and improve the quality and continuity of care provided for this population.

Disability case management is defined as a process of managing occupational and nonoccupational diseases with the aim of returning the disabled person to a productive work schedule and employment. Occupational diseases are the result of injury on the job or illness caused by the work environment. Nonoccupational diseases are health conditions (e.g., trauma caused by an automobile accident) that are not related to the work environment but result in short- or long-term disability that prevents return to work for a period of time and sometimes indefinitely (DiBenedetto, 2001). The disability case management process involves the application of the concepts and strategies of workers' compensation case management and the rehabilitation treatment modality. Case managers in disability case management models focus on limiting the disability by coordinating and facilitating immediate medical interventions once an injury or illness occurs and by facilitating the referral process to rehabilitation providers and specialists. The ultimate goal of care and services is to return the patients to work and to restore optimal level of functioning and independence as soon as possible.

Disability case managers possess special training and expertise in the management of short- and long-term financial, psychological, sexual, physical, social, and vocational consequences of an illness or injury. Successful rehabilitation and cost-effectiveness result from the use of case managers who are specialized in the care of catastrophic injuries and disability insurance and claims management. Many employers and disability insurance companies employ the services of this type of case manager as soon as a catastrophic injury occurs because the earlier the case management services start, the better the financial and medical care outcomes.

Because of the benefits of disability and rehabilitation case management services, we find case managers today working in almost every catastrophic injury specialty center. The focus of case management in these centers is similar to that of external case managers (i.e., private and independent) in the following areas:

- Developing care and projecting short- and long-term outcomes
- Planning the return-to-work plan
- Encouraging family involvement in the care of the injured person
- Coordinating necessary services and durable medical equipment
- Planning transitions
- Managing benefits and claims
- Communicating with the employer, insurance company, occupational health and risk management staff, medical and rehabilitation care team, and lawyers
- Ensuring compliance with the law

3.16. DESIGNING CASE MANAGEMENT MODELS

Whether introduced in the inpatient, outpatient, or any other care setting across the continuum of care, case management models can be adapted to meet the goals of quality patient care in a fiscally responsible manner. Selection of the most appropriate model will depend on the needs of the organization, the available resources, and the expected goals and outcomes. When designing a case management model, healthcare executives must consider the following:

1. *Operationalization of the model at the patient level.* It must be easy to implement the model at the individual patient level, and patients must be able to realize its impact on their care and outcomes. Some models have been designed in a global, abstract, conceptual sense without any effort to explain how they apply to the individual patient. This leaves the healthcare providers and the case management staff in a struggle, trying to make sense of the model. To eliminate confusion, the conceptual framework of the model must be first redefined at the individual patient or patient care unit level before it is implemented.

2. *System-wide perspective.* Refrain from implementing a model that does not apply to all services and to the care of the different patient populations served. It is appropriate and acceptable to slightly modify the model to meet the needs of the different services; however, the basic concepts of the model must be maintained regardless of the patient population (e.g., the presence of a case manager in every service or a case manager/social worker dyad). Another example is the integrative role of the case manager; if it is integrated in one specialty, you may need to integrate it in others.

However, an acceptable variation is the criteria used to identify patients who benefit from case management services.

3. *Redesign of the administrative, clinical, financial, and quality management processes.* Because the implementation of case management models means a change in the patient care delivery processes (i.e., clinical management), it behooves the healthcare executives who design and apply these models to redesign the other processes and align them with case management. The processes affected the most are those related to the role of the case manager: transitional/discharge planning, resource allocation and utilization management, and quality and outcomes measurement. This redesign is important because it determines and ensures cost effectiveness and efficiency in the delivery of patient care.

4. *Sources of accountability and empowerment.* A clear definition of the case manager's role with identified role boundaries, scope of responsibility, and power is an important factor for success in case management. Case managers who are arbitrarily placed in their roles are set up to fail. Communicating the accountability and responsibility of case managers to all of the departments and staff in an organization is essential for promoting the case manager's power. One way of achieving this is by explicitly identifying the presence of case management as a department, and case managers as a staff, on the table of organization for every staff member to see.

5. *Integration of service delivery.* Cost savings are achieved by examining the number of departments an organization has and evaluating how each is impacted by the creation of the case management model/department. Almost always this results in merging and consolidation of departments. If an organization does not merge efforts, fragmentation and duplication will continue to exist and cost savings will not be accomplished. The departments affected the most by case management are social work, utilization review, discharge planning, and quality management. Some level of integration must be done as a result of case management (Box 3.16).

6. *Measurement systems.* Before implementing case management models, it is advisable to have a measurement system in place. The system must include the outcomes to be measured and must identify the process of data collection, aggregation, analysis, and reporting. A prospective approach to

Box 3.16 Integration of Departments in Case Management Model Design

Integration of departments (e.g., utilization management, discharge/transitional planning and social work, clinical care management, and quality management) in the design and implementation of case management may be of three levels:

1. *Simple*: No integration at all and the focus of case management is on any one core activity. Most organizations focus on either clinical care management or utilization management. This type of model fragments care delivery, is expensive, and presents a potential for overuse or underuse of resources.

2. *Moderate*: Partial integration that focuses on merging two of the core activities. The most commonly integrated core activities are either clinical care management and transitional planning or clinical care management and utilization management. This level of integration results in better outcomes of cost effectiveness and efficiency in care delivery.

3. *Complex*: Full integration that includes all of the core activities. This type of integration is the most forward-thinking approach and results in best outcomes of cost effectiveness and efficiency in care delivery. However, one must balance the case manager's responsibilities and the patient caseload.

evaluating the effectiveness of the model assists in keeping all involved focused. It also prevents mistakes or unnecessary efforts from being made. The outcomes to be measured must always be driven by the goals and expectations of the model. One should maximize data collection from already existing automated systems, such as electronic medical records and data repositories, cost accounting systems, admitting, discharge, and transfer systems, and so on.

3.17. SETTING UP THE CASE MANAGEMENT PROGRAM

The following can be used when setting up a program in any setting across the continuum. As you move forward with your design and implementation, be sure you have addressed each of these points. Keep a running list for yourself and/or the committee working on the project to ensure that all relevant questions have been addressed. Each point can be addressed in any order, but be sure that each question is answered before the implementation of the program (Case Manager's Tip 3.17).

 CASE MANAGER'S TIP 3.17

Issues to Consider When Creating the Case Management Department

- Quality, safety, accreditation and regulatory mandates
- Cost implications/budget
- Staff (professional/secretarial/clerical support) and job descriptions
- Salaries and compensation
- Equipment and supplies
- Table of organization
- Hours of operation
- Reporting structure
- Relationships to other departments
- Policies and procedures
- Information technology/systems
- Educating the organization

3.17.1. Creating the Department

3.17.1.1. Quality, Safety, Accreditation, and Regulatory Mandates

With the advent of the Patient Protection and Affordable Care Act of 2010, there are a number of mandates the case management department must be involved in which impact adherence. For example, Value-based Purchasing Program, Hospital Readmissions Reduction Program, and Meaningful Use. Case managers are able to focus on reducing financial risk and enhancing revenue. Additionally, case management and case management departments, through special focus on quality and accreditation standards, are able to enhance performance and outcomes. They also are able to assure patient's safety and optimal care experience while transitioning across the various settings of the healthcare continuum.

3.17.1.2. Cost Implications/Budget

Develop a business plan. The plan should include both personnel and nonpersonnel costs needed to run the department. Consider all staff needed, including professional staff and support staff such as secretarial and clerical staff.

Also consider equipment needed, such as fax machines, photocopiers, and computers. Cost this out as part of the business plan. Set up a budget with the annualized cost of running the department.

3.17.1.3. Staff (Professional/Secretarial/Clerical Support) and Job Descriptions

Staffing should be based on the role functions to be performed. For example, RN case manager to patient ratios will be driven by the functions the RN is performing. If the RN case manager is performing clinical coordination/facilitation, transitional planning, and utilization/quality management functions, an appropriate caseload in the hospital setting would be 1:15–1:20. The number of case managers needed can then be calculated based on the bed capacity of the hospital.

Other staffing ratios should also be driven by the size of the organization and the functions to be performed.

3.17.1.4. Salaries and Compensation

The case management market is competetive and the demand for case managers outweighs the supply. Experienced case managers may not be always available to fill vacant positions. Before determining the salary and compensation you offer candidates for the case manager role, conducting a market salary analysis is important to then be able to allocate appropriate and competetive salaries and compensation packages.

3.17.1.5. Equipment and Supplies

The time to budget for equipment and supplies is before the implementation while the budgetary costs are being determined. Consider all functions being performed and the hardware and software needed to support those functions. Also consider the management needs and report writing capability when selecting a software package. Other supplies that should be budgeted for include stationery, paper, telephone lines, transportation, and conferences.

3.17.1.6. Table of Organization/Reporting Structure

Develop a table of organization for the department with a clearly differentiated reporting structure. Also consider where the department will fit into the organization and to whom the director of the department will report. Of significant importance is the case manager. The table of organization must clearly state where the case manager's position is and to whom he or she reports. This statement is essential for empowering those who assume the case manager's role.

3.17.1.7. Hours of Operation

The hours of operation of the department may be driven by budgetary constraints. Decisions will need to be made as to whether the department will operate 7 days a week or will function 5 or 6 days. Perhaps you will consider having the ED staff working longer shifts (such as 12 hours) while the inpatient staff work 8-hour shifts. Consider the clinical needs of the organization and the goals of the department when making these decisions. If there is a considerable amount of activity on the weekends, operations on the weekends must be planned for.

3.17.1.8. Relationships to Other Departments

The department may have either formal or informal relationships with other departments in the organization. Consideration should be given to how these relationships will be defined. You may want to consider an oversight committee that would be composed of leadership staff from related departments, such as admitting, medical records, patient accounts/billing, radiology, pharmacy, and so on.

3.17.1.9. Policies and Procedures

A policy and procedure manual should be developed and should include all policies and procedures needed to define the functions of the staff. For example, if utilization management is one of the functions of the department, then all appropriate utilization review policies should be included. Consider requirements and standards of accreditation agencies such as those of TJC, National Commission for Quality Assurance, and URAC when developing the manual. Include the table of organization and the staff job descriptions, training, and competencies in the manual. Also important to have on hand for use by case managers is a resource manual that has contact information readily available, particularly for community resources, volunteer agencies, charity and shelter services, transportation services, and skilled nursing/long-term facilities.

3.17.1.10. Information Technology/Systems

If the budget permits, select computer hardware and case management software applications that are state-of-the-art and that will support the functions you are performing both now and in the future. For example, if one of the goals of the department is to eventually become paperless, be sure that your system will support this goal. In terms of case management software products, try to view and test several products before making your selection. Be sure that the software can store and manipulate all of the data needed, especially variance data, for reporting purposes for the department. Other important features of the software applications are ability for electronic documentation and case management tools which focus on clinical care documentation, utilization management, transitional and discharge planning, and reporting.

3.17.1.11. Educating the Organization

Before implementation, set up a series of educational programs. Programs should be conducted for case management staff at an in-depth level and for other staff on a less detailed level. Provide additional focused education to the medical staff and administrative staff as needed. Educational programs should be geared toward the needs of the different nursing, medical, and allied health staff (see Chapter 9 for more details).

3.17.1.12. Developing the Case Manager's Role

The issues presented in Case Manager's Tip 3.18

 CASE MANAGER'S TIP 3.18

Issues to Consider When Developing the Case Manager's Role

- Role and functions
- Integration with other departments/disciplines
- Job descriptions
- Management versus union level (exempt or nonexempt; preferably exempt)
- Service line versus unit-based
- Across the continuum or care setting or level of care specific
- Reporting structure
- Staffing patterns
- Caseloads
- Hours of operation
- Clinical practice guidelines
- Variances/delays
- Documentation (paper or electronic; general or specialized case management software application)
- Orientation
- Goals and objectives
- Cost
- Quality, safety, accreditation, and regulatory mandates

should be considered when designing the role of the case manager.

3.17.1.12.1. Roles and Functions. Careful consideration must be taken when defining the role functions of the case manager. Depending on the role functions selected, other departments may need to be restructured or eliminated. Consider all of the functions discussed in this chapter and match these to the goals and objectives of the department and the organization. If staff members from restructured or eliminated departments are used as case managers, they should be provided with special training. In addition, conducting team-building sessions for these staff members is advisable to work out any concerns they may have.

3.17.1.12.2. Integration with Other Departments/Disciplines. In some instances, other departments may become integrated with the case management department. Typically these may include social work and/or quality management. A physician staff member may also need to be integrated, such as a physician advisor. All related departments should be consulted as these decisions are being made, and appropriate staff should be trained accordingly.

3.17.1.12.3. Job Descriptions. Job descriptions should be completed before the implementation of the department. As staff are interviewed and hired for these new positions, they should have an opportunity to review the job description and expectations for the position for which they are interviewing. Be sure to include all job functions, skills, performance expectations, and expected outcomes of the position. A job clarification exercise is usually helpful in determining who is best suited to assume responsibility for what functions.

3.17.1.12.4. Management Versus Union (Exempt or Nonexempt Status). If your organization is unionized, a decision will need to be made as to whether the case manager position will be in or out of the union. There are pros and cons to each position, but the ultimate decision will probably be dependent on the structure of your organization and its relationship with the union. It may be difficult to justify keeping the position out of the union if the case managers do not perform any of the functions typically considered as management functions, such as hiring/firing and evaluation of other staff.

3.17.1.12.5. Service Line Versus Unit-Based. The case managers can be assigned to specific product/service lines, or clinical areas, or be unit-based. They may also be assigned to physician groups or geographical areas, depending on whether your department is in the hospital or in the community. This decision will ultimately drive your staffing patterns and needs. Decisions must be made carefully because of their impact on performance, productivity, and the possibility of ending up with unnecessary unproductive time such as travel time between units, departments, or different locations.

3.17.1.12.6. Specific Level of Care or Across the Continuum. Similar to service line or unit-based, it is important to decide whether the case manager is to follow patients across settings of the continuum of care. If so, you need to consider nonproductive time. As case managers travel across settings they will waste time that otherwise would have been spent with patients. If across the continuum, the caseload per case manager is usually smaller. There are advantages and disadvantages to both approaches; you just need to examine what is best for the organization and the patient population served.

3.17.1.12.7. Reporting Structure. A strong infrastructure is important to the success of a case management department. Be sure that the case managers have a clear line of authority and are well supported as they perform their functions.

3.17.1.12.8. Staffing Patterns/Case Loads. A typical mistake made when designing case management departments is to not provide the proper staffing patterns to support the role functions selected. Be sure that the caseloads are not so great that the case managers cannot perform their functions effectively or efficiently. This will surely be a formula for failure. Staffing patterns should also depend on whether you go with service line case managers or unit-based case managers, patient acuity levels, and length of stay.

3.17.1.12.9. Hours of Operation. Select hours of operation that best meet the operational needs of the department and the patients. Increase the number of staff at busier times, and decrease the number of staff at quieter times. Consider evening, weekend, and holiday needs. Hours of operation should be adjusted to the needs of different care settings and patient populations.

3.17.1.12.10. Clinical Practice Guidelines. The format for the organization's clinical practice guidelines should be determined before startup of the department. In this way the case management staff can begin developing the guidelines as soon as the department is implemented.

3.17.1.12.11. Variances/Delays. A variance identification system should be developed before implementation. Categories of variances such as patient, system, and practitioner should be selected, as well as a methodology for collecting, coding, aggregating, analyzing, and reporting of variances.

3.17.1.12.12. Documentation. Frequency of case management documentation and expected content should be determined and included as a policy and procedure for the case managers. Each organization needs to determine its own specific expectations for documentation while considering TJC, NCQA, Commission on Accreditation and Rehabilitation Facilities (CARF), URAC, and other regulatory requirements for documentation. Also special consideration should be made whether electronic documentation is used or a traditional manual system.

3.17.1.12.13. Orientation. Curricula for orientation of case management staff, other departments, physicians, and administrative staff should be developed, and education should take place before implementation. This will ensure greater organizational support because the reason for the changes will be understood by all involved (see Chapter 9 for details).

3.17.1.12.14. Goals and Objectives. Departmental goals and objectives should be identified before implementation and included in the educational programs. The goals and objectives selected should be consistent with the vision and mission of the organization. These may include measures of cost such as cost per day/cost per case and measures of quality patient outcomes. All should be prospectively identified and should drive the evaluation of the program.

3.18. KEY POINTS

1. There are four basic types of case management programs using RNs, physicians, or social workers as case managers.
2. Hospital-based models generally use the RN as the case manager, but the RN can be a primary nurse, CNS or nurse practitioner, or utilization review nurse. In some cases the case manager may be a social worker.
3. In some hospital-based models, the RN case manager performs the function of utilization management; in others this may be the responsibility of a dedicated case management associate.

4. In RN/social work dyad models, the two disciplines work as an integrated team.

5. Outpatient case management models can be applied in home care, the community, or along the continuum.

6. Some models focus on management of the chronically ill.

7. Long-term case management can take place in the subacute setting, rehabilitation facility, or chronic nursing home setting.

8. Health insurance plans and managed care organizations-based models use the case manager as either a utilization manager or clinical manager acting on behalf of the MCO.

9. Telephonic and independent/private case management are considered "external" case management services.

10. All case management models must be designed to promote quality and safe care in a fiscally responsible manner.

3.19. REFERENCES

American Academy of Family Physicians, American Academy of Pediatrics, American College of Physicians, and American Osteopathic Assocaition. (2007). Joint Principles of the patient-centered medical home. www.acponline.org

Buckley, J. (2008). *Palliative care: An integrated approach*, Wiley-Blackwell, Somerset.

DiBenedetto, D. (2001). Navigating workers' compensation, *Continuing Care 20*(6):12, 14.

Matzo, M. & Sherman D.W. (2014). *Palliative care nursing*, Springer, New York, NY.

McAllister, J.W., Cooley, W.C., VanCleave, J., Boudreau, A.A., & Kuhlthau, K. (2013). Medical home transformation in pedistric care: what drives change, *Annals of Family Medicine 11*: S90-S98, May/June.

Patient Centered Promary Care Collaborative. (2000). An overview to patient centered medical homes for patients. www.pcpcc.net/content/pcmh-videos

Rutenberg, C. (2000). Telephone triage, *Am J Nurs 100*(3):77–81.

Stam, H.J., Buyruk, H.M., Melvin, J.L., & Stucki, G. (2012). *Acute Medical Rehabilitation*, VitalMed Medical Book Publishers, Northbrook.

4

Role of the Case Manager

The advent of the case manager's role has improved healthcare delivery. It changed the provision of care from a multidisciplinary to an interdisciplinary or interprofessional focus with heightened interdependencies. The old days of "parallel play" in providing healthcare, in which the different professional disciplines involved in patient care worked in isolation, are outdated. Today's customers demand high-quality care that can be best achieved through "interactive play," where ongoing interaction and cooperation among members of the various disciplines is key. With the creation of the case manager's role as the focal point of the care coordination hub characterized by an interdisciplinary and collaborative approach to care, the age of isolation, territoriality, fragmentation, redundancy, duplication, lack of communication, and the use of unnecessary tests or procedures is gone and no longer affordable. The new age of patient care is characterized by collaboration, cooperation, integration, coordination, continuity, consistency, interaction, and open communication. Most importantly, however, is the active engagement of the patient and family in their own care. These shifts have contributed to making today's healthcare consumers happier and more satisfied with the care received and case managers play an integral role in this accomplishment (Case Manager's Tip 4.1)

The role of the *case manager* is designed to maximize interdisciplinary collaboration within and across healthcare settings and providers. When effectively executed, it without a doubt contributes to better quality, safety, and cost-effective outcomes. The role has been implemented in all care settings across the healthcare continuum and in almost every healthcare organization. Currently, case managers are found working

 CASE MANAGER'S TIP 4.1

Case Managers Play a Pivotal Role

Case managers play an integral role in care delivery to individuals where they ensure it is patient-centered, focuses on value rather than volume, ensures quality and safe outcomes, reduces unnecessary cost, improves provider's reimbursement for services rendered, and contributes to a rewarding patient experience.

in health insurance plans/commercial insurance and MCOs; acute, intensive, and ambulatory care settings (including emergency departments, nursing centers, outpatient clinics, patient centered medical homes); long-term care facilities, nursing and group homes; hospice and palliative care; senior citizen centers; assisted living and home care. Their job description may vary from one setting to another, but the roles, functions, responsibilities, and qualifications or skills required for success in the role are very similar. Chapter 4 describes the *case management* process through which the various roles, functions, and responsibilities case managers assume are discussed.

The extent of responsibilities provided for case managers is dictated by the job description defined by each healthcare organization. Factors which affect the description of the role include, but may not be limited to the following:

- The operations of the organization
- Placement of the case management department/program and the case manager in the table of organization and reporting structure

- Power and authority embedded in the role
- The role type and degree of integration of the main case management functions such as transitional planning and utilization management
- Cost incurred by the role: salary and other than personnel expenses
- Goals of the case management model or program
- Organizational vision, philosophy, objectives, and strategic goals

The focus of the role of the case manager is determined by the area of practice or the care setting in which it is implemented. Although the common theme is patient care management, there still exist some differences that are reflected by the type of services needed in relation to the care setting.

4.1. CASE MANAGEMENT PROCESS

The case management process is a set of steps and activities applied by case managers in their approach to patient care management. It delineates the roles and responsibilities of case managers toward patient care from the time of admission to a care setting or a care encounter until discharge and in some instances after discharge. One may describe the case management process as a modified version of the nursing process (Table 4.1). Both the case management and nursing processes are similar in that they identify the plan of care of patients by assessing needs, diagnosing the

TABLE 4.1. Comparison of the Nursing and the Case Management Processes.

Nursing Process Activities	Case Management Process Activities
	Case finding/screening and intake
Assessment	Assessment of needs
Diagnosis	Identification of actual and potential problems
Planning	Interdisciplinary care planning
Implementation	Implementation of interdisciplinary plan of care
	Monitoring of delivery of care and services
Evaluation	Evaluating outcomes of care/patient responses to treatments and interventions
	Discharge/disposition
	Repeating the case management process
	Following-up on patient post-discharge or transition

problem(s), planning and implementing the care, and monitoring and evaluating outcomes. The nursing process is applied to the care of every patient by all nurses in any care setting regardless of the patient care delivery model followed by the organization. However, the case management process is used by case managers in an environment in which case management is the patient care delivery model, and in some organizations it may be applied only to a select group of patients who meet specific predetermined criteria that identify them as elegible for case management services.

The case management process is a systematic approach to patient care delivery and management (Figure 4.1). It identifies what the case manager should do at what time during the patient's hospitalization or course of care. The process provides the framework for the role of the case manager. It also helps organize and simplify the case management work. Each step in the process requires the case manager to be astute, use particular knowledge, and exhibit specific skills. The combination of these skills is the token for success in the role.

The case management process is discussed in Chapter 4 in a linear fashion; however, in reality this process is not linear. The case manager may go back and forth or skip some of the steps depending on the patient and family's situation or care aspect at hand and the needs of the patient. Similar to the role of the case manager, the case management process focuses on four major functions: clinical care management, utilization management, and transition/ discharge. For the purpose of clarification, these functions are presented as separate processes in Table 4.2. However, in real patient care situations, case managers approach the delivery of case management services in an integrated way; that is seemlessly integrating these three functions. Additionally and at every step of the process, case managers engage in monitoring and evaluation of patient care goals and outcomes.

Case managers are active members of interdisciplinary healthcare teams which consist of providers from various professional backgrounds working toward a common goal (i.e., provision and management of cost-effective, efficient, safe, and high-quality patient care). Membership of the interdisciplinary team varies based on the care setting, the patient's problems, and the plan of care. Today however, due to the complexity of care provision and the need to transition patients to the appropriate level of care, collaboration and involvement of healthcare providers spans from the various settings within and across the care continuum (Figure 4.2).

Interdisciplinary healthcare team members can be described in three groups based on the degree of in-

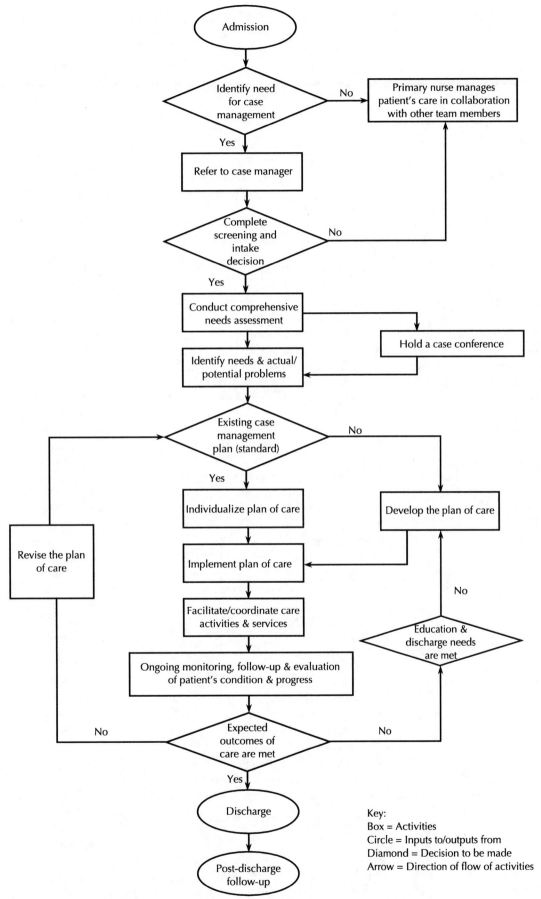

Figure 4.1 Flow diagram: the case management process.

TABLE 4.2. The Relationship Between the Case Management, Utilization Management, and Transitional/Discharge Planning Processes.

Case Management Process	Utilization Management Process	Transitional/Discharge Planning Process
1. Case finding/screening and intake • Select patients who would benefit from case management services 2. Assessment of needs • Identify care and services needed during episode of care • Idetify post-discharge care needs 3. Identification of actual and potential problems 4. Interdisciplinary care planning • Conduct case conference with interdisciplinary care team as needed • Establish goals of treatment and expected outcomes of care 5. Implementation of interdisciplinary plan of care • Facilitate/coordinate patient care activities including post-discharge services 6. Monitoring the delivery of patient care services 7. Evaluation of outcomes of care/patient responses to treatments and interventions 8. Patient discharge and disposition 9. Repeating the case management process 10. Following up on patient post-discharge or transition	1. Patient's admission/encounter • Evaluate appropriateness for care and level of care using predetermined guidelines 2. Assessment of resources • Assess patient's needs for healthcare resources based on medical condition • Assess patient's financial status and health insurance plan benefits 3. Development of resource management plan • Identify patient's problems and need for resource management • Identify services that require authorizations/certifications • Identify criteria for discharge (i.e., discharge outcomes) • Identify postdischarge needs that require payer's approval 4. Implementing the resource management plan • Conduct concurrent review with MCO • Obtain authorizations for services provided during the care encounter or to be provided post-transition • Discuss need for extended length of stay as needed • Transition patient to next level of care 5. Evaluation of resource management plan • Identify potential denial areas and implement action • Monitor outcomes and appropriateness of plan • Determine patient's readiness for transfer to next level of care • Confer with healthcare team, patient and family, and payer 6. Discharging patient • Identify patient's readiness for discharge based on discharge outcomes determined earlier in process • Confirm discharge with patient and family and healthcare team 7. Repeating the process • Re-examine resource management process and revise based on patient's needs, conditions, and treatment plan	1. Patient's admission/encounter • Screen patient for post-discharge needs • Identify need for discharge services 2. Assessment of discharge/ transitional planning needs • Agree on post-discharge needs with patient, family, healthcare team • Assess type and availability of needed resources 3. Development of transitional/ discharge plan • Design action plan for meeting patient's post-discharge needs • Agree on goals of plan and expected outcomes 4. Implementation of the transitional plan • Put plan into action • Coordinate necessary activities • Broker services with community agencies, etc. • Educate patient and family regarding healthcare needs 5. Evaluation of the transitional plan • Monitor appropriateness of plan • Examine outcomes of plan • Exchange information with post-discharge agencies as needed 6. Preparing patient for discharge • Confirm patient's discharge • Confirm post-discharge services 7. Patient's discharge • Complete actual patient's discharge • Transfer patient to another facility 8. Repeating the process • Reapply transitional planning process based on changes in patient's condition 9. Following-up on patient and family post-discharge or transition • Call patient or family within 48–72 hours post-discharge • Ensure post-discharge care and services are optimal

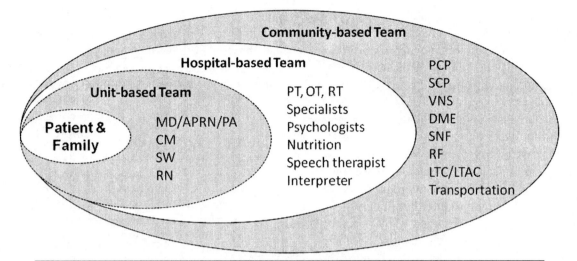

Figure 4.2 Members of contemporary interdisciplinary healthcare teams. APRN: advanced practice registered nurse; CM: case manager; DME: durable medical equipment; LTAC: long-term acute care; OT: occupational therapist; PCP: primary care provider; PT: physical therapist; RF: rehabilitation facility; RT: respiratory therapist; SCP: specialty care provider; SW: social worker; VNS: visiting nurse service.

volvement in patient's care including the discharge/ transitional plan. Some members are always represented, such as the case manager, physician, housestaff, nurse practitioners, physician assistants, RNs, and patients and their families. Other members are called upon in consultation, such as the social worker, physical therapist, occupational therapist, respiratory therapist, and nutritionist. The groups are as follows:

- *Always present*: healthcare professionals who are necessary in care provision regardless of who the individual patient is. They play an active role in assisting the patient and team in meeting care goals and treatment plan objectives. They include the case manager, physician, housestaff, advanced practice registered nurse (APRN), physician assistant (PA), RNs, and patients and their families/ caregivers.
- *Called upon in consultation as needed*: those whose involvement is dictated by the patient's condition, needs, and specifics of the plan of care. These may include the social worker, physical therapist, occupational therapist, respiratory therapist, pharmacist, pschologist, and registrered nutritionist.
- *Called upon on an ad hoc basis*: representatives of agencies external to the healthcare setting or organization where the patient is receiving care. They are mostly brought in based on the patient's

post-discharge service needs. These may include transportantion agencies, community resource organizations, and durable medical equipment vendors.

4.1.1. Case Finding/Screening and Intake

The initial step in the case management process is case finding (i.e., identifying the patients who require and would benefit from case management services). The purposes of case finding/screening are to identify the patient problems, determine the needs for and value of case management services, and confirm the patient's eligibility for these services. Case managers may identify such patients in four different ways. They may:

1. Screen all admissions to select those who are in need of case management services
2. Screen some, for example, only those patients who are referred for services by other healthcare providers
3. Not screen any patients but consider them all in need of some sort of case management services
4. Respond to a referral or request made by the patients or families themselves or any other member of the interdisciplinary healthcare team.

It is important, however, for each healthcare organization to define the method of patient referrals and identification for such services. *Guidelines* or policies must be established at the same time that case management systems are implemented and case manager roles are defined and established. The clearer the system for case finding, the easier the role of the case manager becomes and the faster the patients are referred to or identified for case management services. The efficiency of the system impacts the cost and increases the effectiveness of the case management program.

To expedite case finding, interdisciplinary healthcare team members are encouraged to make referrals to case managers as early as the time of admission but no later than 24 hours of patients' admission to a hospital, *sub-acute care facility*, or long-term care facility. In other care settings such as clinics or emergency departments, patients should be referred as soon as their needs for case management services are identified and is best referred by the healthcare professional who identifies such need. In home care settings, patients are referred for case management services in the home while still on the premises of a healthcare facility or within a few days of discharge from a hospital setting. It is a best practice today that a case manager in the home health agency, the skilled care facility, and rehabilitation centers reviews new patients at high risk for readmission to acute care setting.

Private physicians, housestaff, primary nurses/RNs, social workers, utilization managers/reviewers, discharge planners, APRNs, PAs, physical therapists, and nutritionists can refer patients to the case manager. Generally each case manager is responsible for identifying patients in his or her clinical service or area of responsibility. Healthcare organizations may need to prospectively define the patient selection criteria to make this responsibility easier. It is important to establish patient referral criteria, especially if the case management model followed identifies patient referrals as the major source for selection of patients for case management services rather than waiting for case managers to screen every admission to the hospital. These criteria eliminate any confusion that may arise when a member of the interdisciplinary team evaluates whether a patient needs to be referred to the case manager.

Box 4.1 presents a list of examples of patient selection criteria for case management services. Some of these criteria are generic; can be applied to any care setting; and are based on issues that may affect the patient in terms of quality of care, length of stay, risk for acute care readmission or unanticipated access to emergency services, and/or cost of care. Other criteria are based on the service/setting and are only appropri-

ate to that specific service/setting. The list serves as a guide for case managers to use to establish the criteria specific to their area of responsibility.

Whatever the case finding method is, case managers still have to evaluate the appropriateness of patients for

---

Box 4.1   Criteria for Case Management Services

This is a list of examples of criteria for referral and/or acceptance of patients for case management services. It is not an exhaustive list. However, healthcare organizations may adopt some of these criteria into their guidelines.

Generic Criteria applicable regardless of patient population or level of care

- High risk for readmission to acute care setting
- Physiological instability and complexity
- Inability to assume self-care as a result of physical dependencies and/or neurological status
- Mobility impairment/disability/functional dependence
- Lack of social support system or disengaged caregiver or significant other
- History of nonadherence with medical/surgical regimen (e.g., medications, follow-up care)
- Chronic pain management problems
- Complexity of diagnosis and multiple comorbidities or chronic illnesses
- Complex medication regimen and polypharmacy
- Fluctuating emotional status
- Prone to problems/complications
- Involvement of several disciplines in the care
- Multiple readmissions to acute care or frequent emergency department visits in a short period
- Complex discharge needs, need for placement in a particular facility
- Need for intensive healthcare education of patient/family
- Death and dying/end-of-life issues, palliative care, hospice care
- Managed care insurance carrier
- Medicare or Medicaid managed care carrier/Advantge health plans
- Financial risk to the hospital (i.e., inadequate healthcare coverage/financial support)
- At risk for prolonged length of stay
- Required treatment in various care settings in one hospitalization (e.g., intensive care unit, telemetry, regular unit) and by multiple care providers (i.e., medical, surgical, and other specialists)
- Pre-existing problems accessing healthcare
- Need for durable medical equipment
- Guardianship issues
- Interinstitutional transfer; acute to acute or sub-acute transfer
- Potential or suspected abuse

Service/Unit-Specific Criteria

Emergency department/clinic/medical home

- Homelessness
- Lack of primary care physician
- Inconsistency in medical follow-up including no show for appointments
- Disengagement in follow-up care
- Requiring admission into the hospital
- Multiple or frequent visits in a short period
- Substance use/abuse
- Dual diagnoses
- Psychiatric and mental health problems
- Multiple chronic conditions and complex medications regimen (polypharmacy)

Neonate/pediatric

- Age
- Chronic illness (e.g., asthma, croup, HIV/AIDS)
- Prematurity, less than 32 weeks' gestation
- Vaccination
- Child abuse
- Newborn weighing less than 1,500 g
- Requiring individualized instructions such as CPR
- More than three medications on discharge
- Requiring a home care referral for post-discharge services and follow-up
- Needing durable medical equipment at home, such as a glucometer

Obstetrics/gynecology

- First pregnancy
- First baby, multiple newborns
- High risk/complicated pregnancy (e.g., gestational diabetes, preeclampsia)
- No prenatal follow-up
- Substance abuse during pregnancy
- Delivery of a premature baby
- Teenage pregnancy
- Perinatal grief

Geriatric

- Elderly, lives alone, with functional impairment and/or exhibiting mental status changes
- Requiring placement in a nursing home, rehabilitation, or assisted living facility
- Dementia/Alzheimer's disease
- Medically complex condition and requiring multiple services
- Frail elderly
- No social support system
- Elder abuse
- Frequent emergency department visits or hospital admissions in short period
- Extended length of hospital (or other facilities such as subacute care) stay
- Potential discharge problems such as inadequate financial status, living arrangements, or caregiver support

Intensive care unit(s)

- Ventilator dependency/weaning
- Organ transplant
- Multisystem failure
- End-of-life issues or withdrawal of treatments including life support
- Ethical issues
- Transfer to another acute care facility
- Need for psychosocial counseling for patient or family

Regular/medical-surgical unit

- Diagnosis specific (e.g., stroke, heart failure)
- First-time diagnosis
- Leaving (or history of leaving) against medical advice
- Complex discharge plan and post-discharge services
- Medical complications
- Physiological instability
- Functional dependence
- Three or more physicians actively involved in care
- Requiring multiple services and community resources post-discharge

Renal

- Complications with dialysis access: thrombosed access, infection
- Newly diagnosed end-stage renal disease
- Newly placed on dialysis treatments
- Decision making regarding dialysis treatment modality
- Candidate for organ transplantation
- Complex educational needs
- Need to establish diet and exercise regimens
- No insurance coverage
- Inadequate home environment
- Lack of psychosocial support
- Frequent readmissions
- Need for transportation services
- End-of-life decision making/termination of treatment

HIV/AIDS

- Newly diagnosed HIV (6 months or less)
- Medical complexity, more than one opportunistic disease
- Repeated hospitalizations
- Lack of insurance or inadequate coverage
- No housing or suboptimal home environment
- Counseling and psychosocial support
- Termination of treatment
- Lack of or inadequate social support system

Neuroscience

- Ischemic stroke or intracranial hemorrhage
- Brain and spinal cord diseases: brain tumors, traumatic spinal cord injury
- Tracheostomy
- Cerebrospinal fluid drainage
- Deficit requiring intensive postdischarge services and resources
- Multiple providers/services involved in care provision
- Complex discharge/transitional plan
- Transfer to another facility

Psychiatry/behavioral health

- Complex medication therapy
- Complex medical condition including dual diagnoses
- Compromised behavioral condition requiring one-to-one therapy
- Legal risk
- Acute depression and suicide
- Homicidal behavior
- Need for extended hospitalization
- Coordination of postdischarge services and community resources
- Increased frequency of hospitalizations and recidivism
- Lack of or inadequate social support system
- Complex discharge/transitional plan
- Seclusion

Oncology

- Metastasis
- Complex chemotherapy and radiation therapy protocols
- Terminal stage
- Withdrawal of treatment including life support
- Hospice, palliative care, or end-of-life care
- Complex discharge/transitional plan
- Lack of or inadequate social support system
- Pain management
- Extended hospital stay
- Multiple physicians/services involved in care provision

case management services and determine the necessity for "intake." The decision of whether a patient requires case management services (i.e., intake) is made based on screening (initial assessment) of the patient's needs, review of the medical record, and a discussion with the referring personnel. It is then determined whether the patient meets any of the selection criteria for case management. When the intake decision is made, the case manager flags the medical record, identifying that the patient is accepted for case management services, and writes an intake note in the patient's record. Most case

management programs have designated a specific location in the patient's medical record where to document involvement of the case manager. This is made clear and easy to locate by any member of the interdisciplinary healthcare team.

4.1.2. Assessment of Needs of the Patient and Family

Once the case manager has identified patients who meet and would benefit from the predetermined selection criteria, a case management assessment must take place. This assessment is comprehensive and covers a wide range of areas, including the following:

- The chief complaint that required the patient to seek medical attention
- The physical, behavioral, emotional, mental, spiritual, psychosocial, and financial status of the patient
- The healthcare insurance coverage, benefits, and, when needed, whether the patient's admission has been approved (i.e., precertification) by the MCO
- The patient's social support system and coping mechanisms
- Adjustment to illness and hospitalization
- Health literacy and the health education needs of the patient and family
- The projected discharge planning needs
- Services and resources the patient was using prior to the admission
- The resources required for caring for the patient and family

The assessment data that case managers collect and analyze fall into two important categories:

- *Subjective data.* The information told by the patient and family is the subjective data. It is related to the chief complaint and the history of the problem(s) that made the patient seek medical attention in a clinic, emergency department, or hospital. Case managers should be careful when interpreting such data because of its subjectivity.
- *Objective data.* This type of information is usually observable, concrete, and sometimes quantifiable. It includes findings from the physical examination, laboratory test results, and other diagnostic tests. The objective data are important because they help validate the subjective data and interpret the patient's history more accurately by providing a basis for comparison.

The subjective and objective information case managers collect when interviewing the patient and family, the physical examination, the results of laboratory tests, and the results of the diagnostic procedures make up the assessment database, which is necessary for better identification of the patient's actual and potential problems. The goal of the "assessment of needs" step of the case management process is to gather and record information that is most helpful in designing the most appropriate plan of care for the individual patient.

Assessment data collection can be extensive, and some of it may not be necessary at times. Case managers may limit the type of assessment data they collect by answering the following questions:

- What data should I collect?
- How should I collect data?
- How best should I organize the data for effective care planning decisions?
- What data is most relevant for me to identify the necessity for case management services and actions?
- How far back in time should I cover in my data collection?
- What should I verify with the patient, family, and/ or other members of the healthcare team?
- What is the value of contacting members of the healthcare team from the facility or agency where the patient was transitioned from? What information should I ask for?
- What information should I get from the patient's primary care provider? From the case manager at the health insurance plan?

Case managers may elect not to perform a physical assessment of the patient. However, they should review the medical record, particularly the admission history and assessment completed by the primary nurse, the physician, and other providers such as social workers and physical therapists, and the paperwork from transferring facilities. The assessment of needs requires collecting and synthesizing data from multiple sources across providers and various care settings and/ or services, including the patient and family. The initial encounter of the case manager with the patient and family is the beginning of an unwritten contract that dictates the rest of the relationship. It also is essential to the case management process because it helps establish rapport and promotes trust in the relationship. This is maximized through the case manager's professional attitude and effective and skillful communication and interviewing techniques. Performing an assessment of needs that is accurate and relevant to the patient's presenting problem(s) requires case managers to possess interviewing and technical skills that are invaluable,

especially motivational interviewing (Case Manager's Tip 4.2).

Other important aspects of the initial assessment are appropriateness of the patient's admission to that level of care and the post-discharge needs. As the case manager interviews the patient and family and reviews the medical record and any information available from the care setting prior to current encounter, he or she evaluates the appropriateness of the level of care the patient is to receive, using certain criteria such as InterQual or Milliman Guidelines (see Chapter 5). If the

CASE MANAGER'S TIP 4.2

Effective Interviewing of Patients and Families

1. Review the medical record before you approach the patient.
2. Discuss the reasons for case management services with the person referring the patient before you conduct the interview.
3. Obtain as much information as possible about the patient and family before you interview them.
4. Introduce yourself, indicating your full name, your title and role responsibility, and what you prefer to be called.
5. Make them aware of what you can do to help them survive and cope well with the current episode of illness.
6. Inform the patient and family of the reasons for your visit.
7. During the interview, ask open-ended questions to obtain an appropriate history of the problem/chief complaint. Also, ask direct questions based on the needs you may have identified during the chart review and the discussion with the person who referred the patient.
8. Use motivational interviewing skills especially when discussing a challenging or a sensitive matter or seeking information from an uncooperative patient/ family.
9. Maintain privacy and confidentiality during the interview.
10. Obtain information related to the patient's social support system, healthcare insurance coverage, education needs, prior services, and needs after discharge. These questions are important in evaluating appropriateness for case management services.
11. Discuss with the patient and family the next step(s) regarding the plan of care and case management.
12. Provide the patient and family, in writing (e.g., on a business card), your name and how you can be reached.

case manager finds that the admission or the level of care is inappropriate (i.e., above or below what the patient's current care requires), he or she will initiate some action to correct the situation. This may require the case manager to discuss the situation and negotiate a better plan with the physician and other members of the healthcare team. This is also important for ensuring reimbursement for the services provided and avoiding unnecessary financial risk.

At the same time the case manager assesses the appropriateness of the admission, he or she identifies the patient's and/or family's post-discharge healthcare needs. This assessment acts as the beginning of the transitional/discharge planning process (see Chapter 6). The utilization management and transitional planning assessments are important because they affect the follow-up actions and determine the most appropriate plan of care for the patient.

4.1.3. Identification of Actual and Potential Problems

A thorough assessment of the needs of the patient and family provides the basis for identifying the actual and potential problems (e.g., nursing diagnoses, health problems). Identifying these problems dictates the types of interventions and treatments necessary to achieve the desired outcomes. Accurate and comprehensive identification of these problems has a significant effect on the quality of care, patient safety, incurred cost/expense, reimbursement, course of care, and length of stay or treatment. Case managers are always advised to seek the collaboration of the interdisciplinary healthcare team and the patient and family in identifying the actual and potential problems. This strategy improves outcomes and promotes agreement on the plan of care. It also increases consistency and continuity in the provision of care among the various disciplines involved and across care settings as applicable.

Regardless of the patient's clinical condition, case managers should always identify any needs or problems the patient and family may have related to healthcare teaching, discharge/transitional planning, and social support systems. The earlier such problems are identified, the sooner they are incorporated into the plan of care. This results in better control over the length of stay and ensures that patients' needs and preferences are met. It also expedites the process of resolving the problems.

During the time case managers identify the patient's actual and potential problems, they elect to reassess the patient's current and post-discharge needs to validate

uncertain or incomplete areas that existed in the previous assessment. It is important for case managers to be certain of the patient's needs before finalizing the problems list or sharing it with members of the interdisciplinary team or confirming it with the patient and family/caregiver.

4.1.4. Interdisciplinary Care Planning

Interdisciplinary care planning helps establish a seamless approach to patient care. It requires the involvement of members of the various disciplines that will be caring for the patient (refer to Figure 4.2). In addition, it is important to involve the patient and family. The first activity in this step of the case management process is case conferencing, which can be completed in either of two ways:

- Formal sit down forum using a prescheduled time and location, specific to one patient
- Informal as an interdisciplinary discussion about the plans of care for a number of patients (e.g., daily patient care rounds)

Regardless of the degree of formality, the case manager presents the findings of the assessment of patient's needs and the identified actual and potential problems to the interdisciplinary team. The team then prioritizes the patient problems, selects appropriate intervention/treatment modalities to resolve these problems, and establishes the expected outcomes of care. During this discussion the plan of care is developed.

A care plan that is interdisciplinary and well developed helps decrease the risk of incomplete tasks or incorrect/inappropriate care. It also provides a seamless approach to care that supports the standards of care of regulatory (e.g., CMS) and accreditation agencies (e.g., TJC, fomerly known as the Joint Commission on Accreditation of Healthcare Organizations [JCAHO]). Such a plan provides direction to all the disciplines involved in the care of the patient, opens the lines of communication among these disciplines and the patient and family, and ensures continuity and consistency of the care provided, especially post-discharge.

During this step of the case management process, case managers establish the goals of treatment and the projected/desired outcomes of care (Case Manager's Tip 4.3). They also include goals for utilization management and transitional planning. It is important to establish these goals and desired outcomes in collaboration with members of the interdisciplinary team as well as with the patient and family. An interdisciplinary approach to setting the goals and expected out-

CASE MANAGER'S TIP 4.3

Planning Care and Value-Based Purchasing

Case managers play an integral role in focusing the team on integrating the applicable process measures based on the value-based purchasing mandate into the patient's interdisciplinary plan of care, goals, expected outcomes, and interventions. In this regard, case managers ensure that the process measures are part of the milestones of care (i.e., intermediate and discharge outcomes) and that these are monitored and evaluated throughout the hospital stay and appropriate interventions instituted to lead the team to meeting the value-based purchasing expectations.

comes is the key to cost-effective, safe, and quality care.

With their assessment skills, clinical expertise, and holistic approach to patient care, case managers ensure that a comprehensive interdisciplinary plan of care is developed and that it is synchronized with the patient's and family's goals and preferences. They also verify that it contains the identified patient's actual and potential problems, the mutually determined and agreed-on goals with the interdisciplinary team members and the patient and family, the required patient care activities that reflect all of the involved disciplines (specifically the nursing interventions and medical treatments), and the preventive measures for complications or undesired outcomes. In addition, the plan should always include patient and family teaching and discharge planning components.

The interdisciplinary plan of care developed is the case management plan (CMP) (see Chapter 12) to be followed by all disciplines in the care of individual patients. If a CMP (specific to the patient's diagnosis/procedure) already exists, the case manager presents it to the interdisciplinary team during case conferencing or interdisciplinary care rounds for review and individualization to meet the patient's and family's needs. The CMP then becomes the tool used to identify, monitor, and evaluate the treatments and interventions and the care activities and outcomes. It is constantly evaluated and revised to reflect the changing needs of the patient and family.

Planning an appropriate patient's course of care is a skill required by case managers. To be effective in their role, they should be knowledgeable about the available hospital and community resources necessary for the care of patients, the various care settings, management of resources, cost, and reimbursement, and they should be clinically astute.

4.1.5. Implementation of the Interdisciplinary Plan of Care

In this step of the case management process, the interdisciplinary plan of care/CMP is put into action. Each member of the interdisciplinary team ensures that his or her responsibilities, as indicated in the CMP, are met within the projected timeframes. Implementation encompasses all of the interventions (medical, nursing, and others) that are directed toward meeting the pre-established goals, resolving the patient's problems, and meeting the patient's healthcare needs and predetermined care outcomes.

Reassessment skills possessed by case managers are the key to success in this role. When reassessing the patient and the care, case managers usually answer questions such as the following:

- Does the patient have any new needs?
- Does the interdisciplinary plan of care/CMP meet the patient's needs?
- Does the plan need to be revised?
- Are the projected patient care activities indicated in the plan appropriate and timely?
- Will the patient's problems be resolved during this episode of care?
- What is the appropriate timeframe for resolving the identified problems?
- Does the transitional plan meet (or continue to meet) the patient's and family's needs?
- Are authorizations/certifications obtained from managed care companies for the treatments instituted or to be implemented?
- Are the patient and family or caregiver aware of and in agreement with the plan of care, including the potential transitional plan?

Answers to these questions help case managers to confirm that the planned interventions remain appropriate to the patient's condition and projected/desired outcomes. When case managers identify any problems, they are responsible for bringing them to the attention of the interdisciplinary team, discussing them, recommending necessary changes in the CMP, and ensuring that the plan is revised to meet the patient's latest condition.

Case managers are pivotal in facilitating and coordinating patient care activities. They informally direct the work of the interdisciplinary team members in an effort to promote cost-effective and appropriate care and to ensure that services are provided in a timely manner and patients are well informed and advocated for.

Case managers facilitate and coordinate patient care activities related to required tests, procedures, interventions and treatments; patient and family teaching; and discharge planning and the need for community resources. They are responsible for confirming that tests, procedures, treatments, and interventions coincide with those recommended in the CMP, are preauthorized/certified by the patient's health insurance plan, and are scheduled and completed in a timely fashion. They also make certain that changes in these activities are dictated by the patient's condition and are not arbitrary.

Case managers act as gatekeepers of the interdisciplinary teams they belong to. With their continuous follow-up on the implementation of the patient care activities and evaluation of outcomes and reassessment of the patient's condition and needs, they keep tabs on all of the interventions in order and ensure that what is supposed to occur is taking place. They may remind members of the team of any incomplete or inaccurate activities; expedite tests and procedures; eliminate or prevent any fragmentation, duplication, or unnecessary services; and prevent any confusion or misunderstanding. When case managers identify delays, variations, or deviations in the care from the CMP, they immediately act on the issue and attempt to correct it; in some cases they may call upon another member of the interdisciplinary healthcare team to address the concern.

Because of their understanding of the total picture of the care of the patient, they are invaluable in coordinating the scheduling of the different tests and procedures required for a patient's workup and treatment. They ensure that these tests or procedures are not scheduled at the same time. Their careful attention to such situations prevents the occurrence of any conflict, delays, duplication, or fragmentation of care. Case managers are also instrumental in facilitating timely reporting of the results of diagnostic and therapeutic tests or procedures. This function allows the interdisciplinary healthcare team to make timely decisions pertaining to the appropriateness of care, to change interventions and treatments to more effective ones as indicated by the clinical status of patients and supported by objective data (i.e., results of tests and procedures), and to validate that the recommended patient care activities outlined in the CMP or interdisciplinary plan of care are achieved in a timely fashion.

Facilitating and coordinating the patient and family teaching activities are important functions of case managers. They are able to manage these activities efficiently and effectively because of their extensive knowledge of the healthcare system, their clinical experience and skills, and their familiarity with the adult learning theory and the health-belief model. Case managers may be directly or indirectly involved in patient and family teaching activities. They are more likely to be directly involved in teaching in situations such as the following:

- Patients with complex diagnoses that lead to complicated teaching needs (e.g., patients with multiple problems such as chronic renal failure, diabetes, hypertension, and heart failure): Patients with such conditions require intensive teaching plans. Case managers may elect to develop such plans in collaboration with others from the interdisciplinary team, including the patient and family and the primary nurse. They may conduct some teaching sessions pertaining to specific topics or needs (e.g., insulin self-injection) or supervise and/or ensure the completion of teaching activities related to other topics (disease process, signs and symptoms, or medications) by the primary nurse or other members of the interdisciplinary healthcare team.

- Patients with multiple admissions in a short period of time: These patients may have problems that are beyond the understanding of the disease process and signs and symptoms. After careful assessment of the patient's and family's teaching needs, case managers may find that the real problems of repeated admissions are inconsistent clinical follow-up, nonadherence to the medical/surgical regimen, or an inappropriate social support system. In such situations, active involvement of the case manager is essential. The case manager then concentrates on the real issue and works closely with the patient and family to prevent readmission to the hospital and improve adherence to the post-discharge plan of care.

The role of patient and family educator can be challenging to most case managers as hospital length of stay decreases and patient acuity increases and the shift to providing healthcare services in the home, sub-acute care, patient centered medical home, and ambulatory settings become more popular. This role is important in maximizing patient care outcomes, minimizing cost, and promoting the patient/family independence in care. Case managers can function as role models and experts in patient and family teaching and counseling to other interdisciplinary team members such as the primary nurses and social worker. Their responsibility toward patient and family teaching starts at the time of admission in assessing the patient's health literacy and teaching needs and initiating the teaching plan that helps meet these needs. They also coordinate the teaching activities, based on the plan, to be completed by the different members of the healthcare team, including the primary nurse.

The patient and family education role requires case managers to be astute in assessing patient teaching needs and readiness, identifying any existing barriers and limitations to teaching, and selecting the appropriate methodology. They are also required to be sensitive to the patient condition, culture, values, and belief system. Case managers should demonstrate competency in how to incorporate these factors into the patient and family teaching plan and help members of the interdisciplinary team choose the most effective method and plan for teaching.

Case managers are key players in effective discharge/transitional planning. They play an important role in coordinating and facilitating the patient's discharge. Their role in discharge planning starts with admission of the patient to the hospital, or at the time the patient seeks medical attention, and during the first encounter with the patient and family. They are responsible for assessing the patient's needs for safe and appropriate discharge and coordinating the process of getting these services approved and perhaps instituted before the patient is discharged.

Case managers collaborate with the patient and family, physician, primary nurse, social worker, home care planner, and other members of the healthcare team in establishing the patient's most appropriate discharge plan and work closely with them to achieve this plan. Case managers update and revise the plan as needed based on their ongoing reassessment of the patient's condition and needs. They also discuss and communicate any changes in the discharge plan to the members of the team informally or formally during case conference meetings.

Facilitation and coordination of discharge planning activities may require case managers to communicate with external services such as medical equipment providers, home care agencies, or representatives from other healthcare facilities. They may also need to contact case managers in MCOs or health insurance plans seeking certifications for the post-discharge services or transfers to other facilities as required by patients. These functions demand that case managers be skillful in negotiation techniques and brokerage of services. They also need to possess excellent communication skills and be knowledgeable in managed care contracts, health benefits, entitlements, federal and third-party payers, other reimbursement methods, laws and regulations, policies and procedures, and the variety of available community services and agencies. Seasoned case managers can be found to have established successful business relationships with key people in the different agencies they contact on a regular basis. Such relationships are instrumental in providing case managers with a wide networking circle and expediting the process of approval, certification, and delivery of post-discharge services.

4.1.6. Evaluation of Patient Care Outcomes

In the evaluation of the patient care outcomes step of the case management process, case managers evaluate the effectiveness of the interdisciplinary plan of care/CMP and the patient care activities, interventions, and outcomes. They are also responsible, in collaboration with members of the interdisciplinary healthcare team, to continuously monitor the patient's condition, responses to interventions, and progress toward recovery or stablility in health condition. Ongoing communication with the healthcare team regarding the appropriateness of the plan of care in relation to the patient's changing condition and needs, and whether the plan is realistic, is important for timely revision of the plan and implementation of new interventions and treatments.

When evaluating patient care interventions and outcomes, case managers should answer the following questions:

- Were the patient care decisions, activities, interventions, and resources accurate and timely?
- Were the goals of the patient and family and the healthcare team accomplished?
- Have the patient and family needs been met?
- Has the patient's condition progressed toward recovery/stability, deteriorated, or remained the same?
- How is the patient progressing relevant to the intermedicate and discharge outcomes or milestones?
- Are the interdisciplinary care team and patient's plan of care meeting the applicable core measures based on the value-based purchasing expectations?
- Which interventions or treatments need to be changed or added?
- Should patient care outcomes, activities, and/or goals be reprioritized?
- Is the care being delivered in the appropriate setting or at the right level?
- Is the transitional/discharge plan relevant and does it clearly identify the post-discharge services needed?
- Have certifications been obtained for services and resources before their delivery as indicated in the managed care contract or health insurance plan?
- Are the patient, family, and/or caregiver in agreement with the plan of care, including the discharge/transitional plan?

Answers to these questions by the interdisciplinary team members at case conferences and patient care management rounds, or by case managers when reviewing medical records and evaluating the appropriateness of patient care activities and outcomes help the healthcare team remain focused and make timely revisions to the plan of care. This function of case managers is important in ensuring that high quality, safe, and cost-effective care is delivered at all times. Additionally, such efforts help reduce the care provider's financial risk.

Case managers are responsible for monitoring and evaluating delays and variances of care on a continuing basis. They identify and track deviations from the CMP (i.e., variances of care) as they relate to the following:

- *Patient* (e.g., refusal of test or procedure, deterioration in condition)
- *Practitioner* (e.g., medication errors, delay in scheduling or performing a certain test, visiting nurse not showing up for postdischarge care, certifications for services and treatments not obtained)
- *System* (e.g., unable to complete a test because the machine is broken, no physical therapy available on weekends, MCO not certifying/approving home care services). (See Chapters 9 and 14 for more detailed discussion on variances.)

Case managers also keep members of the interdisciplinary healthcare team well informed of the presence/occurrence of variances and together attempt to resolve these variances. Early detection and resolution of such variances are essential to prevent complications or undesired outcomes, delays or ommissions of care activities or services, avoidable prolonged length of stay, increased cost, and deterioration in patient and family satisfaction.

Case managers are also made accountable for evaluating the fiscal, quality, and clinical outcomes of care. These outcomes are interrelated, and a deficit in one usually affects the others negatively.

- *Fiscal outcomes* are those related to the organizational goals rather than the patient's health. Examples of fiscal outcomes are cost and revenue of care, resource use, length of stay, inappropriate admissions, and system-related variances.
- *Traditional quality outcomes* have been those directly related to a patient's health and functioning. Examples of quality outcomes are nosocomial infection rates, patient's functional independence, health perception, readmissions, inappropriate dis-

charges, complications, and patient and family satisfaction with care.

- *Clinical outcomes* are those directly related to patient care activities. These outcomes are identified proactively by members of the interdisciplinary team and included in the CMP, and they are expected to be achieved while caring for the patient and family. Some examples are the intermediate and discharge outcomes (see Chapters 9 and 14). Through timely facilitation and coordination of patient care activities, patient and family teaching, and discharge planning, case managers are able to maintain a delicate balance of these outcomes.

While monitoring and evaluating care; reviewing medical records; or communicating with the patient and family, primary nurses, members of the interdisciplinary healthcare team, and ancillary departments, case managers continually collect data related to variances and outcomes of care. They then aggregate the data based on similarities in issues and diagnoses, conduct a trending and analysis review, and finally generate reports to be shared with appropriate personnel (e.g., quality improvement department, case management department, interdisciplinary team members, chiefs of services/clinical departments [nursing, medical, and ancillary], and administration). Case managers are instrumental in their feedback related to the critical issues, particularly system problems that require administrative attention and initiation of quality improvement task forces for resolution.

Throughout the evaluation of the patient care outcomes step of the case management process, case managers exhibit certain skills that are essential to the role. These skills are problem solving, decision making, critical thinking, clinical reasoning, consensus building, quality improvement, leadership abilities, networking, partnership, collaboration, interviewing, communication and feedback, and negotiation. It is through these effective skills that case managers are able to make a difference in patient care management and to meet the goals of the case management model and the organization.

4.1.7. Patient's Discharge and Disposition

At some point when appropriate, it is important for case managers to bring their relationship with the patient and family to closure. Discontinuation of case management services, whether it is due to the patient's discharge or transition from the hospital/facility or because case management services are deemed no longer required by the patient, is the last step in the case management process. During this phase case managers hold a "case closing" conference with the patient and family and the interdisciplinary team, during which the plan of care is evaluated for its completion, particularly the appropriateness of the discharge plan including post-discharge services and the effectiveness of patient and family teaching. This is the time when case managers confirm that the transitional plan is appropriate and that all post-discharge services required by the patient are in place and the necessary paperwork has been completed. If a problem is identified, it should be resolved before the time of the patient's actual discharge.

Case managers ensure that all discharge activities are completed effectively before the time of discharge or transfer to another facility for follow-up care such as rehabilitation. They evaluate the patient's readiness by making sure that the discharge outcomes are met and that all of the required interdisciplinary activities have been successfully achieved or the receiving facility has already accepted the transfer and arranged for a bed for the patient. It is essential to answer the patient's and family's last questions regarding care after discharge and provide them with emotional support and counseling as necessary. Sometimes it is helpful for them to have the case manager's phone number; this is a safety or reassurance mechanism for patients and families that reduces their anxiety and fear of discharge and being responsible for self-care while at home. It is also important for case managers to provide them with written instructions pertaining, but not limited, to the following:

- Care after discharge
- Scheduled follow-up appointment(s)
- Pending or necessary ambulatory tests
- Detailed information about the prescribed medications
- Summary of care explaining the course of treatment during the episode of care

4.1.8. Repeating the Case Management Process

Case managers usually repeat the case management process every time they are in contact with the patient and family. This function is not considered a true or direct step in the case management process. Reassessment of patients, ongoing evaluation of patient care activities and outcomes, and constant checking and ensuring that care is delivered as scheduled in a timely fashion are all examples of tasks that require going through every step of the case management process. Case managers are constantly repeating the process whether formally or informally, sometimes focusing

on the most relevant and essential steps rather than the whole case management process.

Repeating the case management process is one way of ensuring that the provision of care is appropriate, the quality is not compromised in the name of cost containment, and the patient is discharged safely and post-discharge services and resources are secured. Case managers have the opportunity and obligation to repeat the case management process every time a task is not completed effectively, a delay in any care activity is identified, an expected outcome is not met, or the patient or a family member are in disagreement with the plan. When repeating the process, case managers implement new interventions and activities to resolve the identified problem(s). They also may modify the goals of care accordingly and obtain the support of the interdisciplinary team about the changes and the approval of the patient and family/caregiver of the modified priorities and interventions. Repeating the case management process functions as a safety net for ensuring that appropriate care is delivered and as a method for developing an action plan for problem solving that assures quality, safe and cost-effective outcomes.

4.1.9. Following Up on Patient Post-Discharge

Some institutions require case managers to make follow-up phone calls to the patients, patients' families, or caregivers within 48–72 hours after discharge. These calls aim to evaluate the patients' level of functioning, engagement in self-care, and adherence to the medical regimen and follow-up appointments. Case managers may spend a considerable amount of time asking about whether patients have secured the medications and are administering them as prescribed, understand their indications, precautions, and side effects. They also review the patients' understanding of red flags, which are symptoms and experiences the patient must watch out for and seek the support of a healthcare provider when they occur, and inquire whether any were experienced recently. In addition, they answer any questions the patients or caregivers may have.

The use of this evidence-based practice has been on the rise because it has demonstrated its ability to prevent avoidable and unplanned readmissions of patients for the same problems (chief complaint or diagnosis) that caused the recent admission to acute care. This reduces financial risk imposed by the Medicare Hospital Readmission Reduction Program on the acute care organization. Another added benefit to post-discharge calls is an increase in the patient's and family's satisfaction with care and faith in the healthcare team and organization.

CASE MANAGER'S TIP 4.4

Post-Discharge Follow-up Calls

Those who conduct post-discharge follow-up calls with the patient, family, or caregiver must have access to the patient's medical record. This allows the caller to have at his/her fingertips key information about the care of the patient while in the acute care setting, the plan of care, and the discharge instructions. At a minimum, the care summary and discharge instructions must be made available to facilitate effective conversation with the patient/family. This is necessary since the caller may not always be the same person who cared for the patient while hospitalized.

Post-discharge calls are an opportunity to ensure continuity of care and prevent unnecessary readmissions or access to emergency services. If a concern is identified during the call, the caller must attempt to resolve the issue or refer it to someone else who can and inform the patient of such referral.

There may be a need to attempt post-discharge follow-up calls multiple times for each patient until a call completion is achieved. Often patients may agree on a certain day and time prior to the discharge or transition from the episode of care and then daily living demands get in the way and the patient/family are no longer available. When reporting on calls completion, it is advisable to track the number of attempts until completion is achieved. Reporting on both attempts and completions allows for a better estimation of the resource requirements of a post-discharge follow-up call program.

To effectively connect with the patient or family post-discharge, case managers or other healthcare team members formally discuss the post-discharge calls with the patient prior to discharge or transition to another setting. Most healthcare organizations have formally incoporated this into the discharge planning process, discharge instructions, and documentation. These team members ask the patient about preferred day, time, and contact approach (e.g., video conference, telephone, e-mail, text message), obtain the contact information, and document the outcomes of such conversations in the patient's medical record or another system such as a dedicated post-discharge call manager (Case Manager's Tip 4.4).

4.2. VARIOUS ROLES PLAYED BY CASE MANAGERS

The roles described below apply to case managers regardless of the setting in which they are working. They are universal to the roles of the case manager whether that case manager is a social worker or a registered nurse. As such, case managers are involved in many different situations throughout their day. They may provide a patient and/or a family with care instructions and may teach staff members about new trends in patient care. They may also ensure approval/certification of services by MCOs/health insurance plans or negotiate home care services with a visiting nurse agency. The varied scope of roles, functions, and activities they may provide increases their challenge for ensuring that high-quality, safe, and cost-effective care has been delivered.

This wide range of responsibilities requires case managers to put more than one role or function into action at the same time. The interrelatedness of these roles is the key to success. Case managers may be found assessing or reassessing patients while monitoring and evaluating outcomes. They may be scheduling a test while trying to resolve delays related to tests or procedures. Their diverse roles are important for timely patient care delivery and outcomes. The various responsibilities and roles of case managers and their ongoing planning and prioritization of the tasks to be

 CASE MANAGER'S TIP 4.5

Time Wasters Case Managers Should Avoid

- Lack of or ineffective attempts at ongoing prioritization and planning
- Unrealistic goals and time estimates
- Overambition and desire to impress superiors
- Inattentiveness and insufficient communication and feedback
- Tendency to be perfectionists
- Confusion with regard to responsibilities, functions, and boundaries
- Insecurity, fear of failure, and lack of confidence and self-esteem
- Failure to follow up on incomplete tasks
- Ego and feeling of overimportance
- Sense of unnecessary obligation
- Inability to say no when needed
- Failure to obtain important information when it is required to do so, or collecting unnecessary information
- Being an "extra pair of hands" to everyone
- Inability to delegate
- Treating every problem as a crisis (overreaction)
- Procrastination
- Leaving tasks unfinished
- Being unaware of importance of things
- Socializing
- Being hands-off when delegating some tasks as if you are no longer responsible

CASE MANAGER'S TIP 4.6

Strategies for Effective Time Management

- Set realistic and clear objectives, goals, priorities, and deadlines.
- Use "to do" lists for the day. List activities in order of priority/importance based on the number of tasks to be completed. Update your list continually. Keep your priority list current.
- Distinguish the urgent from the truly important.
- Delegate the activities and tasks that can be delegated. Be clear about expectations and follow-up when you delegate.
- Avoid being a perfectionist. Lower your standards to what is reasonable and acceptable.
- Communicate effectively, accurately, and in a timely manner.
- Collect appropriate data and necessary information only. Determine what is needed for planning activities, making decisions, and providing feedback.
- Clarify your job responsibilities, power, and boundaries with your supervisor.
- Constantly check progress and follow up on unfinished tasks.
- Refuse to spread yourself too thin. Say no, give reasons, and provide alternatives. You may say, "Sorry, I cannot. I do not have the time, but I have a suggestion." or "Thanks for the compliment, but I am afraid I have to decline."
- Make no assumptions, and avoid being critical.
- Recognize that things may take longer to complete than planned. Accept this fact. Impose realistic deadlines on tasks.
- Seek the help and guidance of your superior as needed. Avoid struggling with uncertainties on your own.
- Avoid socializing, distractions, or unnecessary interruptions.
- Respect deadlines. Avoid procrastination. Be urgent when appropriate.
- Use technology, especially mobile devices, to their fullest capabilities.

 CASE MANAGER'S TIP 4.7

Maintaining Clinical Expertise

- Become a member in professional organizations and/ or nursing societies.
- Subscribe to journals that pertain to clinical practice.
- Stay abreast of the healthcare literature and the changes in technology.
- Attend organization-based continuing education sessions.
- Participate in conferences, particularly those related to case management.
- Seek the help of other experts when faced with a situation that is uncertain or unfamiliar.
- Make every effort to learn new skills and gain new knowledge when opportunities arise.
- Participate in clinical activities such as case study presentations, case conference, evidence-based practice review, or clinical research.
- Spend some time in the library or on line (at least 1 hour a week) searching for new knowledge.
- Attend medical staff/student teaching rounds.
- Seek higher education.

patient and family needs while establishing the actual and potential health problems, goals for treatment, and desired outcomes; applying the nursing process; planning, implementing, evaluating, and coordinating the care activities to meet the patient and family goals and expected outcomes; using advanced treatment modalities and technologies; and dealing with patients as biopsychosocial systems with the treatment plan directed toward the system as a whole rather than just the disease.

4.2.2. Consultant

Because of their clinical experience and knowledge of the institutional operations/systems, policies and procedures, and standards of care and practice, case managers can be called on as consultants by physicians, nurses, and other case managers and members of the interdisciplinary healthcare team. They are helpful in solving clinical and administrative issues when members of the interdisciplinary team are in doubt.

Case managers, particularly those who work in an ambulatory care setting, may provide telephone consultations to MCOs/health insurance plans or other healthcare insurance companies, patients and families, and home care agencies. They may also operate advice lines aimed to triage patients and guide them through their navigation of the complex healthcare system or answering questions they may have regarding medications and post-discharge treatment or plan of care.

completed require them to be astute in time management, which is integral to the effectiveness of their role (Case Manager's Tips 4.5 and 4.6).

4.2.1. Clinical Expert

Case managers are chosen for their role because of extensive clinical experience, skills, and knowledge of patient care. They bring excellence in clinical practice to the role (Case Manager's Tip 4.7). They act as role models and resources to nursing, medical, and other staff members. They exhibit clinical competence in assessing

4.2.3. Coordinator and Facilitator of Patient Care—Patient Flow

Case managers spend a great deal of their time coordinating and facilitating patient care activities and expediting the completion of diagnostic and therapeutic tests and procedures. They also ensure that results of the tests and procedures are available within a reasonable turnaround time. This role provides the foundation for patient flow as it facilitates the movement of the patient through the acute care continuum. This function is important in reducing length of stay, enhancing treatment progression, and eliminating delays and variances in patient care activities or outcomes. In collaboration with members of the healthcare team, they help patients move smoothly and safely through the hospital and healthcare systems.

In this role function, case managers prevent any fragmentation or duplication in the delivery of care. Their timely intervention when a patient's condition changes increases the efficiency and effectiveness of care and promotes safe and qaulity care outcomes. When necessary, they ensure that authorizations for services are obtained before initiation of treatment. In addition, they coordinate the patient's teaching and discharge plans and ensure the completion of all discharge activities in a timely fashion to prevent unnecessary hospital stays or readmissions. This role is important in controlling the use of resources, enhancing safety and quality of care, and containing cost. (See Chapter 3 for more information on the role of the case manager in patient flow).

4.2.4. Manager of Patient Care

Case managers function as managers of healthcare services by controlling the use of resources to achieve the desired outcomes. They act as gatekeepers of the interdisciplinary healthcare team to ensure that all patient care activities are accomplished by each team member within the projected timeframes. In addition, especially in the acute care setting, they assure that appropriate members of the healthcare team participate in the daily patient care management rounds.

One of their main responsibilities is direct supervision of the process of patient care to ensure quality outcomes. Case Manager's Tip 4.8 lists some strategies for managing patient care.

4.2.5. Educator

The role of educator is two-fold. Case managers are involved in patient and family education and staff

CASE MANAGER'S TIP 4.8

Strategies for Better Patient Care Management

- Maintain constant knowledge of the patient's plan of care. Update your information as indicated by changes in the patient's condition.
- Prevent delays in patient care activities.
- Ensure that tests and procedures are prescheduled.
- Obtain timely results of tests and procedures, and adjust the plan of care accordingly.
- Become knowledgeable about the contracts of managed care companies and federal and third-party reimbursement procedures.
- Encourage patients' timely discharge.
- Maximize the use of outpatient testing and same day of admission procedures.
- Communicate with the interdisciplinary team on an ongoing basis. Participate in (and lead) patient care managemrent rounds. Assure they occur on the days you are off duty.
- Ensure the involvement of the members of the interdisciplinary team in patient care-related decisions and problem solving.
- Maximize the involvement of the patient and family in such decisions.
- Prevent redundancy, duplication, or fragmentation of patient care activities.
- Eliminate any unnecessary or inappropriate tests or procedures.
- Seek administrative support as needed.
- Seek the guidance of experts when uncertain in a particular situation.

education. Regarding patient and family, they ensure that all healthcare needs are met within a reasonable timeframe during the hospital stay. They usually incorporate the teaching plan as part of the CMP and transitional plan as early as the time of admission or care encounter. They may provide direct patient teaching activities or supervise their completion by the primary nurses and/or other team members. Case managers may also be involved in developing patient and family teaching materials and planning and conducting patient teaching classes (Case Manager's Tip 4.9) especially pertaining to discharge instructions and postdischarge services and follow-up care.

Regarding nursing and other staff members, case managers are instrumental in mentoring the less experienced staff. They participate in in-service sessions related to case management and new trends and advances in patient care, including case management operations, community-based services and resources, new regulations (e.g., Patient Protection and

CASE MANAGER'S TIP 4.9

Strategies for Effective Patient/Family Education

- Educate patients and families only when they are ready.
- Identify the barriers or limitations to learning before you conduct a patient's education session and address them as necessary..
- Maximize the family's/caregiver's involvement.
- Use visual aids such as handouts, drawings, audiotapes, and videotapes. Record the teaching session and make available online for the patient/family, especially if the patient has a web-accessible personal health record.
- Assess health literacy and the need for low-level reading materials. At the same time, avoid being "cutesy." Adult learners might feel insulted.
- Apply the concepts of adult learning theory in your teaching sessions/activities.
- Encourage the patient's/family's participation in the decision-making process regarding learning needs.
- Apply the teach back method in the evaluation of learning. Include return demonstrations or verbalization of material shared.
- Adapt the teaching strategy to the patient's level of understanding, capabilities, or preferences.
- Involve other professionals (e.g., pharmacists, staff nurses, clinical nurse specialists) in educating patients/families.
- Limit the material to be taught to what the patient is able to grasp in one session. Always start with understanding what the patient already knows.
- If possible, schedule the next teaching session with the patient/family.
- Evaluate the ability of the patient/family to retain the information taught.
- Be consistent in the information provided, especially if other professionals are involved in teaching or reinforcing patient/family education.
- Put special emphasis on the postdischarge care needs and services.
- Conduct small group education sessions when appropriate.
- Allow for questions and answers.
- Avoid the use of medical jargon. Speak a language the patient understands.
- Clearly indicate the patient's teaching plan in the medical record.
- Use patient and family education materials written in the patient's language. Employ the help of an interpreter as needed.
- Use Internet resources as appropriate, especially with patients who are familiar with how to navigate the Internet.

Affordable Care Act), reimbursement methods, and core measures. Their staff teaching activities may be done as unit-based sessions or formal classes planned and held in collaboration with staff education departments. Either way, they are actively involved in the dissemination of new patient care knowledge and delivery systems.

4.2.6. Negotiator/Broker

Among the other roles assumed by case managers is the role of negotiator and broker of care and services. They are instrumental in getting necessary tests and procedures completed on time. They also negotiate the best treatment plan possible with the healthcare team, patient and family, and most importantly, the MCO/ health insurance plan. In addition, case managers negotiate with healthcare agencies for the community services needed for patients' support after discharge from the hospital such as home care and Meals on Wheels. Moreover, they negotiate with managed care companies for approval of the patient's hospitalization, the need for durable medical equipment, or the necessary services needed after discharge. Case Manager's Tip 4.10 lists strategies for effective negotiation.

4.2.7. Patient and Family Advocate

One of the important responsibilities of case managers is patient and family advocacy (Case Manager's Tip 4.11). Case managers assume a liaison role between the patient and family and the healthcare team. They assure that care decisions, plans of care, and post-discharge services remain patient-centered at all times. With their relationship with the patient and family/ caregiver at the time of admission (sometimes from before the admission), case managers are able to build trust and establish rapport to help facilitate the implementation of the plan of care. They keep the patient and family constantly informed of the plan of care, tests and procedures, and condition, which makes them the best vehicle through which the care is advocated, negotiated, agreed on, facilitated, and coordinated.

Case managers advocate for patients in case conferences and healthcare team meetings held throughout the patient's hospitalization or care encounter, during which they communicate the needs and wishes of the patient and family. They also advocate for the patient when reviewing plans of care with case managers of MCOs/health insurance plans for purposes of obtaining authorizations/certifications and when negotiating with agencies for community services or informing them of a patient's care needs after discharge.

CASE MANAGER'S TIP 4.10

Successful Negotiation

The strategies discussed in this section could be applied when the case manager negotiates services with outside agencies, physicians, consultants, and professional and ancillary staff, as well as when attempting to facilitate and coordinate patient care activities and prevent delays in patient care within and outside the boundaries of the institution.

- Separate people from positions.
- Negotiate for agreements—not winning or losing.
- Establish mutual trust and respect.
- Avoid one-sided or personal gains.
- Allow time for expressing the interests of each side/party.
- Listen actively during the process, and acknowledge what is being said.
- Use data/evidence to strengthen your position.
- Focus on interests—patient care interests. Remain patient-centered at all times.
- Always remember that the process is a problem-solving one, and the benefit is for the patient and family first.
- Never forget that patient care is the priority.
- Avoid using pressure.
- Be knowledgeable of the institutional policies, procedures, systems, standards, and the law. Apply this knowledge in the process.
- Try to understand the other side well. Ask questions and seek clarifications when unsure or uncertain.
- Avoid emotional outbursts. Do not overreact if the other party exhibits such behavior.
- Avoid premature judgments.
- Be concrete and flexible when presenting your stand.
- Use reason and be reasonable.
- Be fair.
- Make sure you have all the necessary information. If unsure, do not make it up.

4.2.8. Outcomes and Quality Manager

Monitoring and evaluating patient care quality and outcomes are integral to the role of case managers (Case Manager's Tip 4.12). They are important because they link case management to quality improvement and help determine whether the patient and organizational goals are met. Case managers monitor the occurrence of variances and outcomes of care as they relate to the CMP. The results of this monitoring process provide important data for quality improvement efforts and evaluating the effectiveness sand efficiency of the case management model and the use of CMPs. Case man-

 CASE MANAGER'S TIP 4.11

Advocating Effectively for Patients/Families

- Know the plan of care of your patients well, including the minute details.
- Spend enough time discussing the care with the patient and family and understand their concerns. Encourage informed decision and allow them to consider various options.
- Be familiar with the Patient's Bill of Rights.
- Take the time to address issues, concerns, and conflicts or assure they are addressed.
- Be knowledgeable of the law and the standards of regulatory agencies regarding certain patient care issues such as informed consent and do not resuscitate (DNR) orders.
- Be honest with the patient and family. Admit when you do not know the answers to their questions.
- Convey patient/family concerns to the appropriate personnel, obtain answers, and report results back to the patient and family.
- Identify ethical dilemmas and refer them to the ethics committee in a timely fashion.
- Provide the patient and family with emotional support as needed. Alleviate their anxieties and apprehension.

agers also investigate the reasons of variances and attempt to resolve them as soon as they are identified.

Case managers communicate variances, delays, and undesired patient care outcomes to members of the interdisciplinary healthcare team so that the team can revise the CMP as necessary. Together as a team they are better able to convince administration of the need for quality improvement task forces to have a closer look at certain system issues and nonvalue-adding processes, particularly those that require immediate attention. Case Manager's Tip 4.13 lists actions to help improve patient care quality.

 CASE MANAGER'S TIP 4.12

Role in Value-Based Purchasing

Case managers spend a considerable amount of time evaluating whether the interdisciplinary healthcare team has achieved the expected outcomes of care, especially in the area of measures that are part of value-based purchasing such as readmisisons to acute care, patient's experience with care, the care transition measure which is part of the Hospitals Consumer Assessment of Healthcare Providers and Systems, and other quality outcomes associated with specific conditons such as heart failure, pneumonia, and total hip replacement.

CASE MANAGER'S TIP 4.13

Strategies for Improving Patient Care Quality

- Focus on the process, not the people.
- Listen to patient and family concerns.
- Identify patient care problems (variances and delays) early and attempt to resolve them in a timely fashion.
- Attend to patient problems as an interdisciplinary team, rather than individually.
- Keep lines of communication open at all levels. Discuss the issues as they arise with the patient/family, superiors, subordinates, and whoever is deemed appropriate.
- Ensure that the desired/projected outcomes of care are met.
- Ensure patient's safe discharge.
- Provide care that is patient focused.
- Attend customer relations classes. Apply strategies learned in practice.
- Obtain and read the results of patient satisfaction surveys and quality improvement monitors. Change behavior and practice as indicated by the results.
- Conduct concurrent or retrospective chart reviews on an ongoing basis.

4.2.9. Scientist/Researcher

Research and evidence-based practice have been made a part of the case manager's role in institutions in which the required educational background of case managers is a master's degree. In this role, case managers are expected to participate as active members of institution-based research committees. They are also expected to write grant and research proposals, collect research data, and evaluate patient care activities. As advanced practice registered nurses, case managers are excellent at knowledge development and dissemination and utilization of research.

Case managers help nursing, social work, and other departments establish a research-based clinical practice, policies, procedures, and standards of care. Case Manager's Tip 4.14 lists some strategies to help in becoming involved in research and evidence-based practice.

4.2.10. Risk Manager

Because of their proximity to the bedside and involvement in direct patient care activities, case managers are at the forefront of identifying patient care issues that are considered legal risk. They are good at ensuring that the care delivered is in compliance with the standards of regulatory agencies, such as the U.S. Department of Health and Human Services and accreditation

 CASE MANAGER'S TIP 4.14

Strategies for Getting Involved In Research and Evidence-Based Practice

- Learn the processes of research and evidence-based practice. Take courses in research or seek the help of research experts.
- Apply research outcomes to practice.
- Conduct research and evidence-based projects on topics relevant to case management.
- Obtain funding; write grants.
- Participate in institutional research efforts: collect data, identify potential subjects, and so on.
- Become a member of the research committee.
- Get involved in evidence-based practice, research utilization, and dissemination programs.

agencies such as TJC, and the internal/institution's policies, procedures, standards of care, and standards of practice. Their role in assessment and monitoring of the delivery of patient care activities and evaluation of outcomes makes them crucial in identifying risk management issues and bringing them to the attention of the legal department in a timely fashion.

Case managers are able to establish a trusting relationship with the patient and family. Because of this relationship, they are able to prevent problems from escalating and becoming potential legal risk issues (Case Manager's Tip 4.15). Their advocacy of patient care helps them reduce the seriousness of any problem and makes patients view them as "God-sent angels." They are also helpful to members of the healthcare team. They provide them with answers to their clinical dilemmas and act as resource people to the team when faced with administrative problems. Case managers are excellent in this role because of their knowledge of the institution's administrative and clinical policies and procedures.

4.2.11. Change Agent

Case managers are the *champions of change*. They are the most helpful change agents an institution may have while implementing a new case management model (Case Manager's Tip 4.16). Case managers act as role models, resource people, and experts in case management to all staff during the transition into case management care delivery and thereafter. They are knowledgeable in the subject matter, which makes them well versed in case management and able to educate other staff members such as physicians, staff nurses, and ancillary staff.

CASE MANAGER'S TIP 4.15

Reducing Legal Risk

- Always know the law. Seek the help/advice of the legal and risk management department and specialists in your institution when uncertain.
- Familiarize yourself with the standards of care and practice of regulatory and accreditation agencies, especially those most applicable to case management.
- Familiarize yourself with institutional policies and procedures and standards of care and practice.
- Refer to the experts or the available reference manuals when unsure of a situation or a decision. Seek advice, counsel and support
- Attend to problems immediately as they arise. Do not wait for them to escalate.
- Do anything possible to prevent problems from occurring.
- Advocate for patients/families as opportunities arise.
- Know the details of the Patient's Bill of Rights. Ensure that patients are also educated about their rights—and duties.
- Obtain knowledge of the requirements of federal and third-party payers.
- Understand well the managed care contracts and their impact and relation to patient care.
- Monitor and observe patients constantly. Make sure you are aware of the latest changes in your patient's condition and that the plan of care, including the transional plan and postdischarge reources, are modified accordingly.
- Communicate changes in the plan of care to the patient and family in a timely fashion.
- Apply the scientific method to the development of CMPs. Use evidence-based practice.
- Base CMPs on the latest therapies, research outcomes, expert opinion, and recommendations/standards of professional societies.
- Use CMPs as standards of care. Develop and apply one CMP for each diagnosis or procedure.
- Use checklists or standardized tools to guide your work. This assures consistency and that quality and safety obligations are met.
- Include a disclaimer in the CMP explaining that it is only a recommended treatment plan and needs to be individualized to the patient's needs when applied. For example, a disclaimer might read: *"This case management plan is a suggested interdisciplinary plan of care. It is a guideline that may be changed and individualized according to patient condition and needs."*

In their training, case managers are prepared to handle resistance to change and change-resistant people. Their coaching, mentoring, and teaching approach to staff when facing resistance makes them able to conquer problems. They are well aware that resistance is a normal coping mechanism some people choose to follow when experiencing change and uncertainty. Their professional and mature approach to such situations makes it easier to convince staff to support the change. Case managers are also trained in problem solving, conflict resolution, and negotiation. These skills help

CASE MANAGER'S TIP 4.16

Instituting Effective Change

- Become familiar with change theories and processes.
- Recognize and foster the attitude that change is inevitable.
- Learn the goals and objectives of the change happening at your institution. Communicate them to all those involved.
- Give special consideration to all the aspects of change: physical, emotional, conceptual, perceptual, individual, organizational, and financial.
- Acknowledge that an organization cannot change unless most of the staff buy into the change, and that there will always be some who resist change.
- Reduce turf battles.
- Educate all staff about the change, reasons, goals, benefits, new processes/systems, mission, and philosophy.
- As a case manager, act as a change agent, champion, coach, and mentor.
- Identify and communicate the benefits of change.
- Avoid surprises. Be as open and transparent as possible.
- Keep lines of communication open. Invite questions and provide answers.
- Invite participation of all those interested. Encourage and support them in promoting the change.
- Admit to difficulties. Seek support and assistance.
- Attend to those resistant to change. Investigate their reasons and concerns. Consider their recommendations for improving the situation.
- Recognize and reward everybody's efforts regardless of their position in the organization or degree of participation. Every little effort is important.
- Involve informal leaders and those who are powerful.
- Maintain ongoing follow-up and reinforcement.
- Establish/clarify new policies, procedures, and standards.
- Establish an open forum for communication and dissemination of information.

improve their outlook and their strategies for preventing resistance. They also help them to build a better response to staff concerns.

Case managers are the main advocates for case management systems an institution is lucky to have. Case managers' commitment to their role and their hard work make them successful and help them to attain excellence in their practice.

4.2.12. Holistic Care Provider

Case managers attend to their patients as whole systems (i.e., biopsychosocial systems). They assess patients and families for any actual or potential health problems regardless of the chief complaint or the disease for which they are being treated (Case Manager's Tip 4.17). They are savvy in their evaluation of the patient's condition; they identify the physical, psychological, financial, and spiritual needs and make sure that these needs are incorporated into the CMP/ interdisciplinary plan of care. For example, when a patient is admitted to the hospital for uncontrolled diabetes, case managers not only assess dietary habits, blood glucose levels, and compliance with insulin and follow-up visits, but they also assess the patient for complications of diabetes such as deficiency in vision and foot ulcers. In addition, they assess footwear, skin care, support systems, adjustment to the disease, and insurance and benefits.

Case managers ensure that disease prevention and lifestyle changes are addressed with their patients and families. They work with them closely to identify the best strategies to improve compliance with the medical/surgical regimen and disease risk reduction. For example, they may counsel a cardiac patient on strategies for quitting smoking and consuming alcohol or beginning a physical exercise program. They may provide patients and families with important information regarding community services and support groups for the same purpose.

4.2.13. Counselor

Another role of case managers is counseling and support of patients and families (Case Manager's Tip 4.18). Case managers are attentive to the emotional and spiritual needs of patients. They are astute at providing patients with emotional support, and they counsel them regarding adjustment to hospitalization and their coping skills and mechanisms with the disease—particularly if patients are suffering from a chronic disease that requires frequent hospitalization, such as cancer.

Case managers may also work closely with victims of domestic violence and sexual and physical abuse. Their counseling skills and emotional support to these groups of vulnerable patients are highly appreciated. They also ensure that these patients are well educated regarding availability of crisis teams and how they can be accessed, and they direct them to local agencies or

 CASE MANAGER'S TIP 4.17

Providing Holistic Patient Care

- Deal with the patient as a biopsychosocial being.
- Develop an action plan that meets all of the patient's symptoms, preferences, and needs rather than just the disease.
- Attend not only to the patient's actual needs but also to the potential ones.
- Educate the patient about health promotion activities and strategies for disease risk reduction.
- Promote a healthy lifestyle.
- Incorporate complimentary and alternative care modalities into the case management plan of care.
- When dealing with the patient, do not forget about the family or the caregiver.
- Evaluate the impact of the patient's illness on the patient-family system and relationship, not just the patient.
- Encourage a healthy adjustment to illness (patient and family related).
- Include health promotion activities in the CMP.

 CASE MANAGER'S TIP 4.18

Effective Counseling

- Evaluate the patient's and family's ability to cope with and respond and adjust to illness.
- Alleviate anxieties and apprehension.
- Address the patient's and family's spiritual, emotional, social, and psychological needs.
- Conduct or arrange for therapy/counseling sessions.
- Communicate therapeutically, patiently, compassionately, and effectively.
- Allow for questions and provide answers.
- Attend to patient and family concerns.
- Alleviate the patient's fears and concerns regarding care after discharge.
- Coach and guide patients in problem solving and coflict resolution rather than attempting to resolve their concerns independent of them.
- Apply motivational interviewing techniques in your counseling efforts.
- Avoid being judgmental or critical.

support groups for further follow-up and support after discharge from the hospital or emergency department.

4.2.14. Utilization Manager

Utilization management (see Chapter 5) is an integral component of case management. It helps contain cost and ensures the provision of appropriate care at the right level and in the appropriate setting. It is a technique used by case managers to ensure that the patient meets predefined criteria to support the level of care being delivered. These criteria are national guidelines applied particularly by MCOs/health insurance plans and are agreed on with the providers and payers during managed care contract negotiations. Examples of these guidelines are InterQual criteria, which are mostly used for Medicare and Medicaid populations; and Milliman Guidelines, which are mainly used for patients with managed care or commercial health insurance plans. By applying the criteria present in these guidelines, the case manager ensures reimbursement for services provided.

Utilization management is a predominant function in hospital-based case management models. Case managers usually collaborate with members of the interdisciplinary team in transitioning the patient to the appropriate level of care to prevent reimbursement *denials*. Case managers also communicate with other case managers in the MCOs/health insurance plans either daily or periodically regarding the services being rendered and based on the contractual agreement which usually includes a specific clause(s) about utilization management procedures. This communication is called *concurrent review*, and its purpose is to obtain certifications/authorizations for the plan of care before delivering the necessary services. This process is important because it reviews, monitors, evaluates, and certifies the allocation of healthcare resources and services. Case managers apply the utilization management process for the following purposes:

- Examining the patient's *severity of illness*
- Identifying the *intensity of services*
- Precertification of services
- Authorizations for continued/extended length of stay
- Transitional planning and approval of post-discharge services
- Transitioning patients from one level of care to another of lesser intensity
- Transferring patients from one healthcare facility to another
- Timely delivery of services
- Reimbursement

Case managers in commercial health insurance plans/MCOs get involved in utilization management mainly because of their role in telephone triage. In this role, they direct patients to access healthcare services at the appropriate setting; that is, they act as gatekeepers. They also certify the delivery of services requested by other case managers who work for the provider. They do this during the patient care review process, before or during the delivery of care.

4.2.15. Transitional Planner

Transitional planning (see Chapter 6), also sometimes referred to as *discharge planning*, is another predominant function of case managers in the hospital-based setting. It focuses on brokering post-discharge services for patients and their families or caregivers. These services apply to the varied settings across the *continuum of care*. Transitional planning also involves a team approach to care planning, delivery, monitoring, and evaluation. Similar to utilization management, it is integrated with the case management process. Case managers design the transitional plan in collaboration with the interdisciplinary healthcare team and based on the patient's:

- Treatment plan
- Clinical condition
- Financial status and health insurance plan
- Support system
- Ability for self-care management
- Post-discharge services and medical regimen
- Need for rehabilitative services
- Discharge location

Case managers engage in ongoing assessment and reassessment of the patient's condition, progress and needs. They identify any changes and incorporate them in the transitional plan as necessary. They make these efforts to ensure timely, safe, cost-effective, and quality discharge. As they exercise this function of their role, case managers apply the laws and regulations (federal and state) and the standards of accreditation agencies and ensure adherence to these expectations. If they identify any issues, concerns, or problems, they address them accordingly. Sometimes they conduct case conferences with the patient and family and the team for this purpose.

Pursuant to transitional planning, case managers refer patients for evaluation by specialist providers such as physical therapy, nutrition, home care, and social services. These referrals are essential for the development of an appropriate and safe discharge plan and to maintain compliance with the regulations. However, the case manager remains responsible for ensuring that referrals and evaluations are completed in a timely manner and that recommendations from the specialist providers are discussed by the healthcare team and incorporated in the transitional/discharge plan as deemed necessary.

4.2.16. Ethicist

Case managers have long defined themselves as patient advocates. In this role they constantly face ethical dilemmas and challenges. Today's managed care environment has brought about new ethical problems such as inaccessibility to care and denials of services. As coordinators and managers of patient care, case managers are obliged to address and resolve these issues. However, they are not expected to resolve them alone; they do consult with ethics specialists for this purpose.

Case managers usually bring ethical dilemmas to the attention of the healthcare team and facilitate their resolution by looking out and advocating for patients and their families and by assisting the team in making decisions that are in the best interest of the patient. Because these deliberations are usually challenging, case managers rely on the guidance of ethicists.

In dealing with ethical dilemmas, case managers apply the principles of autonomy, beneficence, justice, veracity, and nonmaleficence. They also apply the code of ethics of their profession (e.g., nursing, social work) and that of the Commission for Case Manager Certification, especially if certified and hold the Certified Case Manager credential. These codes guide the case managers in the process of ethical decision making and problem solving (see Chapter 18).

4.3. ROLES OF THE CASE MANAGER IN VARIED SETTINGS

Case management models have been implemented in every setting along the continuum of care. This makes the case manager's role available in all settings as well. Although the care settings are different, the basic functions and responsibilities of case managers are essentially the same. The case management process discussed previously acts as a generic process for all settings and shares the important elements of case management that can be slightly modified and individualized to the specific care setting. The main focus of case management services differs between settings. These differences explain the variations of the role.

Case managers apply different iterations of the case management process depending on the setting they are employed in and the focus of the case management model. For example:

- Acute care focuses on *utilization review* and transitional planning.
- Admitting department focuses on appropriateness and patients' eligibility for admission to the hospital.
- Emergency department focuses on gatekeeping and appropriateness of patients' admission to the hospital.
- Peri-operative care focuses on patients' readiness and eligibility for surgery, appropriateness for ambulatiory surgery, and ability to meet criteria for inpatient hospital stay if they are to be admitted.
- Community-based care focuses on primary care, wellness, prevention, and health maintenance.
- Home care focuses on chronic care management and self-care management while in the home.
- Subacute care focuses on restoration and rehabilitation of function.
- Long-term care focuses on chronic and supportive care management.
- Disease management focuses on population risk stratification and reduction and chronic care management.
- Ambulatory care clinics and patient centered medical homes focus on wellness, illness prevention, management of chronic illnesses with the aim to prevent deterioration in condition, and the need for admission to acute care setting.
- Managed care focuses on utilization management, *demand management*, and gatekeeping.
- *Telephonic case management* focuses on giving advice, triage, and gatekeeping.
- Independent/private case management focuses on disability and rehabilitation care management.
- *Workers' compensation* focuses on rehabilitation and vocational services and return-to-work planning.

Case management activities in all of these settings include aspects of clinical care management, utilization management, and transitional planning. However, the main focus may differ depending on the setting. For example, in MCOs, the main aspect of the case manager's role is utilization management. Table 4.3 presents examples of these functions as they relate to the specific setting. The list is not exhaustive, and further descriptions of the varied models can be found in Chapter 3.

TABLE 4.3. Examples of Case Manager Roles in Varied Settings.

Care Setting	Examples of Case Management Roles and Activities
Acute Care	■ Obtain authorizations for services and resources ■ Develop and implement plan of care and discharge/transitional plan ■ Conduct concurrent utilization reviews with commercial hesalth insurance plans/MCOs ■ Facilitate interdisciplinary plan of care and communication ■ Educate patient and family regarding care and post-dischrge needs ■ Transition patients across necessary levels of care and based on patient's condition and needs ■ Expedite diagnostic and therapeutic tests and procedures ■ Conduct case conferences and patient/ family counseling ■ Complete post-discharge follow-up call/check on patient/family ■ Communciate with primary care provider or medical home
Admitting Department	■ Assess patients for eligibility of admission ■ Obtain authorization for services ■ Initiate the assessment of preadmission services and potential post-discharge needs ■ Develop preliminary transitional plan ■ Suggest use of alternate level of care
Emergency Department	■ Provide timely care and services ■ Arrange for community resources ■ Provide counseling for patients and families ■ Plan patient's admission or discharge ■ Suggest use of alternate level of care ■ Expedite tests and procedures ■ Assure follow-up care appoints scheduled ■ Communicate with primary care provider or medical home
Perioperative	■ Complete preadmission tests ■ Evaluate post-discharge needs and establish transitional plan ■ Discuss discharge options with patient, family, caregiver, and healthcare team ■ Provide psychosocial counseling to patient and family ■ Obtain authorization for services ■ Ensure patient's readiness for surgery: tests, medical clearance, insurance, approval, consent ■ Adjust operating room schedule ■ Address operating room delays and cancellations ■ Facilitate patient's tranfer to an inpatient bed or discharge home
Ambulatory Care/ Patient Centered Medcal Home	■ Support patient and family to achieve optimal state of wellness and functioning ■ Provide primary care and primary prevention services ■ Conduct patient and family education and counseling sessions ■ Implement strategies that aim to enhance patient engagement and self-care management ■ Coordinate use of community-based resources ■ Prevent need for acute care and services ■ Stratify patients/population into risk groups and provide case management services accordingly ■ Focus on strategies for health risk reduction ■ Engage in telephonic case management ■ Promote healthy lifestyle and behavior ■ Implement case management strategies for patients with multiple chronic illnesses and polypharmacy ■ Oversee the role of community health worker

(continued)

TABLE 4.3 (continued). Examples of Case Manager Roles in Varied Settings.

Care Setting	Examples of Case Management Roles and Activities
Home Care	■ Provide postacute care services such as wound care, dressing changes, administration of IV antibiotics, infusion therapy ■ Prevent unplanned readmission to hospitals or emergency department ■ Promote self-care management skills ■ Provide patient and family education regarding healthcare needs and services ■ Coordinate care from home setting with physician and other specialty providers such as physical therapist ■ Monitor treatments rendered by other providers such as infusion therapy, home health aide, social worker ■ Evaluate safety of home environment ■ Coordinate use of durable medical equipment ■ Communicate with health insurance plan/MCOs
Subacute	■ Provide services such as weaning from respirators, IV antibiotic therapy, extensive wound management ■ Provide restorative and rehabilitative services ■ Coordinate care and services with physician and other providers/interdisciplinary team ■ Obtain authorizations for services ■ Establish and implement transitional plan ■ Handle end-of-life issues and decisions, palliative, and hospice care
Long-Term Care	■ Provide skilled care ■ Provide supportive care and services ■ Communicate and follow-up with physicians and other providers on ongoing basis, considering that primary care provider may not examine patient on daily basis ■ Counsel patients and families as needed
Disease Management	■ Ensure safety in delivery of care and management environment ■ Conduct risk stratification surveys for population served ■ Stratify patients into risk categories ■ Provide case management services based on needs of each risk group ■ Provide telephone support services ■ Educate patients and families regarding medical regimen, self-care management, risk reduction strategies ■ Manage populations with chronic diseases such as asthma, renal failure, HIV/AIDS, heart failure, premature babies ■ Transition patients across continuum of care as needed ■ Coordinate care in collaboration with interdisciplinary healthcare team ■ Facilitate and expedite care and services
Managed Care and Commercial Health Insurance	■ Coordinate demand management services ■ Conduct health surveys ■ Provide preventive screening services such as mammography, hypertension, cholesterol ■ Distribute patient and family education newsletter and materials ■ Provide gatekeeping services ■ Authorize/certify services ■ Engage in managed care contract preparation and negotiation
Telephonic	■ Triage patients according to need ■ Facilitate access to healthcare services ■ Act as gatekeeper ■ Provide advice over the telephone ■ Assess patient's condition and needs and coordinate care accordingly ■ Communicate patient's needs to physician and other providers ■ Use algorithms to help in decision making ■ Provide psychosocial counseling services

(continued)

TABLE 4.3 (continued). Examples of Case Manager Roles in Varied Settings.

Care Setting	Examples of Case Management Roles and Activities
Independent/Private	■ Provide case management services to MCOs and providers of healthcare facilities ■ Manage patient's plan of care and clinical and financial services ■ Obtain authorizations for services ■ Advocate for patient and family ■ Coordinate rehabilitative and restorative services ■ Transition patient along continuum of care ■ Facilitate return-to-work plan ■ Represent patient, provider, or payer, depending on contractual agreement ■ Facilitate communication among different providers ■ Implement complex plan of care and services
Workers' Compensation	■ Manage care of on-the-job injured patients ■ Collaborate with occupational health department, risk management, human resources, and lawyers ■ Establish and implement plan of care and transitional plan ■ Coordinate complex plan of care and services and return-to-work plan ■ Obtain authorizations for services ■ Expedite diagnostic and therapeutic procedures ■ Manage patient's benefits ■ Facilitate provision of disability and rehabilitation services ■ Provide psychosocial counseling to patient and family

4.4. THE SOCIAL WORKER AS CASE MANAGER

As in most clinical arenas, the role of the social work case manager varies greatly from one care delivery setting to the next and is based on the patient population served. Nevertheless, certain elements are considered fundamental to the differentiation of social work case management from that performed by other professionals, in particular, nurse case managers. The National Association of Social Workers, in its social work case management standards (NASW, 2013) explains the work of social work case managers based on how the healthcare organization perceives the role case management plays in a patient's care, thus influencing organizational culture, service provision, the patient's experience, and ultimately outcomes. NASW defines case management as a process that highlights the roles a social work case manager assumes while caring for patients. These include planning care for the patient and seeking, advocating for, and monitoring the services a patient may need from different healthcare organizations and at various care settings (NASW, 2013).

One can then describe social work case management as a method of providing services to patients within and outside a specific healthcare setting, whereby a professional social worker assesses the needs of the patient and the patient's family/caregiver when appropriate and arranges for what the patient needs especially postdischarge from an episode of care. The social worker arranges, coordinates, monitors, evaluates, and advocates for a package of multiple services to meet the specific complex needs of clients. Social workers may be found to practice case management in a broad-range of specialties and settings (Box 4.2).

Box 4.2 Social Work Case Management

Specialties and settings of social work case managers

Specialties

■ Aging
■ Behavioral health including mental health and substance use
■ Child welfare and other youth and family oriented services
■ Patients with disabilities: cognitive, developmental, physical, and psychiatric
■ Disease specific
■ Palliative and hospice/end-of-life care
■ Income support services

Settings

■ Corrections facilities
■ Schools, especially at early childhood
■ Employee assistance programs (organization-based)
■ Healthcare settings: acute, rehabilitative, ambulatory, community, long-term care
■ Public health
■ Shelter and temporary housing, group homes
■ Veterans and active duty, military
■ Tribal

Social work case managers distinguish themselves from other case management professionals by addressing the client's biopsychosocial status and the state of the social system in which case management operates. Social work case managers develop therapeutic relationships with their clients and may link them to other services that they may require.

Nurse case managers and social workers collaborate to ensure a patient's safe and quality care including post-discharge services. Often they work as dyads especially in the acute care setting. When found together on a interdisciplinary care team, they each assume clearly defined responsibilities, yet at the same time shared responsibility for some functions.

- *Nurse case manager responsibilities*: tend to be driven by the nursing scope of practice, education, and professional background of the nurse in the role. These may include coordination and facilitation of care activities , resources, services, and interventions, clinical discharge/transitional planning, utlization review and management, readmissions assessments, and management of care delays or variances.

- *Social worker responsibilities*: tend to be driven by the social work scope of practice, education, and professional background of the social worker. These may include psychosocial counseling, crisis intervention, social discharge/transitional planning, financial assistance (e.g., Medicaid application and charity care).

- *Shared responsibilities*: these are broad activities or functions that are common to both nursing and social work scope of practice and therefore can be assumed by either the nurse case manager, social worker, or both. Examples are patient and family eductaion and health behavior counseling and the evaluation of safe and quality outcomes including addressing discharge or transition delays.

Perhaps the most fundamental difference between the social worker as case manager and the nurse as case manager is the deeper focus on the patient's entire social system. Examples in Table 4.4 and Table 4.5 clarify this difference. The other steps in the case management process are consistent to both groups. In addition, social workers have certain values unique to their profession. These include the primacy of the cli-

TABLE 4.4. Guidelines for Referrals: Case Managers and Social Workers, Emergency Department.

RN Case Manager	Shared Responsibilities: RN Case Manager/Social Worker	Social Worker
■ Admission utilization review: Intake assessment of admitted patients ■ Utilization/insurance calls ■ Coordinate/facilitate plans of care for admitted patients ■ Screening/assessments of patients for psychosocial needs in conjunction with plan of care ■ Discharge planning including equipment, home care, infusion treatment ■ Initiate inpatient discharge planning ■ Participates in the development of ED guidelines for care ■ Tracks data (e.g., variances in patient care standards, systems standards) ■ Clinical resource for staff ■ Facilitates patients' progress through the ED to disposition ■ Oversees/facilitates transfers from institution to institution	■ Coordinate/facilitate plans of care for discharged patients ■ Transportation ■ Patient education (e.g., reinforcement regarding follow-up with medical appointments, medical regimen) ■ Crisis intervention needed for patient/family having difficulty coping with illness, family dysfunction, trauma, death, accidents, injuries, substance abuse ■ Referrals for nursing homes, adult homes, shelters	■ Patient/family having difficulty understanding/ accepting and/or following through on medical plans of care and continuing care options ■ Interventions regarding issues impacting the ability to access the continuum of care (e.g., immigration problem, primary caregiver, or disabled person) ■ Advocacy and counseling around entitlements or other essential services (e.g., Medicaid, food stamps, housing, medications) ■ Suspicion or evidence of domestic violence, elder abuse or neglect, child abuse or neglect, sexual assault ■ Ethical or legal concerns (e.g., patient, family, team conflicts related to medical plan of care, guardianship or APS cases, end-of-life issues around Advance Directives) ■ Referrals for home supports for psychosocially complex patients ■ Referrals needed for marital, individual, or family treatment ■ Assistance needed in locating families of unidentified, seriously ill patients ■ Tracking difficult to locate patients for follow-up medical care

APS, Adult Protective Services

TABLE 4.5. RN Case Managers and Social Workers, Maternal Child Inpatient Units.

RN Case Manager	Social Worker
▪ Performs admission and concurrent utilization management, including insurance calls ▪ Coordinates/facilitates plans of care ▪ Facilitates daily rounds and team meetings ▪ Assesses all patients for psychosocial needs ▪ Discharge planning, including equipment, home care, rehabilitation, and long-term care facilities ▪ Orders transportation ▪ Discharge planning forms ▪ Oversight of clinical guidelines ▪ Tracks data (e.g., variances in patient care, and systems standards) ▪ Provides alternate level of care notification	▪ Patient/family difficulty coping with diagnosis, lifestyle changes; difficulty understanding/accepting decision making with long-term discharge planning and/or continuing care options ▪ Psychiatric, cognitive, or behavioral factors that may impede delivery of care and discharge planning process ▪ Inadequate supports that may impact on compliance with continuing care needs (social workers can offer information to case managers regarding entitlements for patients/families) ▪ Ethical or legal concerns (e.g., patient, family, team conflicts related to medical plan of care, guardianship cases, or end-of-life issues around Advance Directives such as DNR) ▪ Suspicion or evidence of domestic violence, abuse or neglect, rape, sexual assault ▪ History of poor medical compliance (e.g., lack of prenatal care, late registration, late immunizations) ▪ Advocacy around entitlements and community social services ▪ Drug or alcohol abuse ▪ Cannot afford medications and no plan for access in near future ▪ Bereavement (e.g., terminally ill child, fetal demise) ▪ Homelessness or unable to return to prior living situation ▪ Questionable parenting skills or interactions among family members ▪ Community referrals

ent's interests, respect for diversity, culture, and psychosocial dynamics; confidentiality, client self-determination; and respect.

Most acute care organizations have designed their case management program where the nurse case manager is the person of primary responsibility for overseeing a patient's case management services including coordination of the interdisciplinary plan of care. Social workers are then brought in when a patient/family has complex care planning needs (e.g., homeless, counseling for a life changing disease situation, psychosocial complexities, Medicaid application) and post-discharge services (e.g., placement in a skilled care facility, sub-acute rehabilitation, charity care). In these situations social workers and nurse case managers work collaboratively to meet the patient/family needs. In some specialties or settings, such as those described in Box 4.2, social workers may be found to function as the case manager with primary responsibility for case management services. This is true in the case of behavioral and mental health specialties including the acute care setting.

4.5. THE ADVANCED PRACTICE REGISTERED NURSE AS CASE MANAGER

Advanced practice registered nurses assuming the role of the case manager are both CNSs and nurse practitioners (NPs). Because of their educational backgrounds and training, each brings a different set of skills to the role and enhances it in specific ways. For example, NPs as case managers are more autonomous and independent in their practice compared with CNSs because of their prescriptive privileges and roles in primary care. Although in some states CNSs may have precriptive privileges, this is not a common practice throughout the United States. Both professionals bring special aspects of their preparation into the case manager's role as follows:

▪ *CNS*: expert clinician, educator, consultant, and researcher, with a main focus in acute care
▪ *NP*: expert clinician, health promotion and disease prevention, referrals to other services, reimbursement for care, and prescribing treatments, with

main focus on primary care in inpatient and outpatient settings

With their advanced education (i.e., master's degree or doctor in nursing practice), NPs and CNSs can effectively implement managed care and case management strategies for cost control and the provision of safe, cost-effective, and quality care. They can also function as change agents and care decision-makers. The success of the case management program/model relies heavily on the person who assumes the pivotal role of case manager. The CNS or NP as case manager ensures that the critical link between the patient, the payer, and the provider in the context of complex healthcare systems is kept as simple as possible and at a manageable level. Because of their advanced educational preparation, they are better able to tolerate the challenges of patient care management presented to them as case managers compared to those with a bachelor's degree. Their graduate education allows them to be more confident, knowledgeable, and skillful. Moreover, they demonstrate better skills than those prepared at the undergraduate educational level in problem solving, delegation, critical thinking, clinical judgment, negotiation, interdisciplinary collaboration, and outcomes evaluation.

The case manager role assumed by CNSs and NPs is not any different from the role discussed in this chapter. However, one challenge of the use of advanced practice nurses in the role of the case manager is the area of financial management. Educational programs of both NPs and CNSs lack courses in financial management, cost accounting, and cost-benefit analysis. Because of this limitation, cost control as an aspect of the case manager's role presents some challenges. Therefore healthcare organizations using CNSs or NPs as case managers must prepare them in this area. Suggested focus is training in cost of care, charges, expenses, revenue and loss analysis, and reimbursement methods. Although case managers may spend 5%–10% of their time in financial management, this aspect makes their role more powerful.

4.6. A DAY IN THE LIFE OF THE CASE MANAGER

In their various roles, functions, and responsibilities, it is highly important for case managers to be able to work efficiently and effectively with the interdisciplinary healthcare team members. Teamwork, cooperation, collaboration, and accountability are essential at all times and in all situations. In addition, case managers are expected to be skilled in time man-

agement, organization, prioritization of work and responsibilities, and follow-up on issues until closure or resolution. Their role is a challenging one, particularly because their priorities change throughout the day as a result of changes in patients' conditions, priorities of the interdisciplinary team, or priorities of the healthcare organization.

Box 4.3 provides a generic example of a day in the life of a hospital-based case manager. This example is a concise version of what needs to be accomplished daily by case managers. It can be used by those who are new to the role or struggling with how to survive their busy day. It can also be used as a structure for prioritizing what needs to be done on a certain day and as a tool for time management and improving productivity. When electing to apply this example in their daily activities, case managers are advised to adjust the example to meet the constantly changing needs of their patients. In addition, they are urged to reprioritize their task lists to meet the changing demands of their patients.

4.7. ORGANIZING YOUR DAY AS A CASE MANAGER

It seems that every year case managers are asked to take on more and more roles and functions. Every time a new rule or regulation comes out from the CMS, administrators turn to case management as the group to take the new problem or task on. This translates to more work! How many of us have heard the age-old phrase "give it to the case managers. They're already in the charts!" This kind of logic is a throwback to the time when case management was actually utilization review, and utilization review managers (case managers) spent their work days reviewing medical records. But times have changed and now case managers are an integral part of the interdisciplinary care team. As with any professional group or specialty, there is a finite amount of work that case managers can do, and do effectively with positive outcomes for their patients and the organization they work for.

4.7.1. A Routine for the Hospital Case Manager

In order to understand the workflow for a case manager, we need to first understand that the work we perform in the case management process is not linear. Linear work, such as that performed in a factory for example, follows a course that is not deviated from. As Toyota builds a car, the process of car building follows a strict algorithm and any deviation is considered a failure in terms of quality. In our work as case managers, we

Box 4.3   A Day in the Life of a Case Manager

To be able to provide efficient and effective case management services for an entire group of patients, case managers may elect to follow the daily routine presented here as a guide.

This routine is only one example of how an acute care/hospital-based case manager may spend his or her day to ensure that the important tasks for the day are completed. When adopting this schedule of activities, one should be careful not to be rigid about the timeframes suggested. One should also be able to adjust this schedule to the specific organization, area of practice, specialty, and responsibilities of the role as delineated in the case manager's job description of the individual healthcare organization.

An important function of the case manager is priority setting. This function is essential for time management, organization of activities and responsibilities, and completing the most important tasks first. A case manager may decide to prioritize his/her activities based on quality, safety, and cost-effectiveness criteria. Case managers adopting this schedule of activities should factor in the need to revise their "to do" lists throughout their day based on the significant changes in the conditions of their patients and the constantly changing priorities. They ought to understand that the key here is flexibility and fluidity.

8:00 A.M.–9:30 A.M.

- Report to your assigned unit or area.
- Print and check the patient census for your unit or assigned beds. You should have your case management software configured so that you can print out your assigned area with little difficulty every morning. If you don't have case management software, then your admission/discharge /transfer (ADT) system should be able to create a similar census report for you daily.
- Review the patients in your assigned area. Identify which patients were newly admitted or transferred to your unit since yesterday, and which patients were discharged since yesterday.
- Print face sheets for new admissions or transfers and place them in your binder as discussed above.
- For patients transferred to your unit, request report from the transferring case manager.
- Review your notes from the day before to see what tasks you left for completion today on existing patients.
- Review the medical records of any patients new to you, including transfers and new admissions. As you read the medical record review the following data sets:
    —What brought the patient to the hospital?
    —Was this a 30 day readmission?
    —Is the patient insured—by whom?
    —What are the patient's support systems?
    —Where does the patient live?
    —What is the expected length of stay?
    —If available, review laboratory, diagnostic, and other tests results.
    —Review physician and nursing notes.
    —Identify the patient's route of entry to the hospital.
- Jot down any questions or points of clarification you may have for the interdisciplinary care rounds.

9:30 A.M.–10:30 A.M.

- Interdisciplinary care rounds take place during this time slot. They should occur daily at the same time.
- Rounds may take place in a conference room or you may have walking rounds. Walking rounds are considered best practice and are a much more efficient and effective way to conduct rounds.
- If you are conducting walking rounds, bring your notebook with the face sheets in it. Have your questions ready for the interdisciplinary team. Core team members should be on rounds including the physician, the staff nurse, the nurse manager, the case manager, and the social worker if possible. As discussed in prior months, the case manager and social worker should provide relevant information on rounds including the expected length of stay, the anticipated discharge plan, and any barriers to care or discharge such as insurance issues or family dynamics. This is also your opportunity to gather additional information on the patient and ask any questions of the rest of the team. Rounds are an opportunity to give as well as receive information.
- Once the patient information has been reviewed in the hall, the team should go into the patient's room and introduce themselves. Allow the patient to ask any questions, but set time limits. If the patient needs additional time, tell the patient that you will come back after rounds are completed.
- Review the patient and their environment visibly. Check the patient's affect and mental status. Check for intravenous lines, Foley catheters, or other drains or devices. Ask them if they have gotten out of bed, and if they have eaten. This will help you when you do your clinical review later.

- Make a note of any additional information you may need or referrals you may need to make.
- Request any discharge orders for the day that have not been written.
- Request any physician orders that need to be written.
- Complete your admission documentation on newly admitted patients. Use your case management admission form.
- Refer any cases that meet psychosocial high risk criteria to the social worker.

10:30 A.M.–10:45 A.M.

- This may be a good time to take a 15 minute break, if possible.

10:45 A.M.–12:00 P.M.

This can be the busiest time of the day for case managers. Both discharging of patients and clinical reviews will need to be completed.

- Begin the discharge process for patients leaving today. Be sure that you have discharge orders for the day's discharges.
- Ensure transportation has been arranged and ask nursing to complete discharge paperwork. Discuss any last discharge issues with the patient/family.
- Your goal should be to have today's discharges out of the hospital by 12 P.M. whenever possible. Some patients may have to stay later if a diagnostic test result is pending. Facilitate obtaining those results so that the discharge can be expedited.
- During this time slot you will need to complete clinical reviews for those third party payers who require their review by 12 P.M. You should know what your cut-off times are for each payer and adjust your work accordingly. If you do not complete the clinical review by the expected time, as per your contracts, you risk a denial of payment to the hospital.
- Based on your admission assessment and/or daily assessment, make referrals to home care as appropriate.
- If any patients are going to other levels of care such as acute rehab, subacute or long-term care, discuss their options with them. For skilled nursing facilities and home care, give them the list of choices of agencies and facilities and let them know that you will come back later in the day to discuss their choices and answer any questions they may have.

12:00 P.M.–1:00 P.M.: Lunch break

1:00 P.M.–2:30 P.M.

- If any tests, treatments, consults or other referrals are delayed, expedite these by contacting the appropriate department or discipline.
- Identify tomorrow's discharges and obtain discharge orders and prescriptions when possible.
- Conduct any discharge education needed to prepare patients who are pending discharges.
- Alert the staff nurse to pending discharges so that clinical education can be completed.
- Order transportation as needed and/or notify the family of the time they should arrive to pick up the patient.
- Provide a verbal as well as written hand-off to the next level of care.
- Complete any additional clinical reviews, particularly Medicare patients.
- Review the "choice list" with any patients who received the list that morning and/or provide a list to any patients newly identified.
- Document progress notes in medical record.

2:30 P.M.–2:45 P.M.: 15 minute break

2:45 P.M.–3:00 P.M.: Conduct "mini-rounds"

This is a good time in the afternoon to conduct mini-rounds. Mini-rounds are a quicker, less detailed version of the morning rounds with a smaller number of team members. The purpose of these rounds is to follow up on any issues that arose during morning rounds that needed a quick intervention and resolution. For example, a patient may have needed to have an MRI expedited. During rounds whoever was responsible for this can report on the outcome.

The case manager, social worker, staff nurse, and case manager should participate in these rounds. They can be done quickly and informally. Only the patients who had issues from the morning are discussed, so this is a small sub-set of all your patients. Mini-rounds help to save time because by planning to have them every day, you do not need to chase after team members throughout the day to give or receive updates. You can wait until mini-rounds to close the loop on any of these issues.

3:00 P.M.–4:00 P.M.

This is the time to wrap up your day. Any remaining issues should be completed at this time.

- Review your caseload and be sure that you have completed everything you needed to for the day.
- Be sure that you have documented in your patient's medical records where necessary.
- Continue with any needed patient education regarding the discharge plan.
- Talk with any family members who may be present at the patient's bedside.

- Make any needed follow up phone calls to patents discharged on the prior day. Ensure that they received any planned for services and answer any questions they may have. Ask the following questions:
  —Did home care arrive?
  —Did durable medical equipment arrive (DME)?
  —Did you fill your prescriptions?
  —Are you taking your medications as prescribed?
  —Do you have any questions regarding your medications?
  —When is your next doctor's appointment?
  —Do you have a way to get to that appointment?
  —Do you have any questions?

In addition, case managers conduct patient care rounds informally with the attending physicians when they visit their patients, and they discuss the plans of care. They attend to emergency situations as they arise. They also collect data about core measures and track patient care variances/delays in care and follow-up on resolutions of problems identified. Case managers are also expected to collaborate with other disciplines (e.g., utilization review, social work, nutrition, physical therapy) as needed. They may also attend certain meetings (e.g., case management departmental meetings, patient/family teaching committee, CMP development teams, grandrounds) and conduct staff inservice education regarding case management as needed.

need to follow a process but we also need to appreciate that sometimes work has to be repeated. This means that we sometimes have to circle back to functions we have already performed and either repeat them again or perform them in a different way or in a different order.

Despite the fact that our work is not linear, we still need to have structure to it. A work structure is important because it ensures that we don't forget anything or unnecessarily repeat work. So, organization is the name of the game. Keeping yourself organized is the surest way to complete your work and get satisfaction from completing it.

4.7.2. Overall Structure for the Day

As healthcare professionals, we know that every day will be different and that each day may bring new and different challenges. By organizing your day, you will allow room for the unexpected snags that will invariably come up. When you were a staff nurse, your day was organized around medication administration, treatments, and paperwork. As a case manager, the work functions are different and do not immediately lend themselves to a time structure. Nevertheless, some of what we do is time limited. This means that some routine work must be completed by a certain time of the day. Examples of this include clinical reviews, today's discharges, and daily rounds as some examples.

4.7.3. Organizing the Patient Assignment/Caseload: Use a Binder!

One of the tools that can be very helpful to you is a binder with your patient's "face sheets" in it. Depend-

ing on the case management software that you use, there may be a different name for this document. The document should include the patient's demographics such as address, insurance information, next of kin, and so forth. The binder should be organized with a section for each of your patient's face sheets. Each section should represent a bed number. You can use this face sheet in the binder to jot down anything you need to remind yourself to do for that day or during the course of the hospitalization. You can take it on rounds with you and refer to it. You can refer to it when asked a question about one of your patients. It is impossible to remember everything and things move very quickly. By jotting down notes to yourself, you don't need to spend wasted time trying to remember things or running back to the electronic medical record (EMR) every time you need to refresh your memory. Once the patient is discharged, you can simply discard the form as it is not a permanent part of the medical record.

4.7.4. Organizing Your Day

Let's plan our day around an eight hour shift. If your day is longer or shorter than this, you can adjust accordingly. Let's also assume that you have some version of case management software. If you do not have case management software, then you can still obtain the data sets mentioned here through your information technology (IT) systems (see Box 4.3).

4.8. INTERDISCIPLINARY PATIENT CARE MANAGEMENT ROUNDS

Interdisciplinary patient care management rounds, in-

TABLE 4.6. Sample Daily Patient Care Management Rounds Checklist.

Key aspects of Rounds	Person/Role Responsible for Reporting	Status	Action Plan/Follow Up Items
Patient name			
Date and day of week			
Attending in charge and team	MD/PA/NP		
Identified surrogate/caregiver (if needed)	MD/PA/NP		
Goals of care (aggressive/palliative/unknown/other)	MD/PA/NP		
Expected discharge disposition place (e.g., home, rehabilitation)	CM/SW		
Out of bed in prior 24 hours? Walking? If not, why not?	RN		
Catheters/IVs/pressure ulcers injuries/nutritional status/other devices	RN		
Working DRG/diagnosis	MD/PA/NP		
Expected LOS	MD/PA/NP		
Day of hospitalization (e.g., day 1, 2, 3, . . .)	CM/SW		
Expected discharge date	MD/PA/NP		
What happened in past 24 hours?	MD/RN		
Plan for next 24 hours. What can the team expedite? What can be done as an outpatient?	MD/PA/NP		
Pending results of tests and consults? How will they impact the plan of care?	MD/PA/NP		
Medications review: All current medication. Convert to PO? Discontinue? Home infusion?	MD/PA/NP/ Pharmacist		
Barriers to next level of care/discharge (clinical, functional, social, economic)?	MD/SW/CM/RN/ PA/ NP		

CM, Case Manager; DRG, Diagnosis Related Group; IV, Intravenous; LOS, Length of Stay; NP, Nurse Practitioner; PA, Physician Assistant; PO, Given Orally; RN, Registered Nurse; SW, Social Worker

cluding bedside rounds, have become a key component of any contemporary case management department or nursing department. They are considered best practice by both the Institute for Healthcare Improvement (IHI) (Institute for Healthcare Improvement, 2015) and the TJC. Rounds should occur at the same time each morning and should be considered mandatory for all members of the interdisciplinary healthcare team. Each member is able to contribute to patient care planning and progress toward achieving care goals. Table 4.6 provides a checklist case managers and other members of the team may use to guide them through having successful rounds. The checklist provides important aspects of patient care the team should address, the primary responsible party, and a way to document whether a need for follow-up arises.

4.8.1. The Rounding Process

The process includes a combination of reporting with the team in the hall outside the patient's room followed by a visit to the patient's bedside. While outside the patient's room the team can discuss issues of a clinical nature in more detail than they might at the patient's bedside. Each team member can provide insights and information from their point of view as well as patient care updates. When the team visits the patient at the bedside they can then introduce themselves and share the plan for the day as well as the discharge plan with the patient and family (if present). The team should use a structured approach for both the hall discussion as well as the bedside discussion with the patient and family.

CASE MANAGER'S TIP 4.19

The structure for the rounds discussion should look like this:

- What happened yesterday?
- What needs to happen today?
- What needs to happen to move the patient to discharge home or transition to another level of care?

The rounds leader can be any member of the interdisciplinary care team but should be the same person every day. This person's role is to keep the discussion on-point and to keep the process moving forward. The leader is typically the nurse manager, case manager, or physician (Case Manager's Tip 4.19).

By structuring the discussion in this way, each patient can be covered in approximately 60 seconds. Some patients may take a bit longer while others may be a bit shorter. The team does not need to discuss the patient's prior medical history unless it is relevant to the day's discussion. Only issues relevant to the clinical plan of care and discharge plan should be discussed in any detail. Should more detailed discussion be necessary, the team can return to that patient once the rounds have concluded.

The staff nurse is an integral part of rounds. Once her patients have been rounded on she can return to her patients and the next staff nurse can join in. The physician should also be an integral part of the rounds and should be in attendance if possible. This is easier in hosptials with hospitalists, interns, and residents. Even if a physician is not present the rounds should be conducted anyway (Case Manager's Tip 4.20).

4.8.2. Mini-Rounds

In the afternoon, a lighter version of the morning rounds should take place. These rounds should include the case manager, staff nurse, and nurse manager. The social worker should also be included if the patients to be discussed have been assigned to the social worker. Only patients that had outstanding issues in the morning need to be included in the mini-rounds discussion. Mini-rounds should take place at the same time each afternoon, just like morning rounds. They do not need to take place at the bedside.

4.9. SUCCESS IN THE ROLE OF CASE MANAGER

The role of the case manager is essential to the success

CASE MANAGER'S TIP 4.20

Talking Points for Interdisciplinary Rounds

Physician/staff nurse should discuss:

- The plan of care
- The expected outcomes of care
- The expected length of stay
- Discharge plan
- Barriers to care

Case manager should discuss:

- Status of discharge plan
- Barriers to care and to discharge
- Any reimbursement issues
- The expected length of stay (if different from above)

Social worker should discuss:

- Any psychosocial issues
- Any barriers to discharge or post-discharge services
- Any follow-up on discharge paperwork or concerns

Respiratory therapy/physical therapy/nutrition should discuss:

- Any interventions and goals of care
- Any barriers to care

---

of the case management system. It is the key to ensuring that cost-effective and high-quality, safe patient care is provided. This role is designed to maximize collaboration among all members of the healthcare team; integration of the services required for the care of each patient; coordination and facilitation of tests, procedures, and other patient care activities; continuity and consistency in the provision of care across care settings and services; and most importantly, the openness of lines of communication among all disciplines and on all levels. In addition, it is important for integrating the patient's, provider's, and payer's perspectives and interests in healthcare delivery and management.

The case manager's role is successful only when full support and commitment of healthcare executives and departmental leaders (e.g., nursing administrators, chief quality officers, chief financial officers) are evidenced and their belief in case management becomes part of the culture and values of the healthcare organization. The description of the role presented in Chapter 4 is extensive and could seem to be overwhelming in terms of the amount of responsibility that goes with the case manager's role. However, it is important to keep in mind when studying this role description that it is a thorough approach to the functions and responsibilities of case managers, while the reality is that the role may be limited to some of these functions or organized somewhat differently and based on the individual healthcare organization's interest. Healthcare executives are urged to evaluate this description and only adapt to their institution what seems to be appropriate to their needs based on their systems, procedures, policies, standards, operations, financial status, care settings, and, most importantly, the goals of their case management program, system, or model and what they are attempting to achieve through this role.

4.10. KEY POINTS

1. Case managers function as an integral part of the interdisciplinary healthcare team.
2. Case managers usually manage, coordinate, and facilitate patient care. They ensure timely patient and family teaching and discharge/transitional planning.
3. Case managers perform their role functions in virtually all healthcare settings across the continuum.
4. Case managers have many different roles and responsibilities, which are defined differently in each institution. Sometimes their responsibilities cross the boundaries of a particular care setting.
5. Social workers, in collaboration with case managers, play an important role in case managing the biopsychosocial needs of patients. Social workers may be found to assume the case manager role in the behavioral and mental health/psychiatric population.
6. Advanced practice nurses are emerging as case managers in a variety of care delivery settings.
7. Today, case managers work in all patient care settings. They are found to be effective in reducing length of stay and avoidable readmissions, assuring the delivery of quality, safe and cost-effective care, and improving performance on value-based purchasing measures including patient and family satisfaction/experience with care.
8. Case managers should be clinically competent and astute in time management, problem solving, negotiation, and teamwork.

4.11. REFERENCES

Ballew, J.R. & Mink, G. (1996). *Case management in social work*, Charles C. Thomas, Springfield, IL.

Institute for Healthcare Improvement. (2015). *How-To Guide: Multidisciplinary Rounds*, Cambridge, MA.

National Association of Social Workers. (2013). *NASW standards for social work case management*, Washington, DC.

5

Utilization Management

5.1. RELATIONSHIP BETWEEN UTILIZATION MANAGEMENT AND CASE MANAGEMENT

Utilization management is a technique used by case managers to ensure that the patient meets pre-established criteria to support the level of care being delivered. Criteria that guide the process of determining the appropriate level of care and setting have been established for acute, sub-acute, home care, and virtually all levels of service across the continuum. A match between the patient's clinical picture and needed care interventions and the level of service being provided will greatly increase the likelihood that the provider will be reimbursed for the services rendered. When a match cannot be achieved, the case manager is responsible for working with the interdisciplinary team to transition the patient to the appropriate level. This may mean that the patient will either need a higher level or a lower level of service. For example, the patient may be receiving care in the acute care setting, but after intervention and stabilization, the patient may be appropriate for transition to a subacute setting. Conversely, a patient in a nursing home may become acutely ill and require a transfer to an acute care setting to receive acute care services.

Before the introduction of case management in acute care settings, utilization management was a discrete function generally performed by RNs. More commonly known as utilization review (UR), it was introduced as a function in the 1960s for matching patient needs to necessary care interventions with the goal of reducing waste and overutilization of resources. At the time, UR was limited to acute care settings. The UR nurse was responsible for reviewing the patients' medical re-

cords and for communicating with physicians when there were delays in care delivery or when a patient did not meet the criteria for the level of service being provided.

Although the terms utilization management and utilization review are used somewhat interchangeably, they are not the same. Table 5.1 summarizes the differences between these two terms. Both UR and utilization management describe activities or programs used by healthcare providers, review agencies, and MCOs to ensure medical necessity, appropriateness, efficiency, and cost-effectiveness of the healthcare services being provided. The process also includes a review of services to ensure that they are being provided in the most appropriate setting.

Utilization management is the term used to describe programs that focus on planning, organizing, directing, and controlling healthcare resources and services in an effort to ensure the provision of cost-effective, appropriate, and high-quality care. UR, however, describes the process, technique, or method by which a healthcare organization reviews, monitors, and evaluates its use and allocation of resources and services. UR is subsumed under the umbrella of utilization management. It enhances an organization's ability to meet the standards of regulatory and accreditation agencies and the policies and procedures of MCOs.

For example, a UR nurse might try to intervene when it is noted in the medical record that the patient had been waiting for an extended period for a computed axial tomography (CAT) scan or other diagnostic tests. In this case, the UR nurse might contact the department responsible for performing the test and facilitate its completion. The UR nurse also might communicate

TABLE 5.1. The Differences Between Utilization Review and Utilization Management.

	Utilization Review	Utilization Management
Medical record review	Yes	Yes
Process	Retrospective	Prospective/concurrent
Use of criteria	Yes	Yes
Patient contact	No	Yes
Monitoring of resources	Allocation	Necessity/appropriateness
Authorization of services	No	Yes
Scope of responsibility/service	Limited	Wide
Providers contact	Indirect	Direct
Cost	Containment	Effectiveness
Care setting	Acute care	Across the continuum of care
Focus on transitional planning or level of care	Minimal	Maximal
Interaction with MCOs	No	Yes
Contribution to the plan	No	Yes of care
Case conferencing with	No	Yes providers
Case conferencing with	No	Yes patient/family
Reimbursement appeals	Minor	Major function

with the discharge planner when there are perceived delays in discharging the patient from the hospital.

There were inherent problems with this type of review process, which became more obvious after the inception of the acute care prospective payment system in the mid-1980s. The UR nurse performed chart reviews and seldom actually interviewed, assessed, or met with a patient. In some organizations, the UR nurse was not allowed to speak directly to a patient. It was believed that such interactions would prohibit the UR nurse from being completely objective in her analysis of whether the patient was meeting the criteria for the level of service being provided. The lack of direct patient contact limited the UR nurse's review and analysis to only what was documented in the medical record. If certain assessments, interventions, or outcomes were not documented, the UR nurse would have no way of knowing that they existed or had occurred.

After the inception of prospective payment, the need for better management of these UR processes became increasingly evident. Reimbursement was limited to the DRG payment, and excessive use of resources would mean that the total case rate reimbursement would be chipped away by the excessive or redundant use of resources. In addition, it was clear that the UR nurse was, by design, disconnected from the patient, the healthcare team, and the other care processes. This was particularly problematic as it related to the discharge planning process. In some instances the UR and discharge planning functions overlapped and the prac-

titioners found themselves "bumping into" each other. In other instances, lack of communication might mean that issues "fell through the cracks" and were either addressed late or not at all. This led to system inefficiencies, higher cost, and poorer quality of care.

As the 1980s waned, higher and higher managed care penetration in various parts of the country heightened the need for more efficient utilization management. Most MCOs required "reviews," meaning that communication of clinical and service delivery interventions be given to the company on a regular basis while the patient was in the hospital or under the care of a healthcare provider in another setting. It became evident that the clinician providing this information needed to have a working knowledge of the factors related to that patient's hospital stay. If the UR nurse had to rely on others to continuously obtain that information, the process was delayed and was clearly less efficient. If he or she referred the MCO to another clinician, this made it more challenging for the MCO to navigate the hospital system and added to the inefficiencies.

In the early 1990s these "passing of the baton" models of care no longer met the needs of a changing healthcare delivery system. These models required some drastic modifications to be more relevant to the changing marketplace. Many acute care hospitals realized that economies of scale would need to be designed to respond to the changing needs of the environment and to make their organizations more productive and efficient.

CASE MANAGER'S TIP 5.1

Utilization management is one of the typical role functions of a hospital-based case manager.

5.1.1. The Move Toward Case Management

In an effort to improve efficiency and optimize dwindling resources, many acute care settings began to integrate some functions that previously had been disconnected in hospital settings. Many of the early case management models in acute care settings were designed to integrate the functions of clinical coordination/facilitation, discharge planning, and utilization management. The new care providers to take on these integrated functions were titled case managers (Case Manager's Tip 5.1).

Some argued that integrating the utilization management function with the other case management functions would switch the focus of the role to a solely

CASE MANAGER'S TIP 5.2

Added Responsibilities to the Case Manager's Role as a Result of Utilization Management

- Review the medical record for appropriateness of documentation that reflects intensity of service and severity of illness (i.e., necessity for care provision in the specific care setting).
- Obtain authorizations/certifications for services before providing care regardless of setting (e.g., operative procedures, home care).
- Conduct ongoing medical record reviews and communicate results to appropriate members of the healthcare team, staff of MCOs, or other third-party payers.
- Ensure timely discharge from acute care settings, efficient transfer/transition to a different level of care, or termination of treatments/services.
- Ensure the provision of cost-effective services as reflective of the patient's healthcare benefits package or health plan.
- Appeal reimbursement denials or denied services based on necessity and appropriateness and within specific timeframes.
- Collect quality assurance data related to resource utilization and reimbursement for services rendered.
- Collaborate with medical director or physician advisor as needed (e.g., when reviewing or addressing challenging situations/cases).
- Report on outcomes of reviews and identify opportunities for improvement.

financial one. However, forward-thinking organizations recognized the benefits to such an approach.

By integrating these previously disconnected functions, the case manager would manage all functions indirectly related to patient care. This concept of "one stop shopping" enabled the case manager to coordinate all aspects of care from clinical coordination and facilitation to resource management, to ensuring reimbursement, to transitioning the patient to the next care setting when appropriate. By having this "big picture" focus, the new acute care case manager could successfully assist the hospital in becoming more streamlined, efficient, and consumer-focused. Adding the utilization management function to the case manager's role resulted in added responsibilities. These additional responsibilities are outlined in Case Manager's Tip 5.2.

5.2. THE REVIEW AND CERTIFICATION PROCESS

The majority of today's third-party payers require that the hospital provide information from which a decision to approve reimbursement for the stay, or a portion of the stay, is made. This review includes three processes: precertification, continued stay, and discharge planning.

5.2.1. Precertification (Also Known as Prior Authorization)

Patients whose care is being reimbursed by an MCO are required, as per their contract, to obtain precertification before rendering any nonemergent care. Therefore a patient being admitted for elective surgery (or in the case of a planned medical admission) will require that the MCO be notified and a "precert" number be obtained. For elective surgical patients, this process is generally completed by the physician's office staff. The hospital may need to verify the precertification number with the third-party payer. In some situations the third-party may request additional clinical information. The actual process of precertifying a patient is strictly a clerical function and does not require an RN or other clinician to perform it. When MCOs request additional clinical information, a clinical person should be identified to provide this information. This may be a case manager, the physician, or his or her designee. It is clearly a waste of resources to have an RN case manager obtain all precerts. Generally this function should remain with either the admitting department or the finance department. Under any circumstance, it is important to remember that failure to ob-

CASE MANAGER'S TIP 5.3

The Sharing of Utilization Management Functions

Not all utilization management functions need to be performed by a registered nurse. Functions such as precertification can be delegated to clerical support staff. Controversial situations that may result in reimbursement denials must be handled by clinicians such as case managers.

tain precertification before the service is rendered can result in partial or full denial/lack of payment (Case Manager's Tip 5.3).

5.2.2. First-Level Reviews

First-level reviews are conducted while the patient is in the hospital. Care is reviewed for its appropriateness and may include the following:

- *Medical necessity on admission*: to determine that the hospital admission is appropriate, clinically necessary, justified, and reimbursable.
- *Continued stay*: to determine that each day of the hospital stay is necessary and that care is being rendered at the appropriate level. Examples include acute care, critical care, and subacute care.
- *Overutilization and underutilization of resources*: Using a clinical practice guideline, clinical pathway, or other established criteria as a guide, determination is made as to whether the patient is receiving all appropriate services, or those services that are redundant or overused.
- *Appropriateness of setting*: to determine if the care needed is being delivered in the most appropriate and cost-effective setting possible.
- *Delay in service*: to identify delays in the delivery of needed services and to facilitate and expedite such services when necessary.
- *Levels of service*: to identify and verify, based on the patient's condition and the needed level of service, that the patient is receiving care at the appropriate level.
- *Quality monitoring*: to ensure that care is being delivered at or above acceptable quality standards and as identified by the organization or national guidelines.

5.2.3. The Process

The insurance company requesting or receiving infor-

mation regarding the patient's condition and the delivery of services will do so either by telephone, by fax, or electronically, depending on the specific system in the hospital. The turnaround time for responding to a request for a review will depend on the organization's contracts with the MCO. Generally the information will need to be provided by the end of the business day and usually by a specific predetermined time of day. The case manager must provide the MCO representative (e.g., case manager) with the clinical evidence that supports the level of service being provided. The case manager must provide supportive evidence that the patient's plan of care is reflective of the clinical condition and that the interventions/treatments support the level of service. Pre-established and nationally acceptable criteria are usually used for this purpose. Examples are InterQual and Milliman.

5.3. CRITERIA USED FOR UTILIZATION REVIEW

One of the more commonly used sets of criteria, particularly for the Medicare and Medicaid populations, are the InterQual criteria (InterQual, 1998). The InterQual criteria were developed in 1978 by a physician and an RN to assist in identifying and supporting the level of care and services provided to patients to ensure reimbursement. Consistent with the healthcare environment of the time, the criteria were strictly hospital-based.

The criteria help to support the intensity of service (IS) and severity of illness (SI) of the patient; they also identify discharge criteria. They have been updated over the years and now address the continuum of care and include observation, critical care, telemetry, acute care, subacute care, rehabilitation, and home care. The criteria are used as a tool to facilitate appropriate admissions, transfers, and discharges. The case manager should know which criteria the third-party payer is using (Case Manager's Tip 5.4) and should apply the criteria by asking the following questions:

- Is the patient a candidate for the requested level of care?
- How sick is the patient? (SI)
- What treatments/services is the patient receiving? (SI)
- What resources does the patient require? (IS)
- Is the patient stable and ready for discharge?

As discussed in Case Manager's Tip 5.5, the functions of coordination/facilitation and utilization management are interrelated. Combining them is efficient and effective.

CASE MANAGER'S TIP 5.4

Criteria for Utilization Review

As a case manager performing UR functions, you have a right to know what criteria the third-party payer uses for certification purposes. These criteria should be made accessible and you must apply them to the reviews you conduct.

5.4. CRITERIA USED FOR UTILIZATION REVIEW—INTERQUAL

The InterQual criteria (McKesson, 2010) is used as a guide in assisting the case manager in determining a patient's appropriateness for admission, continued stay, or discharge. It identifies the patient fitting into one of two levels of care: acute adult or acute pediatric patient. The level of care answers a number of questions:

- Is the patient's illness severe enough to require the current or proposed level of care?
- Are the services provided appropriate to the patient's current or proposed level of care?
- Is the patient clinically stable. Can the patient's needs be met at an alternative level of care?

Determining the patient's SI is completed through the use of objective indicators reflective of the patient's illness. The SI criteria include clinical, imaging, ECG, and laboratory findings. Time definitions are also included as part of the criteria for each category of findings. For example, acute onset would be within the past 24 hours, recent onset would be within the past week, and newly discovered would be at the present episode of illness.

Clinical findings are composed of chief complaints, vital signs, and working diagnoses as identified by the physical examination and patient interview.

Findings related to imaging include the results of di-

agnostic radiology procedures such as x-ray, ultrasound, MRI, or positron emission tomography (PET) scanning, echocardiography, and nuclear medicine studies.

Laboratory findings include blood gases, pulse oximetry, and arterial blood gas measurements; hematology, which are tests related to blood and blood-forming organs; chemistry, which includes chemical analysis of blood, tissue, secretions, and excretions; microbiology, which includes analysis of blood, tissue, secretions, and excretions for identification of microorganisms; and cerebrospinal fluid analysis.

The criteria include clinical parameters for each of the findings. The parameters are based on abnormal states/values indicating the need for care. For example:

Blood Gases:

- Arterial PO_2 59 mmHg (7.9 kPa)
- Arterial $P_{CO_2} \geq 51$ mmHg (6.8 kPa)
- Arterial pH ≥ 7.50

The InterQual criteria includes three stages:

- Primary
- Secondary
- Appeal

The primary review, or initial review, is performed to determine if a medical intervention is or was appropriate for a patient. It must be conducted by a clinician reviewer. As a result of the review the reviewer may find that the criteria are met and approve the level of care. If the reviewer finds the the criteria are not met, he/she obtains additional information. If, based on that additional information, the level of care is found not to be met, the reviewer may ask for a secondary review. Box 5.1 lists some of the common reasons for a secondary review.

A secondary review can be performed by another designated nurse reviewer, a physician, or a third party/outside reviewer.

When doing an acute care review, there are important elements the review must include to be considered comprehensive (Box 5.2).

CASE MANAGER'S TIP 5.5

Logic for Combining Coordination/Facilitation with Utilization Management Functions

Through the process of clinical coordination and facilitation, case managers can familiarize themselves with the criteria sets being used in their hospital. By combining the functions of coordination/facilitation and utilization management, the processes become more streamlined and efficient.

Box 5.1   Common Reasons for Secondary Reviews

- Criteria not met
- Service delays
- Case manager/social worker delays
- Alternate level of care not available
- Patient has comorbidities
- Patient choice/delays
- Other delays that may be organizationally specific

Box 5.2   Elements of Comprehensive Acute Care Review

Products

- Acute Adult (≥ 18 years)
- Acute Pediatric (< 18 years)

Categories

- Medical
  —Condition specific
  —General
  —Extended stay
- Surgical
  —General surgery
  —Transplant surgery

Criteria subsets

- Vary by product (see Table 5.2)

Episode days

- Day 1: first day in episode of care for the patient, and for that condition
- Includes all appropriate levels of care for the condition
- Episode Day 2, 3, etc.
- Extended stay subsets do not include specific episode days

Levels of care

- Observation
- Acute
- Intermediate
- Critical
- Nursery
  —NICU Level IV
  —NICU Level III
  —Special Care II
  —Newborn Level I
  —Transitional Care

Responder type criteria (see Table 5.3)

Criteria points:

- Rules
- Time requirements
- Notes

The criteria points are clinical statements that refer to the various aspects of patient care provision and care planning. These may include the following:

- Test results
- Medications
- Symptoms
- Findings
- Monitoring
- Medical management
- Functional status
- Prescribed therapies

These criteria points can also be stand-alone or can be organized in a decision tree. The rules specify how many of the next level of care criteria are required. Examples would be the following:

- One
- ≥ One
- Both
- All

5.4.1. Applying the Criteria

Selection of the patient's level of care and the criteria subset is based on the patient's clinical findings and actual treatments/medications. For example, available clinical information indicates that the patient is scheduled for cardiac surgery and requires cardiac monitoring postoperatively. The case manager would select and apply the critical-cardiac subset.

5.5. THE CONTINUUM OF CARE

The case manager must always be cognizant of the continuum of care and be sure to apply the appropriate criteria to the patient's current setting or review the criteria to determine the appropriateness of transitioning the patient to another setting (Case Manager's Tip 5.6).

TABLE 5.2. InterQual Criteria Subsets.

Criteria Subsets	Descriptions	Use When
General	Addresses one or more conditions	A patient's primary condition or DX corresponds to a condition specific subset
	Includes general medical, general trauma and nursery	A patient's primary condition, symptom, or finding does not correspond to a condition specific subset
Extended Stay	Addresses the conditions, DX, and symptoms that necessitate an extended stay	Until the designated end points are fulfilled; the patient's condition or symptoms resolve and responder criteria are met or until a condition specific or general subset would be more appropriate
Surgical	Addresses one or more surgical procedures	A patient requires an inpatient surgical procedure or management of complications related to an ambulatory procedure

TABLE 5.3. InterQual Responder Type Criteria.

Responder Type	Indicates
Responder	Patient is clinically stable (in the last 12–24 hours) and discharge is expected
Partial Responder	For this condition and episode day, the patient is clinically appropriate for continued stay at this level of care
Nonresponder	Patient requires continued stay or episode days, or level of care within the current sub-set have been exhausted

5.5.1. Subacute Care

To qualify for subacute level of service, there must be an expectation for continued recovery. The patient must be cleared medically for less than acute care. Finally, there must be a need for more IS than a skilled nursing facility or home care would provide. Examples would include concomitant conditions, post-major acute conditions, and medical complications. Patients who are end stage and who need complex care, comfort, and dignity would also qualify for this level of service.

5.5.2. Example

A 55-year-old male with a history of angina has been treated with nitroglycerin for approximately 3 months. He arrives at the ED via ambulance after a 2-day history of shortness of breath. On physical examination, he has rales one-third up bilaterally, his chest film reveals pulmonary edema, and his ECG shows uncontrolled atrial fibrillation. Based on this information, the case manager should set an expectation of care and search the record for such therapies as IV inotropics, continu-

 CASE MANAGER'S TIP 5.6

Criteria Must be Applied to the Appropriate Setting

Criteria are available for all levels of service along the continuum of care and must be applied by the case manager appropriately. Criteria designed for a particular care setting (e.g., acute care) must be applied to that setting only. However, case managers need to be familiar with and knowledgeable about the criteria for all levels of service so that they can effectively and efficiently transfer patients to other levels of care as their medical conditions warrant transfer.

ous cardiac monitoring, continuous oxygen therapy, serial ECGs, pulse oximetry, and intravenous/sublingual (IV/SL) nitroglycerin.

5.5.3. Rehabilitation Care

Rehabilitation care is defined as coordinated, goal-oriented, multidisciplinary programs for individuals who have had an illness/injury or exacerbation of known disease with resulting functional deficits and whose expectation for improvement is reasonable. Rehabilitation programs are designed to meet the patient's physical, social, psychological, and environmental needs. They require that the patient actively participate in rehabilitation activities/exercises and that there is an expectation of functional improvement. Patients are often medically frail and on-site physician presence is expected. This is in contrast to subacute care, in which treatments are provided for the patient but there is not necessarily an expectation that a level of patient's participation be present. Physician presence may be more sporadic as well.

5.5.4. Home Care

Home care is considered a comprehensive approach to healthcare services for individuals who have experienced an episode of acute illness, injury, or exacerbation of a disease process and where the potential for complications and/or deterioration exists. Both professional and paraprofessional services are provided in this level of care.

The case manager should always consider that home care is a cost-effective alternative to inpatient care when the patient's clinical needs can be appropriately met in the home setting.

5.6. MCG (MILLIMAN CARE GUIDELINES)

In addition to the InterQual criteria, another set of commonly used criteria are the MCG (Hearst Health, 2015). These guidelines, commonly known as the Milliman Care Guidelines, are most typically used by managed care companies for UR purposes. The guidelines have been designed based on a commercial population and to the exclusion of the Medicare and Medicaid populations.

Therefore it is important for the case manager to remember that the MCG may not strictly apply to the Medicare and Medicaid populations. They are intended to be applied as the most efficient practices for "ideal" patients supported by an "ideal" infrastructure. Unfortunately, many insurance companies do not adhere to this application but instead follow the guidelines to the letter of the law, even when a guideline clearly is not a good match with either the patient or the healthcare delivery system.

The MCG are also called Optimal Recovery Guidelines (ORG) and follow a specific format and apply to specific diseases and surgical procedures. The elements of each ORG include the ORG description, International Classification of Diseases, Ninth Revision, Clinical Modification (ICD-9-CM), and/or Current Procedural Terminology (CPT) code. As ICD-10-CM goes fully into effect, the guidelines will use the ICD-10-CM codes instead of ICD-9-CM.

The use of the ORGs also include specifications about case management actions based on the clinical review and use of criteria. The actions may consist of the following:

- Adequate reasons for admission
- Inadequate reasons for admission
- Alternatives to admission
- Day 1 (expected patient progress in best practice)
- Day 2
- Day 3
- Goal length of stay in days

The MCG can be matched to the patient's specific diagnosis, while the InterQual criteria are applied using categories and criteria subsets.

There are certain assumptions made concerning the application of the guidelines. The case manager must have an understanding of these assumptions to work with the insurance company and to optimize reimbursement for the provider. The first assumption is that the patient has an uncomplicated course of treatment. The patient does as well clinically as the physician hoped he or she would. The second assumption is that all necessary continuum of care infrastructures are in place and available. The third and final assumption pertains to an expectation that there exists the cooperation of the patient, the family, and any other caregivers.

Milliman research indicates that 80% of commercial HMO members and 50% of Medicare HMO members fit the definition of uncomplicated patients (Schibanoff, 1999).

The structural requirements needed to fulfill the MCR requirements are as follows:

- A rapid treatment site (and/or observation)
- Ambulatory surgery access
- Ancillary services 24 hours a day/7 days a week
- Discharges 7 days a week
- Home infusion and healthcare
- Skilled nursing facility and rehabilitation availability

Because the MCG are based on clinical diagnoses and/or surgical procedures, it may become more difficult to apply a single guideline that will single-handedly manage the length of stay and clinical outcomes. Case managers must use their best clinical judgment when selecting and applying a guideline and must work with the third-party payer to ensure that the patient's other clinical needs are addressed as well. In general, the guideline most closely matching the primary reason for hospitalization should be used as the best guide for that hospital stay.

In addition to adequate reasons, inadequate reasons for hospitalization are also outlined in the guidelines. This data can be a powerful tool used by the ED and admitting department's case managers to assist in the identification of other treatment modalities when hospitalization may not be the most appropriate option. Like InterQual, Milliman provides the case manager with care interventions for other care delivery sites across the continuum, such as home care, skilled care, and subacute care. As in the case of acute care, the guidelines provide clinical interventions and outcomes appropriate to those settings.

5.6.1. Proper Use of the MCG

The guidelines are based on clinical outcomes that are expected to be achieved during a predetermined timeframe; for example, daily in acute care settings. The acute care case manager should be well skilled in the use of these designated timeframes. For example, day three of the Community Acquired Pneumonia Guideline calls for the patient to have a declining temperature, to be breathing comfortably at rest, to have microbiology culture reports completed, and to be discharged. Although it may indeed be day three of the hospital stay, the patient may not have achieved all of these outcomes and therefore discharge would be clinically inappropriate. Perhaps the patient's temperature has not declined significantly. The acute care case manager should discuss this clinical outcome with the case manager at the MCO/health plan the patient is enrolled in. Negotiations should be made for an additional day of hospital reimbursement because the patient was not clinically ready to move to the next phase of care. In this case, the acute care case manager should indicate to the insurance-based case manager that day three will be repeated until the patient has met the expected clinical outcomes and is then ready for discharge. This extension of the hospital stay is appropriate and should be approved for reimbursement. The acute care case manager should think of the expected outcomes in terms of "phases" of care rather than as true days, as some

CASE MANAGER'S TIP 5.7

Strategies for Using the MCG

When following the MCG, the case manager may need to request a continued stay authorization when the outcomes for that day have not been met. Each set of outcomes can be considered in terms of phases rather than days.

patients may not achieve these outcomes in perfect 24-hour intervals. If the managed care case manager (i.e., the acute care case manager) you are providing the review to does not understand this, then you should ask to speak to that individual's supervisor or to the medical director (Case Manager's Tip 5.7).

The acute care case manager should also use this logic when reviewing the criteria for discharge. If the patient cannot meet the clinical outcomes necessary for a safe and appropriate discharge as per the guidelines, the discharge should be held until they are met. Box 5.3 suggests some success factors for the role of the case manager in utilization management. Case managers must apply these strategies in their case management departments and use them in their day-to-day UR and case management activities.

As an acute care case manager, be sure that you have access to copies of any criteria you are being asked to use by any third-party payer. You cannot adequately do your job without having access to the same criteria being looked at by the third party. The third-party payer should tell you which criteria they are using so

Box 5.3   Success Factors in the Case Manager's Utilization Review/Management Role

- Use of established criteria such as MCG and InterQual
- Clearly defined job description and responsibilities
- Clearly defined and well-communicated process for UR and utilization management
- Availability of a medical director or physician advisor for consultation and help when needed
- Clear identification of scope of responsibilities, role boundaries, and collaboration with other departments (e.g., admitting office, finance, patient accounts, medical records, managed care contracts, information technology, and management)
- Appropriate caseload and staffing patterns
- Automation and electronic communication and exchange of information including financial and quality performance/productivity reports
- Formal denials and appeals process in place with clear delineation of responsibilities of personnel

that you are able to make the review as efficient and complete as possible. You have a right to know which standards you are being held to and you should expect to be told which criteria are in use and to have copies of these criteria.

5.7. DENIALS AND APPEALS

During the concurrent review process, the third-party payer's case manager will either approve or deny payment for the hospital stay or a portion of the hospital stay. You will most likely be informed of this information during the review, or by an "end of day" report. You may also be informed at a later point in time by letter. Once a denial of payment has occurred, an appeal should take place. As per the hospital's contracts, as well as the insurance and public health laws (Table 5.4), there will be time limits to this process. You will generally have between 30 and 60 days to appeal a denial of payment. The insurance company must respond to your appeal within similar parameters. An appeal may result in the entire denial being upheld, a portion of the stay being denied, or a complete reversal of the denial. As an acute care case manager, you may or may not be directly involved in the written formulation of an appeal. This function may be performed by the admitting physician or by designated nurses in the case management department who take responsibility for writing letters of appeal.

5.7.1. Writing Letters of Appeal

Whenever possible, the individual writing the appeal should be the attending physician of record (Case Manager's Tip 5.8). If this is not possible or realistic in your organization, the case should, at a minimum, be reviewed with the physician of record before the appeal letter is written and submitted. The physician of record is in the best position to argue for why he or she cared for the patient in the manner that he or she did and why the hospital should be reimbursed for the services provided. Regardless of who is writing the appeal, the appeal should use the criteria of the third-party payer

CASE MANAGER'S TIP 5.8

The Physician of Record

Whenever possible, the attending physician of record should participate in writing the letter of appeal because the physician is in the best position to make a case for why reimbursement for the care provided is appropriate.

as the basis for its argument. Information as to which criteria are used is usually found in the managed care contractual agreement. If the third-party payer follows MCG guidelines, the person writing the appeal should refer to the appropriate criteria for the case and match the criteria and outcomes in the guideline against the patient's care interventions. This increases the chances of reversal.

5.7.2. Reasons for Denial

Each organization may categorize its denials in various ways (Box 5.4). Broadly speaking, though, the categories will fall into either clinical or nonclinical groupings. Clinical denials are related to the patient's condition and decided on based on appropriateness and necessity of the clinical care delivered. An example is denying reimbursement for a diagnostic or therapeutic procedure such as endoscopy that is not justified or precertified as an inpatient procedure. The nonclinical reasons for denials refer to those that have nothing to do with the patient's clinical situation or need for care. They usually indicate factors in the organization's contracts that were not met such as delays in submitting claims.

5.7.3. Appealing Nonclinical Denials

Nonclinical denials tend to be much more difficult to appeal. Because the reason for the denial is generally based on the contract with that insurance company, the basis of an appeal may be rather limited. Your own department must decide whether it will or will not take the time to appeal such denials. One must weigh the odds of winning such an appeal against the cost of generating the appeal in the first place. It is very difficult and rare to win nonclinical appeals.

5.7.4. Appealing Clinical Denials

The case manager, or whoever is writing the appeal, should review the case against the established review criteria in use. Whenever possible, the criteria should frame the argument for the appeal. In writing the appeal, it should refer directly to how the patient did meet the criteria if this is indeed true. These criteria will form the greatest likelihood of a reversal of the denial. If the criteria are truly not met, the appeal may be much more difficult to win. Other arguments may need to be introduced, such as the unavailability of subacute care beds or home care services. These sorts of arguments do not generally win an appeal. The case manager in the acute care setting needs to know the "philosophy"

Box 5.4 Denial Reasons

Nonclinical (Administrative) Reasons for Denial

1. *Technical*—Medical record not produced by requested deadline.
2. *Appropriateness of setting*—Procedures that should be performed in outpatient setting (e.g., ambulatory surgery, ED). These cases can be billed to these settings.
3. *Delay in service/treatment*—Primarily on weekend days when patients are waiting for tests.
4. *Initial noncovered services*—Services usually not covered by payer (e.g., cosmetic surgery, dental care for Medicare FFS patients).
5. *Precertification*—No prior authorization from third-party payer. Emergency admissions require notification to payer within 24 hours.
6. *DRG*—Payment for a different DRG than originally billed.
7. *Untimely billing*—Bill submitted greater than 60 days after discharge.
8. *HINN issued incorrectly*—HINN letter given to Medicare patients when services are no longer covered by Medicare (e.g., custodial care or awaiting home care). PRO decides if patient is still covered by Medicare.
9. *Preop/preprocedure days*—All elective cases should be admitted on the day of surgery/procedure.
10. *Pass day*—When a patient is discharged and later readmitted for treatment of the same medical condition within 60 days, hospitals are to bill the two admissions as one (e.g., the patient was either admitted with or develops an infection that must be resolved before surgery).
11. *Payment inconsistent with service*—Payment is determined contractually (i.e., case rate, HIV or psychiatric per diem rate, when such contractual billing agreements are not followed).

Clinical Reasons for Denial

1. *Continued stay*—Patient should have been discharged—no longer meeting acute care criteria.
2. *Medical necessity on admission*—Admissions and treatments that do not meet inpatient care criteria.
3. *Necessity of procedure*—No documentation to support need for surgical procedure.
4. *Premature discharge*—Patient readmitted within 31 days—PRO denies second admission—if they decide patient discharged prematurely on first admission.
5. *Alternate level of care*—Patient no longer meets acute care criteria but could not be discharged without continued services (e.g., nursing home, home care).
6. *Level of care reduction*—Payer decreases payment to subacute rate for inability to meet acute care criteria.

TABLE 5.4. Utilization Review and Payment Provisions, Timeframes, and Accompanying Sections of Law.

Law	Major Revisions	Section(s) of Law
	Insurers must make payment to healthcare providers within 45 days of receipt of claims for services rendered.	§ 3224-a (a) Insurance Law
	Insurers must abide by the 45-day rule except in instances when their obligation to pay it is not reasonably clear.	§ 3224-a (a) Insurance Law
Prompt Payment	In instances when the obligation of the insurer is not reasonably clear due to a good faith dispute, the insurer shall pay any undisputed portion of the claim and notify the healthcare provider within 30 days of receipt of the claim that:	§ 3224-a (a) Insurance Law
	It is not obligated to make payment, stating the specific reasons why it is not liable, or	§ 3224-a (b) (1) Insurance Law
	To request all additional information needed to determine liability to pay the claim	§ 3224-a (b) (2) Insurance Law
	Each claim in violation of this section of Law constitutes a separate violation, and insurers are obligated to pay the full settlement of the claim plus interest.	§ 3224-a (c) Insurance Law
Utilization Review Determination	UR agents must make a UR determination involving healthcare and services that require preauthorization and provide notice of a determination to the healthcare provider by telephone and in writing within 3 business days of receipt of the necessary information.	§ 4903 (b) Insurance Law and § 4903 (2) Public Health Law
	UR agents must make a determination involving continued and/or extended healthcare services or additional services in connection with a course of continued treatment and provide notice of such determination by telephone and in writing within 1 business day of receipt of the necessary information.	§ 4903 (c) Insurance Law and § 4903 (3) Public Health Law
	A UR agent must make a UR determination involving healthcare services that have been delivered within 30 days of receipt of the necessary information.	§ 4903 (d) Insurance Law and § 4903 (4) Public Health Law
Internal Appeals of Adverse Determinations	Expedited appeals must be determined within 2 business days of receipt of necessary information to conduct such an appeal.	§ 4904 Insurance Law (b) and § 4904 (2) (b) Public Health Law
	A UR agent must establish a period of no less than 45 days after receipt of notification by the insured of the initial UR determination and receipt of all information to file the appeal from said determination. The UR agent must provide written acknowledgement of the filing of the appeal to the appealing party within 15 days of such filing and make a determination with regard to the appeal within 60 days of the receipt of necessary information to conduct the appeal.	§ 4904 (c) Insurance Law and § 4904 (3) Public Health Law
	Failure by the UR agent to make a determination within the applicable time periods shall be deemed to be a reversal of the UR agent's adverse determination.	§ 4904 (e) Insurance Law and § 4904 (5) Public Health Law

(continued)

TABLE 5.4 (Continued). Utilization Review and Payment Provisions, Timeframes, and Accompanying Sections of Law.

Law	Major Revisions	Section(s) of Law
External Appeals	Healthcare providers acting in connection with retrospective adverse determinations have the right to request an external appeal when services were denied on the basis of medical necessity or services were denied on the basis that they were experimental in nature.	§ 4910 (b) Insurance Law and § 4910 (2) Public Health Law
	Providers have 45 days to initiate an appeal after a final adverse determination is issued.	§ 4914 (b) (1) Insurance Law and § 4914 (2) (a) Public Health Law
	The external appeal agent must make a determination on a standard appeal within 30 days of receipt of the insured's request. The external appeals agent has the opportunity to request additional information within the 30-day period, in which case the agent has up to 5 days if necessary to make such determination.	§ 4914 (b) (2) Insurance Law and § 4914 (2) (b) Public Health Law
	The external appeal agent must make a determination on an expedited appeal within 3 days of the request.	§ 4914 (b) (3) Insurance Law and § 4914 (2) (c) Public Health Law

of the organization to know whether there is an expectation that such appeals will be written. Once again, the likelihood of winning such an appeal must be weighed against the cost of the labor spent on writing it when those resources might be better spent on writing an appeal with a greater likelihood of being won.

See Box 5.5 for a template of a sample appeal letter that includes all the information necessary to include when writing an appeal. As mentioned in Case Manager's Tip 5.9, using a template can streamline and expedite the appeal writing process.

5.8. GOVERNMENT CONTRACTORS

The CMS has implemented a variety of initiatives to prevent improper payments from the CMS by identifying and addressing coverage and billing errors. It is doing so by using contractors to process and review claims using the Medicare rules and regulations (Table 5.5).

5.8.1. Pre- and Postpayment Reviews

Some Medicare claims reviewers perform postpayment reviews using samples of records that are selected using statistically valid sampling processes. The sampling review allows the reviewer to estimate underpayments or overpayments without reviewing all records of the provider in question (see Table 5.5). Additionally, Medicare Administrative Contractor (MAC) may place providers on prepayment reviews. This typically happens when a particular provider is identified as having a disproportionally high rate of error. In the prepay-

ments process, a percentage of claims will go through prepayment review. This delays the rate at which the provider will be paid for claims and negatively affects the revenue cycle. The process continues in a specific facility until the MAC deems that the billing practice has been corrected. At that point the prepayment reviews end.

The Recovery Audit program reviews past Medicare fee-for-service claims for potential over- or underpayment. The auditors use the Medicare rules and regulations including national and local coverage determinations, billing instructions, and other coverage provisions. They analyze claims data using software that helps to identify claims that may contain over or underpayments and then request the records accordingly.

Providers have to respond to an auditors request for medical records within 45 days of receiving a letter from them or be subject to a denial. The provider has the right to appeal these and other other Medicare program overpayment denials.

Each of the reviewer programs listed above are subject to change by CMS.

 CASE MANAGER'S TIP 5.9

Templates Make Writing Appeals More Efficient

By creating a template for letters of appeal, the process can be greatly streamlined. Whenever possible, the criteria (Milliman Care Guidelines or InterQual) should be referred to in the letter.

Box 5.5   Template for Appeal Letter

Organization Name

Address

Patient Name [Organization Reference Number]

Date

Dear: [Name of Third-Party Payer]

We are writing to appeal your decision to [concurrently or retrospectively] deny payment of medical benefits for [Patient Name]. Your decision to deny [level of care] [type of service] from [start date] to [end date] for reasons described in your denial letter as [content from denial letter] is not supported by [basic evidence].

[Describe the particular services rendered]

Below, we present the application of [state your hospital] medical necessity criteria* to the services that your organization has denied. We believe that our criteria are consistent with managed care industry standards and that the evidence to substantiate our claim to cover services is compelling.

Medically necessary means a service or supply that the physician has determined to be: _____
{Following this, state why the service provided fits this criteria} _____ OR state that the service is {reasonably expected to improve the patient's illness, condition}

{Following this, state why the service provided fits this criteria} _____ OR state that the service is {safe and effective according to nationally accepted standards as recognized by professionals or publications}

{Following this, state why the service provided fits this criteria} _____ OR state that it is {the appropriate and cost-effective level of care that can safely be provided for the patient's diagnosed condition}

{Following this, state why the service provided fits this criteria.}

We appreciate your careful consideration of this information and prompt reversal of your earlier determination. Should this not be your conclusion, we will expect you to communicate to us the reasoning behind your decision at a level of detail that substantiates the application of your specific criteria to this specific case.

If you have any questions, please call [name] at [number].

Sincerely,

*An adequate and essential therapeutic response provided for evaluation or treatment consistent with the symptoms. Proper diagnosis and treatment appropriate for the patient's illness, disease, or condition as defined by standard diagnostic nomenclature.

TABLE 5.5. Medicare Contract Reviewers (www.cms.gov).

Type of Contractor	Responsibilties
Medicare Administrative Contractors (MAC)	Process claims submitted by physicians, hospitals, and other healthcare professionals. Submit payment to those providers following the Medicare rules and regulations including the identification of under and overpayments.
Zone Program Integrity Contractors (ZPICs)	Identify cases of suspected fraud and take corrective actions.
Supplemental Medical Review Contractor (SMRC)	Conduct nationwide medical review as directed by CMS including identification of under and overpayments.
Comprehensive Error Rate Testing (CERT) Contractors	Collect documentation and perform reviews on a statiscally significant random sample of records of Medicare fee-for-service claims and produce an annual improper error rate.
Recovery Auditors	Identify under and overpayments as part of the Recovery Audit Program.

5.9. QUALITY IMPROVEMENT ORGANIZATIONS

Your hospital will most likely have contracts with one or more quality improvement organizations (QIOs) formerly known as peer review organizations (PROs). The QIOs are in place to monitor the effectiveness, appropriateness, and quality of care that is being provided to Medicare patients. They are privately contracted by CMS in 3-year cycles. During each cycle a "statements of work" (SOW) is published which details the theme of that time period. The QIOs are contracted to perform a number of functions. In recent years the QIOs have taken on the role of facilitator of continous quality improvement of healthcare services within their constituent hospitals and less of a role in UR.

Less frequently than in the past they may be the reviewer of selected medical records for the purpose of UR. This function is most commonly performed for Medicare and Medicaid. As with any denial and appeal process, the case manager needs to know which criteria the QIO is using and to frame the appeal against those criteria. Once your QIO has requested some medical records for review, it will also review the record for quality issues and anything else it deems necessary. Because the hospital's exposure is greatly increased during an appeal process, some consideration should be taken as to whether the organization wants to conduct the appeal. If other issues are obvious in the record, it may be more prudent for the hospital to skip that particular appeal rather than open the organization up to an audit.

5.9.1. Hospital Issued Notice of Noncoverage for Medicare—Fee for Service

Hospital-issued notices of noncoverage (HINNs) are issued when Medicare no longer maintains the financial responsibility for a hospital admission and financial responsibility is being transferred to the patient. Preadmission reviews may reveal that the inpatient setting is not the appropriate setting for the particular level of service that the patient requires, or the hospital may determine that the level of care is custodial. A HINN may also be issued when the patient is at a skilled level of care and the patient or representative has refused the first available bed in a nursing home. The hospital may also issue a HINN when the medical record clearly documents a discharge plan and the patient/representative is not compliant with the hospital's attempts to execute the discharge plan in a timely manner.

Before issuing a HINN, the case manager should be sure that the medical record contains the following:

- Discharge planning process, clearly documented
- Documentation of all conversations with the patient/representative regarding the discharge planning process
- Evidence of repeated noncompliance by patient/ representative, clearly documented
- Evidence that at least three skilled facilities are contacted at least twice weekly
- If a behavioral health patient, clear documentation that the patient/representative is competent to understand the regulations concerning his or her Medicare benefits
- Clear documentation of all conversations between the hospital and patient concerning the patient's financial liability when the first available nursing home bed is refused
- Finally, a copy of the HINN, signed by the patient, should be placed in the medical record.

HINNs can be issued before or at the time of admission. The attending physician does not have to agree to the issuance. If the HINN is being issued for continued hospital stay, if the admission was appropriate then the attending physician may or may not agree. If the attending physician disagrees, the hospital can issue the HINN once the case has been reviewed by the PRO and it agrees with the issuance.

An admission HINN should be issued before 3:00 P.M. on the day of admission. Continued stay HINNs issued and appealed to the QIO by the patient or representative before noon on the first working day after receipt of the HINN entitles the patient protection from financial liability until noon of the day after notification of the QIO's determination.

5.10. WHAT CASE MANAGERS NEED TO KNOW ABOUT MANAGED CARE CONTRACTS

Organizations contracting as providers for a specific MCO usually negotiate contracts that include elements such as rates and types of reimbursement per case and UR activities and functions (may also be referred to as case management). Once the specific contract has been signed by both the provider and payer, the provider becomes responsible for following all of the agreed on elements in the contract. If not followed precisely, the MCO has the right to deny payment for services rendered, even if those services were medically necessary and appropriate. For example, if a patient is admitted for cardiac surgery but the admission was not precertified as per the contract, it is possible that payment will be denied for part or all of the admission (Case Manager's Tip 5.10).

The functions of utilization or case management are fundamental to any contract. Whenever possible, a case management representative from the provider organization should be present during contract negotiations. When this is not possible, the contract, once written, should be reviewed by the UR or case management department. This process will ensure that the agreed-on elements are realistic and achievable. For example, the contract may call for reviews to be

 CASE MANAGER'S TIP 5.10

Case Managers and Managed Care Contracts

A case management representative should be given an opportunity to review the utilization management portion of any managed care contract before it is signed. The review should focus on the appropriateness of the demands made by the MCO and the likelihood that the provider/agency (i.e., hospital) is able to comply with the contract and deliver the agreed-on services within the agreed-on timeframe.

performed 7 days a week. The case management department may not be staffed 7 days a week and therefore would not be able to meet the requirements of the contract, thus resulting in denials of payment for services rendered, especially those provided on days when the department is closed.

A case manager working in a hospital setting needs to know the reimbursement elements of the contract. For example, the case manager should know whether a particular case type is being reimbursed as discounted billed charges, a per diem rate, a case or DRG rate, or a capitated rate. Some contracts may include certain case types that may be reimbursed under any of these methods. Therefore a single contract may include per diem and case rates within it. The risks assumed by the organization change as the reimbursement changes.

A discounted FFS structure is least risky to the provider. Because reimbursement may be between 20% and 50% below the nondiscounted rates, the case manager will need to ensure that all provided services are reasonable and necessary so that resources are not overutilized.

Per diem rates are daily reimbursement amounts that are agreed to as part of the contract. Once again, the case manager will need to know that a per diem rate is in effect. In a per diem rate methodology, the MCO may deploy continued stay denials when it believes that the patient is no longer meeting acute care criteria and should be downgraded to a lower level of service. This method creates higher financial risk to the provider.

Case rates or DRG rates may apply to particular types of patients as identified in the contract. When a case rate is applied, the provider should not receive continued stay denials or denials for delays in service because the financial burden of a length of stay extension becomes that of the provider.

Finally, the contract may call for capitated rates. In capitated arrangements the entire financial burden falls on the provider. In these circumstances the provider is incentivized to reduce the inappropriate use of resources and to aggressively manage the length of stay.

Other elements of the contract that should be communicated to case management would include clinical review criteria. These criteria should include the frequency and type of reviews, as well as the expected turnaround time. Finally, case management should be aware of all precertification and authorization processes.

5.11. WORKING WITH PATIENT ACCOUNTS

The patient accounts or billing department is the department that submits the hospital's bills for reim-

bursement. The patient accounts department must work closely with case management or the denial/appeals staff if they are separate from the case management staff. Patient accounts receives third-party payments and should be electronically interfaced with the case management department.

The case management department should keep a database of all denial and appeal activities. This database should be supported by the actual dollar amounts denied or reimbursed by third-party payers. In this way case management can keep accurate statistics as to days and dollars denied, appealed, won on appeal, or lost on appeal. When it is time for the organization to renegotiate its contracts, the performance of the MCO in terms of its denial rate relative to other payers should be considered. Patterns and types of denials should also be tracked and trended by payer. For example, does one payer routinely deny for precertification at a higher rate than another, and on appeal is it often determined that the precertification number had indeed been obtained? Does another MCO deny for continued stay at a higher rate than the others?

The case manager should stay informed and up-to-date on the organization's contract status and the expectations of both organizations as it relates to case management and utilization management functions. When possible, the case managers should have timely access to this information and be kept informed as specific elements change.

5.12. REPORTING UTILIZATION MANAGEMENT DATA

Utilization management data can be reported in a variety of ways, depending on the focus and needs of the organization. Regardless of the data reported, it should be tracked and trended over time and used for quality improvement opportunities when the data shows a downward trend. The case management department should be able to show a relationship between the data and the department's interventions to improve the processes that the data represents. For example, if it is noted that continued stay denials have consistently increased for two quarters of a given year, case management will need to show that a process improvement plan was initiated to identify the reasons for the negative trend and the processes put into place to correct it.

Table 5.6 demonstrates one way of reporting aggregated denial and appeal data for discreet periods. The table shows denial and appeal activity and data for a 3-year period. In this example, the organization received a total of $11,767,300 in denials of payment be-

TABLE 5.6. Denial Summary 2013–2015 as of December 31, 2015).

	Amount	Percent
Denials	$11,767,300	—
Recoveries	$3,231,665	27.5%
Denials Net Recoveries	$8,535,635	72.5%

Note: Financial amounts shown are for demonstration purpose only and do not represent the actual performance of any organization.

TABLE 5.7. Recovery Rate for Cases Closed in 2015.

	Amount	Percent
Cases Closed	$3,889,000	—
Recoveries	$1,680,000	43.2%
Final Denials	$2,209,000	56.8%

tween 2013 and 2015. Of those initial denials received, the organization recovered $3,231,665 or 27.5% after appealing the denials. Another 72.5%, or $8,535,635 is pending appeal or has been lost following the appeal process. This number represents monies currently outstanding or not available to the organization.

Table 5.7 reports a subset of the previously mentioned data for one specific year. It also reports the cases recovered (43.2%) and the cases lost on final appeal (56.8%).

Another way to reference the data might be by reason for the denial. This data can be reported in days denied or in dollars denied. It can also be reported based on the date the denial is received. Table 5.8 represents denials received regardless of when the patient was admitted to the hospital.

Denial can also be reported based on when the patient was in the hospital. This data indicates the performance of the organization at a particular point in time. In the case of Medicare or Medicaid denials, the denial may be received months or even years after the patient was in the hospital. This data can be reported as a percentage of patient days because it correlates to all of the patients who were in the hospital at that point in time. Table 5.9 demonstrates how an organization might report this type of data. Organizations will want to keep their denials as a percentage of total patient days as low as possible because this statistic directly relates to the organization's financial performance at that point in time.

5.13. CONDITIONS OF PARTICIPATION—UTILIZATION REVIEW

Hospitals that are participating in the Medicare and Medicaid programs, meaning that they receive reimbursement from Medicare and/or Medicaid, are required to participate in Medicare's Conditions of Participation (CoP) (CMS.gov). The CoP includes the actions that hospitals are required to perform in order to continue to participate in the Medicare and Medicaid programs. They are required and are not optional.

As discussed, case managers are bound to two of the components of the CoP. These are the discharge planning sections and the UR sections. The discharge planning section will be discussed in Chapter 6.

5.13.1. The First Role of Case Managers

UR was the first role assumed by hospital case managers. It was a stand-alone role and was performed as a requirement under the Medicare program. As the case management models evolved, UR was subsumed as one of many roles performed by hospital case managers. Whether your case management model applies UR as a stand-alone role, or whether it is part of an integrated approach, your hospital is bound by the components of the CoP for UR. It is critical that case managers are aware of what these requirements are and that they are also included in the hospital's UR plan.

TABLE 5.8. Denials Based on Reason—Reported in Total Days Denied.

	1Q 2015	2Q 2015	3Q 2015	4Q 2015	2015 Total	2015 Percentage
Continued Stay	466	414	390	459	1,729	31.7%
Precertification	245	370	235	272	1,122	20.6%
Medical Necessity	256	230	298	242	1,026	18.8%
Care Level Reduction	98	148	106	174	526	9.6%
Other	159	290	345	254	1,048	19.2%
Total	**1,224**	**1,452**	**1,374**	**1,401**	**5,451**	**100%**

TABLE 5.9. Initial Denials as Percentage of Total Patient Days—Based on Date of Service.

	2014	2015	Variance
Initial Denial Days	4,687	3,500	(1,187)
Patient Days	163,438	165,536	2,098
Percent of Patient Days	2.87%	2.11%	−0.76%

5.13.2 Section 482.30 Issued and Effective on October 17, 2008

The section on UR starts with the basic requirement of the section. It states the following: "The hospital must have in effect a utilization review (UR) plan that provides for review of services furnished by the institution and by members of the medical staff to patients entitled to benefits under the Medicare and Medicaid programs. "

The hospital's UR plan should include the following:

- A delineation of the responsibilities and authority for those involved in the performance of UR activities
- Procedures for the review of the medical necessity of admissions
- The appropriateness of the setting
- The medical necessity of extended stays
- The medical necessity of professional services

5.13.3. The Utilization Review Committee

The composition of the UR committee must include two or more practitioners who carry out the UR functions. At least two members of the committee must be doctors of medicine or osteopathy. The other members can be any type of practitioner (Box 5.6).

Box 5.6   Utilization Review Committee

The UR committee must be in one of the following forms:

- A staff committee of the institution that has delegated to the UR committee the authority and responsibility to carry out the UR functions.

OR

- A group outside the institution
  —Established by the local medical society and some or all of the hospitals in the locality; or
  —Established in a manner as approved by CMS.

If your hospital is too small to practically have a functioning UR committee, then a committee must be established as per above.

The UR committee's reviews cannot be conducted by any individual who have any of the following:

- A direct financial interest in the hospital (an example would be an ownership interest)
- A professional involvement in the care of the patient whose case is being reviewed

5.13.4. Section 482.30(c) Standard: Scope and Frequency of Review

This section discusses the manner in which clinical reviews must be conducted. The following information must also be included in the UR plan.

- The UR plan must provide for review for Medicare and Medicaid patients with respect to the medical necessity of:
  —Admissions to the institution
  —Duration of stays
  —Professional services furnished including drugs and biologicals
- Review of admissions may be performed before, at or after admission to the hospital.
- Reviews may be conducted on a sample basis.
- Hospitals that are paid for inpatient hospital services under the prospective payment system must conduct review of duration of stays and review of professional services for:
  —For duration of stays, these hospitals are only required to review cases that they reasonably assume to be outlier cases based on extended length of stay.
  —For professional services, these hospitals need only review cases that they reasonably assume to be outlier cases based on extraordinarily high costs.

5.13.5. Implementing Review Frequency

While the CoP states that reviews may be conducted on a sample basis, except for extended stays, most contemporary case management departments review all admissions to the hospital. Due to the changes in Medicare payments including the two-midnight rule, reductions in payment for readmissions and so forth, it has become necessary to look at all admissions at the start of the stay and daily thereafter. In the case of extended stays, less frequent reviews may be appropriate.

The UR plan should include the hospital's expectations concerning reviews for medical necessity with respect to admission, duration of stay, and the professional services furnished. If your hospital is not paid under the prospective payment system, then these rules are not applicable.

5.13.6. Section 482.30(d) Standard: Determination Regarding Admissions or Continued Stays

The CoP tells us that the determination that an admission or continued stay is not medically necessary:

- May be made by one member of the UR committee if the practitioner or practitioners responsible for the care of the patient concur with the determination or fail to present their views when afforded the opportunity.
- Must be made by at least two members of the UR committee in all other cases.
- Before making a determination that an admission or continued stay is not medically necessary, the UR committee must consult the practitioner or practitioners responsible for the care of the patient and afford the practitioner or practitioners the opportunity to present their views.
- If the committee decides that admission to, or continued stay, in the hospital is not medically necessary, written notification must be given. This notification must be given no later than 2 days after the determination, and must be given to the hospital, the patient, and the practitioner, or practitioners responsible for the care of the patient.

5.13.7. Applying the Rules for Admission and Continued Stay Reviews

When someone other than a physician makes an initial finding that an admission or continued stay does not meet criteria, the CoP gives specific instructions as to how the process should be conducted. Generally, it is the case manager who is making these initial determinations and the case manager is usually a registered nurse. However, the CoP requires that, if the criteria are not met, that the case be referred to the UR committee of sub-group of the UR committee. This sub-group must contain at least one physician. In most hospitals, this would be the physician advisor.

The committee or physician advisor is then required to review the case. If the physician advisor agrees that the case does not meet the hospital's criteria for admission or continued stay, then the attending physician must be notified. The attending physician must be given an opportunity to present his or her views and any additional information relating to the patient's needs for admission or extended stay.

5.13.8. Clinical Criteria and Utilization Review

It is important to apply the role of the clinical documentation improvement specialist (CDI) into this process. For example, if you, as the case manager reviewing the record, determine that the documentation does not support medical necessity for admission or continued stay, you may also note that the patient's clinical condition and other factors seem to support the admission. Before contacting the physician advisor, you should consider contacting the CDI specialist to review the record and query the physician if additional documentation is warranted and would support the admission. In some cases, it is strictly the addition of more comprehensive documentation that is needed to support the admission or continued stay. This step should always be considered so that the physician advisor is only contacted when no other solution is available at that point in time.

5.13.9. The Physician Advisor

Once the documentation is in order, and the case still does not meet clinical criteria for admission or continued stay, then the physician advisor must be contacted. The physician advisor, after reviewing the case, may determine that the stay does not meet medical necessity. If the attending of record does not respond or does not contest the findings of the physician advisor, then the findings are final.

If the attending physician contests the decision of the UR committee or the physician advisor or if the physician of record presents additional information related to the patient's stay, then at least one additional physician of the UR committee must review the case. If the two physician members agree that the patient's stay is not medically necessary or appropriate after considering all the evidence, then their determination becomes final. Written notification of this determination must be sent to the attending physician, the patient (or next of kin), the hospital administrator, and the state agency (if a Medicaid patient) no longer than 2 days after the final decision, and no more than 3 working days after the end of the assigned extended stay period.

The CoP also points out the schedule that they expect hospitals to follow. They state that there are 5 working days in a week and that normally these days are Monday through Friday. They go on to say that if the hospital prefers to use a different 5 days, for example Tuesday through Saturday, they are welcomed to establish this in their UR plan and operations. When a holiday falls on one of those days, then the holiday is not counted as one of the 5 working days.

If the case manager makes a referral to the physician advisor questioning the medical necessity of an admission or continued stay, and the physician advisor determines that the admission or continued stay is justified, the attending physician is then notified. An appropriate date for subsequent review, if appropriate, is then determined and noted in the patient's medical record.

This notification must also be sent to the attending physician in writing, the patient (or next of kin), the hospital administrator and the single state agency (in the case of Medicaid) no later than 2 working days after the final determination is made, and in no event longer than 3 working days after the end of the assigned continued stay period. For example, if the physician advisor reviews that case and determines that continued stay is approved for 2 days, then another review and determination must be made by the end of those 2 days.

5.13.10. Who May Make Final Determinations

The CoP for UR are very clear as to who in the hospital can make final determinations as to a patient's level of care. They state "in no case may a nonphysician make a final determination that a patient's stay is not medically necessary or appropriate." This point clearly requires that the hospital have an active physician advisor in place and that all cases deemed not meeting medical necessity by the case manager are referred to the physician advisor. Many hospitals do not have this process in place and therefore would be out of compliance if audited on this CoP.

5.13.11. Ensuring Compliance

It is prudent to conduct chart reviews on a random sample basis to ensure that you are in compliance with the CoP. Elements to records review would include the following:

- Review a sample of records found to be medically unnecessary (not meeting clinical criteria for admission or continued stay) and determine if these decision were made by:
  —One member of the UR committee, if the practitioner responsible for the patient's care concurs with the determination or fails to present his or her views.
  —At least two members of the UR committee in all cases not qualified in the above bullet.
- Review a sample of records found to be medically unnecessary (not meeting clinical criteria for admission or continued stay) and verify that the phy-

sician was informed of the committee's expected decision and was given an opportunity to comment.
- Review a sample of records found to be medically unnecessary (not meeting clinical criteria for admission or continued stay) and verify that all involved parties were notified of the decision that care was not medically necessary no later than 2 days following the decision.

5.13.12. Section 482.30(e) Standard: Extended Stay Review

The CoP refers to long stay patients as extended stay. They define extended stay as patients whose length of stay has reasonably exceeded the threshold criteria for the diagnosis as determined by the hospital. This threshold is determined by the prospective payment system's expected length of stay for the diagnosis related group and then the hospital can define what it considers to be extended beyond that. The hospital is not required to review an extended stay that does not exceed the outlier threshold for the diagnosis.

The UR committee must review the record no later than 7 days after the day required in the UR plan. Therefore the UR plan must include the hospital's own definition of what an outlier patient is.

This section of the CoP is dependent on a definition in the UR plan that specifies what the hospital considers an extended stay. Most hospitals use this definition to review cases for medical necessity but also for delays related to discharge planning issues.

5.13.13. Defining Long Length of Stay (Extended Stay)

Most hospitals define long length of stay as cases that exceed a predetermined length of stay. For the majority of hospitals this is patient stays with a length of stay greater than 7 days. If however, you find that this length of stay leaves too many cases to review, you can change your definition to greater than 10 days. The frequency of review of these cases should also be defined in the UR plan (Case Manager's Tip 5.11). Best practice calls for weekly review of these cases to ensure that progress is being made and interventions are happening as needed.

  CASE MANAGER'S TIP 5.11

The review of the cases with long length of stay should be included in the minutes of the UR committee.

While not common, some hospitals may use different thresholds for different diagnoses. If your hospital chooses to do this, then there must be a written list of the lengths of stay for each diagnosis. Clearly this can be a cumbersome and difficult process to operationalize and is why most hospitals choose to have one extended stay threshold that applies to all patients.

5.14. NATIONAL AND LOCAL COVERAGE DETERMINATIONS

Case managers should be familiar with both the national and local coverage determinations. Medicare's National Coverage Determinations (NCDs) is a nationwide determination as to whether or not Medicare will pay for an item or service. Medicare covers only those services they deem to be "reasonable and necessary" to treat the diagnosis related to an illness or injury. It applies to the medical necessity of specific procedures, such as total hip and knee replacements, bariatric surgery, specific pacemakers, spine surgery, and others. This medical necessity differs from the clinical medical necessity to meet admission and continued stay criteria, as it is appropriateness criteria. Medicare is denying for lack of supporting documentation in the medical record for the medical necessity of the procedure.

Local coverage determinations (LCDs) are made by the local Medicare contractor or MAC. They apply to the local jurisdiction in which the MAC operates. As with the NCDs they specify under what clinical circumstances a service is considered to be reasonable and necessary. Their guidance is used to assist providers in submitting correct claims for payment. NCD decisions are binding for all Medicare contractors, and LCDs can be no more restrictive than an NCD.

5.15. THE TWO-MIDNIGHT RULE

The two-midnight rule went into effect on October 1, 2013. CMS enacted this new rule as part of the 2014 Hospital IPPS Final Rules as a way of reducing or eliminating short stay admissions, specifically 1-day stays.

5.15.1. A Time-Based System

Known as the Medicare Utilization Day (MUD), CMS has applied language and logic in a new way as it redefines a 24-hour benchmark process. The 24 hours no longer refer to the amount of time a patient *needs* hospital care but rather refers to the 24 hours (that begin at midnight) of the first calendar day that a patient is in a bed and continues until the following midnight. While CMS states that this is still a 24-hour benchmark, it goes on to say that "the relevant 24 hours are those encompassed by two midnights." This leaves the potential for the MUD to last up to 48 hours when patients are admitted just after the first midnight benchmark.

The rule requires that when a physician expects that a patient's hospital stay will encompass at least two midnights that the patient be admitted to the hospital as an inpatient. The time that the patient spends in the emergency department receiving treatment, and/or the time that that patient spends in surgery, is counted as part of this time period. Therefore the patient's time of presentation will affect whether or not they get admitted, rather than their medical condition in some instances. It also requires that physicians be able to anticipate and project the expected treatment duration, something that can often be quite difficult. The physician must have a reasonable expectation that the patient's stay will cross two midnights and admit the patient based on that expectation.

5.15.2. Out-Patient and Observation Status

In addition to delineating what an admission requires, the rule also clarifies what is inappropriate for an inpatient hospital stay. It stipulates that surgical procedures, diagnostic tests, and other treatments that require that the patient be in the hospital for a more limited time period, and do not cross two midnights, are generally not appropriate for admission to the inpatient setting.

Our view of observation status, as providers, also changes with this new rule. Observation had been used as a "time-extender," allowing the physician additional time following care in the emergency department, to determine if the patient needed to be admitted to the hospital. Now CMS is directing hospitals to place any patient whose stay will not span two midnights into observation status. It goes on to say that once the physician has additional information, the status may be changed to inpatient or the patient may be discharged.

This distinction between the previous use of observation and the 2014 use of observation warrants further explanation. In the 2014 use of observation status, the physician's selection of inpatient versus observation status is strictly based on his anticipated duration of care and not on the patient's level of illness or needed services.

CMS further explains that even a patient requiring care in a critical care bed or telemetry, but whose stay will not span at least two midnights, should be placed in observation status. CMS explains that the majority of patient stays under two midnights will generally not be appropriate for an inpatient admission, with the following exceptions: death, transfer, patients leaving against medical advice, unforeseen recovery, and election of hospice care. Should patients fall under any of these categories, the hospital will be able to bill the stay as an inpatient admission. It is important that your hospital check its policies regarding the use of certain specialty hospital beds, such as critical care beds, to ensure that observation patients placed in these beds are not outside the hospital's own policies about use of these beds.

Under very limited circumstances the physician may admit the patient to the inpatient setting even though the expectation is that that stay will not span at least two midnights. These include: medically necessary procedures on the inpatient only list, new onset mechanical ventilation (not including intubations expected as part of a surgical procedure), others approved by CMS and outlined in sub regulatory guidance.

5.15.3. Physician Documentation

In addition to changes in the use of observation status, there are changes in the final rules as they apply to physician documentation expectations. The new rule requires that every inpatient admission is certified by the physician of record, that is, the physician who is most familiar with the patient's needs and reason for hospitalization. Certification is fulfilled when there is a valid order for admission that is authenticated prior to discharge and is in compliance with the two-midnight rule. In addition the medical record must also include a history and physical outlining the diagnosis and treatment plans for the patient, and a documented discharge plan at the time of discharge. The physician must also be sure to document other complex medical factors such as comorbidities, the severity of the signs and symptoms, current medical needs, and the risk of adverse events. The physician does not need to include a separate attestation for the expected length of stay. Rather this information is inferred from the physician's standard medical documentation. Examples of this include the plan of care, treatments orders, and physician's notes.

Case managers must be sure that they discuss the discharge plan with the physician of record and the agreement with the discharge plan is clearly documented in the medical record by the physician of record. CMS does not require that the physician complete a "certification form," although some hospitals have chosen to use a form or template in their electronic medical record. Whether a form is used or the hospital depends solely on the presence of the physician's documentation in the medical record is a choice that each hospital must make.

5.15.4. The Use of Screening Criteria: A Change for Case Managers

CMS, in the final rules, explains their take on the use of inpatient level UR screening criteria. While the hospital may continue to use existing UR criteria, these criteria are not binding on the hospital, CMS, or outside review contractors. When a Medicare external review contractor reviews the medical record, the review entails an assessment of the following:

- The reasonableness of the physician's expectation of the need for and duration of care based on complex medical factors such as history and comorbidities
- The severity of the signs and symptoms
- Current medical needs
- Risk of an adverse event

This is a change from the traditional use of UR criteria to determine the medical necessity of admission. In the past, case managers in the ED have used commercial screening criteria to determine whether or not the patient should be admitted to the hospital. When the patient did not meet these criteria, the case manager would have a conversation with the admitting physician to see if an alternative plan could be created, thereby preventing the admission to the hospital. While CMS does not direct hospitals to stop doing this, clearly the decision to admit will now be based on the expected duration of the stay and not on whether or not the patient meets the medical necessity criteria for admission. This is a significant change in the approach of UR in the emergency department. ED case managers will now need to review the patient's expected length of stay and guide the physician in determining whether or not the patient should be admitted to the hospital.

5.15.5. Care Following Surgical Procedures

CMS explains how to manage patients who may need additional recovery time following a minor surgical procedure. When the determination is made that the patient needs additional recovery time, the physician should reassess the expected length of stay. Generally speaking, if the expected length of stay is unclear, and/or the physician can determine that the patient's expected length of stay will not span two midnights, then the physician should continue to treat the patient as an outpatient. If additional information is obtained during that time that suggests that the patient's stay will span greater than two midnights, then the physician may admit the patient to the hospital as an inpatient.

5.15.6. Other Roles for the Hospital Case Manager

When the patient is placed in observation status, the patient should be notified in writing of this decision. It is prudent to have the patient sign the written notice and the case manager should place a copy of the signed document in the medical record.

The case manager should explain the differences between inpatient admission and observation status to the patient in a manner that they can understand. The implications of the increase in out-of-pocket expenses that may be incurred by the patient if they remain in observation status throughout the stay should also be explained. These expenses may include a co-pay as well as a deductible. In some instances, the patient may also be billed for medications that are not related to the reason for the period of observation such as diabetic or anti-hypertensive medications.

5.15.7. Review of Claims

Contract reviewers audit medical records. Contractors will include the time the beneficiary spends receiving outpatient care in their review decision. Refer to Case Manager's Tip 5.12 for determination of time of the two-midnight rule. If the total time that the patient is expected to spend receiving medically necessary hospital care (includes out-patient care and inpatient care) the mechanism for review will look like this:

- *Zero to one midnight*: Review contractor will review to see if the beneficiary was admitted for an inpatient-only procedure or if other circumstances justify inpatient admission per CMS guidelines (new onset ventilation).
- *Two or more midnights*: Review contractor will generally find Part A payment to be appropriate.

 CASE MANAGER'S TIP 5.12

The two-midnight benchmark "clock" starts:
- When hospital care begins
  —Observation care
  —Emergency department, operating room, and other treatment areas
- The start of care after registration and initial triaging activities such as vital signs
- Excessive wait times are excluded

One point of clarification is important to note. While the total time in the hospital will be taken into consideration when the physician is making an admission decision (expectation of hospital care for two or more midnights), the inpatient admission does not begin until the inpatient order and formal admission occur.

For additional information on the two-midnight rule visit www.cms.gov and search for CMS-1599-F.

5.16. ROLE OF THE PHYSICIAN ADVISOR

The Physician Advisor is a medical doctor or doctor of osteopathy who performs a number of UR functions on behalf of the hospital. He or she can be fully employed, part-time employed, or sub-contracted outside of the hospital. The physician advisor may be notified of cases that meet any of the issues listed below. It is the Physician Advisors role to intervene where appropriate and necessary.

1. Patients who do not meet medical necessity and are in the hospital.
   - This could include two sets of circumstances. First, the patient clearly does not meet medical necessity. Second, the patient seems to possibly meet medical necessity, but the physician has not documented such medical necessity. After discussing the case with the attending physician and the physician either having no medical necessity to document, or refusing to document medical necessity, the case manager escalates the case to the physician advisor. The attending physician is always communicated with before an escalation to the physician advisor. At that time the physician contacts the attending (or consulting) physician for further understanding of the case.
2. There are actual or potential third party payer denials when the case manager has already escalated the denial to the attending physician.
   - If the attending physician agrees to either document appropriately in the medical record and/or to contact the payer medical director, there is no need to refer to the physician advisor. However if the physician does not document and/or will not contact the payer, the physician advisor reviews the medical record and confers with members of the team and the attending physician to perform an assessment of the issues surrounding the denial and the potential to correct these issues.

The hospital's own clinical criteria in conjunction with medical discretion should be the driver for making determinations as to whether or not to appeal the case.

5.16.1. The Physician Advisor Process

5.16.1.1. What Cases are Referred to the Physician Advisor (PA)?

The case managers refer all concurrent denials for review by the PA if the attending physician will not participate in the denial process. The appeals coordinator refers all retrospective medical necessity denials for review.

5.16.1.2. How Is the Appeal of Cases Prioritized?

All concurrent denials are attended to immediately upon, or soon after, referral. A determination by the payer is most often rendered by the close of the same day. Retrospective denials are prioritized for completion based on the date by which the appeal must be submitted to the payer.

5.16.1.3. How Are Cases Chosen to Be Appealed or Not Appealed?

A data worksheet form is filled out for every case reviewed. It includes patient demographic information as well as pertinent clinical information. Standardized clinical criteria (e.g., Milliman Care Guidelines) are applied to prepare an appeal to refute the payer denial. All cases meeting standardized clinical criteria are appealed.

- Those concurrent cases felt to be medically justified despite lacking adherence to standardized criteria also will be pursued by utilizing the concurrent appeal process.
- Those retrospective cases felt to be medically justified despite lacking adherence to standardized criteria also will be pursued by preparing a clinical justification appeal letter to be included in the appeal packet sent to the payer.
- For cases that are felt not to fit into one of the above scenarios, the reasons are included on the data worksheet form. The concurrent cases in this group are not pursued with the payer, but are pursued with the attending physician of record. This is done for a number of reasons (Case Manager's Tip 5.13).
- The retrospective cases in this group are appealed but without a clinical justification appeal letter by the physician advisor.

 CASE MANAGER'S TIP 5.13

Reasons for Pursuing Reviews of Denied Cases by Attending Physicians of Record

- To obtain clinical information about the patient that may not be apparent from a review of the chart but that may be sufficient to justify an acute care stay.
- To educate the physician on the criteria used to determine the necessity of an acute care stay.
- To ensure that the patient is in the most appropriate setting for the level of care needed

 5.17. KEY POINTS

1. Effective utilization management techniques as performed by the case manager can increase the percentage of reimbursed services for a healthcare provider.
2. Case managers must be very familiar with the criteria used by the third-party payers they interact with.
3. Commonly used criteria include the InterQual criteria and the Milliman & Robertson Health Care Management Guidelines.
4. The criteria used should always match the patient's location along the continuum of care.
5. Denials can be cataloged as either nonclinical (administrative) or clinical.
6. Case managers should be familiar with the managed care contracts negotiated in their organization.
7. Utilization management data should be collected, tracked, and trended on a regular basis and reported through the organization's internal structure.

5.18. REFERENCES

Heart Health. (2015). MCG, Seattle, WA.

InterQual, Inc. (1998). *System administrator's guide*, InterQual, Marlborough, MA.

McKesson Health Solutions. (2010). *InterQual*, Newtpon, MA.

Schibanoff, J.M., (Ed). (1999). *Health care management guidelines*, Milliman & Robertson, New York, NY.

6 Transitional and Discharge Planning

In these times of fixed payments and increased financial risk, whether they are the result of prospective payment systems, managed care reimbursement systems, bundled payment methods, or value-based purchasing, healthcare organizations no longer can afford to keep patients at one level of care for an extended period of time, especially one that is of high acuity, intesity, and cost. Without ongoing assessments for timely transfer to a more appropriate level of care, these organizations risk either no reimbursement for services rendered or denial of payments for all or a portion of these services. Transitional planning, traditionally known as discharge planning, is the process case managers apply daily, in conjunction with utilization and clinical care management. This process ensures that the interdisciplinary healthcare team provides patients with appropriate services in the most appropriate setting (i.e., level of care) as delineated in the standards and guidelines of regulatory and accreditation agencies (federal and private). Chapter 6 focuses on the transitional planning process and its relationship to case management. Utilization management is discussed in Chapter 5.

Transitional planning places the case manager in a pivotal position in the patient care delivery process, especially where decisions are made to ensure quality, safe, efficient, cost-effective, fair, equitable, patient-focused, and continuous care. Transitional planning is defined as a dynamic, interactive, collaborative, and interdisciplinary process of assessment and evaluation of the healthcare needs of patients and their families or caregivers during and after a phase/episode of illness. Transitional planning also includes planning and brokering of necessary services and resources (e.g., durable medical equipment) identified as needed based on

the patient's condition. In addition, it ensures that these services are delivered in the patient's next level of care (i.e., setting) or after discharge from a hospital. This process is systematic and aims to facilitate the transition of patients from one level of care to another more appropriate, necessary, and reimbursable level without compromising the quality and continuity of care or the services being provided.

Transitional planning is a team effort. There are three distinct groups of individuals involved in a patient's transitional planning process. These are:

1. The patient and the patient's family, caregiver, or designated healthcare proxy;
2. An interdisciplinary team of healthcare providers from within the healthcare organization caring for the patient: the case manager and other relevant providers such as the physician(s), nurse(s), social worker, physical therapist, occupational therapist, speech pathologist/therapist, pharmacist, psychologist, nutritionist, and financial counselor/ screener or reviewer;
3. Representatives from agencies that are external to the organization caring for the patient such as payer-based case manager or other payer representative, home care, skilled nursing facilities, hospice, durable medical equipment, and transportation.

Not every member of the transitional planning team is involved to the same degree in every patient's care. This is true for individuals internal or external to the organization caring for the patient. Some members may only be involved based on their specialization and as they relate to the needs of patients and/or patient's family. For example, a patient with cardiovascular disease would not routinely require the services of a speech pathologist/therapist, whereas a patient who had suffered a stroke would. The case manager usually ensures that the appropriate members of the healthcare team are involved in the transitional planning process as warranted by the condition of the patient and needed resources.

6.1. TRANSITIONAL PLANNING OR DISCHARGE PLANNING

Transitional planning was not born by happenstance. Over the years and as in any evolutionary process, some sociopolitical and economic factors contributed to the advent of discharge planning and later to its evolution into transitional planning. Discharge planning was not a component of case management until the late 1980s when healthcare organizations began to view unnecessary use, fragmentation, and duplication of resources as wasteful and cost-ineffective. In addition, certain pressures such as the prospective payment system in acute care settings forced hospitals to reduce the patients' length of stay, which was accomplished through discharging patients expeditiously either to home or another less acute care setting.

The shift to transitional planning did not occur until legislative changes in reimbursement and care delivery (i.e., the Omnibus Budget Reconciliation Act [OBRA] of 1986 and the Balanced Budget Act of 1997 and most recently the Patient Protection and Affordable Care Act [PPACA]) of 2010) took place, coupled with the increased incidence of managed care in the 1990s, bundled payment methods of the 2010s, and value-based purchasing and the PPACA of the late 2000s. Only then did transitional/discharge planning evolve to a necessary function of every acute care hospital, every case management program, and ultimately every healthcare setting across the continuum of healthcare delivery.

Rather than discharge planning, the term transitional planning better demonstrates the essence of this process and its intent. This can be substantiated in three ways. First, transitional planning describes the act of transitioning patients from one level of care into another within or outside the acute care organization (i.e., from intensive care to intermediate step-down, or regular floor, and then discharge), whereas discharge planning focuses on discharging patients from acute care settings to another facility or to home, discounting the different levels of care within the acute care setting. Second, transitional planning means the beginning of a new phase of care, whereas discharge planning denotes

ending care. The use of the term discharge planning, then, is not truly reflective of case management because case management also includes the act of managing patients' transitions across the healthcare continuum and services instead of focusing on the care provided in a single episode, setting, or level of care. Third, transitional planning, as terminology, reflects the way managed care and value-based purchasing reimbursement function, that is, reimbursement based on the level of care provided, the outcomes of that care, and the transitioning of patients from one level. This process continues until the patient is ready for discharge from the service or the setting without encountering any complications.

6.1.1. Driving Forces for Transitional Planning

Transitional planning as a function performed by case managers is important for several reasons, some of which follow.

- Existing pressures and limits on hospital length of stay
- Shift in reimbursement methods, with FFS being the least used mechanism
- Focus on improved and cost-effective resource management and allocation methods
- Demand on healthcare providers and agencies to justify why the care is provided in a certain setting and at a specific level of care
- MCOs denying reimbursement for a portion of or all services provided
- Ensuring the identification of the patient's and family's potential needs for referrals to specialty healthcare providers and for community resources after hospital discharge or transition from an acute care setting to another of lesser acuity
- Availability of varied and numerous options for patients after discharge from an acute care setting such as subacute care, acute rehabilitation, home care, skilled nursing facilities, assisted living facilities, Meals on Wheels, day care centers, and so on
- Physicians are no longer the sole decision-makers as to what types of services a patient may require and in what setting
- Heightened awareness and knowledge of healthcare consumers of their benefits and entitlements and their demand for patient-centered care
- Scrutiny by MCOs and accreditation and regulatory agencies
- The current perception of utilization management and discharge planning as "real" and essential clin-

ical work and not a "nuisance" that is external to patient care delivery and management

■ Managing patients in an increasingly complex environment characterized by multiple payers, providers, sites, and settings

■ Value-based purchasing where performance on specific measures (e.g., patient experience of care, readmission to acute care for same condition within 30 days of discharge) may result in reimbursement penalties and loss of revenue for the provider

■ Transparency of how a provider or healthcare organization performs on specific quality, safety, and cost measures. Today such measures are available on the internet in the public domain and easily accessed by potential consumers of healthcare services, resulting in their ability to compare providers and organizations and ultimately decide where to go for care. Such ease of access to important information is also placing pressure on healthcare insurance plans to associate with providers with competitive performance

6.1.2. Mandates of Regulatory Agencies and Professional Societies

Transitional planning has been mandated or advocated for by federal agencies in the form of legislation, by accreditation agencies in the form of accreditation or performance standards, and by professional organizations/associations in the form of policies or best practice guidelines (Box 6.1). For example, OBRA mandates that hospitals have a transitional planning program in place to meet the Medicare's conditions of participation or to be eligible for providing services to Medicare patients (OBRA, 1986).

The continuum of care standard of the TJC calls for hospitals to have explicit policies and procedures for discharge planning that ensure early identification of patients' needs for post-discharge services and to have a process in place for the coordination and arrangement of these needs. TJC also requires hospitals to establish a process for the assessment of available and appropriate resources for this purpose. This process entails gaining knowledge of the resources available for patients within the internal and external healthcare environments (TJC, 2015).

To assist in meeting the requirements of federal and accreditation agencies and to help hospitals develop solid discharge/transitional planning programs, the American Hospital Association (AHA) published its guidelines for discharge planning in 1984. These guidelines apply mainly to acute care settings. They

---

> **Box 6.1   Examples of Legislation and Entities That Mandate or Advocate for Transitional Planning**
>
> **Legislation**
> ■ The Omnibus Budget Reconciliation Act (OBRA) of 1986
> ■ The Social Security Act
> ■ Balanced Budget Act of 1997
> ■ Patient Protection and Affordable Care Act of 2010
> ■ American Recovery and Reinvestment Act of 2009
> ■ Medicare Conditions of Participation
>
> **Accreditation Agencies**
> ■ The Joint Commission (TJC), formerly known as the Joint Commission on Accreditation of **Healthcare Organizations (JCAHO)**
> ■ Commission on Accreditation of Rehabilitation Facilities (CARF)
> ■ National Committee of Quality Assurance (NCQA)
> ■ URAC
>
> **Professional Associations/Organization**
> ■ American Hospital Association (AHA)
> ■ American Nurses Association (ANA)
> ■ American Geriatrics Society (AGS)
> ■ Case Management Society of America (CMSA)
> ■ Society of Hospital Medicine (SHM)
> ■ National Transitions of Care Coalition (NTOCC)

---

explain the essential elements of discharge planning: early identification of patients in need for post-discharge services, patient/family education, assessment and counseling, development of the discharge plan, coordination and implementation of the discharge plan, and follow-up after hospital discharge (AHA, 1984). Today, however, the views of the AHA on discharge/transitional planning have extended beyond the acute care and hospital setting. For example, AHA emphasizes the need to:

■ Identify the most appropriate post-acute care setting to minimize the patient experiencing unnecessary multiple transitions.

■ Use discharge and transition tools that avoid imposing additional burden on the provider and healthcare organization.

■ Actively engage physicians and other providers in the transitional planning process and related activities.

■ Reconcile redundancy and counteract fragmentation. It is necessary to involve patients and their families in the planning process and to ensure interdisciplinary collaboration so that every member of the team is well aware of the plans, status of the transition, and appropriateness of the care setting the patient is transitioning to relevant to the patient's healthcare needs.

The American Nurses Association (ANA) in its nursing scope and standards of practice described the role and responsibilities of the professional nurse in discharge planning and continuity of care (ANA, 2010). According to these standards, the nurse is expected to collaborate and consult with other providers in the delivery of safe and quality patient care. This entails the assessment of patients' needs, making referrals to other providers, identifying and securing appropriate services available to address patients' health-related needs, ensuring continuity of care, and educating patients and their families regarding health needs and the patient's condition. More specifically, the ANA emphasizes the role of the nurse in the:

- Coordination of the patient's transition between healthcare systems and settings such as moving from the hospital to rehabilitation and home settings.
- Maintaining open communciation with the patient, patient's family or cargiver, and other members of the interdisciplinary healthcare team at all times regarding the transition.
- Involving the patient and family in the decision regarding care and transition options.

The AHA guidelines and the ANA standards function as resources for healthcare organizations and providers to use in the development, implementation, and enhancement of their discharge planning programs and processes. Today there are specific case management standards and guidelines available that explain the role and responsibilities of case managers in discharge/transitional planning. These are advocated for by the Case Management Society of America (CMSA) (Box 6.2). In addition, certifying bodies for case manager's certification, such as the Commission for Case Manager Certification (CCMC) and the American Nursing Credentialing Center, include transitional planning as a topic or dimension of the certification examination (Box 6.3). This makes it necessary for case managers to assume the role of transitional planner and be knowledgeable in this function.

With the advent of case management, healthcare organizations, particularly acute care hospitals, re-examined who is best to assume the role of the discharge planner. The traditional method of having either a social worker or a RN designated solely to this function/aspect of patient care became no longer acceptable.

Box 6.2 Case Management Society of America's Standards on Discharge/Transitional Planning

Although not exactly phrased as discharge planning standards, the Case Management Standards of Practice (CMSA, 2010) identify some roles and responsibilities of the case manager regarding discharge planning. These are as follows:

1. The case management plan identifies immediate, short-term, and ongoing needs, as well as where and how these care needs can be met.
2. The case management plan sets goals and timeframes for achieved goals that are appropriate to the individual or his or her family and agreed to by the client/family and treatment team and ensures that funding and/or community resources are available to implement the plan.
3. Plan with client/family a goal-oriented care process that analyzes and gives direction to a treatment plan that moves the client toward health, wellness, adaptation, and/or rehabilitation. Involve the client in decision-making regarding care options.
4. Focus on accountability for quality care and cost or benefit to clients consistent with payer, provider, and consumer expectations.
5. Be knowledgeable and educated with regard to the roles and capabilities of various professionals and research the various resources for determining the type and quality of these resources.
6. Assist client with navigating the healthcare system to achieve successful care, especially during transitions.
7. Refer, broker, and/or deliver care based on the ongoing healthcare needs of the client and the ability, knowledge, and skill of the health and human services providers.
8. In conjunction with the client/family, link the client/family with the most appropriate institutional or community resources.
9. Procure and coordinate healthcare services.
10. Collaborate with other providers and the client/family or support system on moving the client to self-care whenever possible.
11. Focus on transitions of care and ensure a complete transfer of the client from one level of care to the next where the next provider assumes full responsibility, as appropriate, and the transition is necessary, effective, safe, timely, and complete.
12. Document the collaboration and communication with other healthcare providers and the client, especially during each transition to another level of care within or outside the client's current care setting.

Box 6.3   Discharge/Transitional Planning as Evident in Case Manager's Certification Tests

Topics included in the Commission for Case Manager Certification's certification exam (CCMC, 2015) that refer to discharge/transitional planning are as follows:

1. Transitions of care/transitional care
2. Continuum of care/continuum of health and human services
3. Levels of care and care settings
4. Alternative care facilities
5. Community resources and support programs
6. Rehabilitation service and delivery systems
7. Public benefit programs such as Medicare, Medicaid, and Social Security Income
8. Assistive technologies and devices
9. Healthcare benefits and insurance principles

Topics included in the American Nurses Association's certification exam that refer to discharge/transitional planning (ANA, 2015) are as follows:

1. Linking client to available resources
2. Determining level of care using utilization review criteria
3. Planning for transition of care
4. Community and support services
5. Negotiating for support services (e.g., medical options, durable medical equipment)
6. Utilization of management concepts—discharge planning
7. Collaborating with key stakeholders

The pressures for efficient, quality, safe, and cost-effective care delivery processes influenced healthcare executives to design models of practice and patient care delivery that eliminated the problems of fragmentation and duplication of services, roles, and responsibilities. Case management programs and delivery models became most popular because of their focus on addressing these pressures through consolidation of departments such as utilization management; quality improvement and management; clinical care management; social services; and most importantly, discharge planning. Hence this became the beginning of an integrated case manager's role. Today this role most commonly integrates transitional planning, clinical care management, and utilization management (Case Manager's Tip 6.1). Such integration has demonstrated the best cost, quality, efficiency, and consumer-related outcomes.

 CASE MANAGER'S TIP 6.1

Integrating Transitional Planning in the Case Manager's Role

When integrating transitional planning into the role of the case manager, you must consider the following:

- The cost incurred since expanding the scope of responsibility of the case manager may require adding more case managers to the department and perhaps limit the number of patients (i.e., case load) seen by each
- Clearly defined roles and boundaries; of particular interest must be clarifying the difference between the role of the social worker and the case manager
- The impact on the relationship of the case manager with other staff in the organization such as the primary nurse, physician, APRNs, admitting office staff, ED staff, and others
- The impact on the relationships of the case manager with outside agencies such as MCOs, skilled nursing facilities, home care, durable medical equipment vendors, and transportation
- Reassessment of the role of the primary nurse, especially relevant to discharge planning and transitions of care
- Making clerical staff available to assist case managers in clerical/secretarial functions so that case managers can spend the majority of their time in the clinical area and with their patients or the healthcare team. This may result in establishing the role of a "case management associate"
- Assigning case managers to the clinical areas in a way that maximizes productivity and reduces downtime/unproductive time
- Use of automation and technology (e.g., electronic communication; electronic transitional planning systems across care settings and organizations)

6.2. THE CONTINUUM OF CARE

Before the role of the case manager in transitional planning is explained, it is important to review the continuum of care. A focus on the continuum of care is instrumental for success in transitional planning and case management. To simplify the discussion, we decided to divide the continuum of care into three types of services and settings: pre-acute, acute, and post-acute care and services. These are distinct in terms of scope, type, intensity, and cost of services (Table 6.1). The services provided in each of these settings are highly regulated and warrant that case managers be knowledgeable of the clinical, reimbursement, and eligibility guidelines for the provision of services in each setting. In addition,

TABLE 6.1. Characteristics of the Continuum of Care.

Settings	Preacute	Acute	Post-Acute
Cost	Low and in some instances free	High	Moderate to high
Complexity of care	Least complexity Proactive Self-directed care	Most complex Reactive Total/assisted	Moderate complexity Reactive Assisted
Type of services	Primary care Primary care/patient centered medical home Prevention of illness Risk assessment Screening for illness and risk lifestyle behavior Fitness Health promotion Self-care management Counseling Behavior modification Population health Diagnostic testing	Secondary/tertiary Acute care Intensive care Surgical and operative procedures Emergency care Specialty care	Long-term care Rehabilitative Maintenance Restorative Custodial Palliative End of life Supportive Home care Skilled care Medical or health home
Institutionalization	Rare Ambulatory Community-based	Always Hospital Ambulatory surgery centers Urgent or emergent care centers	May be necessary depending on type of care (e.g., inpatient hospice)
Case management services	Minimal Telephonic Health appraisals Risk reduction strategies Health and wellness education	Intensive Comprehensive In-person care provision Management of risk for avoidable readmission to acute care	Transitions of care Moderate to intensive Self-care management Prevention of avoidable readmissions to acute care Chronic disease care management

they must apply these guidelines when they collaborate with the members of the healthcare team in the development of the transitional plans for their patients (Case Manager's Tip 6.2). Moreover, case managers must be able to match the patient's condition to the appropriate next level of care with adequate consideration of the patient's health insurance plan and its related benefits (Case Manager's Tips 6.3 and 6.4).

■ Pre-acute services are those offered to prevent illness or deterioration/changes in the patient's health condition that may warrant the need for acute care or hospitalization. Examples of these services are health risk assessment and screening (e.g., cholesterol and blood pressure/hypertension screening, mammography, prostate screening, risk assessment questionnaires focusing on degree of healthy lifestyle), patient and family education materials for wellness, health promotion and illness prevention, health advice lines, triage services, and counseling. Settings

included in this type of services are MCOs, ambulatory/clinics, physician offices or group practices, and community-based health centers.

■ Acute services are those provided during an acute episode of illness and in a hospital setting. Examples are emergency and trauma care and operative procedures such as coronary artery bypass graft surgery. Settings included in these types of services are hospitals, acute rehabilitation facilities, post-anesthesia and intensive care units, and EDs.

■ Post-acute services are those provided for patients after an acute episode of care whether in a facility setting or at home. They usually aim at rehabilitation and health maintenance. Examples include sub-acute care, geriatric rehabilitation services, skilled care, and visiting nurse services. Settings included in these types of services are long-term care facilities, skilled nursing facilities, assisted living facilities, palliative and hospice care, and home care.

CASE MANAGER'S TIP 6.2

Determining the Level of Care

As a rule of thumb, case managers must deliver care that is patient-centered. Focusing on the patient's condition rather than the level of care provides the most desired benefits for both the patient and the healthcare provider and organization. It is the patient's condition that drives the decision as to the level of care that is appropriate. For example, a home care case manager may transfer a patient to an acute care hospital when the patient experiences an acute hyperglycemic episode, or a case manager may transfer a patient from an intensive care setting to a regular inpatient unit when the patient's signs, symptoms, and treatments are able to be managed in a lower level of care setting compared to current level.

Case managers are responsible for matching patients to the next appropriate level of care, which in most instances requires either the discharge or the transfer of a patient to another institution or care site. Tables 6.2, 6.3, and 6.4 provide examples of the types of patients and services that are cared for in the different pre-acute, acute, and post-acute settings, respectively. As case managers assess the conditions of their patients to make decisions pertaining to transitional planning, they apply the criteria of admission and discharge to and from the various care settings. In the case of Medicare- and Medicaid-participating organizations, these criteria are usually driven by federal reimbursement regulations (i.e., InterQual guidelines). For example, to transition a patient into an acute rehabilitation facility, the patient must be able to tolerate and participate in therapy for a minimum of 3 hours per day.

There is no need for one to be ill to access the services offered in any of these settings. They are provided for both healthy and ill persons and are aimed at maintaining health and functioning.

Case managers also apply the criteria used by commercial health insurance plans and managed care agen-

CASE MANAGER'S TIP 6.3

Matching Patients to the Level of Care

It is important for the case manager to understand what constitutes the different levels of care and settings (e.g., skilled nursing facilities, acute rehabilitation, home care) and the different health insurance plan coverage for these settings when matching patients for the most appropriate next level of care.

CASE MANAGER'S TIP 6.4

Managed Care and the Level of Care

It is imperative that the case manager to be aware of the rules for coverage as delineated by the MCO/health insurance plan and to obtain authorizations/certifications before rendering the services according to the procedures indicated by the health insurance plan. The case manager must also be aware of what the patients have already exhausted from their benefits and determine whether what is left is adequate to cover the next needed service.

cies (i.e., Milliman Guidelines) when indicated by the patient's insurance or health plan. In a practical or operational sense, criteria of the InterQual and Milliman Guidelines are usually referred to as either of the following:

1. *Intermediate outcomes*; that is, outcome measures or indicators when met by the patient's condition indicate the need to transition the patient to the next level of care. For example, a cardiology patient in an intensive care setting is transferred to the telemetry unit when the patient's condition no longer requires invasive hemodynamic monitoring.
2. *Discharge outcomes or criteria*; that is, outcome measures or indicators when met by the patient's condition indicate the discharge of the patient completely from the healthcare organization/setting. Usually these criteria are applied for transitioning a patient from a hospital/acute care setting to another of less acuity and intensity. For example, a pediatric patient admitted for acute exacerbation of asthma is discharged home when he or she is breathing comfortably and shows adequate oxygenation or improvement in peak expiratory flow.

The TJC has greatly influenced the healthcare organizations' view of and focus on the continuum of care and services in its accreditation standards. According to JCAHO (2001), case management services must aim at coordinating care and services across the continuum of care. This is necessary especially because patients may need to receive a range of services in multiple settings and from multiple healthcare providers. This makes it essential for hospitals to view the care they provide to patients as part of an integrated system of settings, services, healthcare providers, and care levels. These characteristics make up the continuum of care. Therefore it is in the best interest of hospitals to ensure that they have a process in place that addresses com-

TABLE 6.2. Types of Services and Patients in Preacute Service Settings.

Settings	Types of Services and Patients
Telephonic/triage	Offering advice regarding care, triage services, provision of authorization to pursue access to healthcare services, crisis intervention
Managed care organization/private or commercial health insurance plans	In addition to telephonic and triage services, offering health risk assessment and screening; counseling; identifying at-risk health behavior; instituting an action plan for behavior modification; patient/family education and counseling using materials, fact sheets, newsletters, electronic communications, and support groups
Ambulatory/clinic/community health centers/medical or health homes	Medical follow-up services, disease management services, routine health appraisals, health behavior counseling such as nutrition counseling, smoke cessation, exercise and fitness services, crisis intervention, patient/family education

pliance with the continuum of care standard described by the TJC. This process is the transitional planning process and must be applied for all patients and at every encounter. It is best practice for case managers to assume responsibility for transitional planning, especially because they are better prepared for this function as compared with other providers (Case Manager's Tip 6.5).

The TJC defines the continuum of care, focusing on the role healthcare organizations (e.g., hospitals) play in transitional planning and transitions of care. The continuum of care according to the TJC entails care provided over time in various settings, programs, or services and spanning the illness-to-wellness continuum (TJC, 2015). Case management programs and delivery models enhance compliance with the provision of care standard which also includes expectations about the continuum of care and transitions of care. These standards naturally focus on care coordination and transitions of care activities which delineate stan-

dards in terms of the process of patients' admission, discharge, and transfer or transition to another care setting from a hospital (Box 6.4). Not surprisingly, these activities are essential components not only of general delivery of care to patients but of the transitional planning process as well.

In addition to the care coordination and transitions of care activities, the TJC identifies six standards with which hospitals must adhere at all times to meet the requirements of the provision of care functions. These standards are as follows:

1. The hospital must have a process in place to ensure that patients access the appropriate level of care and services they require based on their assessed needs.
2. The hospital must accept patients to an appropriate level of care and services based on a completed assessment of needs. This assessment must be completed based on pre-defined criteria with regard to the patient information necessary to make

TABLE 6.3. Types of Services and Patients in Acute Care Settings.

Settings	Types of Services and Patients
Acute care	Inpatient/in-hospital care, operative procedures, invasive diagnostic and therapeutic procedures, invasive monitoring and supervision, intensive care
Acute rehabilitation	Acute rehabilitation such as geriatric rehabilitation services (however, patient must be able to tolerate 3 hours of rehabilitation activities per day), recent functional loss, trauma victims, dependence on the assistance of another person, expected significant improvement in condition
Emergency department	Conditions requiring urgent care such as myocardial infarction, new onset stroke, life and death situations, trauma, unclear condition requiring complex and immediate workup
Transitional hospitals	Complex medical conditions that do not require an acute phase of care and are too complex to be in a skilled nursing facility, mechanical ventilation dependency or requiring weaning, use of total parenteral nutrition, extensive wound management, coma recovery, complex intravenous medication management

TABLE 6.4. Types of Services and Patients in Post-Acute Care Settings

Settings	Types of Services and Patients
Sub-Acute care	Skilled nursing, physical therapy, occupational therapy, speech therapy, respiratory therapy, restorative care, social services and activities
	Examples of patient types:
	Requiring intravenous therapy and antibiotics, daily injections, tube feedings, tube, drain and catheter care, ventilator monitoring and weaning, wound care and more frequent dressing change, peritoneal dialysis, maximum assistance in ADLs, building self-care activities, skilled therapies, total bladder and bowel incontinence
Patient centered medical home	Chronic illness and disease management, healthy behavior lifestyle modification, prevention of readmission to acute care, prevention of need for emergency services, population health management, health education and counseling, patient engagement, monitoring of health conditions
	Examples of patient types:
	Presence of one or more chronic illnesses, polypharmacy, mental and physical disability
Home care	Skilled nursing, physical therapy, occupational therapy, home health aide, companion, hospice, social services and activities, respiratory therapy, durable medical equipment, intravenous infusion therapy, and chemotherapy
	Examples of patient types:
	Homebound, requiring assistance with ADLs, intermittent and skilled care, wound care, ostomy care, Foley catheter, tube feeding, patient teaching for self-care management, phlebotomy, vital signs monitoring, medication supervision, death and dying support
Long-term care	Custodial care, oxygen therapy/administration, tube feedings, skilled nursing, social services and activities, hospice care, respite care
	Examples of patient types:
	Requiring skilled nursing, complex or chronic medical conditions, severe mental retardation, lives alone and cannot care for self, cognitive or functional impairment, lack of social support, unsafe home environment, chronic illness and deteriorating, 24-hour supervision, long-term/unweanable ventilator
Respite care	Custodial care, social services, and activities
	Examples of patient types:
	Patients are appropriate for long-term care facilities but wish to stay at home or with family members, caregivers needing a rest
Residential facilities/ custodial	Assisted living, assistance with ADLs, medications supervision, social interactions and activities, transient/intermittent episodes of confusion or impaired judgment
	Examples of patient types:
	Requiring skilled nursing, 24-hour supervision, stand-by assistance in ADLs, bowel and bladder incontinence, assistance with grocery shopping, cooking, and housekeeping

appropriate decisions regarding the level of care, service, and setting.

3. The hospital must have a process in place to ensure continuity and coordination of care and services over time.

4. The hospital assesses and reassesses the patient's condition, needs, and readiness for discharge, referral, or transfer to another level of care, setting, or provider. Such a decision must be made based on the hospital's and other facility's (e.g., skilled care facility) or agency's (e.g., home care) ability to meet the patient's needs. The hospital is obligated to inform the patient in a timely manner of the plan of discharge or transfer and obtain the patient's consent.

5. The hospital must exchange appropriate and neces-

CASE MANAGER'S TIP 6.5

Success of Case Managers

The success of case managers in providing care across the continuum is dependent on their knowledge, skills, and ability to do the following:

- Provide the right care
- In the right quantity or amount
- At the right time
- In the right place/setting
- The right provider
- With the right cost and health insurance benefits
- The right outcomes
- The right quality

---

sary information with other facilities and providers when transferring patients. This information is usually related to the services required for a patient's care to ensure continuity and enhance safety.

6. The hospital must have a clearly defined procedure for resolving complaints, and denials of care con-

flicts. Such procedures must take into account the needs of patients as they are (re)assessed on an ongoing basis.

These standards are relevant to case management and transitional planning. It is natural then to design a case manager's role that incorporates these functions. For example, standards one and two can be incorporated in the screening and case identification function of case managers, standard two can be addressed in the planning care function, standard three relates to the care coordination and facilitation function, standards four and five are appropriate components of the discharge/transitional planning function, and standard six can be incorporated in the utilization management function.

The CMS is the federal agency that defines the standards of discharge planning in the form of Medicare's Conditions of Participation. These standards are available online in the State Operations Manual, Interpretive Guidelines for Hospitals, Medicare CoP–Discharge Planning §482.43, a through e (CMS, 2014). Similar to TJC's provision of care standards, they focus on the process of care coordination for discharge and transi-

---

Box 6.4   Care Coordination and Transitions of Care Activities Based on The Joint Commission Standards (TJC, 2015)

1. *Before admission*: The hospital must identify and use available information sources about the patient's needs and communicate with other care settings for this purpose.
2. *During admission*: The hospital provides services that are consistent with its mission and the population it serves. It must make arrangements with other facilities to facilitate patients' admission or transfer as indicated by their needs and based on intensity, risk, and staffing levels. In addition, it must refer patients to clinical consultants and providers of contractual agencies as appropriate.
3. *While in the hospital*: Continuity of services must be maintained through the phases of assessment, treatment, and reassessment of patients, and the care provided must be coordinated among all providers. Before discharge or transition: The patient's post-discharge needs must be evaluated and arrangements made to meet these needs, including patient/family teaching regarding such care. The hospital must assess and reassess the patient's needs on an ongoing basis and confirm or modify the discharge/transitional plan accordingly and keep patient informed of the plan.
4. *At time of discharge or transition*: The patient must be referred to other providers or agencies to provide the post-discharge services needed. Such arrangements must also be reassessed and confirmed before discharge. The hospital is required to communicate relevant information to the agency that will assume responsibility for continuing care after the patient's discharge.
5. *Any time during care provision or transition*: The hospital must inform the patient or the patient's family about the freedom to choose any participating providers of services needed post-discharge such as home healthcare, skilled care, and infusion therapy and when possible respects the patient's choice. If the patient belongs to the Medicare benefit program, the hospital must give the patient a list of Medicare participating home care, skilled care, or infusion therapy providers available in the geographical area where the patient lives. If the patient belongs to a commercial health insurance or managed care plan, the hospital must provide the patient with a list of the contracted providers for the commercial insurance or managed care organization.
6. *Before discharge or transition*: The hospital must educate the patient and the patient's family about the discharge, transfer, or transition including the treatments, services, and follow-up care. The hospital also must complete all the required paperwork to adhere to the law and accreditation standards such as notice of discharge or transition.

tional planning. A summary of these standards follows. More detailed information is available in Table 6.5. According to these regulations, hospitals are expected to do the following:

- Have a discharge planning process applicable to all patients, and the related policies and procedures must be made available in writing.
- Identify the patients in need of discharge planning and post-discharge services at an early stage of hospitalization.
- Provide a timely discharge planning evaluation for patients who require it and those who request it regardless of need.
- Have a licensed professional, such as an RN, social worker, or other appropriately qualified professional develop or supervise the development of the discharge planning evaluation.

- Include a timely evaluation of the patient's likelihood of needing post-hospital services, and arranging for the availability of the services before discharge avoiding unnecessary delay.
- Evaluate the likelihood of the patient's capacity for self-care or the possibility of returning to the pre-hospital environment.
- Document the patient's discharge plan in the medical record.
- Share the discharge plan with the patient or designee for approval and counseling.
- Assess the patient's discharge needs on an ongoing basis while hospitalized, revise the plan when necessary, and prevent a delay in the patient's discharge.
- Refer or transfer the patient to other facilities and providers as needed for follow-up care and share the necessary information for that purpose.

TABLE 6.5. Centers for Medicare and Medicaid Services' Regulations and Interpretive Guidelines for Hospitals: Discharge/Transitional Planning.

Regulations	Interpretive Guidelines
§482.43: Discharge Planning The hospital must have in effect a discharge planning process that applies to all patients. The hospital's policies and procedures must be specified in writing.	This CoP applies to all types of hospitals and requires them to conduct appropriate discharge planning activities for all patients who are admitted to the hospital as inpatients, except for those who are cared for in the emergency department but are not admitted as hospital inpatients. The written discharge planning process must reveal a thorough, clear, comprehensive process that is understood by the hospital staff. Adequate discharge planning is essential to the health and safety of all patients. Patients may suffer adverse health consequences upon discharge without benefit of appropriate planning. Such planning is vital to mapping a course of treatment aimed at minimizing the likelihood of having any patient rehospitalized for reasons that could have been prevented.
§482.43(a): Identification of Patients in Need of Discharge Planning The hospital must identify at an early stage of hospitalization all patients who are likely to suffer adverse health consequences upon discharge if there is no adequate discharge planning.	The hospital must set the criteria for identifying patients who are likely to suffer adverse health consequences upon discharge without adequate discharge planning. The following factors have been identified as important: functional status, cognitive ability of the patient, and family support. Patients at high-risk of requiring post-hospital services must be identified through a screening process. The hospital should re-evaluate the needs of the patients on an ongoing basis, and prior to discharge, as they may change based on the individual's status. There is no set time frame for identification of patients requiring a discharge planning evaluation other than it must be done as early as possible. The timing is left up to the hospital and its staff.
§482.43(b): Discharge Planning Evaluation	The post-discharge needs assessment can be formal or informal and generally includes an assessment of factors that impact a patient's needs for care after discharge from the acute care setting. These may include assessment of biopsychosocial needs, the patient's and caregiver's understanding of discharge needs, and identification of post-hospital care resources.

(Continued)

TABLE 6.5 (continued). Centers for Medicare and Medicaid Services' Regulations and Interpretive Guidelines for Hospitals: Discharge/Transitional Planning.

Regulations	Interpretive Guidelines
§482.43(b)(1): The hospital must provide a discharge planning evaluation to the patients identified in paragraph (a) of this section, and to other patients upon the patient's request, the request of a person acting on the patient's behalf, or the request of the physician.	The purpose of a discharge planning evaluation is to determine continuing care needs after the patient leaves the hospital setting.
§482.43(b)(2): A registered nurse, social worker, or other appropriately qualified personnel must develop, or supervise the development of, the evaluation.	The responsibility for discharge planning is multidisciplinary and not restricted to a particular discipline. The hospital has flexibility in designating the responsibilities of the registered nurse, social worker, or other appropriate qualified personnel for discharge planning. The responsible personnel should have experience in discharge planning, knowledge of social and physical factors that affect functional status at discharge, and knowledge of community resources to meet post-discharge clinical and social needs.
§482.43(b)(3): The discharge planning evaluation must include an evaluation of the likelihood of a patient needing post-hospital services and of the availability of the services.	The hospital is responsible for developing the discharge plan for patients who need a plan and for arranging its initial implementation. The hospital's ability to meet discharge planning requirements is based on the following: ▪ Implementation of a needs assessment process with identified high risk criteria; ▪ Evidence of a complete, timely, and accurate assessment; ▪ Maintenance of a complete and accurate file on community-based services and facilities including long term care, sub-acute care, home care or other appropriate levels of care to which patients can be referred; and ▪ Coordination of the discharge planning evaluation among various disciplines responsible for patient care.
§482.43(b)(4): The discharge planning evaluation must include an evaluation of the likelihood of a patient's capacity for self-care or of the possibility of the patient being cared for in the environment from which he or she entered the hospital.	The capacity for self-care includes the ability and willingness for such care. The choice of a continuing care provider depends on the self-care components, as well as, availability, willingness, and ability of family/caregivers and the availability of resources. The hospital must inform the patient or family as to their freedom to choose among providers of post-hospital care. Patient preferences should also be considered; however, preferences are not necessarily congruent with the capacity for self-care. Patients should be evaluated for return to the pre-hospital environment, but also should be offered a range of realistic options to consider for post-hospital care. Hospital staff should incorporate information provided by the patient and/or caregivers to implement the process.
§482.43(b)(5): The hospital personnel must complete the evaluation on a timely basis so that appropriate arrangements for post-hospital care are made before discharge, and to avoid unnecessary delays in discharge.	The timing of the discharge evaluation should be relative to the patient's clinical condition and anticipated length of stay. Assessment should start as soon after admission as possible and be updated periodically during the episode of care. Information about the patient's age and sex could be collected on admission while functional ability data is best collected closer to discharge, indicating more accurately a patient's continuing care requirements. The hospital must demonstrate its development of discharge plan evaluation for patients in need and then must discuss the results of the evaluation with the patient or individual acting on his/her behalf.

(Continued)

TABLE 6.5 (continued). Centers for Medicare and Medicaid Services' Regulations and Interpretive Guidelines for Hospitals: Discharge/Transitional Planning.

Regulations	Interpretive Guidelines
§482.43(b)(6): The hospital must include the discharge planning evaluation in the patient's medical record for use in establishing an appropriate discharge plan and must discuss the results of the evaluation with the patient or individual acting on his or her behalf.	The discharge plan evaluation must be documented in the patient's record. The hospital is expected to document its decision about the need for a plan, the existence of plans when needed, and indicate what steps were taken to implement the plans. Evidence of an ongoing evaluation of the discharge planning needs of the patient is an important factor of documentation. Documented evidence of discussion of the discharge planning evaluation with the patient, if possible, and interested persons should exist in the medical record. It is preferable that the hospital staff seek information from the patient and family to make the discharge planning evaluation as realistic and viable as possible. The hospital CoP at §482.13(b): Patients' Rights states that "the patient has the right to participate in the development and implementation of his or her plan of care." (CMS views discharge planning as part of the patient's plan of care). "The patient or his/her representative (as allowed under State law) has the right to make informed decisions regarding his/her care," and "The patient's rights include . . . being involved in care planning and treatment."
§482.43(c): Discharge Plan The hospital must ensure that the discharge plan requirements are met.	It is a management function of the hospital to ensure proper supervision of its employees. Existing training and licensing requirements of a registered nurse and social worker in discharge planning are sufficient. "Other appropriately qualified personnel" may include a physician.
§482.43(c)(1): A registered nurse, social worker, or other appropriately qualified personnel must develop, or supervise the development of a discharge plan if the discharge planning evaluation indicates a need for a discharge plan.	The hospital should determine who has the requisite knowledge and skills to do the job. However, because post-hospital services and, ultimately, the patient's recovery and quality of life can be affected by the discharge plan, the plan should be supervised by qualified personnel to ensure professional accountability.
§482.43(c)(2): In the absence of a finding by the hospital that a patient needs a discharge plan, the patient's physician may request a discharge plan. In such a case, the hospital must develop a discharge plan for the patient.	The physician can make the final decision as to whether a discharge plan is necessary. The hospital will develop a plan if a physician requests one even if the interdisciplinary team had determined one to be unnecessary.
§482.43(c)(3): The hospital must arrange for the initial implementation of the patient's discharge plan.	The hospital is required to arrange for the initial implementation of the discharge plan. This includes arranging for necessary post-hospital services and care, and educating patient, family, caregivers, or community providers about post-hospital care plans.
§482.43(c)(4): The hospital must reassess the patient's discharge plan if there are factors that may affect continuing care needs or the appropriateness of the discharge plan.	The discharge plan should be initiated as soon as possible after admission. As changes in the patient's condition and needs occur, the discharge plan must be reassessed and updated to address those changes.
§482.43(c)(5): As needed, the patient and family members or interested persons must be counseled to prepare them for post-hospital care.	Evidence should exist that the patient and/or family and/or caregiver is/are provided information and instructions in preparation for post-hospital care and kept informed of the progress. It is important that the patient and caregivers who are expected to provide the care know, and as appropriate, can demonstrate or verbalize the care needed by the patient. Use of family caregivers in providing post-hospital care should occur when the family is both willing and able to do so. It is appropriate to use community resources with or without family support whenever necessary.

TABLE 6.5 (continued). Centers for Medicare and Medicaid Services' Regulations and Interpretive Guidelines for Hospitals: Discharge/Transitional Planning.

Regulations	Interpretive Guidelines
§482.43(c)(6): The hospital must include in the discharge plan a list of HHAs or SNFs that are available to the patient, that are participating in the Medicare program, and that serve the geographic area (as defined by the HHA) in which the patient resides, or in the case of a SNF, in the geographic area requested by the patient. HHAs must request to be listed by the hospital as available.	The Social Security Act (SSA) at §1861(ee) requires Medicare participating hospitals, as part of their discharge planning evaluations to: ▪ Share with each patient, as appropriate, a list of Medicare-certified home health agencies (HHAs) that serve the geographic area in which the patient resides and that request to be included on the list. In addition the SSA prohibits hospitals from limiting or steering patients to any particular HHA and must identify those HHA to whom the patient is referred in which the hospital has a disclosable financial interest or which has such an interest in the hospital. ▪ Include an evaluation of the patient's likely need for hospice care and post-hospital extended care services and to provide a list of the available Medicare certified hospice and skilled nursing facilities (SNFs) that serve the geographic area requested by the patient. In addition, the discharge plan shall not specify or limit qualified hospice or SNFs and must identify those entities to whom the patient is referred in which the hospital has a disclosable financial interest or which has such an interest in the hospital. ▪ Develop and maintain its own list of hospices, HHAs, or SNFs; or in the case of SNF, simply print a list from the Nursing Home Compare site on the CMS website, www.medicare.gov/, based on the geographic area that the patient requests.
§482.43(d): Transfer or Referral The hospital must transfer or refer patients, along with necessary medical information, to appropriate facilities, agencies, or outpatient services, as needed, for follow-up or ancillary care.	The hospital must ensure that patients receive proper post-hospital care within the constraints of a hospital's authority under state law and within the limits of a patient's right to refuse discharge-planning services. If a patient exercises the right to refuse discharge planning or to comply with a discharge plan, documentation of the refusal is recommended. "Medical information" may be released only to authorized individuals according to provision §482.24(b)(3). Examples of necessary information include functional capacity of the patient, requirements for healthcare services procedures, discharge summary, and referral forms. "Appropriate facilities" refers to facilities that can meet the patient's assessed needs on a post-discharge basis and that comply with Federal and state health and safety standards.
§483.43(e): Reassessment The hospital must reassess its discharge planning process on an ongoing basis. The reassessment must include a review of discharge plans to ensure that they are responsive to discharge needs.	The hospital's discharge planning process must be integrated into its quality assurance and performance improvement (QAPI) program. The hospital must have a mechanism in place for ongoing reassessment of its discharge planning process. Although specific parameters or measures that would be included in a reassessment are not required, the hospital should ensure the following factors in the reassessment process: ▪ Timely effectiveness of the criteria to identify patients needing discharge plans; ▪ The quality and timeliness for discharge planning evaluations and discharge plans; ▪ The hospital discharge personnel maintain complete and accurate information to advise patients and their representatives of appropriate options; and The hospital has a coordinated discharge planning process that integrates discharge planning with other functional departments, including the quality assurance and utilization review activities of the institution and involves various disciplines.

Compiled from Medicare's Conditions of Participation: Discharge Planning, CMS, 2014.

It is evident in the CMS discharge planning regulations that hospitals must focus on the continuum of care and safe discharge planning and transitions of care in the provision of healthcare services to patients and their families or caregivers. Similar to TJC's standards, each of these requirements can be fit in one or more steps of the transitional/discharge planning process. Therefore case management models and programs in acute care and other settings enhance adherence to Medicare's Conditions of Participation and TJC's standards of accreditation. Moreover, case managers, who are licensed professionals as stipulated in the regulations, are best suited to assume the responsibility for these functions: discharge planners and transition of care coordinators. They can apply the transitional planning process for this purpose.

6.3. THE CASE MANAGER'S ROLE IN TRANSITIONAL PLANNING

Case managers are responsible and accountable for transitional planning in virtually every institution that employs case management delivery services and discharge planning functions. This section discusses the role of the case manager in transitional planning through the application of a systematic process (Figure 6.1) especially designed for that purpose. The goals of the transitional planning process are, but not limited to, the following:

1. Facilitating high-quality, safe, cost-effective, and patient/family-centered care

2. Providing links among the varied providers within and outside the healthcare organization and across the healthcare continuum

3. Assuring timely transition from one level of care to another and based on the patient's health condition and care needs

4. Providing links between healthcare providers, organizations and MCOs/payers

5. Influencing an interdisciplinary healthcare team approach that includes patients and their families or caregiver for the planning of care and service delivery, including services needed post-discharge from the hospital

6. Ensuring optimal services and continuity of care for patients and families, especially after discharge from acute care settings

7. Brokering community services/resources for patients and their families as deemed appropriate based on patient condition

8. Maintaining adherence to guidelines and standards of regulatory and accrediting agencies, health insurance plans, and MCOs

9. Examining the outcomes of the discharge plans and services provided in preparation for or after discharge

As noted in the previous section, a particular focus of the continuum of care is coordination of resources and services provided by a healthcare organization to meet the ongoing identified needs of individuals. This includes referrals to appropriate community resources and liaison with others, such as the individual patient's physician or primary care provider; other healthcare organizations; and community services involved in care or services.

The transitional planning process assists healthcare organizations in the implementation of the plan of care and prevents the use of unnecessary duplication of services. It consists of seven steps or phases in the care of the patient. As noted in Figure 6.1, these are as follows:

1. Assessment of the patient's condition, risks, and needs

2. Development of the discharge/transitional plan, including the goals of treatment and disposition

3. Implementation of the plan

4. Evaluation, ongoing monitoring, and modification of the plan as warranted

5. Confirmation of and final preparation for the patient's discharge or transition

6. Discharge or transition of the patient to another level of care or to home

7. Follow-up communication with patient post-discharge

The steps in this process, although listed in a linear fashion, are not necessarily linear. They are also not limited to an acute care setting focus, even though the patient may be receiving care while in the hospital at this point (Case Manager's Tip 6.6). Case managers usually shift back and forth between the steps while engaged in functions such as assessing/reassessing and monitoring of the patient's condition, changing care needs, and discharge planning services, accounting for the latest changes in the patient's condition when revising the plan of care, attempting to confirm the transitional plan with the insurance plan or MCO, and making the final arrangements for transferring a patient to another facility.

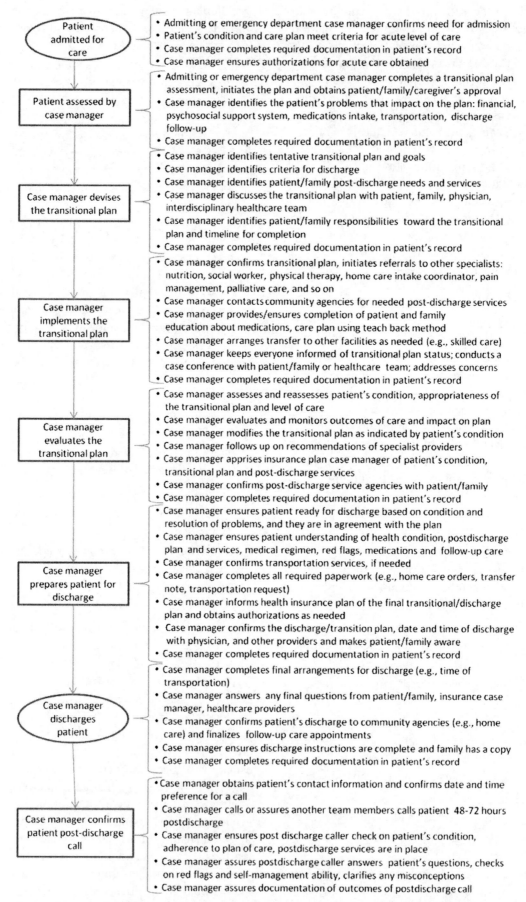

Patient admitted for care
- Admitting or emergency department case manager confirms need for admission
- Patient's condition and care plan meet criteria for acute level of care
- Case manager completes required documentation in patient's record
- Case manager ensures authorizations for acute care obtained

Patient assessed by case manager
- Admitting or emergency department case manager completes a transitional plan assessment, initiates the plan and obtains patient/family/caregiver's approval
- Case manager identifies the patient's problems that impact on the plan: financial, psychosocial support system, medications intake, transportation, discharge follow-up
- Case manager completes required documentation in patient's record

Case manager devises the transitional plan
- Case manager identifies tentative transitional plan and goals
- Case manager identifies criteria for discharge
- Case manager identifies patient/family post-discharge needs and services
- Case manager discusses the transitional plan with patient, family, physician, interdisciplinary healthcare team
- Case manager identifies patient/family responsibilities toward the transitional plan and timeline for completion
- Case manager completes required documentation in patient's record

Case manager implements the transitional plan
- Case manager confirms transitional plan, initiates referrals to other specialists: nutrition, social worker, physical therapy, home care intake coordinator, pain management, palliative care, and so on
- Case manager contacts community agencies for needed post-discharge services
- Case manager provides/ensures completion of patient and family education about medications, care plan using teach back method
- Case manager arranges transfer to other facilities as needed (e.g., skilled care)
- Case manager keeps everyone informed of transitional plan status; conducts a case conference with patient/family or healthcare team; addresses concerns
- Case manager completes required documentation in patient's record

Case manager evaluates the transitional plan
- Case manager assesses and reassesses patient's condition, appropriateness of the transitional plan and level of care
- Case manager evaluates and monitors outcomes of care and impact on plan
- Case manager modifies the transitional plan as indicated by patient's condition
- Case manager follows up on recommendations of specialist providers
- Case manager apprises insurance plan case manager of patient's condition, transitional plan and post-discharge services
- Case manager confirms post-discharge service agencies with patient/family
- Case manager completes required documentation in patient's record

Case manager prepares patient for discharge
- Case manager ensures patient ready for discharge based on condition and resolution of problems, and they are in agreement with the plan
- Case manager ensures patient understanding of health condition, postdischarge plan and services, medical regimen, red flags, medications and follow-up care
- Case manager confirms transportation services, if needed
- Case manager completes all required paperwork (e.g., home care orders, transfer note, transportation request)
- Case manager informs health insurance plan of the final transitional/discharge plan and obtains authorizations as needed
- Case manager confirms the discharge/transition plan, date and time of discharge with physician, and other providers and makes patient/family aware
- Case manager completes required documentation in patient's record

Case manager discharges patient
- Case manager completes final arrangements for discharge (e.g., time of transportation)
- Case manager answers any final questions from patient/family, insurance case manager, healthcare providers
- Case manager confirms patient's discharge to community agencies (e.g., home care) and finalizes follow-up care appointments
- Case manager ensures discharge instructions are complete and family has a copy
- Case manager completes required documentation in patient's record

Case manager confirms patient post-discharge call
- Case manager obtains patient's contact information and confirms date and time preference for a call
- Case manager calls or assures another team members calls patient 48-72 hours postdischarge
- Case manager ensures post discharge caller check on patient's condition, adherence to plan of care, postdischarge services are in place
- Case manager assures postdischarge caller answers patient's questions, checks on red flags and self-management ability, clarifies any misconceptions
- Case manager assures documentation of outcomes of postdischarge call

Figure 6.1 Transitional planning process and the case manager's roles.

CASE MANAGER'S TIP **6.6**

The Continuum of Care

Case managers must always remember that the continuum of care is virtual in perspective and is not limited to a particular setting. It is a state of mind and not a physical place. Case managers are expected to focus their efforts on coordinating the care of their patients across the various settings and healthcare providers, not just the location in which they work. This aspect of care coordination is essential to the success of the transitional plan and usually ensures the safety of the patient's discharge and the continuity of care/services beyond the single care setting where the patient received care before the transition.

6.3.1. Step One: Assessment of the Patient's Condition, Risks, and Needs

On admission to the hospital and as early as possible, case managers should screen patients to determine what their needs are and whether these needs may require case management and post-discharge services. As they complete this assessment, they pay special attention to identifying the discharge planning needs and the conditions that will necessitate the transition of patients from one level of care to another. In this assessment, case managers apply criteria for admission to the hospital as indicated, for example, in the Milliman Guidelines or InterQual criteria. To illustrate this point, let us assume that a patient is seen in the ED with a possible stroke and is admitted to the hospital if he or she meets any of the following criteria (these are select examples):

1. *InterQual Criteria*: inability to move limb(s), unconsciousness, aphasic, need for surgery, uncontrolled seizure activity
2. *Milliman Guidelines*: intracranial hemorrhage, hemiparesis, need for physical therapy and/or speech therapy evaluation as a result of the disease, requiring anticoagulation therapy

Case managers can see in this example that the criteria from InterQual and Milliman Guidelines are essentially the same. In this example, case managers evaluate the appropriateness of the admission to the acute care setting/hospital, which means the transfer of the patient from the ED level of care to the inpatient level of care. Based on the complexity of the patient's condition, that is, the severity of the presenting illness and the intensity of the required resources, the patient may

be transferred to either an intensive care unit or a regular inpatient unit as needed. The case manager initiating the preliminary assessment of this patient can also identify the patient's potential post-discharge/hospital needs and include these needs in the transitional plan for follow-up and ongoing evaluation.

Institutions may have an ED or an admitting office-based case manager complete such assessments and develop an initial transitional/discharge plan for the patient—one that adheres to regulatory and accreditation standards. ED case managers can apply the InterQual or Milliman Guidelines and criteria to determine the need and appropriateness to transition a patient from the ED to an inpatient level of care/setting.

After admission to the inpatient unit/level of care, inpatient case managers can then follow up on the plan already developed in the ED. They first reassess the patient's condition and needs, then revise the plan of care, including the transitional plan. Next they begin the interdisciplinary process for service delivery planning, facilitation, and coordination. Before developing the transitional/ discharge plan, the case manager should complete a thorough assessment and evaluation of the patient's:

- Current treatment plan
- Financial status or health insurance benefits
- Psychosocial status and support system
- Advance directives and healthcare proxy
- Medication intake and management
- Medical and surgical history and previous services
- Need for rehabilitative services
- Need for transportation services at the time of discharge
- Need for community-based post-discharge services
- Potential discharge location (i.e., transfer to another facility)

For patients who access the acute care hospital setting as planned admission (i.e., elective admissions), the discharge/transitional planning process should start in the medical provider's office (i.e., primary care provider or the provider responsible for the admission) prior to the actual admission.

6.3.2. Step Two: Development of the Transitional Plan, Including the Goals of Treatment and Discharge

After completing the initial assessment based on the previous list, case managers can develop the transitional plan in conjunction with the interdisciplinary plan of care. The transitional plan must focus on the identified patient problems or areas of deficit and concern. For example, these may be related to the following:

- Assisting the patient in applying for Medicaid because of lack of insurance and the possibility that the patient meets the eligibility criteria for the Medicaid benefit program
- Lack of psychosocial support system and inability to care for self after discharge
- Complex medication regimen (i.e., polypharmacy) that may require visiting nurse services
- Limited functional ability or mobility that may require home care rehabilitation services, use of assistive devices, or the transfer to an acute or sub-acute care facility
- Eligibility for transportation services to and from the dialysis center or follow-up appointments
- Arranging for community services such as Meals on Wheels, support groups, senior citizen's social activities, and the like

As case managers identify and confirm these needs, they establish the goals of the transitional plan that are reflective of the patient's needs and problems identified. Therefore the transitional plan focuses on the issues case managers intend to resolve in conjunction with the patient and family/caregiver and the healthcare team. Before they initiate their action plans, case managers confer with the patient and family and the appropriate members of the healthcare team such as the physicians to approve and finalize the plan.

Generally speaking, discharge/transitional plans are of three types and classified based on the post-discharge services the patient needs after a hospital stay and the complexity and intensity of the services. These are:

- *Basic discharge*: No post-discharge services needed except for routine follow-up care and written discharge instructions. Patients in this category are fairly healthy, independent, possess optimal health insurance plan, and have adequate psychosocial support system.
- *Moderate discharge*: Post-discharge services needed may include home care, simple durable medical equipment, simple medication regimen, community resource and support services information or referral, out-patient rehabilitation, and follow-up appointments with primary or specialty care provider. Patients in this category have short-term medical care need, are independent, have adequate psychosocial support systems, and are able to manage with minimal intervention or support.
- *Complex discharge*: Post-discharge services need-

ed may include rehabilitation (acute or sub-acute); skilled nursing care; substance use rehabilitation; complex medications regimen (polypharmacy) including infusion therapy, hospice or palliative care, dialysis, mechanical ventilation, and long-term medical care. Patients in this category suffer one or more serious and chronic medical conditions; may also have a serious mental, behavioral, or emotional condition; are homeless or with complex psychosocial support system; are uninsured or underinsured; and may require charity care.

During this step, case managers communicate their expectations of the patient and family and explain their responsibilities to them. For example, case managers may request certain documents that are in the possession of the patient/family and necessary for the Medicaid application. Therefore they may establish a timeline with the patient and family for completing the Medicaid application and follow up with them if they do not meet the timeline.

In addition to the transitional plan, case managers focus on the medical plan of care and its impact on transitioning patients from one level of care to another. They usually evaluate the patient's condition and the treatments being provided for their appropriateness to the level of care/setting the patient is in (Case Manager's Tip 6.7). This is important because of their role in transitioning the patient to the next level in a timely fashion and in accordance with the guidelines of the health insurance plan the patient is carrying. This func-

 CASE MANAGER'S TIP 6.7

Use of Criteria When Transitioning Patients

When considering transferring a patient from one level of care to another, case managers must apply the criteria (usually level of care-based) that guide the transitional planning process.

1. The InterQual Criteria: intensity of service and severity of illness
2. Milliman Guidelines: intermediate outcomes

However, when planning the patient's discharge, case managers must evaluate the patient's condition for discharge readiness. This decision is made based on the discharge criteria that are available for each diagnosis and is in the form of:

1. Discharge screens in InterQual criteria
2. Discharge outcomes in Milliman Guidelines

tion results in preventing reimbursement denials or an unnecessary hospital stay.

In addition, this evaluation facilitates the implementation of the discharge/transitional plan. These activities bring to life the act of integrating utilization management and transitional planning for a seamless approach to case management care delivery. For example, when a patient admitted to the coronary care unit because of acute myocardial infarction undergoes uncomplicated angioplasty or a coronary stent placement, the case manager may ensure the patient's transfer to a telemetry or cardiac unit after the procedure. This is indicated because the patient's stable condition no longer meets the criteria for an intensive care setting/level of care. In this case, the case manager not only is expediting the transition of the patient toward discharge but is preventing inappropriate/unnecessary utilization of a higher level of care that may negatively impact reimbursement.

6.3.3. Step Three: Implementation of the Plan

Before the case managers implement the patient's transitional plan, they may arrange for a case conference(s) with the patient and family or the healthcare team. They may elect to conduct the conference either with all parties together or with the patient and family separate from the team. Such a decision is made based on the complexity of the issues and treatment plan and the concerns to be discussed or by a request from the patient and family, the physician, or the team. Regardless of how the case conference is held, the purpose remains to reach consensus on the plan of care. This includes the transitional or discharge plan, confirming the post-discharge plan for needed services, and to answer any challenging questions regarding care. Some examples of the reasons for holding a case conference include discussing palliative, hospice, or end-of-life issues and decisions about continuing or discontinuing treatment, DNR order, disagreement among family members regarding the plan of care and disposition, managed care denial of continuing services, or merely a patient and family education and counseling session.

To implement the transitional plan, case managers may need to request the involvement of specialists in the care of the patient such as physical therapy, speech therapy, respiratory therapy, occupational therapy, pharmacy, home care, pain management, social services, nutrition, psychology, chaplain, and patient representative/advocate. Following pre-determined referral criteria facilitates this process and enhances consistency in the delivery of quality care. Examples of these criteria are available in Box 6.5.

Consultations with specialist providers are necessary, especially when a confusing situation arises that requires their intervention and input or because of the need to adhere to the regulations that govern the practice of that particular discipline. For example, a patient may not receive home care services unless assessed by the home care staff first and deemed eligible for home care services after discharge. Another example is the requirement of a rehabilitation evaluation by a physiatrist before establishing a physical therapy plan of care for rehabilitation purposes or planning the patient for a transition of acute rehabilitation level of care. Using a list of criteria to clarify the need for referrals is essential for providing better quality of care, eliminating confusion as to when a patient may need the care of a specialist provider, and expediting the implementation of the transitional plan.

Other important case management functions in this step of the transitional planning process are patient and family education, managed care authorizations for discharge services, and brokerage of services from community agencies. Case managers may not always be involved in patient and family education; however, they make sure that other providers such as primary nurses provide this service (Case Manager's Tip 6.8). In some instances it behooves case managers to educate their patients and families or caregivers themselves. Examples of these situations include confusion about aspects of the care such as managed care health plans and how they operate, insurance benefits and entitlements, Med-

CASE MANAGER'S TIP 6.8

Patient and Family Education Is Integral to the Transitional Planning Process

In preparation for discharge, the clinical nurse involved in direct care delivery is responsible for educating patients and their families/caregivers about medication administration and management; wound care and dressing changes; tube care such as a Foley catheter, feeding tube, or any other drainage tubes; and use of equipment such as a glucose monitoring device. Other providers may educate patients about specialty needs such as activity and exercise by a physical therapist, meal preparation and grocery shopping by an occupational therapist, healthy eating or special renal diet by a nutritionist, and oxygen therapy at home by a respiratory therapist.

The case manager is usually responsible for ensuring that these educational interventions are completed before the patient's discharge or transition to the next level of care and to prevent delays in the patient's discharge.

Box 6.5   Sample Criteria for Referral to Other Specialty Healthcare Providers

Sample Referral Criteria to Nutritionist

1. History of unintentional weight loss or gain greater than or equal to 10% in 1 month
2. Inadequate nutrition due to poor oral intake (e.g., less than 25% of meal for 3 days or longer)
3. Nausea, vomiting, or diarrhea for 3 days or longer
4. Difficulty chewing or swallowing
5. Total parenteral nutrition/hyperalimentation
6. Newly initiated enteral feedings
7. Albumin level less than 2.5 gm/dl
8. Stage III or IV pressure ulcer
9. Nonhealing wound
10. Malabsorption
11. Substance abuse: alcohol or drugs
12. New diagnoses such as diabetes, heart failure, pre- or post-organ transplantation, end-stage renal disease/dialysis, hypertension, lipidemia, inflammatory bowel disease

Sample Referral Criteria to Social Work/Services

1. Assistance with coping with illness, hospitalizations
2. Lack of appropriate decision-making skills regarding care
3. Suspicion of patient abuse or neglect
4. Current substance abuse: alcohol and drugs
5. Mental/behavioral health illness
6. Need for placement in a skilled nursing facility, long-term care, hospice, foster care
7. Homelessness
8. Elders who live alone and cannot care for self independently
9. New functional deficit
10. Uninsured
11. Recent confusion, disorientation, cognitive impairment
12. Absent psychosocial/family support system
13. Need for transportation arrangements upon discharge or for follow-up care post-discharge
14. Unsafe home/living conditions
15. Need for guardianship

Sample Referral Criteria to Physical Therapy/Rehabilitation

1. New functional deficit requiring occupational or physical therapy such as retraining in ADLs: grooming, bathing, dressing, feeding, toileting
2. Training on the use of a prosthetic device such as artificial leg or assistive device such as hearing aide
3. Training on the use of durable medical equipment such as a wheelchair, bedside commode, crutches, or other prostheses
4. Building an exercise regimen after surgery
5. Training in transfers from/to bed or chair
6. Chest physiotherapy or pulmonary toileting
7. Training in weight bearing or nonweight bearing movements

Sample Referral Criteria to Home Care Services

1. New or problematic wounds, drains, ostomies, and catheters
2. Multiple and complex medication regimen (polypharmacy)
3. Intravenous fluid therapy and medication therapy
4. Pain management and control (acute and chronic)
5. Peritoneal dialysis
6. Home oxygen therapy including mechanical ventilation
7. Home respiratory therapy
8. Skilled care at home such as physical therapy and exercise, psychosocial counseling, assessment and monitoring of vital signs
9. New diagnoses such as diabetes, heart failure, pre- or post-organ transplantation, end-stage renal disease/dialysis, hypertension, lipidemia, inflammatory bowel disease
10. Home infusion therapy

Sample Referral Criteria to Pain Management Services

1. Chronic pain
2. Oncological conditions
3. Palliative care needs
4. Hospice and end of life care
5. Unrelieved pain regardless of multiple attempts to use different types of pain medications
6. Patient's or family's request
7. Need for alternative therapies for pain management

icaid application process, rights to appealing a service denial by insurance plan, the authorization and certification process, transitioning the patient to another less complex or more complex level of care, and the need to transfer a patient to a long-term care facility. Sometimes case managers are involved in educating the patient and family about complex care situations or treatment regimens that are unusual to other nursing staff members.

As for discharging patients to another care facility such as a nursing home or sub-acute care, case managers coordinate the transitional plan with the rest of the healthcare team, the patient and family, and appropriate representatives from the external facility or agency. Depending on the type of insurance plan, they may also contact the case manager of the commercial health insurance plan/MCO for authorization of this type of transition. In the case of a Medicare or Medicaid patient, they apply the eligibility criteria for such transfer available from the CMS. If the case managers assuming this role are not social workers, they may consult with social workers for collaboration on such transfers as needed. This aspect of the transitional plan highlights the need for case managers to apply utilization management knowledge and skills while making these plans and the integration of utilization manage-

ment and transitional planning into a seamless process of care coordination.

Patients' discharge or transitional plans may sometimes require the coordination of post-discharge services available in the community. These community services are either volunteer and free or reimbursable by the patient's health insurance carrier. Examples include the following:

- Medical supplies
- Durable medical equipment
- Assistive devices
- Transportation
- Lifelines
- Pastoral care
- Meals on Wheels
- Support groups
- Social clubs for senior citizens
- Volunteer agencies/services
- Shelters
- Foster care
- Respite care

If case managers arrange for any reimbursable services, they are required to follow the rules and benefits indicated in the patient's health insurance plan or the requirements of the federal- or state-based benefit plans. For example, in the case of Medicare and Medicaid the eligibility criteria must be consulted when arranging for durable medical equipment. In the case of managed care health plans, case managers must contact the managed care case managers for certification of durable medical equipment before it is arranged for, otherwise reimbursement for such service may be denied.

6.3.4. Step Four: Evaluation and Ongoing Monitoring of the Plan

Evaluation and ongoing monitoring of the transitional plan is important because this aspect of the case manager's role keeps the care delivery process in check. Evaluating the transitional plan is essential because it helps case managers determine the plan's continued appropriateness for the patient and ensures that the patient's changing needs are addressed. However, one cannot evaluate the transitional plan without ongoing reassessment of the patient's health and medical condition and plan of care. In addition, it is as important to keep abreast of the nuances of care by seeking daily feedback from the patient, family, caregiver, healthcare team, primary care provider, specialist providers involved in the patient's care, and the representative of any outside agency the patient is referred to for post-discharge services. Based on the new information, case managers usually revise the transitional plan to reflect the changes in patient's condition or wishes regarding discharge services and place.

Case managers also evaluate the appropriateness of the level of care being provided based on the patient's latest condition. Again, in this function case managers apply the InterQual criteria or Milliman Guidelines for this purpose. If the patient's condition is found to meet the next level of care and the patient is not yet transitioned, then the case manager facilitates such transfer. He or she may need to meet with the healthcare team and the patient and family to discuss the transfer or to ensure that it is carried out safely. Other evaluation and monitoring aspects of the case manager's role in this step of transitional planning are as follows:

- Completeness of the necessary patient and family education efforts
- Authorizations from commercial health insurance plan/MCOs for services to be rendered post-discharge
- Recommendations of specialist providers are implemented or incorporated into the transitional plan
- Patients and their families/caregivers are in agreement with the plan and next level of care

- Community services are arranged for
- Confirmation that the healthcare team at the next level of care or facility are in agreement with the patient's transition, have all the necessary information for safe and continuous care and all their questions are answered
- Transportation services needed upon discharge or for follow-up care are arranged for

Based on the outcomes of these evaluations, the transitional plan is adjusted as needed. To eliminate conflicts or fragmentation in care, sometimes case managers may resort to a case conference so that agreements are reached and concerns of any member of the healthcare team or patient/family are discussed and resolved. Decisions made during the conference are then implemented in the transitional plan or the medical plan of care as necessary.

6.3.5. Step Five: Confirmation of the Plan and Final Preparation for Patient's Discharge

This step of the transitional planning process focuses on the patient's readiness for the next level of care or discharge. Confirmation of the plan is done while the case manager is evaluating the plan. The decision to transition the patient to the next level of care or discharge to home is made based on the patient's health and medical conditions, and resolution of the problems the patient presented with at the time of admission to the hospital. Other factors that influence this decision are the patient's agreement with the transitional plan, the decision regarding disposition and the date and time of discharge, the position of the MCO/health insurance carrier regarding the plan and post-discharge services, readiness of the facility to assume responsibility for the patient's care post-discharge, and views of the healthcare team, particularly the physician, about the plan and the patient's readiness for it (Case Manager's Tip 6.9).

To determine the appropriateness of the time and condition of a patient's discharge, case managers apply the InterQual or Milliman Guidelines using the discharge criteria. An example is presented in Box 6.6. Other criteria are as follows:

- Afebrile during the last 24 hours without antipyretics
- Fluid and food intake tolerated and meet nutritional needs
- Switching from intravenous to oral medications
- Passing of flatus or bowel movement after abdominal surgery

CASE MANAGER'S TIP 6.9

Use of Criteria to Assist in Resolving Transitional Planning Conflicts

Sometimes conflicts may arise between the case manager and the physician overseeing the patient's plan of care as it relates to the timing of discharge, the patient's readiness for discharge, or the next level of care the patient is transitioning to. In these situations, the case manager is advised to use the Milliman Guidelines or InterQual criteria as applicable in addressing the conflict. The case manager must focus on the length of stay, service and reimbursement denials, position of the managed care or health insurance plan case manager, and the state or federal regulations when resolving such conflicts.

- Voiding appropriate amount of urine
- Serum medication levels (e.g., digoxin) within therapeutic range
- Patient or caregiver able to care for patient after discharge
- Refusal of continued inpatient treatment
- Availability of post-discharge services
- Acceptance and readiness of facility or provider at next level of care to receive the patient

To determine the most appropriate disposition for a patient, case managers should consider the discharge possibilities based on regulations and admission and

discharge criteria that may be different for the different facilities or transition options. Case managers are encouraged to be knowledgeable about these regulations or consult with those at their institutions who have access to such information so that appropriate decisions are made and safe, quality, timely, and cost-effective discharge is ensured. Some of the discharge options are as follows:

- Skilled nursing facilities
- Subacute care facilities or units
- Rehabilitation facilities or units
- Intermediate care facilities
- Home care
- Hospice care
- Outpatient care
- Residential care
- Assisted living

In this step, case managers also revisit the patients' and families' responsibilities toward the transitional plan as agreed on initially after the patient's admission to the hospital and while the plan was being finalized. They examine whether the patient or family made the arrangements they were expected to make, and if not, a decision is made about the next expected step and who is responsible for handling the situation. In addition, case managers are expected to provide the patient, family, or caregiver with a written discharge notice confirming the discharge. This notice acts as a formal and documented notification for discharge, a copy of which usually is kept in the patient's medical record. As discussed in Chapter 5, if the patient and/or family disagree with the discharge, they are entitled to appeal the decision by notifying the PRO in their region. If they appeal, the discharge is then held until a decision by the PRO is reached and the patient and the organization providing the care are informed.

A final function of the case managers in this step is confirming the following:

- The final transitional/discharge plan with the physician, patient, and family; the facility the patient is to be transferred to (only in such cases); and the case manager of the health insurance plan/managed care company if appropriate
- The date and time of transfer or discharge
- That any required paperwork is completed, such as transportation request form, home care orders, and interinstitutional transfer and handoff notes
- Date and time of delivery of durable medical equipment and other care supplies
- Follow-up care appointments if indicated

Box 6.6   Sample Discharge Screens

InterQual's Cardiovascular-Related Discharge Criteria

- Last prothrombin time (PT) within therapeutic range with anticoagulants
- Potassium between 3.5 and 5.5 in the last 12 hours
- Controlled anginal pain
- Controlled dysrhythmias
- Controlled dyspnea, edema
- No significant ECG changes

Milliman Guidelines' Discharge Criteria for Unstable Angina

- Pain-free
- No significant ECG changes
- Troponin negative for myocardial injury
- No need for immediate invasive therapy in the next 24 hours
- No parenteral medication therapy such as heparin or nitroglycerine

6.3.6. Step Six: Discharge/Transfer of the Patient to Another Level of Care

On the day of the patient's discharge or transition, the case managers may not be involved in any major activities other than confirming that the discharge takes place as planned. Any change in the patient's condition that may require continued hospitalization is addressed, and the case manager, in consultation with the healthcare team, determines if the discharge should be cancelled. If the discharge is cancelled, then the case manager reapplies the transitional planning process, revises the plan, or develops a new transitional plan reflective of the patient's condition and needs.

In this step of the transitional plan, the case manager may answer any final questions of the patient/family, receiving facility or team at the next level of care, or the health insurance plan. The case manager also provides the facility to be responsible for the post-discharge care (whether a skilled nursing facility, a long-term care facility, or a home care agency) with the appropriate information regarding the patient's condition and the required care. This information is important because it ensures safety and continuity of care and prevents unnecessary readmissions to the acute care setting.

6.3.7. Step Seven: Following-Up on Patient Post-Discharge or Post-Transition

In this step of the discharge/transitional planning process, case managers contact the patient and/or family after discharge from the acute care setting and check on the patient, answering any questions that may arise, and ensuring that patient is continuing the plan of care as was discussed in the discharge or transition instruction. Some organizations may have someone other than the case manager complete such calls. Regardless, the main aspects of the follow-up calls include, but are not limited to, the following:

■ Review the post-discharge plan of care
■ Check on the patient's level of comfort with self-care
■ Examine the patient's understanding of and adherence to the medications prescribed and that prescriptions have been filled
■ Examine patient's understanding of and adherence to the necessary treatments such as simple dressing change, diabetic diet followed
■ Answer any questions the patient may have and clarify any misunderstandings
■ Relieve the patient's anxiety about self-care management

■ Ensure the post-discharge services arranged for are available (e.g., home care, Meals on Wheels)

It is important to complete the follow-up call within 48–72 hours post-discharge but no longer than 7 days after discharge. There is ample evidence in the literature that these timeframes do reduce avoidable readmissions, improve patient's engagement in their own care, prevent medical errors, ensure continuity of care, and enhance patient's satisfaction with care.

In some instances patients may not be reachable or may lack capacity to engage in a telephone conversation. Contacting the patient's care giver or representative is appropriate. What is most important is that a follow-up call is completed and a quality, safe discharge is confirmed. If a patient is transitioned to another healthcare organization (e.g., skilled nursing facility) instead of home, the follow-up call can be made to the healthcare team at the receiving organization instead and focus the call on continuity of care and clarification of any issues or concerns.

As part of every step of the transitional planning process, case managers are responsible for documenting their plans, interventions, outcomes of coordinating the post-discharge services, and next action steps.

It is evident that the transitional planning process is an integral component of case management, and it cannot be completed without consideration of utilization management. Although the discussion presented in this chapter focuses mostly on transitional planning, case managers are advised to be careful in their interpretation of this discussion and to consider the steps presented here within the larger context of case management and their roles and responsibilities. At any time and in any given situation, case managers are always applying the concepts of transitional planning, clinical care management, and utilization management into their action plans and the decisions they make to resolve problems. Table 6.6 summarizes the relationship or correlation between the processes of case management and transitional/discharge planning.

6.4. TRANSFERRING PATIENTS TO OTHER FACILITIES

Not every patient is discharged to the home setting after a hospitalization. Some patients may need to be transferred to another facility such as a skilled nursing facility, whereas others may need to be transferred back to the facility they came from before hospitalization. Case managers play an important role in the process of transferring patients from one hospital or level of care to another. They ensure that the transfer packet

TABLE 6.6. The Relationship Between the Case Management and Transitional/Discharge Planning Processes.

Case Management Process	Transitional/Discharge Planning Process
1. Case finding and intake	▪ Patient's admission ▪ Screening patient for post-discharge needs ▪ Identifying need for discharge and post-discharge services
2. Assessment of patient's needs	▪ Assessment of discharge/transitional planning needs ▪ Agreeing on needs with patient, family, healthcare team ▪ Assessing available resources and type of resources
3. Identification of actual and potential problems and concerns	▪ Identification of the key patient's problems or concerns ▪ Discussing the problems of focus with the patient and family ▪ Discussing the problems of focus with the interdisciplinary care team ▪ Agreeing on the main problems of focus in the transional plan
4. Interdiscplinary care planning	▪ Development of transitional/discharge plan ▪ Designing action plan for meeting patient's discharge and ▪ Post-discharge needs ▪ Agreeing on goals of plan and expected outcomes
5. Implementation of the interdisciplinary plan of care	▪ Implementation of the plan ▪ Putting plan into action ▪ Coordinating necessary activities ▪ Brokering of services with community agencies ▪ Educating patient and family regarding healthcare needs
6. Evaluation of patient care outcomes	▪ Evaluation of transitional plan ▪ Monitoring appropriateness of plan ▪ Examining outcomes of plan ▪ Exchanging information with post-discharge agencies as needed
7. Patient's discharge, transition, or disposition	▪ Preparing patient for discharge ▪ Confirming patient's discharge ▪ Confirming post-discharge services ▪ Patient's discharge ▪ Actual discharge to home ▪ Transferring patient to another facility
8. Repeating the process	▪ Repeating the process ▪ Reapplying transitional planning process based on changes in patient's condition ▪ Ensuring the transitional plan of care reflects the changing patient's needs
9. Following-up on patient post-discharge/transition	▪ Contacting patient and/or family post-discharge or post-transition ▪ Checking on status of post-discharge services arranged for ▪ Checking on patient's condition ▪ Answering any questions the patient/family may have regarding continuity of care

contains the complete information that is necessary for continuity of care and decision-making in the receiving hospital or facility. The transfer information, also referred to as handoff, must include the following:

▪ Copy of the medical record that contains the patient's radiographic reports, blood work, medical history and physical examination, ECG reports, assessments from specialist providers, and social services assessment
▪ Copy of any advance directive, DNR order, healthcare proxy, or living will

▪ Patient's consent for the transfer
▪ Physician transfer orders
▪ Treatment plan and post-discharge care expected to be continued in the new facility
▪ Accepting physician's name and medical service
▪ Transfer note which includes a summary of the care the patient received while under the care of the transferring facility and healthcare team. This includes key diagnostic and therapeutics tests and procedures, plan of care, and care required to ensure safety and enhance continuity.

It is important to arrange for these documents to prevent patients from being returned to the transferring facility. Sometimes, and in some states, it is required that a pretransfer evaluation be completed and that this evaluation documents the appropriateness of the transfer and that the accepting facility and healthcare team approves the transfer before the acutal patient's transfer occurs. Case managers can confirm that such regulations are followed and that such an evaluation is completed before a patient's transfer.

In 1998 the CMS passed a regulation regarding transferring Medicare patients that fall in 10 DRG categories. Since then many more DRGs have been added to the list. The first 10 transfer DRGs are listed in Table 6.7. This regulation was passed to curtail the increased number of transfers of patients to subacute care facilities, especially those who are transferred within a few days of an acute care hospital stay. At the time, subacute care was fairly new and not yet under the prospective payment system structure. Acute care institutions found it a rewarding opportunity to transfer patients such as those with strokes, pneumonia, and orthopedic problems early on during their treatment plan for rehabilitation in subacute care settings. Such transfers left acute care hospitals with more desirable lengths of stay and better fiscal states, considering the pressures of the acute care prospective payment system.

As stated in the regulation, patients in any of these 10 DRGs are considered transfers if (1) they were to receive care in a skilled nursing facility or home care after discharge from the hospital, (2) the services are related to the patient's condition during the hospitalization, and (3) these services are provided within 3 days of hospitalization. The condition of 3 days can be translated into a rule of not transferring any patient in any of the 10 DRGs before the acute care length of stay reaches the geometric mean length of stay identified in the DRG system. If this happens, the acute care facility will be penalized.

Case managers can prevent this penalty from happening and can enhance compliance with this regulation through their role in the transitional/discharge planning process. They can incorporate such a regulation as a criterion of transfer when they evaluate their patients' readiness for discharge or transfer to another facility. They can also educate the rest of the healthcare team about this regulation to improve compliance and prevent the hospital from being penalized by the CMS in case of lack of compliance. Another strategy to increase compliance is for case managers to apply this criterion when they are coordinating post-discharge services for their patients with subacute care facilities or home care agencies. Also refer to tips presented in Case Manager's Tip 6.10 for more information about patient transfers.

TABLE 6.7. The First 10 Transfer Diagnosis-Related Groups.

DRG	MDC	Title
14	M	Specific cerebrovascular disorders except TIAs; examples are subarachnoid hemorrhage, subdural hemorrhage, cerebral aneurysm, nonruptured cerebral aneurysm, CVA
113	S	Amputations for circulatory system disorders except upper limb and toe; examples are lower limb amputation, below knee amputation, above knee amputation, disarticulation of hip
209	S	Major joint and limb reattachment procedures of lower extremity; examples are total hip replacement, total knee replacement, limb reattachment
210	S	Hip and femur procedures except for major joint; examples are open reduction of fracture of the head of femur with various hardware
211	S	Hip and femur procedures except major joint without complications or comorbidities
236	M	Fractures of hip and pelvis; examples are fracture of pelvis such as acetabulum and pelvis, femoral neck fracture such as subtrochanteric or intratrochanteric fractures
263	S	Skin graft and/or debridement for skin ulcer with complications and comorbidity; examples are skin graft for cellulitis (any site), decubitus ulcer, chronic skin ulcer
264	S	Skin graft and/or debridement for skin ulcer or cellulitis without complications or comorbidity; examples are skin graft for cellulitis (any site), decubitus ulcer, chronic skin ulcer
429	M	Organic disturbances and mental retardation; example is organic brain syndrome
483	S	Tracheostomy except for face, mouth, and neck diagnosis

Cerebral vascular accident, CVA; geometric mean length of stay, GMLOS; medical, M; major diagnostic category, MDC; surgical, S; transient ischemic attack, TIA.

CASE MANAGER'S TIP 6.10

Transferring Patients to Other Facilities

The case manager must consider the following three scenarios when transferring patients to other facilities:

1. If a Medicare or Medicaid patient is transferred from one hospital to another, the receiving hospital receives the full DRG payment. The transferring hospital, however, receives a per diem payment for each day of the patient's stay based on the DRG rate applicable. The case manager should examine all cases that are transferred before transfer for appropriateness in an effort to prevent financial loss and maximize reimbursement.

2. If a patient is transferred from one level of care to another within the same hospital (e.g., from an intensive care unit to a medical unit) and the patient is then discharged to home or a skilled care facility as required by patient's condition and according to applicable regulations, the hospital receives one payment. The case manager should evaluate patients as necessary for a timely transfer from one level of care to another less intensive or a complex level or discharged to home or skilled care facility to ensure the delivery of safe, cost-effective, and appropriate level of care.

3. If a patient is transferred from one unit in a Medicare- or Medicaid-participating hospital to another hospital or unit that is exempt, the patient is treated as a discharge. However, the case manager is responsible for ensuring that the transfer is appropriate and meets applicable regulations so that reimbursement is not jeopardized.

6.5. SUCCESSFUL, SAFE, AND QUALITY TRANSITIONS OF CARE

Achieving effective transitions of patients from one healthcare organization, provider, or care setting to another depends on the case management strategies, interventions, and activities implemented to provide for the continuation of safe, quality, and cost-effective care and transitional plans.

Transitions of care refer to the movement of patients between healthcare providers or settings and home as their condition and care needs change to warrant the transition (Figure 6.2). For example, a patient may be receiving care in the primary care provider's office on an ambulatory basis and then a change in condition occurs and indicates the need for care and services in an inpatient acute care setting, during which an interdisciplinary team of healthcare providers gets involved,

and after a number of days the patient is transitioned yet to another healthcare team in an acute rehabilitation facility for 2 weeks of rehabilitation, and ultimately the patient returns to the home setting where the primary care provider resumes responsibility for follow up care. During these transitions the patient encounters different healthcare providers and care settings.

Transitions do not always go smoothly. During each of these transitions, the patient may face increased risks for suboptimal care, unsafe situations, medical errors, or miscommunciations that may result in poor outcomes and/or unpleasant patient experience (Case Manager's Tip 6.11).

Hospitals with unacceptably high readmission rates for Medicare and Medicaid patients now encounter financial reimbursement penalties based on the Patient Protection and Affordable Care Act of 2010 and value-based purchasing. Many factors contribute to ineffective transitions. The root causes of these suboptimal transitions vary across organizations. Regardless however, these can be summarized in three main areas, as follows.

1. *Communuication breakdowns*: These involve communciations among the various members of the healthcare teams within and across care settings as well as with the patient, family, or caregiver. Examples of situations which contribute to miscommunication include differing expectations between the senders and receivers of patients undergoing transitions; lack of teamwork and collaboration; not enough time to ensure safe transmistition; and lack of standardized tools, standards, or procedures for handoff communication.

2. *Patient and family engagement and education breakdowns*: These relate to patients not comfort-

 CASE MANAGER'S TIP 6.11

Transitions of Care

Every transition of care involves a handoff communication including keeping patient and family well informed about the transition. Often serious medical errors that occur during or post the patient's transition are almost always due to miscommunication between the healthcare providers within and/or across care settings. These errors sometimes result in unnecessary and avoidable readmissions to the acute care setting. Case managers can play an important role in preventing miscommunciation, ensuring safe patient transitions.

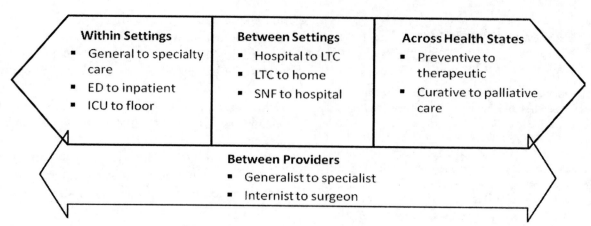

Within Settings	Between Settings	Across Health States
▪ General to specialty care ▪ ED to inpatient ▪ ICU to floor	▪ Hospital to LTC ▪ LTC to home ▪ SNF to hospital	▪ Preventive to therapeutic ▪ Curative to palliative care

Between Providers
- Generalist to specialist
- Internist to surgeon

Figure 6.2 Types of transitions of care.

able with assuming self-care post-discharge and lack of awareness of the treatment plan and follow-up care post-discharge or transition. Examples of circumstances resulting from this breakdown include lack of patient's support system to participate in patient care post-discharge, low health literacy, lack of funds to secure needed medications and monitoring equipment or care supplies, and healthcare providers excluding patient/family from planning the post-discharge care.

3. *Healthcare team or providers accountability breakdowns*: Often these breakdowns result from a lack of one healthcare team member assuming accountability, ownership, and responsibility for ensuring safe and quality patient's transition including complete, accurate, and timely handoff communcation. Examples of when such breakdowns can occur include: multiple specialist providers caring for a patient with no one assuming responsibility for care coordination; primary care provider unavailable for assuming care post-discharge; misplaced or completely absent information regarding the patient's care summary; and plan of care post-discharge.

6.5.1. Strategies, Tools, and Standards for Effective Transitions of Care

Developing ways, tools, and standards to ensure safe transitions of patients across the continuum of care requires effective collaboration among members of the interdisciplinary healthcare team in the care setting the patient is transitioned from and those of the setting transitioned to. Having a case manager as members of these teams is important to facilitate the complete transfer of information from one setting to the next and to answer any questions that arise during and after the patient's transitions. Using tools or checklists to identify patients

at higher risk for unsafe transitions (Case Manager's Tip 6.12) and possible readmissions to the acute care setting is one way to counter ineffective transitions. Box 6.7 lists the factors such tools may include.

Other strategies to ensure effective, quality and safe transitions of care among providers and settings are:

- Support of healthcare leaders including those involved in operations, nursing, case management, quality, and safety programs
- Interdisciplinary collaboration within and across settings of care
- Risk stratification of patients and implementation of specific care interventions appropriate for the risk category
- Early identification of patients at higher risk for transition concerns and avoidable readmissions to acute care
- Case management and discharge/transitional planning programs, standards, checklists, and other tools

 CASE MANAGER'S TIP 6.12

Inadquate Transitions of Care Contribute to Suboptimal Outcomes and Experiences
- Medication errors
- Inefficient, duplicative, or fragmented care and services
- Inadequate patient/caregiver preparation for transition and self-management
- Inadequate follow-up care post-discharge or transition
- Dissatisfaction with the care experience during transition
- Malpractice and litigation
- Unnecessary and preventable cost
- Preventable readmissions to acute care or access to emergency services

---

Box 6.7   Sample Risk Factors Used in Assessing Patient's Risk for Unsafe Transition or Readmission to Acute Care

- Multiple comorbidities
- Diagnoses known to be chronic and are associated with increased and frequent readmissions to acute care such as heart failure, end-stage renal disease, oncologic diseases, chronic obstructive pulmonary disease, chronic pain, and diabetes
- Conditions included in the Medicare Hospital Readmissions Reduction Program (HRRP)
- Polypharmacy
- History of frequent readmissions and access to emergency services; e.g., three times in past 6 months
- Lack of psychosocial support system
- Suboptimal socioeconomic situation
- Issues related to mental and emotional health
- Unengaged in self-care management or inability to assume such role and missing follow-up care
- Age; above 65 years
- Limited or absent financial resources including inadequate or no health insurance coverage
- Suboptimal living situation including home condition
- Multiple care providers involved including primary and specialty providers and across multiple care settings

---

- Medication management and reconciliation, especially for patients on a large number of prescriptions (polypharmacy)
- Active engagement and participation of patients and families including educational programs based on health literacy assessments and use of the teach-back methods
- Use of patient personal health records which include key information about the primary care provider, specialty care provider(s), allergies, medications regimen, health insurance benefits, advance directive or healthcare proxy, red flags to watch out for, follow-up care, and family or caregiver information
- Complete, accurate, and timely handoff and transfer of essential information across settings and providers including detailed summary of care
- Post-episode of care patient call programs which consist of calling patients within 48–72 hours post discharge to follow-up on patient's condition, check whether post-discharge services are in place as was planned, adherence to plan of care, and to answer any questions the patients may have

Similar to using a screening tool upon admission to an acute care setting to assess the patient's risk for un-

necessary and avoidable return to the hospital post-discharge, often acute care organizations also implement a standardized discharge checklist or tool that is evidence-based and thought to ensure a quality and safe patient discharge from the hospital to the home setting, with or without homecare services. Box 6.8 lists a set of the common elements of these tools.

Box 6.8   Sample Elements of Standardized Discharge/Transitional Planning Checklists

- Patient and Family Counseling and Education
  —Smoking cessation counseling
  —Symptom management and red flags
  —Medications administration and management
  —Use of durable medical equipment
  —Treatments post-discharge (e.g., simple wound care) and use of medical supplies
  —Complete discharge instructions given
- Access to Medications
  —Assessment of medication affordability
  —Ability to physically obtain medications or need to arrange for home delivery
- Follow-Up Care
  —Post-discharge calls within 48–72 hours
  —Best contact infiormation and time to call
  —Extended post-discharge calls (e.g., patient with multiple chronic illnesses increasing the risk for avoidable readmissions); calls beyond 72 hours of discharge
  —Scheduling of follow-up care appointments before patient's discharge and ensuring the dates/times are reasonable (e.g., within 7 days of discharge) and meet patient's expectations and ability to adhere to
  —Transportation required for post-discharge follow-up care
  —Home care services
- Referrals
  —Outpatient rehabilitation services including physical and pulmonary therapy
  —Ambulatory specialty care such as podiatry and ophthalmology
- Summary of Care
  —Complete summary of care transmitted to primary care provider and specialty care provider(s)
  —Complete summary of care given to the patient, family, or caregiver
- Enrollment in web-based personal health record tools
  —Initiate access to online personal health record which contains, e.g., a summary of health status, care preferences, information about care providers, plan of care, red flags, medications regimen
  —Access patient and family educational materials
  —Communicate findings from monitoring activities such as blood sugar level, blood pressure, and weight

6.5.2. Interdisciplinary Patient Care Management Rounds in Acute Care Settings

Daily interdisciplinary patient care management rounds in the acute care/hospital settings have recently gained renewed popularity by healthcare executives, case management program leaders, case managers, physicians, social workers, quality management specialists, and other healthcare providers. When completed effectively, they ensure open communication, teamwork, safe, quality, and timely transition of patients from one care setting to another or to home (Case Manager's Tip 6.13). The purposes of interdisciplinary care rounds are described in Box 6.9.

Patients addressed during interdisciplinary care management rounds in the hospital or acute care settings can be categorized into three groups:

1. *Patients being discharged on same day as the rounds*: Confirmation of scheduled discharges for the day and addressing any barriers that may result in discharge delay or cancellation to ensure the discharge stays on schedule and to avoid any potential reimbursement denials. These patients tend to be at the end of their hospital stay and the rounds address primarily, if not completely, the discharge.

 CASE MANAGER'S TIP 6.13

Interdisciplinary Patient Care Management Rounds

Interdisciplinary rounds are popular in the acute care settings, usually occur on a daily basis, and include various members of the healthcare team such as the following:

- Case manager
- Social worker
- Physician(s)
- Physican assistant
- Advanced practice registered nurse
- Therapists (e.g., physical therapist, occupational therapist)
- Pharmacist
- Registered dietician
- Manager or administrator
- Other clinicians involved in patient's care, based on the patient needs and the clinical area

Often the rounds are quick, focused, and may happen in a central location on a patient care unit or at the patient's bedside (preferred) involving the patient and/or family.

Box 6.9 Purpose of Interdisciplinary Patient Care Management Rounds

Interdisciplinary rounds have many purposes and objectives and tend to vary based on the healthcare organization's case management program, policies, procedures, and standards. These may include the following:

- Discuss the patient's plan of care and progress toward achieving care goals.
- Confirm the transitional plan has been developed, is relevant, appropriate, and continues to meet the changing patient's condition and needs.
- Ensure everyone is in agreement regarding the plan of care including the patient and family.
- Improve communication among the interdisciplinary healthcare team members and with patient/family.
- Communicate important information and observations.
- Address concerns such as care delays (e.g., outstanding procedures, laboratory test, barriers to care progression), disagreements and health insurance plan mandates including service denials.
- Assign accountability for specific care follow up activities to healthcare team members.

---

2. *Newly admitted patients*: Identification of goals of care for those recently admitted to the hospital/patient care unit with special focus on developing patient's individualized plans of care and agreeing as a healthcare team on specific care milestones. This type of rounds addresses the needs of patients whose plans of care may not be completely and confidently articulated yet and ensures that the patient, the patient's family/caregiver, and the healthcare team are all on the same page and well aware of the patient's condition and care needs.

3. *Patients hospitalized more than one day and not yet ready for discharge*: Review of the patient's plan of care, clinical milestones, and discharge or transitional plan. Follow up on consults with specialty care providers, tests, procedures, ethical and other care considerations (e.g., advanced directives, palliative care, mental status/competency issues), service denials, and any anticipated discharge challenges such as undocumented status, challenging placement in long term facility, or lack of or limited health insurance benefits. Mostly the rounds for these patients focuses on care progression toward safe discharge or transition to another level of care.

Often and due to value-based purchasing and the

pressure to reduce the length of stay in the hospital/ acute care setting, some healthcare organizations have revised and standardized the conduct of daily interdisciplinary patient care management rounds. These efforts resulted in a streamlined approach to the content and context of rounds for patients who are being discharged on same day as the rounds and those who are not (Table 6.8). Those who are not scheduled for discharge may refer to patients in both the new admission and the not yet ready for discharge categories. Members of the interdisciplinary team may round on all patients at one time or at two different occasions during the day. However, rounding on patients scheduled for discharge should be completed by 10 A.M. at the latest.

Interdisciplinary care rounds have been a tradition in acute care settings, but recently they have gained increasing popularity in the ambulatory and patient centered or primary care medical home setting. In these settings, members of the interdisciplinary healthcare team do not meet daily to discuss patients' plans of care because such frequency is unnecessary. However, they may meet every few weeks or on a monthly basis routinely, and as warranted due to a change in patient condition and need for unanticipated access to services in the emergency or acute care settings (Case Manager's Tip 6.14 and Box 6.10).

6.5.3. Managing Long-Stay Patients in the Acute Care Settings

Case managers always encounter a number of patients hospitalized in the actute care setting who stay longer

TABLE 6.8. Focus of Interdisciplinary Patient Care Management Rounds by Patient Group.

Patients Discharged on Same Day as Rounds (completed early in the morning, preferably before 10 A.M.)	New Patients or Not Ready for Discharge (completed anytime during the day, preferably before 3 P.M.)
▪ Review outstanding/pending laboratory or radiologic tests and procedures ▪ Confirm discharge and post-discharge services (e.g., DME, home care, rehabiltation facility, SNF bed, and infusion therapy) and payor authorization where necessary ▪ Confirm completion of outstanding follow-up items from MD, SW, CM, RN, PT/OT ▪ Confirm completion of discharge summary, prescriptions, and education regarding medications, treatments, and red flags. ▪ Confirm follow-up appointment with primary care provider ▪ Complete patient/family discharge education and enrollment in web-based personal health record ▪ Confirm transportation services	▪ Review active problems and history of present illness ▪ Confirm medical care team and information about patient's primary care provider and/or referring physician ▪ Communicate individual accountability for facilitating discharge or transitional plan of care: CM, SW, RN, or combination ▪ Review estimated length of stay and/or expected discharge date ▪ Confirm patient/family are aware of expected discharge date, discharge destination, and needed post-discharge services ▪ Arrange for all necessary post-discharge services and disposition ▪ Review outstanding follow-up needed from care team: MD, SW, CM, RN, T/OT, etc. ▪ Review results of tests and procedures; implications for care progression, use of clinical pathway or guideline if applicable, whether patient can be taken off isolation, or needing palliative care ▪ Review care aspects: ambulation status, Foley catheter, DVT prophylaxis, pain management, and any other aspects of care that pertain to Value-Based Purchasing measures ▪ Review issues related to patient safety ▪ Review barriers to discharge/transition and relevant psychosocial circumstances ▪ Discuss utilization review and related reimbursement issues(i.e., medical necessity, two-Midnight Rule, PRO or QIO appeals, physician advisor referral) ▪ Decide readiness for conditional discharge order (applies for patients planned for discharged next day, but can not be confirmed in advance)

Case manager, CM; durable medical equipment, DME; deep venin thrombosis, DVT; physician, MD; occupational therapist, OT; peer review organization, PRO; physical therapist, PT; quality improvement organization, QIO; social worker, SW; skilled nursing facility, SNF.

CASE MANAGER'S TIP 6.14

Interdisciplinary Patient Care Management Rounds in Ambulatory Care Settings

Interdisciplinary patient care management rounds in the ambulatory care settings have become an integral part of the operations in patient-centered centered and primary care medical homes. Case managers usually facilitate these rounds and ensure that patients with multiple chronic illnesses and/or on a large number of medications (polypharmacy) are discussed regularly and that they have short- and long-term care goals including a plan of care that is formally reviewed at least semiannually and as indicated by changes in the patient's condition.

than expected; often way beyond the average length of stay at the hospital. Although healthcare professionals and executives traditionally have labeled those hospitalized for 30 days or longer in the acute care setting as long-stay patients, case management experts today define such patient group as those with a length of stay (LOS) that is two standard deviations greater than the hospital's average LOS. For example, if a hospital's LOS is 5 days and the standard deviation is 3 days, then long-stay patients are those with a LOS that exceeds 11 days. More aggressive and proactive case management programs, however, are currently defining long-stay patients as those with a LOS of 7 days or greater. Carefully managing those with such LOS allows case managers and other healthcare professionals to address the barriers to discharge or transition to another level of care before the LOS presents financial risk due to reimbursement concerns and medical necessity criteria for continued acute care stay not being met. Regardless of whether an organization defines the threshold for long-stay patients at 7 days or two standard deviations above the average LOS, interventions and strategies to overcome the challenges of caring for these patients are the same.

Carefully and effectively managing long-stay patients is a necessary component of acute care case management programs. It reduces financial risk and enhances care quality, safety, and the patient's experience of care. This strategic focus is also integral to the discharge/transitional planning process, the role of the case manager, the interdisciplinary team and patient care management rounds, and the role of the physician advisor. These long-stay patients require special management; otherwise they may stay an extended period of time in the hospital unnecessarily, consume a considerable proportion of acute care resources, and

incur added expenses that often place the hospital at increased financial risk as a result of care delays and reimbursement concerns.

Often patients stay longer than expected as a result of challenging discharge/transition plans. For example, when patients are to be discharged to an alternate level of care (e.g., skilled care facility), while the alternative is either not available or difficult to access (i.e., limited number of skilled care beds in the area or region), they may end up waiting in the hospital until the challenge is resolved. As a result, both patients/families and hospitals are disadvantaged in these long-stay situations.

- *Patients are disadvantaged* because they may not be receiving optimum care, and may in fact suffer detrimental effects (e.g., complications) by being hospitalized. An example is hospital acquired healthcare associated infections.
- *Hospitals are disadvantaged* because their resources are not available to other more appropriately hospitalized patients in a timely fashion, resulting in suboptimal and sometimes costly care experiences.

Several factors contribute to long-stay patients: some are patient/family related while others are healthcare providers or systems of care related (Box 6.11).

Box 6.10 Members of Interdisciplinary Teams Who Participate in Patient Care Planning and Management Rounds in the Ambulatory Care Settings

Unlike healthcare teams of the acute care settings, teams in the ambulatory care settings who meet regularly and discuss patients' plans of care are fairly small in size and may include the following:

- Case manager
- Physician/primary care provider
- Specialty care provider(s)
- Advanced practice clinician/provider (e.g., advanced practice registered nurse, physican assistant) if members of care teams
- Clinical nurse
- Pharmacist
- Community health worker
- Health advisor
- Practice administrator

Optional depending on the patient population

- Social worker
- Registered dietician
- Psychologist
- Psychiatrist
- Physical therapist

Box 6.11   Factors That Increase the Risk for Long-Stay Patients in the Acute Care Setting

Factors that contribute to patients experiencing long stays in the hospital or acute care setting can be classified into five broad categories. However, one category alone may not contribute to long-stay; often those who experience extended hospital stays are patients who experience multiple factors from two or more of the following categories.

Patient's Socioeconomic and Demographic Characteristics

- Age: mostly individuals over 65 years old or other ages (e.g., children), however, with medical, developmental, or congenital disabilities
- Gender: females are known to experience long-stay more than males
- Low income or poverty
- Limited or no health insurance coverage
- Poor access to transportation
- Lower educational level

Patient's Health Condition and Illness

- Debilitating illnesses such as stroke, chronic cardiac and circulatory disease, and complex musculoskeletal conditions
- Cognitive impairment, dementia, and sensory disturbances
- Behavioral health illness, especially when present in conjunction with a medical condition
- Requiring close/maximum observation and supervision (e.g., one-to-one care)
- Need for dialysis
- Mechanical ventilator support
- Need for percutaneous endoscopic gastrostomy PEG tube for feeding
- Presence of tracheostomy
- Rehabilitation (acute or sub-acute)
- Total dependence in activities of daily living

Patient's Psychosocial Situation

- Lack of social support system
- Lives alone
- Use of supportive care services or custodial care prior to hospitalization
- Residence prior to hospitalization: suboptimal or unsafe home condition, homeless, floor of residence compared to patient's function abilities
- Need for 24-hour supportive care but not within payor's eligibility criteria or family can not afford
- Guardianship
- Physical abuse by self or others such as a child or next of kin
- Substance use
- Self-isolation

Healthcare Providers (Including Case Managers)

- Mismatching of patient's needs and discharge or transition plan (inappropriate transition plan)
- Delays in care or transition paperwork
- Focusing on one transitional plan with no attention to an alternate plan
- Disagreements among members of the interdisciplinary healthcare team
- Ethical situation not addressed in a timely fashion
- Ineffective communication
- Lack of accountability

Systems of Care

- Awaiting admission to another facility
- Unavilable bed in a nursing home or sub-acute care facility
- Not enough beds in long-term care or rehabilitation facilities
- Unclear regulations or regulatory standards for discharge/transition planning
- Providers or agencies at the next level of care unavailable or unresponsive
- Durable medical equipment and/or care supplies not covered by payer

Long-stay patients may consume greater amounts of time from case managers and tend to distract them from paying closer attention to the care of patients with shorter lengths of stay or those newly admitted to the hospital/acute care setting. This distraction may unintentionally result in care delays including discharge or transition to another less acute level of care which ultimately may lead to health insurance plans denying reimbursement for certain hospital days, and/or a patient and family complaining about delayed services or suboptimal experiences.

Case managers may not be able to control or manage every factor present in a long-stay patient's situation. Some occur naturely, mostly as a result of disease progression, and are considered appropriate. Case managers and/or other healthcare providers may expect that they happen and may not be able to overcome or expedite their resolution. Others appear unexpectedly, are considered variances or deviations from the norm, and are preventable. These often are avoidable and case managers and/or healthcare providers should be able to resolve them or prevent their occurrence altogether. However, system factors that are community-based (e.g., not enough long-term care beds available) and beyond the authority of the hospital-based team may be outside the scope of case managers and require the intervention of case management program leaders and senior executives at the hospital in collaboration with other leaders in the community.

- *Naturally occurring factors* are related to health condition or disease progression pattern and require complex recovery process. For example, weaning from mechanical ventilation.
- *Unexpected or out-of-the-ordinary factors* are related to system characteristics or provider behaviors which result in delays in care or disposition and ultimately an extended LOS. For example, no available beds in long-term care facilities or incomplete discharge or transition planning paperwork.

Most case management programs use a review process that aims to proactively identify and manage long-stay patients, the reason(s) causing the extended LOS, and the intervention(s) recommended to address the identified issue(s). Different healthcare organizations may use different processes and approaches. One example is the process described in Figure 6.3. It first starts with unit-based case managers reviewing the status of all their patients daily as part of their routine workflow and identify those with a LOS that is greater than or nearing the targeted LOS threshold (e.g., 7 days or longer). To make this process efficient and easy to apply and complete, the unit-based case

managers implement the long-stay process while using an automated report that includes all patients admitted to a specific patient care unit. In this approach, case managers collaborate with other members of the interdisciplinary healthcare team directly involved in the care of the patient with actual or potential long-stay concerns and attempt to resolve the factors contributing to the extended hospital stay.

The report case managers apply in the review process is generated based on the patient registration and electronic documentation systems the hospital uses. This report may include important information such as the following:

- Patient's name, location, date and time of admission
- Chief complaint or reason for admission
- Physician and provider team of record
- Calculated LOS to date
- Health insurance plan type

The report may also include other information such as those listed below, but depends on the case management documentation and the electronic systems' ability to compile.

- Number of hospital days authorized by the payer
- Last clinical review with date and decision
- Needed insurance or utilization management follow-up activities
- Disposition plan and status, including alternate plan if one is available
- Physician advisor involvement, reason, and resolution

The initial review can be purposefully embedded in the usual case manager's workflow to allow early identification of long-stay patients and to proactively manage these patients before they present serious financial, safety, or quality of care risks. For those with LOS either approaching or having exceeded the LOS threshold, case managers then identify the factors actually or potentially contributing to the increased LOS. Next case managers stratify the patients into one of the long-stay reason categories (e.g., meeting acute care medical necessity criteria, disposition delays, provider delays, system delays) and attempt to resolve the concern by implementing one or more of the recommended interventions in Figure 6.3 and based on the identfied reason category. For the health condition-related reasons, it is necessary for case managers to complete a clinical review that focuses on medical necessity criteria and appropriateness for continued acute care stay and confirm such, sometimes with the payer/health insurance plan when indicated. The other reasons are considered avoidable or preventable, however they may be of varying complexities and require more specialized interventions such as seeking the counsel of risk management, following the case management program's chain of command, or the attention of a hospital senior executive.

Some case management programs use the services of a specialized long-stay team to manage the complex patients that are known to require highly specialized and intensive interventions, discharge planning activi-ties, and resources. For example, pursuing guardian-ship for a patient or discharging a patient who is an uninsured and undocumented immigrant to the coun-try of origin requires special expertise. Because of the complex nature of the interventions, more time and re-sources are needed to execute successfully. Therefore, unit-based case managers are unable to allocate such time and effort to these patients while still meeting the competing needs of the other patients in their caseload in a timely and safe manner. In situations like this, the unit-

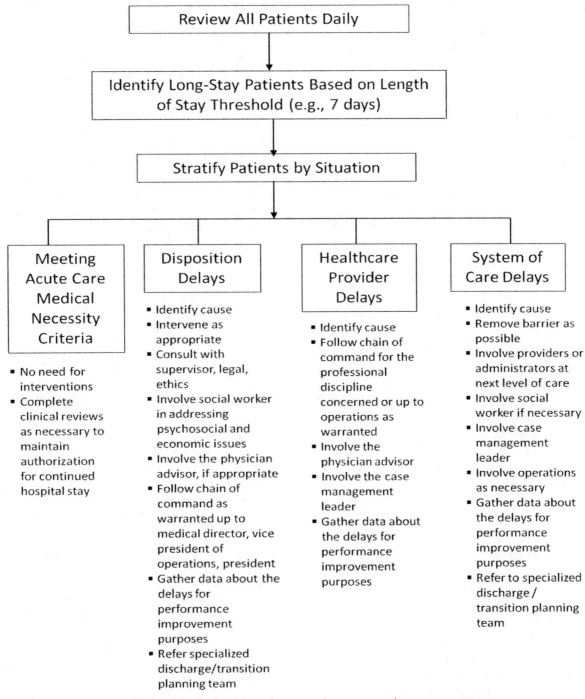

Figure 6.3 Process for identifying and managing long-stay patients.

based case manager refers the long-stay patients with complex needs to the specialized team for follow up.

The specialized long-stay team, sometimes referred to as complex discharge planning team, is an interdisciplinary team that is solely responsible for following up on the long-stay patients. This strategy allows unit-based case managers to pay closer attention to the rest of the patients in their caseloads rather than the overly complex few. When such a team is available, it usually focuses on patients with highly complex discharge or transition needs. Healthcare professionals who participate on these teams may include the following:

- Case manager
- Social worker specialized in complex discharge planning
- Physician advisor
- Case management director or supervisor
- Ethicist or patient and family advocate (optional or ad hoc)
- Risk management representative (optional or ad hoc)

The case manager and social worker act as a dyad to effectively address the clinical, psychosocial, and discharge planning needs of the long-stay patients. The physician advisor supports the case manager and social worker as well as addresses care progression concerns with the medical care providers. The physician advisor may also participate in resolving utilization management issues presented by the health insurance plans (i.e., payers). The ethicist or patient advocate facilitates resolution on ethical dilemmas or end of life care decisions while advocating on behalf of the patient and family. The risk management representative advises the team whether their care decisions may potentially result in any quality of care or malpractice liability risks. The case management director or supervisor addresses any chain of command issues, manages system delays that are beyond the authority of the team, and represents the voice of the senior leadership team.

Case management program leaders and healthcare executives may decide on the number of case managers and social workers to participate on teams of long-stay patients based on the volume of long-stay patients this team is expected to manage. Acute care hospitals may experience 1–2% long-stay patients on an average day. The higher the case mix index of the patient population served, the higher the percentage of long-stay patients. Another factor that impacts the volume of long-stay patients is the health insurance mix. For example, a hospital with a higher number of Medicaid beneficiaries, uninsured, and undocumented immigrants may result in higher long-stay patient volume.

Case management program leaders may determine the necessary composition of the long-stay team based on these factors.

It is important for members of the long-stay team to formally meet once a week, while in between meetings, team members continue to follow-up on their action plans and required interventions. During this meeting, each patient is discussed following the same process as in the interdisciplinary patient care management rounds. However, more time and indepth discussions are dedicated to the issues contributing to the extended acute care stay and status of the related interventions agreed upon during prior meetings. Often these issues are discharge or transitional planning related. The team also designs action plans for addressing the identified concerns of new patients or modify those of existing patients, and agree on who is best among members of the team to assume ownership and accountability for follow-up and communication with the rest of the team and the healthcare providers involved in caring for the patients. The team also documents these plans in the patients' medical records as appropriate. When the team identifies the need to hold a patient and family case conference, one is scheduled accordingly and completed in a timely manner. When there is a need to consult with a healthcare specialized professional who is not part of the patient's routine care team, such consult is sought out and efforts made to advance the care of the patient and progress toward discharge or transition to another level of care.

 CASE MANAGER'S TIP 6.15

Medicare Hospital Readmission Reduction Program

Readmissions to the hospital/acute care setting refer to patients being admitted for care within a certain time interval (usually 30 days) after discharge from an initial hospital stay. Higher readmission rates are an indication of inadequate discharge or transition plans, care, quality, or services while in the hospital or improper or suboptimal post-discharge services.

Medicare hospital readmissions counted in HRRP currently pertain to Medicare patients with five specific diagnoses or conditions, who are readmitted to the same or another acute care hospital within 30 days of discharge and must have at least 25 discharges with each diagnosis to count.

Although the incentive to reduce hospital readmissions refers to Medicare patients with specific diagnoses or conditions, some hospitals have applied their readmission prevention strategies to all patients.

The long-stay team documents its activities for the purpose of evaluating its impact on the quality, safety, and cost of care and reporting on outcomes including return on investment. It is necessary for case management programs which use a specialized team

 CASE MANAGER'S TIP 6.16

Penalties Imposed by the Medicare Hospital Readmission Reduction Program

Penalties are imposed when a hospital's readmissions of patients with the conditions included in HRRP are considered excess readmissions.

Excess readmissions are those that exceed a hospital's expected number of readmissions or rate tracked by HRRP and based on the patient population served in each of the conditions.

A hospital's excess readmission ratio for each HRRP condition is a measure of the hospital's readmission performance compared to the national average for the hospital's set of patients with that applicable condition.

HRRP uses an applicable period of 3 years of discharge data and the minimum of 25 cases to calculate a hospital's excess readmission ratio of each applicable condition.

A hospital's expected readmission rate for each of the HRRP conditions is the national mean of readmissions rate for the condition, risk-adjusted for the demographic characteristics of the patients in that condition served by the hospital, such as age and sex, the severity of illness of the hospital's patients, patient's frailty, and number of comorbidities. This is used to calculate the excess readmissions ratio or factor per condition for each hospital which is the risk-adjusted predicted readmissions divided by the risk-adjusted expected readmissions.

The penalties are calculated applying a complex formula based on the amount of Medicare payments received by the hospital for the excess readmissions. Medicare collects the excess payments from the hospital through a percentage reduction in the base Medicare inpatient claims payments, not to exceed a certain cap. Today the penalty cap has reached 3% of the aggregate inpatient prospective payment system base payment for the hospital.

Not having a readmissions strategy for the conditions inclued in HRRP, the hospital risks up to 3% of the Medicare payments for these conditions. Case management can play an important role in reducing readmissions and therefore enhancing reimbursement by avoiding the HRRP imposed financial risk.

(Details available at www.cms.gov under hospital readmissions program accessible at www.cms.gov/Medicare/Medicare-Fee-for-Service-Payment/AcuteInpatientPPS/Readmissions-Reduction-Program.html)

for long-stay patients to also have representatives from the team participate as members of the utilization review committee. This is one forum where the team can present its report of activities and outcomes, share trends on the types and reasons for long-stay patients, and whether an opportunity exists to launch any performance improvement teams to address the identified trends.

6.5.4. Tools and Standards for Effective Transitions of Care

Health policy makers, executives, providers, consumer advocates, and case management have used patient readmissions to acute care as a proxy for the quality and safety of the discharge or transition plan. The issue of readmissions has gained more attention the past several years due to value-based purchasing, and when CMS began to report hospital readmission rates on its Hospital Compare website in 2009. Although no financial penalty was imposed then, efforts to reduce hospital readmission rates increased and became an integral and necessary focus of case management programs upon passing of the Patient Protection and Affordable Care Act—most importantly when the Medicare Hospital Readmissions Reduction Program (HRRP) went into effect beginning in October 2012 at the start of fiscal year 2013 (Case Manager's Tip 6.15). It is only then when financial incentives went into effect; however this was only related to specific patient populations including Medicare patients 65 years of age or older with the diagnoses of acute myocardial infarction, heart failure, or pneumonia.

In fiscal year 2015, which started in October 2014, the HRRP expanded to include Medicare patients age 65 or older with the diagnoses of elective hip or knee replacement surgery and chronic obstructive pulmonary disease. Although readmissions can be planned

 CASE MANAGER'S TIP 6.17

Improving Medicare Post-Acute Care Transformation (IMPACT) Act

In September 2014 the United States Congress passed the IMPACT Act to go into effect in October 2016. The Act mandates common patient assessment data and quality measure reporting requirements by acute care hospitals to post-acute care providers. This intends to facilitate the flow of patient information to the next healthcare setting. This also may result in changes to the post-acute prospective payment system for Medicare patients.

and unplanned, those which are unplanned present most of the quality and cost risks to providers.

■ Planned readmissions refer to those which require phased care such as patients on chemotherapy treatment. Providers are comfortable with planned readmissions as these are indicated by the plan of care the patient needs.

■ Unplanned readmissions are those which can be avoided or prevented. Unplanned readmissions are perceived to result from inadquate quality of care and poor case management.

TABLE 6.9. Select Transitions of Care Models.

Model	Highlights
Care Transitions Intervention (CTI) www.caretransitions.org Coleman CTI model	<ul><li>A 4-week program designed to foster patient engagement and to promote safe transition from the hospital or skilled nursing facility to home</li><li>Decreases rehospitalizations</li><li>Four pillars for safe transitions: — Medications self-management — Maintenance of a personal health record — Primary care provider follow-up — Alertness to red flags (e.g., management of symptoms or situations of concern)</li><li>Uses a transition coach for the patient who focuses on patient's self-identified goals and helps patient develop comfort with self-care management and engagement in taking care of own health</li><li>Coach does not assume home care or case management responsibilities</li><li>Coach initiates contact while patient in the hospital, obtains patient's consent to participate, and completes a home visit 72 hours post-discharge</li><li>Three phone calls completed after the home visit that focus on follow-up care with primary care provider, medications, and other support services</li></ul>
Transitional Care Model (TCM) http://www.transitionalcare.info/ Naylor TCM model	<ul><li>Involves 1–3 month period of interventions to prevent rehospitalizations</li><li>Focuses on high risk older adults with specific risk factors including cognitive impairment and any of the following: — 80 years or older — Functional deficits — Active psychiatric condition — Four or more comorbidities — Six or more prescribed medications — Two or more hospitalization in the past 6 months — Inadequate social support system — Poor health literacy — Poor adherence to medical regimen</li><li>Employs the role of advanced practice registered nurse (APRN)</li><li>Starts in the hospital setting where a specialized APRN completes a patient's assessment and collaborates with the healthcare team in the development of an effective transitional plan</li><li>APRN: — Visits patients after discharge from the hospital, reaches out to the patients by phone, and follows up on post-discharge care — Accompanies patients on first visit to primary care provider post-discharge — Communicates with the primary care provider and ensures important information has been exchanged — Assists patients in identifying early signs and symptoms of worsening condition</li><li>Model relies on patient engagement, goal setting, and communication with patient, family, and members of healthcare team</li></ul>

(continued)

TABLE 6.9 (continued). Select Transitions of Care Models.

Model	Highlights
Better Outcomes for Older Adults through Safe Transitions (BOOST) www.hospitalmedicine.org Society of Hospital Medicine	• Focuses on hospital discharge process and communication with patients and receiving providers • Enhances quality of transitions and offers tools for the standardization of transitional care • The eight Ps for risk assessment: — Polypharmacy — Psychological comorbidities — Principal diagnosis of cancer, stroke, diabetes, chronic obstructive pulmonary disease, or heart failure — Physical functional limitations — Poor health literacy — Poor social support system — Prior hospitalization in the 6 months before index period — Palliative care needs • Involves discharge planning, medications reconciliation, patient and family communication, discharge instructions, and communication with patient's primary care provider before discharge • Facilitates scheduling of patient's follow-up care appointment and includes post-discharge telephone call to patient • Uses of teachback method in patient education and discharge instructions
Project RED/Re-engineered Discharge https://www.bu.edu/fammed/projectred/index.html Boston University Medical Center	• Improves hospital discharge process, promotes patient safety, reduces rehospitalizations, and enhances patient's experience with care • Twelve interventions: — Language assistance — Scheduling appointments for follow-up care and test — Follow-up on pending test results post-discharge — Organization of post-discharge services and equipment — Medication education and planning to ensure access to medications — Development of discharge plans based on national guidelines — Patient understanding of discharge plan — Patient education regarding diagnosis — What to do in case of problems post-discharge — Sharing of discharge summary of care with providers following up on the patient — Post-discharge telephone follow-up on patient
Interventions to Reduce Acute Care Transfers (INTERACT) http://interact2.net/# Developed by group of experts, supported by a grant from the Commonwealth Fund, located at Florida State University	• Improves care in the LTC setting, SNFs, and ALFs • Reduce preventable hospital readmissions • Includes a number of quality improvement strategies for the management of changing patient's condition in these settings • Offers tools to help healthcare professionals document, communciate, and institute early interventions to avoid worsening patient's condition and hospitalizations. There are three tools: — Communication — Clinical care or pathways — Advance care planning • Enhances communciation among providers in the LTCs, SNFs, ALFs, and hospitals

Note: Detailed descriptions of these programs available online at stated websites

There are many reasons why a readmission to the hospital may occur. These may include, but are not limited to the issues listed below and may result in Medicare reimbursement penalties where applicable (Case Manager's Tip 6.16).

- The patient's
  —Diagnosis(es), severity of illness
  —Lifestyle behavior: activity, exercise, nutrition, smoking, substance use
  —Self-care management ability, engagement in self care, adherence to health regimen
  —Understanding of discharge instruction and post-discharge services
  —Lack of engaged social support system
- Healthcare organization or provider's
  —Implementation of suboptimal discharge and transitional plans
  —Case management program
  —Decision to discharge or transition patient prematuraely

6.5.5. Care Transitions Models to Enhance Care and Reduce Readmissions

There are a number of care transition models developed over the past several years to improve quality of care, assure safe patient transitions, and maximize cost-effectiveness while reducing financial and reimbursement risks. These models have demonstrated such unquestionable value that today they are considered evidence-based and necessary for rewarding patient and provider experiences. They are no longer a luxury and case management programs that do not include a special focus on transitions of care using the evidence these models demonstrated are considered outdated. Table 6.9 highlights some of the most common models and describes their main aspects.

Regardless of the transitional care model or discharge/transitional planning process and tools an organization uses, for these to be effective they must focus on supporting and improving the decision-making process in order to determine the best next level or care setting for the patient and quality, safe patient transition. The tools used for improving the discharge and transitional planning process and outcomes are usually of two types:

- *Patient assessment tools*: focus on assessment of patient needs and determination of most appropriate next level of care that meets these needs. The tools may contain information about the patient's medical (e.g., diagnosis and procedures), functional (e.g.,

---

> **Box 6.12   Common Elements of Discharge or Transitional Planning Models When Applied Decrease Avoidable Readmissions**
>
> Different organizations have used a variety of discharge and transitional planning models. Regardless, the following is a set of elements known to enhance effectiveness of the transition: improve quality, enhance safety, and reduce avoidable acute care readmissions.
>
> - Assessment of patient's risk for readmission to acute care using standardized criteria and tools
> - Interdisciplinary communication, collaboration, at least daily
> - Shared accountability by sending and receiving providers information for ensuring a safe patient's transition or discharge (open communication across care settings and providers)
> - One healthcare professional to coordinate the discharge/transitional plan; usually the case manager
> - Standardized discharge/transitional planning tools, checklists, or procedures
> - Training of members of interdisciplinary healthcare teams in discharge/transitional planning
> - Post-discharge follow-up on the patient; usually between 48 and 72 hours
> - Securing follow-up appointments for the patient with outpatient care provider before discharge from acute care setting; preferred within 7 days of discharge
> - Careful assessment of readmitted patients to understand reason for readmissions and address through quality or performance improvement process
> - Patient and family education regarding care, medications, and red flags; use of the teachback method and health literacy assessment
> - Medication reconciliation and assurance that patient is able to secure the medications post-discharge
> - Providing patient/family with contact information of healthcare provider to call for questions post-discharge
> - Use of a transitions of care coach to guide patients and enhance their engagement
> - Monitoring of outcomes of the discharge or transitional planning process

level of dependence and physical mobility), cognitive (e.g., orientation, competence, or presence of dementia), and social or environmental (e.g., presence and type of health insurance, financial state, and health literacy) conditions. These assessments should assist in determining the patient's post-discharge needs. Refer to Case Manager's Tip 6.17 for a 2016 Medicare regulation.

- *Discharge planning process tools*: although more common in acute care settings, they are increasingly being used in other settings as well, such as skilled care facilities and home care. These focus on the quality and safety of the discharge planning process paying careful attention to assessment of patients' risk for readmission, expected post-discharge needs, and identification of most appropriate next level of care, level of resource use, communication expectations, patterns across care providers and settings (sharing of important patient information), and monitoring of performance during and after

---

Box 6.13   Examples of Discharge/Transitional Planning Tools Used in Case Management Programs

Different case management programs have used a variety of discharge and transitional planning tools to enhance the patient and family experience and effectiveness of the transition: improve quality, enhance safety, and reduce avoidable acute care readmissions.

Post-acute patient placement tools which assist case managers or other healthcare professionals in deciding about the patient's need for post-acute care and type of services. Elements of such tools may include:

- Reason for care or service
- Skilled nursing and specialty care
- Mobility and functional ability and level of dependence
- ADLs and instrumental ADLs
- Rehabilitation and type: acute, subacute
- Patient's cognitive and mental status
- Patient's tolerance of and ability to participate in rehabilitation services
- Estimated LOS
- Frequency of physician or provider supervision for care and services
- Socioeconomic status
- Health insurance benefits
- Age

Tools for the assessment of readmissions to acute care which focus on determining the reasons for readmission then using such information for performance improvement purposes. Elements of such tools may include:

- Reason for readmission; planned or unplanned
- Review of medical and health condition
- Review of socieconomic status including psychosocial support system
- Self-care management and engagement in care
- Healthcare resources needed
- Tests and procedures
- Medications
- Follow-up care from prior admission
- Post-acute services arranged for during previous admission

Personal health record or a guide used to enhance patient engagement in own care. The record or guide can be either electronic or in print form and used to enhance patient's self-management and prevent acute care readmissions. Common elements of the guide are:

- Patient's demographics and contact information
- Patient's next of kin, healthcare proxy, advance directive and care preference: nutrition, life support, do not resuscitate
- Health insurance plan: policy number, type of benefits
- Allergies
- Medical and psychological conditions
- Detailed medications list including reason, strength, dose, route, frequency, over what time period; prescribed and over the counter
- Contact information for primary care provider and other specilists involved in care and reasons for seeing them
- Most recent care summary, results of tests, and discharge instructions
- Services received at home: visiting nurse, physical therapy, home health aide
- Red flags and safety: symptoms and events to watch out for
- Who to reach out to in case of health emergencies: name and contact information
- List of questions to ask healthcare providers

patients' transition or discharge. Refer to Box 6.12 for a list of commonly used elements in discharge/transitional planning models and Box 6.13 for characteristics of discharge/transitional planning tools.

6.6. KEY POINTS

1. Case managers play a pivotal role in ensuring that the discharge and transitional plan is safe, timely, and meets clinical criteria such as InterQual or Milliman Guidelines.

2. The provision of care across the continuum of care can be aggregated into preacute, acute, and post-acute care and services.

3. Matching the patient to the clinically appropriate level of service will ensure reimbursement for care and services rendered to the provider organization.

4. The case manager should use the steps of assessing, planning, implementing, evaluating, confirming, and transitioning the patient through the continuum of care and across appropriate levels of care.

5. Transitional planning is highly regulated. Case managers should stay up-to-date on all relevant regulations, both at the state and federal levels as well as standards of commercial health insurance plans.

6. Following up on patients post-transition out of acute care setting is important for reducing avoidable readmissions and ensuring patients are safe and engaged in own care.

7. Case managers may use evidence-based tools in discharge/transitional planning to reduce readmissions, enhance reimbursement by reducing financial risk, and assuring quality and safe care provision.

6.7. REFERENCES

American Hospital Association. (1984). Guidelines: discharge planning, Chicago, IL.

American Nurses Association. (2010). Nursing–scope and standards of practice, 2nd ed., Kansas City, MO.

American Nurses Credentialing Center (ANCC). (2015). Nursing case management board certification, test content outline. Silver Springs, MD. Available online at www.nursecredentialing.org/NursingCaseMgmt-TCO2015

Case Management Society of America. (2010). Standards of practice for case management, 2nd ed., Little Rock, AR.

Center for Medicare and Medicaid Services (CMS). (2014). Conditions of Participation with Interpretive Statements: Discharge planning. Silver Spring, MD.

Center for Medicare and Medicaid Services (CMS). (2014). State operations manual: Interpretive guidelines for hospitals, Baltimore, MD. Available online at www.cms.gov/Regulations-and-Guidance/Guidance/Transmittals/downloads/R37SOMA.pdf

Commission for Case Manager Certification. (2015). CCM certification guide, Rolling Meadows, IL.

The Joint Commission. (2015). Provision of Care. In: Accreditation manual for hospitals, Oakbrook Terrace, IL.

Joint Commission on Accreditation of Healthcare Organizations (JCAHO). (2001). Continuum of Care. In: Accreditation manual for hospitals, Oakbrook Terrace, IL.

Omnibus Budget Reconciliation Act of 1986. Conference report to accompany H.R. 5300, Section 9305, Washington, DC.

7 Skills for Successful Case Management

Professional nurses, case managers, and social workers have been key advocates in the delivery of quality, safe, and cost-effective healthcare services to patients and their families/caregivers. Their broad skills and training allow them to assess patients' needs and to work well with families and other members of the healthcare team in coordinating the plan of care including the services patients may need after a care encounter. Negotiation, collaboration, communication, advocacy, teambuilding, precepting, educating, and consulting are the basis of what a successful case manager brings to the care setting and patient care delivery each day.

The application of the nursing and case management processes is concerned with the whole person and the full range of patient and family needs, including preferences and interests. This clearly leads to comprehensive and consistent care. Much has been written about the nursing process and its unique qualities. In contrast to the goals of the other members of the health professions, the nurse is involved with human needs that affect the total person rather than one aspect or one problem. Most case managers are nurses who bring a holistic approach to care as they execute their role responsibilities.

Case management is no different in its approach to successful coordination of patient care than that of nursing or those applied by other healthcare professionals. The role of the case manager, by its definition as outlined in the CSMA's Standards of Practice for Case Management (2010), upholds and expounds on the nursing process. "Case management is a collaborative process which assesses, plans, implements, coordinates, [advocates], monitors, and evaluates options

and services to meet individuals' health needs through communication and available resources to promote quality, [safe and] cost-effective outcomes," (CMSA, 2010).

The case manager's expertise is the vital link between the individual (i.e., patient), the provider of care, the payer, and the community. Successful outcomes cannot be achieved without using all the specialized skills and knowledge applied through the case management process. It must be emphasized that not every case manager posseses the skills necessary for success in the role. Case managers need to be clinically astute and competent in their areas of practice. It is important for case managers to be skilled in the application of the case management process and to acquire the assessment skills that make them better able to identify the patient's actual and potential health problems and how best to address them. This allows them to implement the required interventions to successfully resolve these problems and to evaluate the outcomes of care and responses to treatments.

Not all nurses acquire the professional credentials, education, and expertise in the application of the nursing process to succeed as a case manager. Case managers are notoriously consummate organizers, paid to be in control of what many would regard as sheer chaos. Does their skill for organization derive from a compulsive personality, years of experience, mastering the nursing and case management processes, or a balanced blend of all of these components? One would believe the latter to be true. As long as there is a subtle balance in the dynamics a case manager's processes, there will be a positive affect.

How does this overview translate and apply to the

Box 7.1   Functions and Skills for Effective Case Management

Functions Based on the Nursing/Case Management Process

1. Assessment
2. Planning
3. Implementation
4. Coordination
5. Advocacy
6. Monitoring and Evaluation

Leadership Skills

1. Patient advocate
2. Facilitator
3. Negotiator
4. Broker
5. Quality improvement coordinator
6. Utilization manager
7. Educator
8. Financial analyst
9. Consultant
10. Decision-maker
11. Critical thinker
12. Data manager and analyst
13. Evaluater of quality of care
14. Risk manager

Communication/Interpersonal Skills

1. Teamwork and team building
2. Customer relations
3. Public speaking
4. Conflict resolution
5. Delegation
6. Information sharing
7. Systems thinking
8. Emotional intelligence
9. Motivational interviewing

---

required skills necessary for today's successful case managers? The section that follows categorizes and details each function and skill that becomes a critical element when providing the services of an effective case manager (Box 7.1).

7.1. NURSING AND CASE MANAGEMENT PROCESSES

Since the case management and nursing processes are generally similar, the steps in these processes, with special attention to the case manager's skills, will be described as if they were one and the same.

7.1.1. Assessment

Assessment is an ongoing and continuous process occurring with all patient/family-case manager interactions. It is during the assessment phase that the case manager seeks to better understand the patient, the family and caregiver dynamics, and their healthcare beliefs, preferences, and myths. An assessment generally involves three main actions, which at times seem inseparable: gathering data, evaluating data, and determining an appropriate nursing diagnosis or issues of focus to then be included in the case management plan and service delivery. Case managers use multifaceted skills to assess a patient's/family's needs accurately (Box 7.2).

As an assessor, the case manager must obtain relevant data through skillful investigation. All of the information related to the current plan must be evaluated with a critical eye to objectively identifying trends, set and reset realistic goals, and seek viable care alternatives as necessary. At all times, the case manager main-

---

Box 7.2   Various Case Manager's Skills Applied Especially During Patient's Assessment

- *Motivational interviewing skills* that include the ability not only to listen but also to formulate insightful questions and facilitate the patient's sharing of sensitive and important information
- *Interpretation skills* that allow the case manager to understand what patients say about their concerns and symptoms and to transmit this information to other caregivers using concise and appropriate terminology
- *Nonverbal communication skills* that permit the case manager to recognize responses to treatments that reflect the patient's moods, attitudes, and psychosocial needs
- *Relationship skills* that cut across potential social and cultural barriers to promote trust with patients, family members, and professional colleagues
- *Observational skills* that allow the case manager to distinguish normal from abnormal functioning and to recognize subtle changes in patients' responses to treatments
- *Evaluation skills* that permit the case manager to consider the facts about a patient's condition, as well as the interconnection and balance between strengths and weaknesses
- *Goal-setting skills* that help the case manager see beyond the immediate needs to identify intermediate and long-term goals of care
- *Advocacy skills* that allow the case manager to protect the patient's rights and ensure shared decision-making and ability to choose care options

CASE STUDY 7.1 ■ Assessment and Health Balance

Ms. J. Mazure is a 50-year-old professional career woman. She recently noticed excessive vaginal bleeding. A pap smear revealed a malignancy, leading to further tests and ultimately the need for a hysterectomy. As a case manager, you must begin to assess the health needs of the patient and work toward creating balance. You will use a range of skills to help you identify the changes in this patient's health balance as a result of her hysterectomy. In this case, health is not limited to Ms. Mazure's physiologic condition. Your approach must be holistic to create a sustainable balance for Ms. Mazure. For example, self image and coping with the surgery should be part of the assessment and plan of care.

You must also explore Ms. Mazure's strengths and resources, such as psychosocial support systems, health insurance benefits, and employee sick leave policies, as well as evaluate the stresses and demands experienced by Ms. Mazure during this phase of illness and treatment such as the self-imposed pressure of missing work, work responsibilities piling up in her absence, and familial obligations that she temporarily will not be able to handle. By using the health balance approach, you can connect the physical and the psychosocial aspects of the patient's care with the patient's strengths and available resources, ensuring the development of a plan of care for Ms. Mazure applying a holistic approach.

tains an interest in understanding what the patient and family preferences in care are and their perception of their needs and care goals.

Part of being a successful assessor is to find a delicate health balance for each patient. Needs and demands are balanced by strengths and resources. When there is a balance between these factors, there can be positive movement toward achieving care goals. When a patient is in acute distress, patient needs may only be the obvious; however, if a health balance is to occur or to be restored, the case manager must uncover factors that influence the relationships between needs, strengths, and resources. A representation of this health balance approach is shown in Figure 7.1.

Case Study 7.1 presents an example of the use of the health balance model during the assessment of a patient. A vital case management skill used during the patient's assessment is to recognize a patient's health problems and formulate diagnoses based on the subjective and objective data collected during the assessment.

The diagnoses express the case manager's judgment of the patient's clinical condition, functional abilities, responses to treatments, healthcare needs, psychosocial support, financial status, and post-discharge needs.

7.1.2. Planning

Planning is the next step in managing the patient's care. This is accomplished by planning the treatment modalities and interventions necessary for meeting the needs and preferences of patients and families/caregivers. During the planning phase the case manager, in collaboration with the other members of the healthcare team, determines the goals of treatment and the projected length of stay (in the case of acute care settings or facility-based care) and, immediately on admission, initiates the transitional plan of care. The determination of goals is vitally important because it provides a clear timeframe for accomplishing the care activities needed. Case managers must identify immediate short-

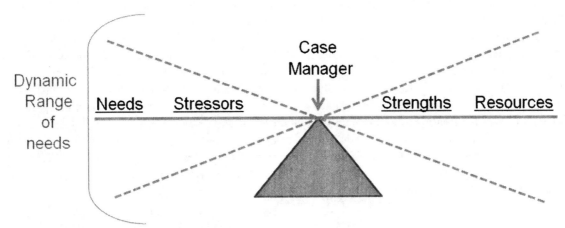

Figure 7.1 The health balance approach (Redrawn from Rorden & Taft, 1990).

CASE STUDY 7.2 ■ Planning

Mrs. Smith is a 25-year-old married woman with a history of three miscarriages and no living children. She is now hospitalized for the second time during her pregnancy. She is admitted with a diagnosis of pre-term labor at 30 weeks gestation with a low-lying placenta. Mrs. Smith was home only 2 days after her first hospitalization before cramping and vaginal bleeding began and she was readmitted to the acute care hospital setting. She is very anxious about delivering early. She lives in an upstairs apartment and has no family support to help her. Her husband cannot take off from work. Financially he can't afford to; for every day not worked, she loses a day's pay. You have assessed her needs to include the following:

■ Pre-term labor requiring medical intervention
■ Teaching about her pre-term labor to reduce her anxiety
■ Motivation to adhere to the probable bedrest regimen that is ahead of her

■ Investigation of the need for home care to follow up on her pregnancy and medical regimen while at home
■ Exploring availability of community resources to support her while at home

You quickly establish that the patient's apartment is a problematic setting and determine the need to include home care in the plan because visits to the physician's office would need to be minimized and bed rest maximized. You also educate Mrs. Smith's husband about pre-term labor and the importance of his wife's maintaining bed rest. The overall plan includes the patient's goal of returning home as soon as possible and ultimately delivering a healthy baby. You plan clear guidelines for patient adherence to the care regimen and establish community resources to meet the goal of leaving the hospital. By using a step-by-step planning process and going beyond the walls of the acute care setting, you are able to meet the needs of this patient while maintaining quality, safe care.

---

and long-term needs and goals, as well as where and how these needs will meet the patient's preferences, interests, and agreed upon care goals.

Planning is initiated as the patient is admitted or before admission to any healthcare setting. The case manager's clinical expertise is quickly tapped into when establishing whether the treatment plan and interventions are appropriate. Data are assimilated, diagnoses are established, and a multidisciplinary plan of care begins to unfold.

Throughout the acute hospital, sub-acute, home care, or long-term care stay, the case manager monitors and re-evaluates the plan for accuracy and relevance as the patient's condition changes. As a planner, the case manager identifies a treatment plan while remaining cognizant of the patient needs, preferences, interests, goals, expected outcomes, and minimization of payer liability. The case manager must include the patient and family in decision-making about care options and must consider the patient's goals as an integral part of the care plan. Alternate plans must always be incorporated in anticipation of sudden shifts in the treatment process or in response to treatments yielding complications. Case Study 7.2 illustrates the principles of successful planning.

7.1.3. Implementation, Coordination, and Advocacy

Implementation and coordination involve building the

case management plan of care, determining the goals of patient care, and deciding what needs to be accomplished to make a viable and realistic plan move toward completion in a safe and cost-efficient manner while meeting the patient's and family's needs. The aim of the case manager at this point is to give the patient and family the knowledge, attitudes, and skills necessary for the implementation of the established plan. Through communication, collaboration, and teaching, the case manager works with the interdisciplinary healthcare team to motivate the patient to succeed in fulfilling the plan of care determined by all of the participants, including the patient and family.

Abraham Maslow (1970), in his theory of the hierarchy of needs, suggested that everyone seeks fulfillment of general needs and that these needs motivate behavior. At a time of high stress or ill health, people seek to fulfill more basic needs, such as survival, food, and safety. The higher needs of self and creativity do not seem as much a priority at this time (Maslow, 1970).

The case manager needs to be aware of this theory of motivation when trying to elicit decisions about discharge/transitional planning or future goals for a patient/family. The patient and family must first reach a level of awareness that enables them to focus on the goals of the care plan, especially those that pertain to post-care encounter needs and services. They must then reach a level of understanding from which they learn in greater depth what the patient's needs and the available

CASE STUDY 7.3 ■ Implementation, Coordination, and Advocacy

You recently thought all steps were taken to provide a safe discharge plan for your cardiac patient, Mr. Johnson. The plan included transportation by an ambulance to bring the patient home from the hospital; Mr. Johnson had no family support or means of transportation and he could not be safely discharged from the hospital alone. Shortly after Mr. Johnson's departure from the hospital, the ambulance driver called the medical unit rather displeased with the lack of assessment and planning done for this patient. Apparently the address given for the patient's home did not exist and was a vacant lot.

Upon carefully investigating the situation, it was discovered that Mr. Johnson's medical record had an address from a previous hospitalization that was no longer valid. No one had verified where the patient lived or reconfirmed his address during the assessment or planning phases of care. This situation could have been

avoided by following the simple steps to implementation, thus avoiding a distressful, embarrassing, and potentially unsafe situation for the patient, you, and the hospital. One should not take information from medical records of prior hospitalizations for granted. The case manager has the obligation to verify the continued accuracy and applicability of the information.

Some, if not most, information available in current or past patient's medical records are necessary for effective implementation and coordination of the plan of care and for advocacy so that the patient/family do not end up facing unsafe situations. The case manager is obliged to review records and verify important information with the patient/family before acting upon such information. Skipping this step may compromise care and potentially increase the patient's risk for readmission to acute care, medical error, and other unsafe experiences.

---

care options and resources are, the likely consequences of these options, and what aspects of self-care and self-management need to be learned. It is at this juncture that motivation will take place and the implementation of the plan will come to fruition.

As the patient nears discharge, the case manager can take three steps to improve the chances of effective implementation of the case management plan of care:

- Clarify the transfer of responsibilities of care
- Review the plan to ensure that nothing has been overlooked
- Make last-minute alterations and arrangements for the immediate discharge period.

Following these steps will confirm the plan for con-

tinuing care (Case Manager's Tip 7.1). Case Study 7.3 presents an example of what can happen to implementation if a step-by-step approach of assessment, diagnosis, planning, and coordination does not take place.

7.1.4. Monitoring and Evaluation

The final step in the nursing process, monitoring and evaluation, is designed to measure the patient's responses to the formulated case management plan of care against the expected goals and outcomes while at the same time ensuring the appropriateness of the plan and the quality of the services being offered to the patient.

To achieve successful evaluation and outcomes, the case manager must routinely assess and reassess on an ongoing basis the patient's status and progress toward reaching the goals set forth in the plan of care. During these reassessments, the case manager monitors and evaluates the patient's condition and responses to the care interventions against the intermediate and discharge outcomes (i.e., milestones of care) that are clearly stated in the plan of care. If the situation is at a halt or regressing rather than moving forward, the case manager must then make appropriate adjustments and alter the plan accordingly.

The following important questions must be asked as the monitoring and evaluation proceed:

- Were the patient's/family's needs identified appropriately early in the hospital stay?

CASE MANAGER'S TIP 7.1

The Importance of Confirming the Case Management Plan of Care

Taking the time and making the effort to confirm the plan of care with the patient, family/caregiver, and members of the interdisciplinary healthcare team greatly increases the probability of the plan's effective and efficient implementation as well as success in meeting the agreed upon care goals. Follow-through on an ongoing basis also helps ensure that the goals are met and the plan of care continues to meet the changing needs of the patient/family.

- Were the patient's/family's interests, preferences, and identified needs appropriately incorporated into the plan of care?
- Were learning goals identified and teaching documented?
- Were referrals to specialty services or post-discharge agencies complete and timely?
- Was the patient/family able to verbalize the goals of the plan of care?
- Were the patient's/family's problems resolved?
- Did the patient/family seem satisfied with the plan of care and the decisions surrounding the plan, services, and resources?
- Did the patient/family adhere to the medical advice and follow the recommendations of the case manager?
- Were the services provided appropriately authorized by the health insurance plan/managed care organization?
- Is the patient progressing toward meeting the intermediate and discharge outcomes of care (i.e., care milestones) as articulated in the plan of care?

These questions will help the case manager to determine if the overall discharge/transitional plan for a particular patient was effective and will assist with quality improvement efforts for future patients. This information is also valuable when evaluating the organization's total case management program. Throughout the monitoring and evaluation processes, all participants in the interdisciplinary healthcare team will identify system, process, clinician, patient, and family variances or delays in care and trend them. These trends will be further analyzed in CQI teams to improve, fine-tune, revamp, and reorganize the processes of care delivery.

The case manager must use many skills and functions of leadership to effectively master the nursing/case management process (Case Manager's Tip 7.2). A more specific and comprehensive breakdown of these skills will add to the role dimensions of the case manager.

7.2. LEADERSHIP SKILLS AND FUNCTIONS

Because case managers function as problem solvers, resource people, and members of the interdisciplinary healthcare team, they should be highly skilled in various leadership qualities. Nursing case managers must be adept at negotiating and contracting and capable of making sound decisions and resolving conflicts. To do this successfully, they should acquire critical thinking and problem-solving skills. Because of their managerial responsibilities, case managers must be involved in

CASE MANAGER'S TIP 7.2

Keep in mind that all of the skills delineated in Chapter 7 are applicable to all forms of case management, including acute care, sub-acute care, post-acute care such as home care, and health insurance plan case management.

quality improvement efforts, speak publicly, and write for publication.

7.2.1. Advocacy and Facilitation of Care Activities

The case manager's work as an advocate (Case Manager's Tip 7.3) for the patient is one of the most criti-

CASE MANAGER'S TIP 7.3

Advocacy Skills

Case managers can best advocate for patients and their families if they apply the following strategies:

- Keeping the patient's best interest paramount in the process of care delivery
- Recommending, coordinating, and facilitating the most effective plan of care
- Protecting the rights of patients and their self-determination
- Communicating to other providers and documenting the patient's care preferences
- Facilitating the patient's and family's decision-making activities by keeping them well informed of their rights, options, etc.
- Clarifying the goals of therapy and treatment
- Determining the appropriateness of the post-discharge (or post-care encounter) services and the discharge/transitional plan
- Ensuring that the interventions are consistent with the patient's needs, interests, preferences, and goals of treatment
- Maintaining the patient's privacy and confidentiality
- Negotiating on behalf of the patient/family with the health insurance plan/managed care organization for authorizations of services, where needed
- Facilitating resolution of ethical conflicts
- Maintaining current knowledge of the legal and ethical requirements and standards of patient care delivery
- Preventing delays and variances in care delivery and progression
- Educating the patient, family, or caregiver in self-care and self-management to ensure safety and continuity of care at all times

cal elements of the role. The patient-case manager relationship is built on the ability of the case manager to be trusted; to foster mutual respect with the patient and family; and to establish a rapport that facilitates communication among the family, caregivers, payers, and other healthcare team members. As case managers gain clear understanding of the patient's needs, care desires, and goals, they communicate this understanding effectively to the members of the healthcare team. They also impact the course of treatment to effect an earlier discharge, negotiate better fees for medical supplies or equipment, or arrange for more efficient home care services and other community resources.

As a facilitator, the case manager can be a catalyst for change by empowering the patient or family members to seek solutions throughout the acute care phase and beyond the hospital setting. The case manager is always on the lookout for quality improvement opportunities that could result in potential cost savings or possibly prolong the healthcare benefits of an individual.

7.2.2. Applicability of Skills to Different Settings

The patient's best interests are always the focal point for the case manager's advocacy and care facilitation efforts, whether for needed funding, treatment options, appropriate and timely home health services, or reassessment, evaluation and modification of care goals. Case managers are concerned with every detail, sifting through the complex array of paths that can easily lead to confusion for any patient. Case managers advocate for their patients/families in three main ways.

1. Defending patients' rights to treatments and options
2. Helping patients to discuss their needs and preferences and to make informed choices that are consistent with their values and beliefs
3. Respecting and honoring patients' values and beliefs and helping them maintain their dignity

7.2.3. Clinical Reasoning and Critical Thinking

In the practice of case management, patient, family, and healthcare provider problems continually arise. Therefore it is important that case managers are able to solve these problems. The ability of case managers to provide safe, efficient, quality, cost-efective, and competent case management services depends heavily on their skills in problem solving, clinical reasoning, and critical thinking. These skills have one thing in common: they all entail the generation of possible solutions to problems, issues, or concerns regarding patient care delivery and options. Case managers use their clinical knowledge and expertise and their leadership skills for this purpose. They capitalize on their role as informal leaders of the healthcare team and facilitators of patient care delivery to solve the problems that may arise.

Case managers are constantly making decisions. They decide what observations should be made in encountered situations, derive meaning from the observations made and data collected, and decide on the actions/interventions to be taken to care for the patient or resolve the situation. The overall goal is the delivery of optimal, cost-effective, safe, and quality care.

Case managers use a framework for decision making and problem solving (Figure 7.2) that bridges the present and the future. They assess the patient's and family's current state and, based on this assessment, they envision the future state by deciding on the goals and expected outcomes of treatment. They apply paradoxical thinking and decision making to confidently articulate the patient's care goals and effect actions accordingly.

Case managers also apply this framework when they implement the action plan to realistically bring the patient and family to the desired future state. This framework enhances an outcomes-based approach to the delivery of case management services. The plan is usually interdisciplinary in nature and implemented

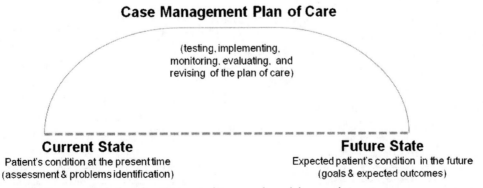

Case Management Plan of Care

(testing, implementing, monitoring, evaluating, and revising of the plan of care)

Current State
Patient's condition at the present time
(assessment & problems identification)

Future State
Expected patient's condition in the future
(goals & expected outcomes)

Figure 7.2 Framework for decision making and problem solving in case management.

only after approval by the healthcare team and consent and agreement by the patient and family.

Understanding that the action plan may not always result in a resolution of the patient's and family's problems, issues, and concerns, case managers engage in constant reassessment, monitoring, evaluation, and revising of the plan until the desired outcomes (i.e., the future state) are achieved (Case Manager's Tip 7.4). Case managers complete these activities using a testing technique applied to examining the appropriateness of the action plan and the relevance of its outcomes.

The case manager's skills in decision making and clinical reasoning and judgment must always help the patient work through the confusion he or she faces in the complex healthcare environment. Case managers operate by answering questions pertinent to the development of the plan of care, actual delivery of care, and evaluation of the discharge/transitional plan, such as those following. These questions are examples of how case managers engage in evaluating the case management action plan using the problem-solving framework shared in Figure 7.2.

- Is the current treatment plan appropriate enough to resolve the patient's problems and meet the patient's needs and preferences?
- Will the current case management action plan prevent the patient from needing readmission to an acute care setting?
- Do the treatments, interventions, and services provide the best possible options for the patient and family?
- Are healthcare team members in agreement with the plan of care including the plan for services after current care encounter?
- Do the patient and family have any issues or disagreements with the plan?
- Should any changes be made to the plan of care or the discharge/transitional plan?
- Will the electricity in the patient's home support a mechanical ventilator?
- Does the patient have safe access to a bathroom on the main floor of the house?
- Is it worth the hospital's financial support to fly a patient out of state rather than incur the cost of an extended length of stay?
- Is the family capable of learning how to perform tracheal suctioning so that their loved one can go home with them rather than to an extended nursing facility?
- Does the patient/family demonstrate ability for self-care and self-management?

Answers to these questions, and many others, influ-

 CASE MANAGER'S TIP 7.4

Current-Future State Thinking

Case managers are aware that not every goal included in the case management plan of care requires its achievement in the setting where the plan was designed and the care is being provided. Some of the goals included in a plan of care that is designed while the patient is in the acute care setting may be dependent on the post-discharge services the patient will be receiving while at home after discharge, perhaps from a home care agency. For example, proficiency in self-administration of insulin and monitoring of blood glucose level. Education may start in the acute care setting but continues while the patient is at home. Therefore, case managers must be realistic about what goals are expected to be achieved and ensure that the patient and family/caregiver are aware of that and are in agreement.

ence the type of care a patient will receive and how it will be accomplished to ensure the best possible outcome for a patient in the most cost-effective and safe manner. Case managers who are able to apply critical thinking and clinical reasoning skills in the decision-making process ensure appropriate, effective, safe, and efficient care delivery. This makes certain that the patient and family will receive the necessary support, potential obstacles to the treatment plan will be avoided, the potential for readmission or need for emergency services will decrease, the educational component of care will be reinforced, and a positive outcome and promotion of health will take place.

7.2.4. Negotiation

Negotiation is a skill that is not primarily taught in nursing or social work educational programs. To be a successful negotiator, a case manager must be a good communicator and time manager. Along with managing their own time, case managers must learn to determine what work others can and should do in assessing a patient's needs when preparing a patient's plan of care. This understanding allows them to negotiate more effectively and keep all members of the interdisciplinary healthcare team, as well as the patient and family, aware of the plan of care and patient's progress toward achieving goals.

Negotiation in case management is an everyday occurrence. It is a skill used with payers and providers, with vendors for durable medical equipment, with the patient and family/caregiver, and even with physicians reluctant to opt for a home care discharge plan

CASE MANAGER'S TIP 7.5

Negotiation Skills

Strategies for better negotiation in case management

- Always have clear, factual, and pertinent data in your possession.
- Do not lose sight of your long-term goal.
- Know the players well, including their values, beliefs, interests, and scope of responsibilities.
- Plan, prepare well, and practice before you start negotiating.
- Always have alternate solutions or options in mind.
- Cultivate an interactive, collaborative relationship rather than an antagonistic one.
- Focus on interests and not positions; on actions or positions and not the person.
- Focus on the exchange of the information.
- Do not give up—persevere.
- Avoid becoming emotional.
- Trust the person you are negotiating with; distrust is destructive.
- Do not miss your chance.
- Focus on negotiation as a process and not an event.
- Ask questions.
- Avoid talking too much.
- Wait for the right moment to make your pitch
- Listen carefully and acknowledge the person you are negotiating with.
- Brainstorm for solutions.
- Be creative.
- Appreciate small wins; they are as important as larger ones.
- Aim for a win-win result.

Strategies to avoid in negotiation

- Make the other side feel guilty.
- Offer options that are only favorable to you.
- Threaten the other side.
- Use sarcasm, cynicism, or putdown statements.
- Play games or tricks.
- Rush the process.
- Jump at the first offer.
- Give away the store.
- Try to score all the points.
- Distort the facts or withhold important information.
- Be emotional.
- Be aggressive.
- Deal with the other person as an enemy.

or placement in a long-term care facility. The purpose of negotiation is to reach an agreement that is in the best interest of the patient and family. Fair negotiation requires trust, rapport, transparency, and complete honesty with regard to a patient's care needs. Successful negotiation (Case Manager's Tip 7.5) is achieved by being well prepared to present the facts clearly and succinctly.

To know if you have negotiated your case well, you must be a good listener who tunes in to verbal and nonverbal cues; otherwise, windows of opportunity could be missed. On the financial side of the equation, we know all too well that healthcare environments are committed to doing more with less and at a lower cost. Financial prowess on the part of the case manager is a must in these times of cost containment. Case managers must work with financial support personnel and help them keep abreast of a patient's insurance health benefit plan, no-fault coverage, or a patient's lack of finances that could lead to Medicaid eligibility.

According to Umiker (1996), negotiation may take three forms. The collaborative form is the most desired approach for negotiation by case managers. It is preferred and known to result in rewarding outcomes when negotiating the plan of care and care options with the patient/family or seeking authorizations for services from a commercial health insurer.

1. *Power play*: assumes that the stronger party will win. The power play process is a form of combat in which one side makes an unfair offer and expects the other side to counter with an equally unfair demand.
2. *Taking positions*: assumes a win-lose outcome. This is a form of haggling wherein each side adopts a fixed position and assumes an inflexible stand.
3. *Collaboration*: assumes a problem-solving approach. This form of negotiation results in a win-win situation wherein each side desires to end up with a good deal while preserving the integrity of the other.

Collaboration is the only one of the three forms of negotiation that allows all parties involved to win and to be pleased with the outcome. It also makes the process more efficient, positive, and amicable. The other two forms must be avoided because they tend to be unproductive and divisive and work against building teams and effective relationships. The power play approach is usually aggressive, intimidating, and condescending; in the taking positions (haggling) approach the process of negotiation becomes a contest of wills.

7.2.5. Utilization Review and Management

Case management plans can be useful tools when determining the allocated resources for a particular diagnosis. Variance analysis or comorbid conditions can help a case manager anticipate extra costs, such as the need for longer hospitalizations, expensive antibiotic treatment, or pain management therapy.

Working alongside the hospital's controller and a managed care/commercial insurance specialist to review the expenses incurred for various diagnoses will serve as a checks-and-balances system of appropriate allocation of funds. The case manager has a key role in being able to communicate the overutilization of laboratory tests or repetitive diagnostics or the under-utilization of less-expensive antibiotics. Thus the case manager can have a major positive impact on the ability of an institution to provide the same quality of care that it is accustomed to while being more cost-efficient and safe in the process.

Another way in which case managers affect the financial balance of an acute care setting while monitoring quality and outcomes is through utilization review and management (see Chapter 5). Participation on a hospital length-of-stay committee or a utilization review committee is one way to monitor utilization of resources. The healthcare team can then be alerted to an inappropriate admission, an unusual length of stay for a given patient, a planned premature discharge with no clear discharge plan and with potential readmission risk, or inappropriate use of resources. It is case managers who are charged with monitoring these potential financial drains on the healthcare organization or value-based purchasing outcomes which potentially compromise reimbursement. It is their high quality and efficiency that provides the organization with a safety gatekeeping mechanism to avoid potential utilization problems. Knowledge of utilization review and management is also effective in other settings such as sub-acute, home care, and health insurance arenas to justify or nullify care requested.

In this ever-shrinking resource environment, it becomes more and more prudent for the case manager to be an instrumental participant in payer contract negotiation, on resource management teams, utilization review committees, clinical pathway or evidence-based practice guidelines development committees, and in any groups designed to promote the delivery of quality and safe care at less cost but with high efficiency and satisfying patient experiences. It is the driving force behind every great case manager to maximize patient outcomes and quality of care while being ever cognizant of the dwindling resources to provide that care.

7.2.6. Patient and Family Education and Engagement

One of the last but certainly not least leadership skills is that of educator. This is a large responsibility within the case manager's role because it covers a broad scope of functions. Being a facilitator of both the patient and the staff is at times a monumental task that brings with it periods of extreme challenge. A good principle to follow is to begin with the end result in mind, similar to the future state-current state framework applied in planning care. First there is the mental picture of the outcome of your patient's plan of care; then you begin to formulate the blueprints and develop your construction plan to get the patient and family to the projected outcome. You do this based on the gaps you identify as you compare the future state against the patient's current state. This idea can be conveyed through the analogy of constructing a house. The blueprint for the house is meticulously designed before any physical creation of the house is begun. Without a developed blueprint, the physical creation will undoubtedly have expensive changes that could double the cost of the house. The case manager, much like the carpenter, must make sure that the blueprint (i.e., patient's plan of care) includes everything needed and that everything has been thought through (Covey, 1989) taking into consideration the current capabilities and resources.

Educating the patient and family is part of the blueprint for success. The clearer the understanding of the disease process and the course of the acute level of care, the better the plan will be. Of utmost importance is that the case manager considers educating the patient and family using language that is understood (Case Manager's Tip 7.6), with consideration for cultural diversity and healthcare beliefs. In our constant awareness of the pressure to reduce lengths of stay, education is sometimes elected to take a back seat.

The healthcare environment can make it hard for patients/families to tell case managers and other healthcare professionals that they do not read well or do not understand healthcare instructions or discussions about care options these professionals have with them. They may feel embarrassed and hide their lack of knowledge and discomfort from the case managers and other teams members. As a result, case managers must be able to assess the patient's health literacy level to determine their readiness for and ability to grasp the health education and instructions for the post-encounter care. This is essential for enhancing patient safety, adherence to care regimens, and self-management ability. If not addressed low health liter-

CASE MANAGER'S TIP 7.6

Health Literacy

Case managers must be able to assess the patient's health literacy level to then design an effective patient education plan that ultimately enhances the patient's self-management skills and abilities.

Health literacy is the degree to which individuals have the capacity to obtain, read, process, understand, and use basic health information and services needed to make appropriate health decisions and follow care instructions. This requires the patient to demonstrate the following skills (AMA, 2015):

- Writing
- Listening
- Speaking
- Numeracy such as calculating and understanding medication dosages
- Critical analysis of information or results of self monitoring on certain care aspects such as blood glucose level, daily weight
- Communication about healthcare needs
- Interaction about healthcare issues such as red flags (symptoms to watch out for) and medications

Some of the factors that limit health literacy include but not limited to the following:

- Use of too much medical jargon
- Severe health conditions (e.g., multiple chronic illnesses and comorbidities) and treatment plan
- Stressful situations
- Feeling vulnerable
- Too much happening at once
- Too many topics discussed at the same time
- Language barriers

---

acy and related concerns may result in the following avoidable situations:

- Less knowledge about health condition and disease process
- Greater risk of preventable rehospitalization and access to emergency services
- Lower chance of receiving preventative services
- Worsened control of chronic illnesses
- Non-adherence to care regimen
- Inability to recognize serious symptoms that warrant immediate attention by a care provider
- Costly care

Timely health literacy assessment and education is crucial, especially as patients experience shorter hospital stays. Placing education at the bottom of the priority list can have devastating effects on outcomes

of care. For example, a family decides to take their loved one, who is dependent on a ventilator, home. All plans appear to be in place: the respiratory company has been arranged, the home is prepared, and the visiting nurse visits are on standby. Everything seems to be ready, but a crucial element is missing. No one thought about the necessity to teach the family how to care for their family member at home, including expertise in ventilator function and resuscitative measures. Without this most important step of early education, the discharge plan runs the risk of failure, costly extra days in the hospital, or potential rehospitalization of the patient as a result of lack of knowledge on the part of family members or the inability to handle the patient's care.

Do the patient and family respond better to verbal or nonverbal communication, audio or video, written word or pictures, discussion or demonstration? It is the case manager who can impact the education process by serving as the resource for staff to develop or select supporting educational materials and define the best method of conveying the information (Case Manager's Tip 7.7). The case manager may also serve as a member of the patient teaching committee or patient and family advisory committee responsible for enhancing the patient and family experience with care and development of educational materials or documentation tools such as the one shown in Figure 7.3.

Ensuring adherence to standards of patient and family teaching as outlined by regulatory and accreditation agencies is also a required facet of the case manager's role. Using the teach-back method is necessary to enhance patient and family educational outcomes. Teach-back is a communication technique that enables clinicians to check patients and families/caregivers understanding of the information conveyed to them (Figure 7.4). It is done by asking them to repeat their understanding of the information shared in their own way, using their own language. This method is not a test of the patient, but rather a test of how well the clinician or healthcare professional (e.g., case manager) explained

CASE MANAGER'S TIP 7.7

Assessing for Readiness to Learn

The case manager must use every possible means of assessing readiness to learn or potential barriers to learning including health literacy and primary language spoken. The preferred and most appropriate method of education must then be determined and applied in health teaching.

PATIENT/FAMILY TEACHING ELEMENTS	SELF ASSESSMENT CHECKLIST	BARRIERS TO TEACHING	DATE TEACHING PROVIDED	METHOD OF TEACHING	EVALUATION OF TEACHING	NOTES	SIGNATURE INITIALS
BABY CARE							
Diaper Change							
Bath: Sponge/Tub							
Temperature							
Dressing							
Umbilical Cord Care							
Skin Care/Rash							
Jaundice							
Circumcision Care							
Uncircumcised Baby Care							
Bulb Syringe							
Crying as Communication							
Car Safety and Car Seat							
Signs of Infection/Illness							
Red Flags and Calling Pediatrician							
Sleep Positions and Pattern							
Vaccinations							
Day Care/Baby Sitting							
Follow-up Care Appointment							
Other:							
BREASTFEEDING							
Positioning							
Latching							
Frequency and Length of Feeding							
Burping							
Feeding Water							
Formula Preparation							
Breast Pump							
Storage of Pumped Milk							
Red Flags and Calling Pediatrician							
Other:							
MOTHER CARE							
Vaginal Discharge/Bleeding							
Incision/Episiotomy Care							
Breast Care							
When Not to Breastfeed							
Bladder/Bowel Functions							
Activity/Rest							
Nutrition/Diet							
Emotions/Coping							
Medications							
When to Call Physician							
Follow-up Care Appointment							
Other							

SELF ASSESSMENT CODES:	1 = Most Important to Learn Before I go Home; 2 = I Would Like to Review; 3 = I Already Know or Comfortable With
BARRIERS TO TEACHING CODES	C = Lack of Confidence; D = Decline to Participate; L = Language; M = Lack of Motivation; T = Lack of Time; O = Other (Specify)
METHOD OF TEACHING MODES:	B = Booklet; C = Class Attendance; D = Demonstration; M = Media (TV, Audio/Video); R = Reinforcement
EVALUATION CODES:	D = Demonstrated Successfully; N = Need Reinforcement/Practice; P = Unable to Perform; T = Teachback; U = Unable to Understand; V = Verbalized Understating

NOTE: Complete the mother's self-assessment before teaching commences. You may use more than one code in each of the sections except in the mother's self-assessment.

Figure 7.3 Example of Patient/Family Teaching and Documentation Checklist: Mother/Baby.

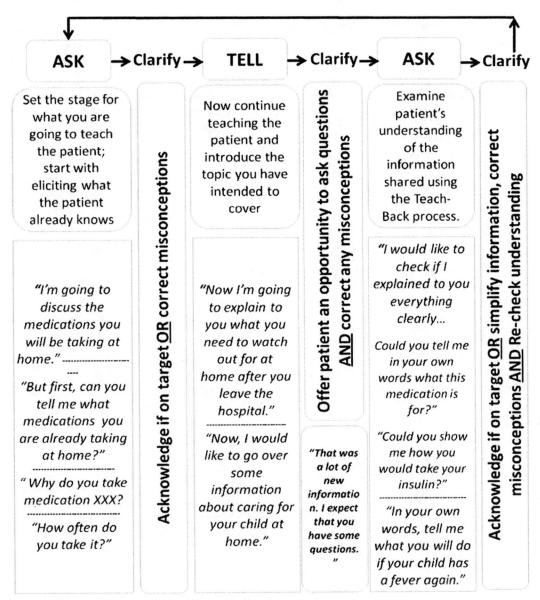

Figure 7.4 Example of a teach-back method.

a concept to the patient/family. Case managers may apply this method to verify that the patient and family:

- Clearly understand the diagnosis, health regimen, and other instructions provided
- Has the key information to effectively complete necessary healthcare tasks at home
- Has the knowledge and skills to participate in the plan of care at home which ultimately assures self-management and adherence

To simplify the patient and family educational activities and to enhance the patient's understanding which ultimely improves adherence to the health regimen, case managers may organize their patient educational activities as follows:

- *The whats*: key topic(s) or issues the patient/fam-

ily must be clear and knowledgeable about; for example red flags (i.e., serious symptoms indicative of derterioration in condition or disease state) to watch out for after discharge
- *The dos*: care activities the patient/family need to master for self-management for example, the act of monitoring blood glucose level or daily weight
- *The whys*: reason for or value of mastering and performing the activities taught; for example, monitoring blood glucose level to avoid hypo- or hypeglycemia and adjust insulin dosage accordingly; daily weights to identify water retention in a heart failure situation

Assessment of health literacy and conduct of patient and family education using the teach-back method enhances the patient engagement and case managers must use such empowering language when interacting with their patients/families.

- *Engagement*: being directly involved in own care and making decisions about care options based on needs and preferences; also acting with full responsibility and accountability
- *Compliance or adherence*: obeying a care directive from a healthcare provider even when sometimes lacking the necessary knowledge or will to effectively follow through on self-care activities.

Engaged patients are also empowered patients (Box 7.3). They are knowledgeable, motivated, and confident about self-care and self-management especially when at home or after an episode of care. They also feel empowered, and demonstrate the ability to effectively manage their own health condition, seek assistance when needed, and assume an active role in avoiding the need for unnecessary or unplanned acute care. Case managers are integral to enhancing patient and family engagement in self-care and self-management when they are knowledgeable, skilled, and demonstrate competence in health literacy assessment, health teaching, the teach-back method, and patient empowerment and engagement.

Case managers may be involved in staff development by enhancing and disseminating new knowledge and skills, especially those related to case management practices. They act as mentors and preceptors of less senior staff. The knowledge of case management itself must also be conveyed across professional lines and levels of hierarchy. In addition, the community is in need of hearing and learning more about case manage-

---

Box 7.3 Examples of Patient Engagement Behaviors

Empowered and actively engaged patients exhibit the following behaviors:

- Finding safe care and services
- Communicating with health professionals when needed without hesitation
- Organizing their own healthcare services and resources
- Paying for care rather than avoiding care due to financial concerns
- Making sound and educated treatment decisions
- Participating in treatment /self-care
- Promoting own health and engaging in healthy lifestyle behaviors
- Getting preventive care
- Planning for end-of-life care
- Seeking health knowledge

---

ment. If a person is hospitalized or offered the option of home care, he or she will have an appropriate expectation of case management and how the case manager will be involved in the plan of care.

7.3. COMMUNICATION AND OTHER INTERPERSONAL SKILLS

Communication and other interpersonal skills are the lifeline that connects each individual in any walk of life and in any organization. As our technological world continues to be fast moving, quality communication becomes essential. Many would claim that communication is the core of leadership and decision-making. Without a doubt, thorough and timely communication is a core managerial function. Therefore as managers and leaders, case managers must master effective communication to be successful in their roles. Communication is the transfer of information, ideas, understanding, or feelings. Case management is working with and through others. Therefore, communication is necessary so that each person knows his or her role and responsibilities in the process of accomplishing goals.

Dash, O'Donnell, Vince-Whitman, and Zarle (1996) define communication as follows:

- A complex, dynamic interchange of verbal and nonverbal messages and meanings between people, the means by which information is transferred
- The process of imparting knowledge
- A social and interactive process
- Something continuous and fluid

We take communication for granted, but in the case of quality job performance—as in the role of a case manager—it should not be treated lightly. A miscommunication or a barrier to effective communication could lead to expensive hardship for a hospital, payer, patient, or family. In fact, it is easier to miscommunicate than to communicate clearly. At any stage in the process of communication something can interfere with its effectiveness, clarity, or accuracy. This interference is called noise. Noise can be physical, such as a cardiac monitor beeping in a patient's ear; psychological, such as the fear of or anxiety as a result of being hospitalized; or anything else that keeps the message from getting from sender to receiver effectively and intact.

A communication model has at least four elements (Figure 7.5). The first element is the sender, as in the case manager, who transmits the communication message. The second element is the message, which includes the verbal (i.e., spoken or written) and nonverbal (i.e., facial expressions and body language). The third component, the receiver, is the person to whom the message is sent. If all goes well, the message received will be the intended message sent. The fourth component, the context, is the surroundings in which the communication takes place. It is the environment which is identified by such factors as the patient's condition, cultural background, health beliefs, and values (Dash et al., 1996).

The channel one chooses is also a factor in effective communication and must be individualized to the patient's readiness to learn and preferred method of communication (e.g., face-to-face, video, group meeting, or written). In addition, the listener's receptivity must be established and maintained if quality communication is to take place. The listener can be either the sender or the receiver of the message depending on the dynamics occurring during the interaction and act of communication.

Because barriers to communication are the pitfalls for any case manager to try to avoid, it is helpful to review some examples in depth.

7.3.1. Physical Interference

The first and most important step in improving communication is to make sure that your intended receiver receives the message. The sender (case manager) must take full responsibility for seeing that the physical barriers to communication are reduced. Case Study 7.4 provides an example of such a situation.

7.3.2. Psychological Noise

The root cause of this interference is distraction (thinking about something else). Accuracy is at stake here. Hunger, anger, depression, medication, worrying about the pets or children at home, and fear all have an impact on the way the receiver understands. Asking for feedback, providing feedback, and verifying the accuracy of the message helps identify the existence of a psychological barrier. See Case Study 7.5 for an example.

7.3.3. Information Processing Barriers

Our brains have the miraculous ability to take in enormous amounts of data but can only process consciously one thought at a time. If information is being sent too fast, the brain and therefore the receiver have trouble taking it in (Case Manager's Tip 7.8). Communication overload is a classic example of a processing barrier. During communication overload too much information is being sent, and the receiver cannot process it all at once. The receiver then becomes overwhelmed and shuts down. You have probably seen this occur numerous times. Picture yourself giving a patient instructions on how to test his or her blood sugar. You go on and on reciting the steps of pricking the finger, dabbing a drop of blood on the glucose test strip, and preparing the glocuse monitoring device to accept the strip for reading. When you suddenly try to make eye contact, what you see is a face staring back at you blankly. The patient is overwhelmed by your instruction, is overloaded, and has shut down.

7.3.4. Perceptual Barriers

Each individual brings a unique set of past experiences to communication. These experiences, good or bad, relevant to the current situation or not, will influence how a person perceives the meaning of your communication. Perception is greatly influenced by our value system, beliefs, rituals, preferences, and habits. We interpret everything we experience through mental images, and we tend to assume that the way we see things is the way that they really are and the way everyone else sees them.

7.3.5. Structural Barriers

There are aspects of organizational structure that can affect the quality of communication. These next barriers to communication, as those previously mentioned, can be applied not only to a case manager's patients but also to a case manager's peers, other members of

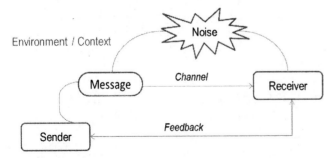

Figure 7.5 Diagram of the communication model (Rawlins, 1992).

 CASE MANAGER'S TIP 7.8

Information Overload and Quality of Communication

Too much information delivered too quickly will result in a poor-quality communication effort. Information about too many topics, especially if unrelated, and shared at the same time may also result in poor-quality communication.

CASE STUDY 7.4 ■ Dealing with Physical Interference

You are a case manager in an acute care hospital setting. You enter room 410 to speak to Ms. Blondin about her discharge/transitional plan. The first thing you notice is that her television is on, she has two visitors by her bedside, housekeeping personnel are emptying the garbage and cleaning around the room, and the lunch meal carts are arriving in the hallway. You immediately gather that very little effective communication will occur if you begin to discuss the discharge/transitional plan with Ms. Blondin. You recognize the need to manage the physical barriers to effective communication. What do you do?

First, you may ask Ms. Blondin if it is the right time to discuss the plan. She has been anxiously waiting for you to visit; she has some questions herself. Next, assuming Ms. Blondin has agreed to discuss the plan, you ask her for permission to turn off the television. Then you

may invite the visitors to participate in the meeting, if Ms. Blondin is agreeable to that and you both feel it is appropriate to do. You can then share the purpose of your meeting with them. You also may ask the houskeeper to perhaps either finish quickly or return in a short time to continue the cleaning. Next, you explain why you are there and make eye contact. You make sure you sit down so that Ms. Blondin and her visitors do not think you are in a rush.

If distractions are still evident, you may wait until the housekeeper has left the room and the dietary cart has passed in the hallway. Then you can proceed because you have taken control of the physical environment and have reduced the physical interference that would have certainly had a negative effect on your communication effort.

---

the interdisciplinary team, payers, and management staff.

The more people involved in a chain of communication, the greater the likelihood that message interruption can occur (Case Manager's Tip 7.9). You may remember the old game of "telephone" in which a message is whispered into the ear of one person who in turn whispers the message to the next person in a group. By the time the message reaches the last person it is substantially different from the initial message. Usually the important details such as times, dates, and names become confused.

7.3.6. Defensive Communication

Defensive communication can also be a barrier to the effective transmission of the message. This type of communication occurs when people attempt to protect

CASE MANAGER'S TIP 7.9

Limiting the Chain of Communication

The fewer people to whom messages must be relayed, the more effective the communication is. The fewer people involved in the communication, the clearer and easier the communication becomes. Communicating with multiple people at the same time (as a group) may compromise the quality of the communication and the openness of those involved due to competing interests of the various parties.

themselves from a real or perceived threat. The threat could be related to the sender or receiver of the message, or it could be present in the message itself. Defensive communication tends to occur when there is a lack of trust—for example, when the receiver of the message is doubtful or suspicious of the sender's motives. Sometimes it also occurs when self-confidence is lacking and the sender or receiver is acting defensively to mask the lack of confidence. Message-related defensive communication takes place when the message being sent contains challenging content or disregard for the receiver's values, beliefs, worth, or feelings or when the sender is doubtful the information is complete, accurate, important, or necessary.

7.3.7. Power

If communication must take place between various levels of authority or power, the differences in status can result in poor-quality communication. This is known as information processing or filtering. Overcoming the communication barrier imposed by status differences is mostly a matter of realizing that it can occur (Case Manager's Tip 7.10). There are generally two types of power:

■ *Directive power*, or power used to affect the behavior of others with the intent of satisfying personal needs
■ *Synergistic power*, or power used to increase the energy and creativity of all participants with the intent of satisfying the needs of all participants

CASE STUDY 7.5 ■ Dealing with Psychological Barriers

You approach Mr. Tumbie, an 80-year-old frail-looking man admitted for dehydration and intractable diarrhea. Your first question, "How are you today, Mr. Tumbie?" You get a nonverbal response of sighs and wringing his hands but a verbal response of feeling fine. You immediately notice that Mr. Tumbie's expressions and actions do not match his verbal reply, and you interpret this as anxiety. As you probe further into his apparent anxiety, you learn that he is tired, has not slept well the night before, and is preoccupied with his daughter and son-in-law, who are "after his money."

Your original goal of offering Mr. Tumbie discharge planning options may be too premature in light of the fact that there is a clear psychological barrier that must be tackled first: his relationship with his daughter and son-in-law. It may be his belief that discussing personal or family problems with a healthcare professional (e.g., a nurse or case maanger) is inappropriate; therefore before discussing his personal life you may first need to establish trust with Mr. Tumbie to help him feel more comfortable. Beginning with a less emotionally charged topic would be advantageous in building rapport and becoming better informed about your patient. You will no doubt be more successful when approaching this sensitive subject with him at a later time.

Knowing how and when to enforce power appropriately, along with having the components of a trusting relationship, will result in a shared sense of responsibility and better outcomes. Possessing a solid power base is crucial, and its appropriateness is essential. As an expert case manager, you must be willing to share expertise, issue directives, follow up on compliance, and attempt to influence as occasions arise (Bass, 1985). Case Study 7.6 provides an example.

7.3.8. Trust

Stress and lack of trust are additional structural barriers to communication. They both interfere with accurate, clear communication, and they both affect the ability to express needs and share information openly and honestly. Building rapport and a trusting relationship with the patient/family and fellow healthcare professionals usually has the added bonus of reducing stress, thereby increasing the chances of accurate communication.

The following sections outline the four basic qualities a case manager should exhibit to initiate a patient–case manager or case manager–colleague relationship in which trust can be developed.

7.3.8.1. Warmth

This quality helps others to feel accepted. Case managers who are willing to extend themselves with openness rather than exhibit cold, expressionless, disapproving behavior will gain trust more quickly. Warmth reflects self-respect, self-acceptance, and genuine concern for others, and people respond to this type of behavior favorably and with much ease.

7.3.8.2. Respect

Treat others as you would want to be treated; take into consideration personality, culture, opinions, customs, values, and beliefs. To respect another person does not necessarily mean that you must like that person; however, you must accept and value him or her for who they are. This becomes important to a case manager when a family's or patient's decisions regarding a discharge plan are not in full agreement with the case manager's recommendation. Keeping patients informed about their care gives them the feeling that they are respected as individuals, not just seen as a bed number or a disease entity.

7.3.8.3. Empathy

Helping people to feel understood means actively tuning in to feelings and thoughts and letting go of stereotypes and prejudices. This is an essential ingredient in trusting relationships and in cultural diversity, competence, and sensitivity. You must really hear, without

CASE MANAGER'S TIP 7.10

Power and Communication

Always keep yourself focused on the goals of your communication and do not get intimidated by hierarchical status of people involved when quality patient care is at stake. Seeking feedback and verifying the information conveyed will help you maintain power and ensure safe and clear communciation.

CASE STUDY 7.6 ■ Appropriate Use of Power on a Patient's Behalf

Mrs. Rose is a resident of Florida who came to visit her elderly sister in Chicago and became ill, requiring hospitalization. Mrs. Rose has remained hospitalized for 9 days and is now ready for discharge. In the course of hospitalization, Mrs. Rose's functional status has deteriorated and the likelihood that she can remain home alone is slim. She requires oxygen therapy and a wheelchair to help her move around safely. The dilemma is how to get Mrs. Rose discharged to a safe care setting when she refuses nursing home placement and wants only to return to Florida where her friends could help her. Many contacts and more hospital days later, it becomes clear to you, Mrs Rose's case manager, that it would be less expensive to arrange for medical air

transport to Florida than to continue to keep Mrs. Rose hospitalized.

You, the case manager in this scenario, have the ability to affect the outcome of Mrs. Rose's hospitalization by using directive power and educating the hospital's administrative body. It is soon realized that it is financially more prudent to send Mrs. Rose back to Florida rather than keep her hospitalized indefinitely. You must clearly communicate to the appropriate executive at your hospital about the cost of a few days in the hospital versus the expense of an ambulance and medical air transport. Besides such arrangements make Mrs. Rose happy as she insists she wants to return to Florida.

---

demanding that someone feel as you think they should in a given situation. In the end it is about the patient and not you.

7.3.8.4. Genuineness

This final component of communication enhances the trust relationship. This quality allows people to feel that they are interacting with a real person who is interested in their well-being. Consistency is a facet of being genuine. If there is inconsistency between verbal and nonverbal behavior, communication will break down. Keep in mind that people who are already stressed by their situation will be more astute to false behavior and inconsistent communication. Armed with the knowledge of the many barriers to communication and the ways in which to avoid or to minimize them, the case manager must be versed in the communication channels that effectively transmit the message from sender to receiver.

7.4. COMMUNICATION PATHS

The path that communication takes, whether it be formal or informal, has an affect on the communication itself. Formal communication takes two forms: downward and upward.

- *Downward communication* is communication about what to do, how to do it, and when it is to be completed. This communication usually takes place when delegating to subordinates. To delegate effectively, all of the aforementioned barriers should be avoided.

- *Upward communciation* is when communciation entails seeking the support, permission, or approval from a superior. An example of upward communication is when a case manager speaks with a chief financial officer (CFO) to request financial approval, as in the previously discussed scenario of flying a patient back to her home state of Florida rather than incurring the cost of an extended hospital stay. The result is a more accurate managerial process.

Informal communication usually takes place between smaller groups, such as the case manager and the social worker. Managers in these two areas may get together after a more formal meeting to discuss a policy that may affect both of their departments. This type of communication must be based on mutual trust, or a more formal communication will need to follow.

Other forms of communciation between healthcare professionals and patients or families/caregivers that have become increasingly popular today are electronic type. Often patients may communciate with their healthcare providers (e.g., primary care provider, case manager) using e-mail, text messaging, or videoconferencing technology. Electronic communications have facilitators and barriers which are similar to verbal and in-person communication methods. Noise, environmental factors, degree of clarity, defensiveness, power, perceptual, and structural factors affect the quality of communication. A sender, receiver, message, feedback channel, and communication paths also apply to electronic communication. However, electronic communication, especially when it is in the form of text messaging or e-mails, may encounter other challenges not ususlly experienced in nonelectronic forms of communication due to the absence of visual and nonverbal cues. This is also complicated by a lack of in-person instantaneous exchange which potentially may result in misunderstanding and confusion of the message. Case managers are advised to avoid the use of electronic communication unless if it is absolutely necessary, otherwise they must make every effort to ensure an effective, safe, quality, timely, accurate, and respectful exchange.

In addition to becoming aware of typical barriers to effective communication and channels of communication, case managers can take additional steps to improve communication competency. How colleagues work together as a team can determine the success or failure of any work environment. Good relationships are fostered when colleagues respect each others' job responsibilities.

7.4.1. Teams

There is a great difference between an effective team and a group of people who have been thrown together with no clear goals or purpose. There are generally 12 elements of an effective team (Box 7.4). While reviewing these elements, think about the members of your organizational team, whether they be social workers, discharge planners, utilization reviewers, nurse managers, payers, or physicians. Rate the effectiveness of your team effort toward a productive case management program and better patient outcomes. You will begin to see that many, if not all, the elements incorporate the communication and interpersonal skills discussed throughout this chapter.

The twelve elements of team effectiveness involve potential attitude adjustment, releasing of power, respect, compromise, cooperation, and conflict resolution.

7.4.2. Conflict

Administrative pressures for cost control and consumer demands for safe and quality care influence case managers in their daily decision-making activities. Now more than ever it is necessary for case managers to work collaboratively with members of the interdisciplinary team to meet the pressures and demands of safe, quality, and cost-effective healthcare delivery. Case managers must keep in mind that conflict is inevitable and that it is not a negative occurrence. Conflict is merely individuals or groups experiencing differences in views, goals, facts, or values that place them at op-

---

Box 7.4   Twelve Elements of Effective Teams

The following are characteristics of effective teams and teamwork. You may use this list to examine whether your team is effective and highly functional.

Team members:

1. Communicate openly and honestly. They listen with understanding.
2. Have common goals and a clear idea of the team's mission and purpose.
3. Support each other. They have assigned duties and are not engaged in turf wars.
4. Take pride in their group's efforts and results.
5. Put the team's interest before one's own.
6. Appreciate and recognize the individual value, belief, diversity, and contribution which ultimately support the team's success.
7. Help make decisions on important issues but when necessary are willing to look for guidance for final decisions.
8. Feel comfortable expressing ideas, opinions, and disagreements.
9. Are encouraged to make the development of new skills a way of life.
10. Are encouraged to use their unique skills and talents.
11. Realize that conflict is normal and that working out differences can lead to new points of view and creativity.
12. Value appropriate humor. Having fun increases openness, enthusiasm, and energy.

---

posite poles. It usually involves areas of differing expertise, practice, or authority.

In most situations conflict falls into one of three categories:

- *Perceived conflict*, the thought that conditions exist between groups that cause the conflict
- *Felt conflict*, when the conflict evokes feelings of threat, hostility, fear, or mistrust
- *Expressed conflict*, which takes the form of debate, assertion, competition, or problem solving

There are five different strategies for resolving conflict (Box 7.5). However, the most often used tactic is the collaborative (i.e., win/win) resolution as explained earlier in this chapter under 'Negotiation'. Groups usually identify solutions that will allow each to maintain their goals and ultimately create a resolution that they are satisfied with. The ability to successfully manage conflict is an important skill for the case manager to master. It can help the case manager to increase the total benefits of the group efforts by becoming more

Box 7.5   Five Strategies for Conflict Resolution

1. *Competing*: An assertive strategy in which an individual's concerns are satisfied at the expense of another's. This strategy is useful in a situation in which the solution is urgently needed and time does not allow waiting for a different strategy to be tried first.
2. *Collaborating*: A cooperative strategy in which individuals work together to find mutually satisfying solutions. This strategy is useful when a solution to a particular conflict is complex and requires that all parties involved be satisfied with the outcome. Usually it results in a win/win outcome.
3. *Compromising*: A strategy in which each of the individuals involved in the conflict must give something up to resolve the conflict. This strategy is useful when the goals of one individual are important or not important enough as compared with the goals of another.
4. *Avoiding*: A passive strategy in which an individual postpones or sidesteps the conflict. This strategy is useful when one party is more powerful than the other and the risk of confrontation outweighs the benefits or the solution.
5. *Accommodating*: A passive strategy in which an individual focuses on the concerns of others and neglects his or her own concerns. This strategy is useful when one individual has a vested interest while the issue is unimportant to the other.

innovative and creative, with the overall outcome of increasing productivity and achieving goals (Case Manager's Tip 7.11).

One member of the multidisciplinary team, the physician, is a vital communication source. If there are conflicts or obstacles to the case manager–physician communication, then the quality of patient care will suffer. Professional and up-front communication regarding the case manager's role is a good place to start in building an effective team among the various disciplines. Case managers must initiate positive dialogue with physicians and address the stereotypes and stresses of a shifting healthcare system. Despite sharing the common goal of the patient's well-being,

CASE MANAGER'S TIP 7.11

Positive Effects of Conflict

If conflict is well-managed, it can actually increase the effectiveness of an organization, teams, and individuals. It also enhances the delivery of timely, safe, quality, and cost-effective care.

physicians and case managers can easily become adversaries when distrust surrounding the case manager's intentions is raised. Comments such as "case managers are the police who work with the insurance payers to deny care" misguide physicians into perceiving case managers as a threat to their medical judgment and their income. As a result of the changing working relationship between case managers and physicians (and others such as nurses, social workers, utilization review coordinators, and discharge planners), the transition to a full cooperative and collaborative relationship is at times awkward and frustrating. Being caught up in past traditional roles hinders the establishment of the collaborative alliance necessary to achieve success in the healthcare of the twenty-first century.

We must constantly remain focused on one goal: delivery of safe, quality, and affordable care to patients. Case managers need to be especially clear on this point—that their interest is in ensuring better quality of care and the best possible outcomes. The physicians (or social workers, utilization review coordinators, discharge planners) must be reassured that case managers are not there to control or dictate practice but are there instead to foster effective, quality communication between members of a multidisciplinary team.

Today's case managers face the challenge of dealing with a diverse patient population. The case manager must be capable of incorporating the communication techniques and skills reviewed in this chapter when communicating with the diversity of groups involved in patient care. For example, a group of growing prominence is the payer source or insurance company. The case manager must listen closely to what the payer is requesting and must clarify any vague communication at the outset. The case manager should not assume that the health insurance claims department has all of the necessary knowledge with regard to a patient's discharge/transitional plan. The case manager, as educator and advocate, becomes vital to the success of the patient's care outcomes by sharing his or her medical knowledge of what the patient needs. Case managers must keep in mind that they are the problem solvers and cannot easily accept a simple "No" or "We don't do that." Case managers must be risk takers when communicating with the payer members of the team, or patients could suffer the consequences. The communication with external members of the multidisciplinary team (e.g., payer, community resources, family members) becomes just as important to the success of the patient's outcome as the communication with internal members.

Much of this chapter has been devoted to communication because it is perhaps the most vital skill

Box 7.6 Communication Styles and Their Characteristics

1. Assertive
   - Pushing hard without attacking
   - Expressive and self-enhancing
   - Influencing results and outcomes
   - Motivated and taking initiative
2. Aggressive
   - Taking advantage of others
   - Self-enhancing at others' expense
   - Intimidating
   - Demand and control
3. Nonassertive
   - Inhibited
   - Self-denying
   - Passive
   - Await direction, permission or approval

that case managers must master. Although different communication styles exist (Box 7.6), case managers must use the assertive style in applying the case management process. However, psychological, physical, and structural barriers can cause turbulence in the information flow. Effective case managers will work tirelessly to reduce these barriers. The more rapidly they receive and communicate information, the better the quality of the decisions they will make (Case Manager's Tip 7.12).

7.4.3. Data Management

The use of data in case management continues to be of great importance. Case managers continually use data for decision-making purposes. They identify, collect, and analyze data when assessing their patients, implementing the required care and monitoring and evaluating the outcomes. This aspect of the case manager's role is important for information management, knowledge development, and enhancing the healthcare delivery system. Therefore case managers must possess appropriate skills in data management to succeed. They also must be able to use certain tools throughout their day for data collection and tracking. Examples of these tools are as follows:

- Variance or care delay data collection tools
- Level of care review tools
- Documentation tools
- Administrative logs and databases
- Quality assessment, insurance, and improvement tools
- Value-based purchasing quality measures

- Information systems and electronic medical records

Case managers must also understand the different methods of data collection and management (i.e., retrospective, prospective, and concurrent), their advantages and disadvantages, and when it is appropriate to use each of the methods. For example, it is best to examine the value-based purchasing measures concurrently so that if an issue is identified it is addressed before it is too late, resulting in financial or reputation risk. In addition, case managers must be knowledgeable in the types of measures used in data analysis, particularly those that are appropriate for use in case management evaluation, such as the following:

- *Numbers*: descriptive statistics
- *Rates*: incidence and occurrence
- *Attributes*: demographics
- *Perceptions*: customer and staff satisfaction
- *Composites*: case mix index

With today's reliance on automation and analytical tools in most data management systems and departments, case managers are expected to be able to access databases, run special reports, prepare graphic reports, conduct statistical analyses, and export or download data. Case managers with these skills are the most desirable and successful. When writing reports, they must be able to summarize the important findings, indicate the outliers and deviations from the norms or standards, and determine whether there is a need for more detailed or different types of data for better decision making or for more accurate interpretations and conclusions. Furthermore, case managers must be capable of writing concise, readable, and easily understood and interpreted reports including meaningful and clear data visualization.

7.4.4. Big Picture/Systems Thinking

Case management delivery models are grounded in systems theory. The delivery of patient care is depen-

 CASE MANAGER'S TIP 7.12

Improving the Effectiveness of Communication

In addition to improving basic communication skills of reading, writing, listening, and speaking, case managers can improve their communication effectiveness by withholding judgment, avoiding inconsistencies, maintaining transparency, and valuing all members of the team, inclusive of the patient and family.

dent on the environment/context in which it is delivered and varies across time and space. For example, intensive care services are not provided in a clinic setting, rather in an acute care setting. Another example is using the emergency department for access to healthcare services at times of emergency and not as a primary care delivery setting. Case managers must understand the differences in the types of services provided in the varied settings across the continuum. If they are not systems focused in their thinking and approach to care delivery and management, they will not be successful and effective.

Case managers are expected to interact with their system at three different levels: the individual, the organization, and the environment at large. They manage the care of the individual patients in the context of the care setting or level of care the patient is at. They also coordinate, facilitate, and arrange for the services their patients may require post-discharge from an episode of care or at the next level of care. This requires case managers to interact with other organizations and community agencies or health insurance plans/managed care organizations, for authorization of services; thus they reach out to other organizations and the environment at large. Regardless of the setting they are in, case managers are expected to employ a systems thinking framework and approach to case management care delivery. This framework assures them success and desirable outcomes.

According to Ridge and Bland Jones (1999), systems thinking is defined as a "powerful problem-solving language that guides the understanding of complex issues within organizations, based on the assumption that organizations are made up of parts with patterns of interaction, rather than discrete structures and components." The complexity of case management models in relation to the scope of services, interdisciplinary approach, and continuum of care focus demands a systems approach to care delivery because of its interdependence on the various disciplines involved in care processes and teams from different settings or levels of care. Case managers must be able to pay careful attention to the environment in which they work and to its related inputs, throughputs, and outputs and the degree to which they interact. The inputs, throughputs, and outputs make up the various functions of case management such as resource utilization, strategic plans, care management activities, roles and job descriptions, goals, objectives, performance, productivity, and outcomes.

Healthcare organizations are systems in which staff members interact and function as interdependent teams to accomplish the goals of the organization. This is true

of case management systems. Case managers must be able to work collaboratively in teams and to facilitate the achievement of the goals of cost-effectiveness and quality outcomes. Case managers must view systems thinking as the desired approach for achieving expected outcomes including those of value-based purchasing and patient experience with care. Systems thinking is a powerful problem-solving strategy and case managers must learn to incorporate it into their daily activities. It helps them focus on the essential interrelationships of the case management model and see and appreciate the "big picture" as well as the interconnectedness of the different components of the case management program, system, or organization. Systems thinking assists case managers in the following ways:

- Managing decision-making
- Managing multiple tasks and functions
- Coping with conflict
- Motivating others
- Managing change
- Facilitating negotiation activities

7.4.5. Emotional Intelligence

Emotional intelligence has surfaced as a necessary skill for effective industry leaders. It has become even more important for those in healthcare; especially for case managers. Emotional intelligence is defined by Cooper and Sawaf (1996) as the "ability to sense, understand, and effectively apply the power and acumen of emotions as a source of human energy, information, connection, and influence." Goleman (1995), however, defined emotional intelligence as the ability to:

- Motivate oneself
- Persist in the face of frustrations
- Control impulsive behavior or decision-making
- Delay gratification
- Regulate one's mood
- Keep distress from swamping the ability to think
- Empathize with others

Both definitions emphasize the importance of self-awareness of emotions and the need to consider these emotions and feelings in the process of making decisions, instituting actions, or dealing with others.

Feelings and emotions, whether positive, negative, or neutral serve as a source of vital information used in making decisions, initiating action, or communicating. They cause case managers to act in a certain way. They also influence how case managers may connect with themselves and others and establish effective relationships. How successful they can be in handling a particular situation or event depends on the following perceptions of emotions:

- Awareness of one's feelings
- Awareness of the emotions and feelings of others
- The effect of these feelings and emotions on the encountered situation or event

Emotions, if used and managed appropriately by case managers, act as a source of power, motivation, feedback, information, influence, innovation, creativity, success, connection, and freedom. Ultimately, emotional intelligence enhances case managers' abilities with regard to the following:

- Making influential decisions
- Resolving conflict effectively
- Communicating openly and honestly with others
- Establishing trusting relationships with patients, their families, and other members of the interdisciplinary healthcare team
- Building rapport with patients and their families
- Creating an environment of care that is centered on the patient and family and is focused on teamwork
- Being present and connected to what is happening at the individual patient level while delivering care

Goleman (1995, 1998) identified five components of emotional intelligence: knowing one's emotions, managing emotions, motivating oneself, recognizing others' emotions, and handling relationships. The first three components are concerned with self-management and regulation skills, whereas the remaining two are associated with building relationships, community, and social skills. These components are described as follows:

1. *Knowing one's emotions* is the state of having a deep understanding of, and insight into, one's feelings, preferences, internal states, and drives, and how they affect self, others, and job performance. Emotionally self-aware case managers are conscious of their capabilities and deficits and have better control over their actions, reactions, and interactions. Their decision-making ability is enhanced and they are more honest and sincere in their practice.

2. *Managing one's emotions* is handling one's feelings, emotions, and internal states appropriately. It is the ability to control one's impulses, delay gratification, and regulate one's moods so that distress is prevented. Case managers who manage their emotions are able to withhold disruptive emotions, reactions, and decision-making until relevant infor-

mation is obtained. In addition, they are able to be flexible in handling change and to be responsible for personal performance. Case managers who manage their emotions are able to self-regulate. They are also able to carry on effective internal conversations about feelings, emotions, and experiences so that they feel free of destructive emotions and thoughts and thus are able to channel emotions in useful ways for themselves, other colleagues, the patient/family, and the job.

3. *Motivating oneself* is the act of taking the initiative for achieving goals and dreams. It is pursuing solutions to problems without waiting for others to take the lead or provide direction. Self-motivated case managers strive for excellence and align with the goals of the interdisciplinary healthcare team and/or the organization. They achieve beyond their own expectations and the expectations of others and what is expected for the job. They are passionate about and take pride in the job they are responsible for. Self-motivated case managers are able to "think outside the box" and to look for nontraditional solutions/approaches to solving problems and improving workflow. Self-motivation enhances their feeling of optimism even after a setback or failure to achieve, or after experiencing frustration.

4. *Recognizing others' emotions* is the ability to recognize the feelings of others and to be more attuned to the subtle signals others send through their behaviors and interactions regarding their needs, wants, and desires. Case managers who have the ability to recognize others' emotions are more aware of others' needs and perspectives. They are able to express their interest in others' concerns and abilities and to work with them on meeting the interdisciplinary team and care goals. The ability to recognize and acknowledge others' emotions is known as empathy. It is essential for understanding and thoughtfully considering the feelings and emotions of others while making decisions or solving problems. Empathy enhances the patient's experience with care and promotes a patient-centered care approach. It also improves teamwork and unity and helps to bring members of the interdisciplinary healthcare team closer together. It also fosters loyalty to the team and the organization.

5. *Handling relationships* is the ability to manage relationships and others' emotions effectively. Case managers who know how to handle relationships make those around them feel welcome, at ease, and an integral part of the team. They are effective on an interpersonal level and adept at inducing desirable

CASE MANAGER'S TIP 7.13

Strategies for Becoming an Emotionally Intelligent Case Manager

1. Knowing one's emotions
   - Identify what information you are using to influence your interpretation of things/events.
   - Identify what influences your mood shifts (i.e., triggers) and the moments you experience them.
   - Know when you are thinking negatively.
   - Know when you are becoming angry or feeling frustrated.
   - Know when you are becoming defensive.
   - Recognize when your verbal and nonverbal communications are conflicting.
   - Be aware of what senses you are currently using.
   - Be able to communicate how you feel or what annoys you.
   - Recognize when you are using defensive communication.
   - Know when you procrastinate or avoid completing a promise or some activity, and the triggers for such behaviors
2. Managing emotions
   - Learn to relax when under pressure.
   - Act productively, especially when you are angry, frustrated, or in anxiety-provoking situations.
   - Attempt to calm quickly before you make decisions or respond to unpleasant situations.
   - Be aware of the relationships between your physiological and emotional states.
   - Remain calm when you are the target of anger or criticism from others.
   - Take some time out.
   - Resort to humor.
   - Accept failure as a learning opportunity.
3. Motivating oneself
   - Regroup quickly after a setback or stressful experience.
   - Change or stop ineffective habits.
   - Develop new patterns of behaviors that are productive and rewarding.
   - Make sure to follow words with actions.
   - Keep the promises you make to yourself and to others.
   - Be persistent.
   - Do not give up.
   - Always attempt to do your best.
   - Complete your responsibilities/duties within the designated timeframes.
4. Recognizing others' emotions
   - Clarify misunderstandings.
   - Ask others how they feel.
   - Validate your perceptions of others.
   - Validate your perceptions of how others think of or feel about you.
   - Recognize when others are feeling distressed, anxious, or distraught.
   - Engage in intimate conversations with others.
   - Manage group emotions appropriately.
   - Help others manage their emotions.
   - Be empathic.
   - Always provide others with the opportunity to express their feelings honestly.
   - Establish common goals.
5. Handling relationships
   - Work out conflicts.
   - Approach problem resolution as a group.
   - Encourage team-building behaviors.
   - Exhibit effective communication skills.
   - Be honest and sincere.
   - Build trust.
   - Build a sense of community.
   - Influence others and allow others to influence you.
   - Make others feel good and welcome.
   - Seek others for support and advice.
   - Avail yourself to others when they need you.
   - Be approachable.

These are only suggestions and do not reflect an exhaustive list.

responses in others. The ability to handle relationships well enhances group work and synergy and nurtures influential relationships. It helps to build social skills. This ability allows case managers to foster a sense of community. It is "friendliness with a purpose," moving people in the right direction. Case managers' effectiveness with regard to social skills depends on other components of emotional intelligence; that is, controlling and understanding their own feelings and emotions and empathizing with the feelings and emotions of others.

The desired qualities of case managers are not limited to their technical, clinical, and interpersonal skills, abilities, knowledge, and expertise. These qualities are deemed most effective if they are coupled with the skill and ability to recognize, understand, manage, master, and appropriately respond to one's own emotions and feelings and those expressed by others, such as nurses, social workers, physicians, administrators, patients, and families (Case Manager's Tip 7.13).

Case management responsibilities and services demand the presence of case managers who are astute and emotionally intelligent; otherwise case managers would not be able to provide efficient, effective, safe, cost-effective, ethical, and quality care. Being emotionally intelligent enhances the case manager's ability to provide a rewarding patient/family care experience (Case Manager's Tip 7.14).

7.5. SUCCESSFUL LEADERS

Successful leaders possess quite an extensive list of skills. This is especially true of case managers as leaders. They must be able to incorporate all of the skills discussed previously into their day-to-day functions with grace.

As stated earlier, not everyone can be or aspires to be a case manager, even with proper education and development. Successful case managers are likely to demonstrate a special ability to operate in peer relationships, lead others in subordinate or peer relationships, resolve interpersonal and decisional conflicts, communicate with the media, make complex interrelated decisions, allocate resources (including their own time), and innovate. Successful case managers must be leaders, not managers. Leadership skills and abilities are more desired in case managers than management skills and abilities. Management has a more narrow focus: How can I accomplish certain things? It is task focused. Leadership, on the other hand, deals with the broader picture: What are the things that I need to change or facilitate? In other words, management is doing things right, whereas leadership is doing the right things. Management is efficiency in climbing the ladder of success; leadership determines whether the ladder is leaning against the right wall.

You can quickly see the important difference between the two if you envision a group of new graduate nurses cutting their way through a jungle. In the front will be the workers cutting through the undergrowth, cleaning it out. The potential managers will be behind them, sharpening their machetes, writing policy and procedure manuals, holding development programs, and setting up work schedules. The potential leader (case manager) is the one who climbs the tallest tree, surveys the entire situation, and yells, "Wrong jungle!" (Covey, 1989).

The metamorphosis taking place in almost every industry, including the healthcare industry, demands professional leadership first and management second. All that has been conveyed in this chapter clearly depicts the leadership qualities needed in today's healthcare environment. Although the title has generally become associated with management, leadership more fully and accurately defines the role of the case manager. Efficient management without effective leadership is "like straightening deck chairs on the Titanic" (Covey, 1989).

 CASE MANAGER'S TIP 7.14

Examples of the Effects of the Case Manager's Emotional Intelligence on the Patient's Care Experience

1. Awareness of your own emotions allows case managers to:
   - Control and avoid engaging in undesirable behaviors such as verbalizing anger
   - Enhance the case manager-patient/family relationship
2. Awareness of others' emotions allows case managers to:
   - Recognize and understand the patient's/family's concerns, interests, and care prefernces
   - Being empathic toward the patient/family enhances the development of a mutually trusting relationship
3. Recognition of the affects of emotions on the situations encountered allows case managers to:
   - Eliminate the patient's/family's anxiety, concerns, or ambivalence about the plan of care and self-management
   - Make the patient/family feel welcome, open, and at ease in sharing sensitive and important information

Effectiveness does not depend solely on how much effort we expend but whether the effort we expend is in the right place. It is irrelevant if a case manager spends days on a discharge/transitional plan, expending much energy, only to find out that as a result of poor leadership vision, the plan was not the right blueprint for the patient.

The pressure for change within our healthcare industry will most definitely continue to intensify rather than diminish in the coming years. This pressure will require case managers and other healthcare professionals to respond with dynamic transformational leadership to cope with future changes. The transformational leader approaches leadership from an entirely different perspective or level of awareness. The transformational leader is one who does the following:

- Raises levels of consciousness about the importance of certain goals or actions
- Encourages others to transcend self-interests for the good of the team and patient care experience and outcomes
- Serves as a role model
- Builds an empowering and inspiring image
- Articulates vision and goals
- Sets high expectations and direction

The case manager of the twenty-first century characteristically has all of these qualities, and any organization interested in building a solid case management program should give consideration to them. As effective leaders, case managers create the future, effect change, welcome risks, see problems and challenges as opportunities for innovation, and inspire others to embrace the higher purpose of safe, quality, and cost-effffective care delivery—the triple aim of better care, better health, and lower cost.

7.5.1. Motivational Interviewing

The work of patient engagement and patient activation is to enhance the patient's self-management skills and ultimately their adherence to complex health regimens and healthy lifestyle behaviors has contributed to motivational interviewing becoming an essential skill for case managers. This to those working in any setting and with any patient popultion. However, most importantly this is true in the patient-centered medical home where patients with multiple chronic illnesses who face increasingly challenging plans of care. These challenges include a restrictive lifestyle especially in the areas of nutrition, exercise, and medication management.

Motivational interviewing assists case managers during all phases of the case management process start-

---

> **Box 7.7   Essence of Motivational Interviewing**
>
> 1. *Patient-centered*: involves interactions that help patients, families/caregivers explore concerns about changing lifestyle and risk behaviors, while respecting their right to self-determination, autonomy, and choice.
> 2. *Bi-directional and collaborative*: strategically and intentionally focuses on interactions that build trust between the patient and the case manager or other healthcare professionals.
> 3. *Change behavior-orientation*: helps case managers and other healthcare professionals to identify one or more preferred strategies for the individual patient/family/caregiver which facilitate achieving targeted change in lifestyle and self-management abilities to ultimately improve the patient's health state.

ing with assessment to planning care and evaluating outcomes. It is a skill or technique in communication that is known to assist case managers in uncovering sensitive and important information about a patient, to gain insight about the patient's situation (i.e., health condition) which ultimately results in better understanding of what is in the way of adherence and effective self-management (Tahan and Sminkey, 2012) (Box 7.7).

Motivational interviewing focuses on the clinical, social, financial, mental, behavioral, and emotional aspects of the patient's status and employs a communication style that is supportive, empathic, and counseling-like. Case managers use this technique as a clinical approach for eliciting the patient's own values and motivations for change. To be effective, they listen to patients and families/caregivers instead of telling them what to do; evoke deep and meaningful self-exploration, identify areas strengths or opportunities for change rather than requiring them to alter unfavorable behavior; and approach them from the perspective of "you have what you need, and together we will find it," rather than "I have what you need and this is what I think you ought to do," (Tahan and Sminkey, 2012).

Motivational interviewing is a highly effective technique case managers apply to improve the patient's care outcomes especially in the degree of engagement in own care, adherence to a recommended plan of care, and active self-management (Box 7.8). To be successful and rewarding, it must involve the following four key activities:

1. Culturally sensitive, patient-centeric, and respectful conversations about lifestyle behavior change(s) where counseling-like comm9nciation,

health teaching, and support facilitate openness to change.

2. Bi-directional communication that is collaborative, goal-oriented, non-judgmental, honors the patient's autonomy, and builds mutual trust.

3. Non-authoritarian interactions that guide patients/families through targeted change and assists them in facing and resolving their ambivalence about the desired change.

4. Negotiation to help patients/families make their own health decisions and encourage them to recognize they are able to change and act upon what they are interested in doing (Tahan and Sminkey, 2012).

When enaged in motivational interviewing, case managers ask their patients/families open-ended questions to not only allow them to share the thoughts, feelings, and concerns they may have about their health condition or plan of care, but to identify areas of strengths and what works (or has worked in the past) for them as well (Box 7.9). During these interactions, case managers are intentional regarding gaining insight about the patient's behavioral, cognitive, and emotional states.

- *Behavioral*: how the patient's health status affects his/her ability to adhere to the medical/health re-

gime (i.e., case management plan of care) and perform all aspects of self-care

- *Cognitive*: whether the patient is able to acquire knowledge and skills that will help him/her to change behaviors and adopt a healthier lifestyle
- *Emotional*: awareness and recognition of emotional issues (e.g., being angry, depressed, panicky, apprehensive, anxious, etc.) triggered by a recent diagnosis or underlying health issue e.g.—how health status is affecting the patient's emotional or affective state

Another purpose of the motivational interview is bringing the patient to a state where he/she is able to recognize the need for change and the benefits to be potentially realized if the change were to occur (Case Manager's Tip 7.15). This is referred to as "awareness of the need to change," which is the beginning of the change talk between the case manager and the patient/family. As soon as awareness occurs, the case manager then moves carefully to assess the patient's *readiness for change*; if readiness is evident, the change talk

---

Box 7.8 Motivational Interviewing and Lifestyle Behavior Change

Case managers rely on the motivational interviewing technique to:

- Move patients, families, and caregivers toward a course of successful, desirable, and sustainable change
- Inspire change and facilitate readiness for it
- Enhance the patient's self-efficacy
- Instill confidence in succeeding

Case managers evaluate the success of the motivational interviewing technique through the patient/family transition from a state of ambivalence, fear, or anxiety to a state of readiness, confidence, and willingness to change, demonstraed through desirable behaviors such as:

- Eating a healthy diet
- Adhering to health regimens including prescribed medications, plan of care, and follow-up care
- Self-management and self-care ability
- Avoidance of health risk behaviors such as smoking and substance use
- Regular exercise and activity which enhance physical function

---

Box 7.9 Examples of Open-Ended Questions

Case managers may ask open-ended questions such as the following questions during a motivational interviewing interaction, as they elicit to understand and know the patient's interest in or struggle with giving-up smoking.

- You indicated you have used tobacco on a regular basis for more than 20 years, but that you recently quit. What motivated you to quit this time? When would you like to try?
- How do you feel today compared to 3 months ago when you were still smoking? How have you changed?
- You recently expressed a desire to quit, what is stopping you from trying?
- Have you tried to quit smoking before? What is different for you this time? What makes you feel that you will be successful this time?
- Do you have any fears or concerns that might affect your ability to remain tobacco-free in the future?
- Are there others in your life who have expressed concerns about your smoking? Since you have recently quit smoking, how do you feel about people smoking around you?
- What resources and support do you think would be helpful for you when you crave a cigarette?
- How might you feel if you "slipped" and had a cigarette? What support would you need in order to recommit to quitting smoking?
- How would you like your life to look in 2–3 years after you've changed your behavior and successfully quit smoking?

CASE MANAGER'S TIP 7.15

The case manager uses motivational interviewing to engage the patient in change talk to ultimately commit to pursue necessary changes in lifestyle behavior including self-management and adherence to their health regimen and plan of care. Key aspects of the change talk and process include recognition of change, verbalizing commitment to change, planning and engaging in change behavior, and sustaining successes. These steps do not happen during one motivational interviewing interaction; rather they occur over time and with repeated motivational interviewing interactions that avoid coersion or judgment. Throughout the process, the case manager counsels and educates the patient/family in the areas of concern, ambivalence, health literacy, and health knowledge (e.g., condition, disease process, and plan of care).

shifts to *engagement in behavior change*. At this stage, the case manager begins to facilitate the patient's acceptance to change by focusing the interaction on exploring the patient's interests and determining his/her desire and will to change. Next comes the *change*

planning and deployment which consists of sharing knowledge about change (i.e., counseling and health instruction) with the patient and obtaining his/her commitment for what, how, and by when. At this stage, the case manager assists the patient/family in acquiring the necessary skills for effective change (Tahan & Sminkey, 2012).

The case manager monitors and evaluates the patient's progress on an ongoing basis. When success is achieved in some areas, the case manager encourages the patient to sustain the change behavior including the tactic(s) that worked in order to avoid relapse in the future. The case manager reinforces the patient's demonstrated desirable behaviors, recognizes the patient's success, and acknowledges the patient's actions

---

Box 7.10 Examples of Strategies to Effect Patient's Change Behavior

1. Express Empathy
   - Convey understanding of the patient's perspective and acceptance of the patient's situation.
   - Approach the patient in a nonjudgmental and non-critical way, especially if he/she is reluctant to change.

2. Recognize Discrepancy
   - Work with the patient to identify the differences between current and future states and specify goals to be achieved.
   - Enhance the patient's ability to recognize desirable behaviors and seek the patient's permission before attempting to move forward.

3. Roll with Resistance
   - Allow the patient to verbalize resistance to change and share the experienced concerns or challenges. Recognize what is important for the patient/support system.
   - Accept the patient's behavior even if it is not positive or indicative of progress toward desired goals.

4. Support Self-Efficacy
   - Affirm the patient's successes and achievements, however small.
   - Identify the patient's strengths to encourage the patient's belief in his/her ability to change.

Box 7.11 Sustaining Change Behavior

Examples of Tactics that Facilitate Change Behavior (Apply)

- Raise the patient's awareness of need/importance of change
- Facilitate the patient's acceptance of need to change by focusing on the patient's interests
- Determine the patient's desire and willingness to change
- Share with the patient knowledge about how to change and obtain commitment
- Enhance patient's acquisition of abilities and skills necessary for success
- Encourage patient's retention of the desired behavior(s)
- Recognize and promote patient's ability/actions to sustain new and favorable behavior(s)

Examples of Tactics that Hinder Change Behavior (Avoid)

- Act in a commanding or authoritative way with the patient
- Communicate or have unrealistic expectations
- Force the issue at a time when the patient is not yet ready
- Take control from the patient
- Commit to goals and expectations the patient did not agree to
- Act in a judgmental or critical manner toward the patient's behavior or inability to change
- Dismiss the patient's culture, values, and/or belief system
- Reprimand the patient in the case of failure or relapse
- Be unavailable to the patient when needed or do not keep promises
- Dismiss the possibility that patient may relapse
- Ignore the patient's concerns when raised
- Avoid active/reflective listening or selective reflection

that confidently will sustain the change. Throughout the change talk process the case manager uses targeted strategies to affect change (Box 7.10) and applies specific tactics that would allow the patient/family to sustain the change (Box 7.11) (Tahan and Sminkey, 2012).

7.6. KEY POINTS

1. Use of the nursing and case management processes—assessment, planning, implementation, coordination, and evaluation—is vital to a successful case manager.

2. Assessment connects the physical and the psychosocial aspects of a patient's care.

3. Planning determines the treatments and interventions necessary for meeting the needs of patients and families during and post-care encounter.

4. Implementation/coordination builds on the plan and determines the goals of patient care, moving the plan to completion.

5. Monitoring and evaluation allow the case manager to measure the patient's response to the case management plan and interventions.

6. Leadership and communication skills such as facilitation, negotiation, utilization management, education, team building, and conflict resolution must be added to the case manager's repertoire and put to use daily.

7. Emotional intelligence and motivational interviewing are two contemporary essential skills the case manager may use to enhance patient and family engagement in self-management and self-care, and to effect adherence to care regimen and change in lifestyle behavior.

8. Teamwork is essential to the success of any patient plan of care. Learn who the members of the team are and develop effective relationships with them.

9. Acquired skills are applicable to all forms of case management, including pre-acute, acute, post-acute (e.g., sub-acute and home care), and health insurance plans.

7.7. REFERENCES

American Medical Association. Health Literacy. Accessed May 25, 2015. Available at www.ama-assn.org/ama/pub/about-ama/ama-foundation/our-programs/public-health/health-literacy-program.page

Bass, B. (1985). *Leadership and performance beyond expectations.* The Free Press, New York.

Case Management Society of America. (2010). Standards of practice for case management, Little Rock, AR.

Cooper, R. & Sawaf, A. (1996). Executive EQ: emotional intelligence in leadership and organizations, Berkley Publishing Group, New York, NY.

Covey, S. (1989). *The 7 habits of highly effective people*, Simon & Schuster, New York, NY.

Dash, K., O'Donnell, L., Vince-Whitman, C., & Zarle N. (1996). *Discharge planning for the elderly: A guide for nurses*, Springer, New York, NY.

Goleman, D. (1995). *Emotional intelligence: Why it can matter more than IQ*, Bantam, New York, NY.

Goleman, D. (1998). *What makes a leader?* Harvard Business Rev 76(12):93–102.

Lancaster, J. & Lancaster, M. (1999). Communicating to manage change. In Lancaster J: *Nursing issues in leading and managing change*, Mosby, St Louis, MO.

Maslow, A.H. (1970). *Motivation and personality*, 2nd ed., Harper & Row, New York, NY.

Mintzberg, H. (1973). *The nature of managerial work*, Harper & Row, New York, NY.

Rawlins, C. (1992). *Harper Collins college outline: Introduction to management*, American Book-Works, New York, NY.

Ridge, R. & Bland Jones, C. (1999). Systems theory and analysis in health care and nursing. In Lancaster J: *Nursing issues in leading and managing change*, Mosby, St Louis, MO.

Rorden, J.W. & Taft, E. (1990). *Discharge planning guide for nurses,* WB Saunders, Philadelphia, PA.

Senge, P. (1990). *The fifth discipline: The art and practice of the learning organization, Doubleday/Currency*, New York, NY.

Tahan, H. & Sminkey, P. (2012). Motivational Interviewing: Building Rapport with Clients to Ensure Desirable Behavioral and Lifestyle Changes. *Professional Case Management, 17*(4): 164–172.

Weisinger. (1998). *Emotional intelligence at work.* Jossey-Bass, San Francisco, CA.

8 Case Manager's Documentation

Greater emphasis has been given to the role case managers play in the delivery of patient care as a result of the redesigning, re-engineering, or restructuring of healthcare delivery systems. These changes have increased the level of importance of documentation. Documentation has become even more important in institutions that developed and implemented new patient care delivery models such as case management, care management, integrated care, and collaborative care. The main reason behind the increased importance of documentation is related to the changes that have occurred in the role of the registered professional nurse and social worker, particularly the introduction of the role of case manager.

The creation of the case manager's role has pressured healthcare providers, nurses, and others to rely more on some of the important functions nurses and social workers play in the delivery of patient care, which have historically been ignored. These functions include but are not limited to the following:

- Coordination of discharge/transitional planning activities
- Facilitation and expedition of patient care activities
- Utilization management and resource allocation
- Psychosocial assessment of needs of patients and families
- Emphasis not only on actual patient/family problems but also on potential problems
- Evaluation of patient care outcomes and responses to treatment
- Counseling of patient/family regarding knowledge of health needs, preventive measures, and coping
- Service monitoring

These functions have been emphasized greatly in the job descriptions and the roles and responsibilities of case managers in a variety of institutions and patient care settings.

8.1. IMPORTANCE OF DOCUMENTATION

Case managers should view documentation as an important aspect of their role (Case Manager's Tip 8.1). Documentation reflects their professional responsibility and accountability toward patient care. In its Standards of Clinical Nursing Practice, the American Nurses Association (1991) identifies documentation as an integral part of its six standards of care (Table 8.1). Bower (1992), Cohen and Cesta (1997), and Tahan (1993) also identified documentation as an important role function of case managers. There are several factors that increase the importance of case manager documentation, including the following:

1. Professional responsibility and accountability to patient care
2. Communication of the case manager's judgments and evaluations
3. Evidence of case managers' plans of care, interventions, and outcomes
4. Legal protection; valuable evidence
5. Standards of regulatory agencies (e.g., the U.S. Department of Health and Human Services, the TJC, the CARF, National Committee of Quality Assurance [NCQA], and the Utilization Review Accreditation Commission [URAC])
6. Healthcare reimbursement (e.g., the DRG system,

managed care organizations, and third-party payers)

7. Supportive evidence of quality of patient care

8.2. ELECTRONIC MEDICAL RECORDS

Due to incentives from the CMS, the use of electronic medical records (EMR) in healthcare has soared in recent years (see Meaninful Use—Section 11.11). EMRs are a digital version of a patient's traditional paper chart. They typically include current as well as prior hospitalizations and encompass physician orders, provider documentation and tests, treatments and procedures. Electronic records streamline work and help to reduce medical errors in documentation by using drop-down menus and standardized formats. Hard-wired processes such as medication orders can reduce the likelihood of wrong doses or other similar errors.

The main concern with today's EMRs is that they sometimes do not interface across the healthcare continuum and are confined to the setting in which they were implemented such as the hospital or ambulatory setting.

Therefore many organizations have moved to electronic health records (EHR) which take a broader view of the patient and their clinical history. They are designed to reach out beyond the original healthcare organization and share information across the continuum including all clinicians involved in the patient's care. The information moves with the patient, allowing the various providers to work as a team (Hamilton, 2012).

For case managers, this is a tool that can be used to understand the patient's clinical status prior to admission. For community-based case managers, including those in home care or ambulatory care, they can review the patient's status and history very comprehensively. Errors and duplication of healthcare resources are reduced in this way.

Some benefits of EHRs include the following examples:

- The information gathered by the primary care provider tells the ED clinician about the patient's life-

threatening allergy so that care can be adjusted appropriately, even if the patient is unconscious.
- A patient can log on to his own record and see the trend of the lab results over the last year, which can help motivate him to take his medications and keep up with the lifestyle changes that have improved the numbers.
- The lab results run last week are already in the record to tell the specialist what she needs to know without running duplicate tests.
- The clinician's notes from the patient's hospital stay can help inform the discharge instructions and follow-up care and enable the patient to move from one care setting to another more smoothly (HealthIT.gov).

8.3. CASE MANAGEMENT SOFTWARE APPLICATIONS

Case management software applications can be embedded in the EMR or can work as stand-alone products. They are specialty products designed to support the work of case managers. These applications perform a variety of functions such as:

- Utilization review and management
- Discharge planning
- Denial management
- Patient flow
- Work lists
- Data repository and report writing

When selecting a system, be sure to understand

TABLE 8.1. Evidence of Documentation in the Standards of Care of the American Nurses Association.

Standard	Measurement Criteria
Assessment	Relevant data are documented in a retrievable form
Diagnosis	Diagnoses are documented in a manner that facilitates the determination of expected outcomes and plan of care
Outcomes Identification	Outcomes are documented as identification of measurable goals
Planning	The plan is documented
Implementation	Interventions are documented
Evaluation	Revisions in diagnoses, outcomes, and plan of care are documented

Modified from the American Nurses Association, 1991.

 CASE MANAGER'S TIP 8.1

The Importance of Documentation

The case manager's documentation is crucial because it is the only evidence of the case manager's role in the delivery of patient care.

which applications your case management department is interested in having and how the software will interface with your EMR. If your hospital system has hospital and community-based case management, be sure to pick a system that can be used across the continuum. Also be sure to look at least three applications before you purchase anything. Include your information technology department in the decision-making process. Some applications charge by the month and some by the user. Your budget should be developed accordingly.

Systems should also support electronic transfer of clinical reviews to third party payers and discharge planning information to home care, skilled nursing facilities, and other post-acute providers. You should also consider what hardware device the case management staff might use such as laptops, tablets, or pcs during the decision-making process.

8.4. ROLE OF CASE MANAGERS IN DOCUMENTATION

Documentation by case managers is extremely important because it is the only concrete evidence of their role in the delivery of patient care. Case managers documentation in the medical record should reflect the case management steps discussed in Chapter 4, the utilization management activities discussed in Chapter 5, and the transitional planning/discharge planning functions discussed in Chapter 6. It should include documentation related to the following areas:

1. Method of patient referral for case management services
2. Patient screening for appropriateness for case management services
3. Assessment of needs
4. Identification of the patient's actual and potential problems
5. Establishment and implementation of the plan of care, including the transitional plan
6. Facilitation and coordination of care activities, including the resource/utilization management activities
7. Patient and family teaching
8. Patient discharge and disposition
9. Evaluation of patient care outcomes
10. Variances in patient care

Appendix 8.1 at the end of this chapter presents an example of a case manager's documentation record.

8.4.1. Modes of Patient Referral for Case Management Services

Patient referrals for case management services may take place in three different ways. The first is a direct referral by a healthcare provider such as the primary nurse, private physician, consulting physician, house staff, nurse practitioner, physician assistant, social worker, or physical therapist. Personnel in the emergency department, doctor's office, or the admitting office could also refer a patient for case management services. The second is referral by the patient/family themselves, particularly if they were familiar with the case management process from previous encounters. The third method of patient referral is not a true referral. The case manager may elect to screen all new admissions and identify those who could benefit from case management. In home care settings and insurance companies, case managers may follow all patients regardless of the seriousness of the episode of illness.

In most institutions the case management referral process is pre-identified by healthcare administrators and nursing executives in a policy, procedure, or protocol and made clear to all healthcare providers through education and training. Referrals are usually made based on prospectively established criteria similar to those discussed in Chapter 4 (see Box 4.1).

The case manager's documentation (Case Manager's Tip 8.2) should include the process used for referal for case management services, who made the referral, the reason(s) for the referral, and the date and time of the referral. If no referral is made and the patient has been identified by the case manager when screening the new admissions, then the case manager's documentation should indicate so.

In some care settings, referrals for case management services by other providers may not exist. Examples are managed care organizations, in which case managers function as gatekeepers and demand managers, and

CASE MANAGER'S TIP 8.2

Elements to Include in Documentation

The case manager's documentation should include the following items:

1. How the patient was referred for case management services
2. Who made the referral
3. Reasons for the referral
4. Date and time of the referral

telephonic case management, in which case managers function as triage nurses. In both settings the patient or family member/caregiver triggers the referral and the case manager completes it by connecting the patient with the appropriate healthcare provider or setting. The interaction between a patient/caller and the case manager in telephone triage/case management is limited in time, assessment process, and interventions given. Documentation in these situations is important for reducing legal risk. It should include a summary of the telephone conversation, the assessment made, the actions taken by the case manager, and the outcomes of the telephone call (Case Manager's Tip 8.3).

8.4.2. Patient Screening for Appropriateness for Case Management Services

However the referral is made, the case manager has to conduct a patient/family screening to determine appropriateness for case management services. A decision regarding the patient's need for case management is made based on the "criteria for patient selection into the case management process" discussed in Chapter 4 (see Box 4.1). Some of these criteria are patient's acu-

CASE MANAGER'S TIP 8.3

Elements of Documentation in Telephonic Triage/Case Management

The telephonic triage/case management note must include the following:

1. Date and time of the call
2. Names of the patient and the caller if other than the patient
3. Relationship of the caller to the patient
4. Age and gender of the patient
5. Patient's/caller's telephone number for the purpose of returning the call
6. Name of primary care provider (PCP)
7. Whether the patient/caller attempted calling the PCP
8. Summary of problem or chief complaint
9. Type of protocol (automated algorithm) used
10. Classification of the problem (emergent, urgent, non-urgent)
11. Actions taken such as calling 911, recommending an emergency department visit, calling crisis team, use of Tylenol, ice packs, and so on
12. Whether the patient/caller agrees with the actions taken
13. Whether there is a need for a follow-up call

ity, age, complexity of diagnosis and medical condition, teaching needs, discharge/transitional planning, noncompliance with treatment regimen, insurance coverage, social complexity, and financial status.

When patient screening is completed and case management services are deemed appropriate, the case manager then writes an intake note in the patient's record explaining that the patient is accepted into the case management process (Case Manager's Tip 8.4).

8.4.3. Assessment of Needs

Screening of the patient/family for case management services and the initial assessment of needs are usually completed concurrently by the case manager because they are interrelated. The assessment of patient/family needs is made during the case manager's first encounter with the patient/family. Careful assessment and documentation of the patient's/family's needs can enhance the effectiveness of case management. Documentation of the initial assessment of needs by the case manager is a more detailed extension of the intake note (Case Manager's Tip 8.5). Both notes are usually completed consecutively, and in most cases one note is written combining both intake and assessment.

The case manager's documentation should not include a thorough health history or a physical examination. A statement indicating that the medical record,

CASE MANAGER'S TIP 8.4

Elements of the Intake Note

The intake note should focus on the following issues:

1. Reason for patient's hospitalization, need for medical attention, need for post-discharge services such as home care or transportation for follow-up appointment
2. Indications for case management services (i.e., which criteria for selection of patients for case management are met) (e.g., age, acuity, complexity of diagnosis, noncompliance)
3. Method of referral (e.g., healthcare provider, patient/family, case manager screening)
4. The date and time patient's screening took place and the time the intake note was written
5. Method of screening (e.g., patient/family interview, discussion with other healthcare providers, review of medical record)
6. Certification/approval of current patient's hospitalization or medical services by the managed care organization

CASE MANAGER'S TIP 8.5

Elements of the Initial Assessment Note

In addition to the elements of documentation mentioned in the patient's screening section, the initial assessment note should include the following:

1. Chief complaint
2. Risk for injury
3. Discharge planning needs
4. Social support system
5. Health education needs
6. Justification for the need of medical services/ attention, treatment

including the patient's history and physical assessment (assessments that are completed and documented by other healthcare professionals, including the primary nurse and the physician), documentation that the case has been reviewed by the case manager is of equal value and importance. However, the initial assessment note should reflect any significant abnormalities and problems identified by the case manager that would dictate the plan of care, the interventions/treatments, and management of the patient's needs.

8.4.4. Identification of the Patient's Actual and Potential Problems

Identification of the patient's actual and potential problems is the starting point for establishing the patient's plan of care. Accurate and comprehensive identification of these problems has a significant affect on patient care outcomes. Thoroughly examining the patient's medical record, in addition to interviewing the patient and family or caregiver, makes it easier for the case manager to prioritize the patient's needs that should be stated in the patient's record as actual or potential problems. Regardless of the patient's condition, needs, and chief complaint, the case manager's documentation of the patient's actual and potential problems almost always includes problems related to the following:

1. Patient/family teaching
2. Discharge planning and disposition
3. Need for post-discharge services
4. Financial status
5. Social support systems
6. Clinical condition (i.e., signs and symptoms)

The problems identified by case managers with

regard to the complexity of patient/family teaching needs, discharge planning, and the absence of a social support system should be clearly and thoroughly documented in the patient's medical record.

For example, an elderly insulin-dependent diabetic patient who is legally blind and unable to self-administer insulin and who is admitted for uncontrolled diabetes cannot be discharged from the hospital before ensuring that he or she has a safe mechanism in place for administration of insulin injections. Another example is a businessman who is newly diagnosed with myocardial infarction and who is going to be started on cardiac medications for the first time. This patient may not be discharged unless patient teaching is completed or home care is arranged for post-discharge follow-up and the patient discharge is deemed safe. Case managers are well trained in how to be proactive planners, particularly in how to meet the discharge planning and teaching needs of their patients before discharge.

The documentation of the case manager's assessment of the needs of the two patients above on admission should include the potential problems regarding discharge planning and complexity of patient teaching and be documented on admission. The plans of care developed should be reflected in the documentation, particularly how the identified needs will be met before the patients' readiness for discharge. Problems similar to the ones discussed in these examples may delay the patient's discharge. Careful documentation of these problems by case managers helps to justify the delay for administrators, insurance companies, and so on. This kind of documentation also justifies the patient's need for services after discharge (i.e., home care). Managed care organizations usually look for such documentation in the medical record, which justifies the need for intensive services, when conducting medical record reviews or making decisions about whether to authorize services.

8.4.5. Establishing and Implementing the Plan of Care

Planning patient care is a key element in the role of case managers. Accurate and careful planning based on the data collected during the initial screening and assessment of patients, as well as the appropriateness of the identified actual and potential problems, enables case managers to provide individualized, efficient, and high-quality care. The plan of care is extremely important because it serves as a communication tool for everyone involved in patient care. Articulating the plan of care in writing and making it clear to all those involved in the provision of care promotes continuity and consistency of care and enhances its efficiency and effectiveness.

Case managers are responsible for making sure that the written plan of care includes the patient's actual and potential problems and/or nursing diagnoses, the expected/desired outcomes of care, and the interventions/treatments needed to meet the expected outcomes (Table 8.2). It is important for case managers to document the patient/family agreement to the plan of care as discussed on admission and at the time the initial assessment of patient's needs is completed. Documenting that the goals of treatment are collaboratively set with the patient/family, the case manager, the attending physician, and others involved in the care is essential. This improves compliance with TJC standard of patient's rights and continuum of care standards.

The case manager should document the goals of care to be met both before and at the time of discharge. These goals are the expected outcomes of care agreed on with the patient and family and the interdisciplinary team. The expected outcomes of care should be documented following a specific format (Box 8.1) and should focus on specific elements (Case Manager's Tip 8.6).

Case managers individualize the treatment plan and nursing interventions based on the signs and symptoms evidenced in the patient's condition. In addition, they include interventions that prevent any undesired symptoms or untoward outcomes. Case managers formulate interventions that are specific, realistic, individualized, patient/family oriented, and based on the signs and symptoms of the disease and the goals of treatment.

Documentation in the plan of care should reflect the case manager's ongoing evaluation of the patient responses to treatment and the required revisions in the plan of care as necessitated by the patient's responses.

Case managers are also required to reassess the patient and family on a continuing basis, evaluate the

 CASE MANAGER'S TIP 8.6

Characteristics of Outcomes

Outcomes should be as follows:

1. Patient- and family-oriented
2. Realistic and practical
3. Clear and concise
4. Measurable and observable
5. Concrete and doable
6. Time- and interval-specific

patient's condition for any improvements or changes, follow up on the appropriateness of the treatment and nursing interventions, identify any new problems that may have arisen and ensure their inclusion in the plan of care. When the patient reassessment is completed, the case manager is expected to write a reassessment note in the patient's record (Box 8.2). It is recommended that case managers who work in acute or sub-acute care settings write a minimum of three reassessment notes for every patient each week of hospitalization. In long-term care settings, one reassessment note every week is considered appropriate. However, in ambulatory care settings such as clinics and home care a note is recommended for every encounter with the patient. In telephonic case management, a reassessment note is completed every time the case manager makes a return or follow-up call to the patient or caller. In addition, a reassessment note is suggested as necessitated by the patient's condition.

8.4.6. Facilitation and Coordination of Care Activities

Because case managers are held responsible for co-

TABLE 8.2. Example of a Patient Problem as Written by a Case Manager in the Plan of Care of a Patient with Fluid Retention Related to Congestive Heart Failure.

Patient Problem/ Nursing Diagnosis	Expected Outcomes of Care (Patient & Family Goals)	Nursing Interventions
Fluid balance; excess	• Stabilized fluid balance • Downward trend in patient's weight; or sudden increase • Balanced intake and output • Adherence to fluid restriction • Electrolytes within normal ranges; no changes in potassium level • Increased urine output • Reduction in severity of peripheral edema	• Weigh patient daily before breakfast • Monitor accurate intake and output • Restrict fluids intake to 1,000 mL per day • Monitor serum electrolytes, notify physician of any abnormal findings • Give diuretics as prescribed and monitor patient's response (urine output) • Assess peripheral edema daily

---

Box 8.1   Examples of Patient Care Outcomes for a Diabetic Patient with a Nursing Diagnosis of Knowledge Deficit

The patient/family will be able to do the following:

1. Describe the signs and symptoms of hypoglycemia
2. Describe the signs and symptoms of hyperglycemia
3. Demonstrate correct insulin injection technique
4. State the appropriate sites for insulin injections
5. Demonstrate appropriate syringe filling technique
6. Describe the preventive measures of diabetes foot care

Box 8.2   Issues to be Addressed by Case Managers in the Reassessment Note

1. Assessment of new needs
2. Follow-up on treatments/interventions
3. Patient and family teaching efforts and progress
4. Facilitation and coordination of tests and procedures
5. Patient/family and interdisciplinary team conferences
6. Referrals to and consults with ancillary or specialized services
7. Discharge planning issues and status of discharge plans
8. Evaluation of patient responses/outcomes
9. Necessary revisions in the plan of care
10. Concurrent reviews with managed care organizations and authorizations for services

---

ordinating and facilitating the delivery of care on a day-to-day basis, their documentation in the patient's record should reflect these functions. Such progress notes include facilitation and coordination of care activities such as the following:

1. Scheduling and expediting tests and procedures and prevention of any delays
2. Patient care—related conferences with the family and the interdisciplinary team
3. Coordination of complex discharge/transitional plans
4. Preparation of patients and families for operative procedures
5. Transition of patients from acute to sub-acute or long-term care settings
6. Consultation with other healthcare providers
7. Ongoing communication with managed care organizations
8. Utilization of resources and related authorizations by managed care organizations
9. Referrals made to other providers or care settings

8.4.7. Patient and Family Teaching

Case managers are responsible for supervising the patient and family teaching activities. This responsibility should be evidenced in their documentation. Case managers make sure that patient/family teaching is included in the plan of care and appropriately documented in the patient's record. They document all of the patient/family teaching activities they conduct (Case Manager's Tip 8.7).

8.4.8. Patient's Discharge and Disposition

Patient's discharge and disposition are important re-

sponsibilities of case managers (Case Manager's Tip 8.8). Assessment of the patient's discharge needs starts at the time of admission and continues throughout the hospitalization until the patient is ready for discharge

 CASE MANAGER'S TIP 8.7

Documentation of Patient and Family Teaching

The case manager's documentation of patient and family teaching, based on the patient's condition and needs, should include the following:

1. Assessment of healthcare teaching needs
2. Review of the disease process, signs and symptoms, risk factors, possible complications, and preventive measures
3. Review of the medical/surgical regimen, compliance with treatment, and importance of continuous medical follow-up
4. Instructions regarding medications intake, dosage, actions, side effects, route, and special observations
5. Pre-operative and post-operative teaching
6. Wound care
7. Pain management
8. Instructions regarding the required use of durable medical equipment (e.g., glucometer)
9. Ongoing review of the plan of care and the discharge plan
10. Availability of and the need for support from community resources after discharge
11. The level of understanding of information taught and whether there is a need for further reinforcement of the information discussed

or transition to another level of care or another facility. Areas of documentation related to the assessment of patient's discharge needs are presented in Box 8.3.

Documentation of discharge planning to support a safe discharge is important because it may be scrutinized by QIOs if the patient is readmitted with the same problem shortly after discharge. Such situations may increase the financial risk of the institution. If the patient is to receive home care services after discharge, the discharge note should then include the reasons for such services and what is expected to take place at home regarding the care of the patient. Because case managers discuss home care needs with home care planners or intake coordinators, it is suggested that such discussions and referrals be included in the discharge documentation.

8.4.9. Evaluation of Patient Care Outcomes

Evaluation of the patient's response to treatment is essential for better decision-making regarding the patient's progress and discharge. Progress notes of case managers should reflect documentation of the patient's status in relation to the desired outcomes established at the time of admission and proactively identified in the plan of care. The frequency with which case managers document patients' progress and responses to treatments depends on the institutional policies and procedures regarding documentation, the charting system, the type of treatments and nursing interventions needed by the patient, the standards of care, and reimbursement requirements.

Case managers are also required to track variances of care and delays in achieving patient care outcomes (see Chapter 14 for a detailed discussion on variance). They are cautioned not to document any subjective

 CASE MANAGER'S TIP 8.8

Documentation of Discharge/Transitional Planning

The case manager documents discharge/transitional planning in the following manner:

1. Actual patient's disposition at the time of discharge in the form of discharge note (Box 8.3)
2. Ongoing assessment of discharge needs because they may change based on changes in the patient's condition
3. Assessment of post-discharge needs in the initial assessment of the patient (i.e., at the time of screening the patient for case management services) (Box 8.4)

Box 8.3   Areas of Documentation Related to Patient's Discharge

1. Disposition (e.g., home, nursing home, group home, rehabilitation facility, hospice)
2. Mode of discharge; transportation provided, if any
3. Person who accompanied the patient on discharge
4. Communication with appropriate personnel regarding confirmation of discharge (e.g., home care agency, managed care organization, patient's family)
5. Confirmation of availability of any equipment needed (e.g., wheelchair, crutches, glucometer, walker)
6. Completion of necessary paperwork related to discharge (e.g., medical request for home care, patient review instrument [for patient's placement in a nursing home])
7. Confirmation of services needed by the patient after discharge (e.g., hemodialysis center, special doctor's clinic)
8. Condition of patient at the time of discharge
9. Discharge instructions

---

judgments or system and practitioner variances because they increase the institutional liabilities.

8.4.10.   Documenting Variances

When documenting the occurrence of a variance, the case manager should describe the event as specifically as possible. The variance should first be categorized at its highest level (e.g., internal system, external system, patient, family, or practitioner) (Box 8.5). Once the highest category has been identified, the case manager

---

Box 8.4   Areas of Documentation Related to the Assessment of Discharge Planning Needs of Patients

1. Services used before hospital admission
2. Projected needs of services after discharge (e.g., home care, physical therapy)
3. Availability of adequate social support systems
4. Need for referrals to specialized personnel/services (e.g., social work, home care intake coordinator)
5. Patient's condition (e.g., mental stability, functional abilities)
6. Financial status and insurance coverage
7. Necessary paperwork when requesting community services after discharge (e.g., medical request for home care services) or nursing home placement (e.g., patient review instrument)

Box 8.5   Sample List of Variances

Internal System Variances

Transfer for procedure that was cancelled
Reasons:
- Cardiac catheterization
- Cardiac surgery
- Clinical complications

Emergency department delay in admission/awaiting bed
Reason:
- Full census

Extended emergency department stay
Reason:
- Observation

Delay in laboratory results
Reasons:
- Equipment failure/malfunction
- Test not available (weekend/holiday)
- Scheduling delay
- Turnaround time (TAT) for reporting > 24 hours

Rehabilitation delay
Reasons:
- Weekend/holiday
- Delay in initiating therapy
- Operating room overbooking

Cancellation of an operative procedure, test, or treatment
Reasons:
- Patient condition
- Physician not available
- Over-booking
- Unavailable messenger/transport services

Pending infectious disease approval for medication
Nonformulary medications
Unavailable beds on telemetry unit
Delay in transfer to inpatient psychiatric facility
Delay in catheter laboratory
Reasons:
- Equipment failure/malfunction
- Test not available (weekend/holiday)
- Scheduling delay
- TAT for reporting > 24 hours

Delay in computed tomography (CT) scan
Reasons:
- Equipment failure/malfunction
- Test not available (weekend/holiday)
- Scheduling delay
- TAT for reporting > 24 hours

Delay in magnetic resonance imaging
Reasons:
- Equipment failure/malfunction
- Test not available (weekend/holiday)
- Scheduling delay
- TAT for reporting > 24 hours

Box 8.5 (continued)   Sample List of Variances

Internal System Variances (continued)

Delay in electroencephalogram (EEG)
Reasons:
- Equipment failure/malfunction
- Test not available (weekend/holiday)
- Scheduling delay
- TAT for reporting > 24 hours

Delay in electrocardiogram (ECG)
Reasons:
- Equipment failure/malfunction
- Test not available (weekend/holiday)
- Scheduling delay
- TAT for reporting > 24 hours

Delay in Haltor monitor
Reasons:
- Equipment failure/malfunction
- Test not available (weekend/holiday)
- Scheduling delay
- TAT for reporting > 24 hours

Delay in adenosine/dobutamine stress test
Reasons:
- Equipment failure/malfunction
- Test not available (weekend/holiday)
- Scheduling delay
- TAT for reporting > 24 hours

Delay in x-ray
Reasons:
- Equipment failure/malfunction
- Test not available (weekend/holiday)
- Scheduling delay
- TAT for reporting > 24 hours

Delay in exercise stress test
Reasons:
- Equipment failure/malfunction
- Test not available (weekend/holiday)
- Scheduling delay
- TAT for reporting > 24 hours

Delay in thallium stress test
Reasons:
- Equipment failure/malfunction
- Test not available (weekend/holiday)
- Scheduling delay
- TAT for reporting > 24 hours

Delay in Doppler/vascular laboratory
Reasons:
- Equipment failure/malfunction
- Test not available (weekend/holiday)
- Scheduling delay
- TAT for reporting > 24 hours

Box 8.5 (continued)   Sample List of Variances

Internal System Variances (continued)

Late discharge
   Reasons:
- Physician delay
- Family delay
- Transportation delay
- Patient delay
- Awaiting procedure
- Awaiting laboratory results
- Prescription not written
- Awaiting result of procedure
- Awaiting physical therapy clearance

External System Variances

No nursing home bed available
   Reasons:
- Weekend
- Patient choice not available
- No beds

Delay in transfer to another institution
   Reasons:
- Awaiting physician orders
- Awaiting family
- Awaiting transportation
- Awaiting approval from receiving facility

Delay in other transportation
No home care available over the weekend
No rehabilitation bed available
Child protective services late to arrive
Medical equipment delivered late
No sub-acute bed available

Patient Variances

Unplanned admission from ambulatory surgery
   Reasons:
- Patient complication
- Delay in recovery
- More extensive surgery than originally planned
- Unplanned conversion to an open procedure

Unplanned admission from outpatient unit
   Reason:
- Patient complication

Readmission within 30 days for surgical wound infection
Readmission within 30 days for surgical complications
Readmission within 30 days for symptoms related to a prior hospital stay
Readmission within 30 days for deep line infection(s)
Readmission within 30 days for exacerbation of chronic illness
Readmission within 30 days planned for staged procedure/chemotherapy
Readmission within 30 days for false labor
Readmission within 30 days for condition unrelated to previous admission
Unplanned return to special care unit
   Reason:
- Clinical complication

Medical complication: Aspiration pneumonia

Box 8.5 (continued)   Sample List of Variances

Patient Variances (continued)

Medical complication: Unexpected cardiac/respiratory distress with intubation
Medical complication: Iatrogenic pneumothorax
Medical complication: Wound dehiscence
Medical complication: Urinary tract infection (UTI) with intravenous antibiotics
Medical complication: Neurologic system
Medical complication: Gastrointestinal system
Medical complication: Cardiovascular system
  Reasons:
  ▪ New deep venous thrombosis (DVT)
  ▪ Other
Medical complication: Genitourinary/renal system
  Reason:
  ▪ Acute renal failure leading to dialysis
Medical complication: Respiratory system
  Reason:
  ▪ New acute pulmonary embolism (PE)
Medical complication: Endocrine system
Medical complication: Musculoskeletal system
Medical complication: Multiple systems
Medical complication: Difficulty/inability to wean
Death: Within 48 hours of surgery
Death: Expected death
Death: Nosocomial infection caused or contributed to death
Death: Autopsy performed
Death: Medical examiner case
Death: Certificate of request for anatomical gift present
Death: Unexpected death
Death: Autopsy requested
Post-operative/procedure complication: Difficulty/inability to wean
Post-operative/procedure complication: Wound dehiscence
Post-operative/procedure complication: Wound infection
Post-operative/procedure complication: Neurological system, including any new peripheral neurological deficit within 48 hours of surgery; any new central nervous system deficit with motor weakness within 48 hours of surgery
Post-operative/procedure complication: Gastrointestinal system
Post-operative/procedure complication: Cardiovascular system, including cardiac arrest, new acute myocardial infarction (AMI) within 48 hours of surgery
Post-operative/procedure complication: Genitourinary/renal system
Post-operative/procedure complication: Respiratory system, including new acute PE
Post-operative/procedure complication: Musculoskeletal system
Post-operative/procedure complication: Unexpected excessive bleeding
Post-operative/procedure complication: Hematoma
Post-operative/procedure complication: Unplanned removal/injury of organ
Post-operative/procedure complication: Multiple systems
Post-operative/procedure complication requiring return to operating room, special procedure, or delivery room: Wound dehiscence
Post-operative/procedure complication requiring return to operating room, special procedure, or delivery room: Wound infection
Post-operative/procedure complication requiring return to operating room, special procedure, or delivery room: Neurologic system
Post-operative/procedure complication requiring return to operating room, special procedure, or delivery room: Gastrointestinal system
Post-operative/procedure complication requiring return to operating room, special procedure, or delivery room: Cardiovascular system

Box 8.5 (continued)   Sample List of Variances

Patient Variances (continued)

Post-operative/procedure complication requiring return to operating room, special procedure, or delivery room: Genitourinary system

Post-operative/procedure complication requiring return to operating room, special procedure, or delivery room: Respiratory system

Post-operative/procedure complication requiring return to operating room, special procedure, or delivery room: Musculoskeletal system

Post-operative/procedure complication requiring return to operating room, special procedure, or delivery room: Unexpected excessive bleeding

Post-operative/procedure complication requiring return to operating room, special procedure, or delivery room: Hematoma

Post-operative/procedure complication requiring return to operating room, special procedure, or delivery room: Unplanned removal/injury of organ

Post-operative/procedure complication requiring return to operating room, special procedure, or delivery room: Multiple systems

Post-operative/procedure complication requiring return to operating room, special procedure, or delivery room: Difficulty/inability to wean

Pre-admission issue: Noncompliance with preadmission procedures

Emergency department issue: Frequent utilization of emergency department services

Treatment of patient: Delay in obtaining therapeutic anticoagulation levels

Patient refusal tests/treatments/procedures

Patient unable to decide on treatment

Patient refusal discharge

Patient noncompliant with medical/surgical regimen, medications, treatment

Unable to wean from respirator (nonsurgical)

Secondary diagnosis with admission

Language barrier

Poor historian

Withholding pertinent information

Signed out against medical advice (AMA)

Refusal discharge due to religious belief, holiday, and/or personal inconvenience

Noncompliant with dietary restrictions

Unable to self-administer medications

Unable to learn about disease

Unable to care for self after discharge

No clothes

No keys for home/apartment

Pressure ulcer present on admission

Hospital-acquired pressure ulcer

Cannot afford to buy medical equipment/medication

Procedure cancelled due to patient illness

Physically unable to progress with treatment plan

Psychologically unable to progress with treatment plan

Financial issues
- Awaiting Medicaid
- No insurance
- No healthcare benefits

Elopement

Family-Related Variances

Unable to pick up patient at discharge

Unable to provide support for care after discharge

Language barrier

Late to pick up patient at discharge

Inadequate level of knowledge regarding patient care

Difficulty with compliance

Unable to learn

Box 8.5 (continued)   Sample List of Variances

Family-Related Variances (continued)

Want another opinion
Unable to bring patient's clothes until after business hours
Cannot be reached
Cannot afford to buy necessary medical equipment, medication
Delay in bringing needed papers for Medicaid application
Guardianship/conservatorship issues

Practitioner Variances

Preadmission issue: No medical necessity
Preadmission issue: No utilization review approval for preoperative day
Preadmission issue: Documentation and plan of care inconsistent with preadmission statement
Preadmission issue: Preoperative day
Preadmission issue: Inappropriate transfer from another institution
Preadmission issue: Transfer requiring day preoperative with questionable acuity
Preadmission issue: Admission requiring day preoperative with questionable acuity
Emergency department issue: Emergency department admission after preadmission denial
Emergency department issue: Emergency department admission for elective procedure
Emergency department issue: Emergency department admission from physician office for test/procedure
Emergency department issue: Social admission
Emergency department issue: Incomplete documentation of emergency department findings/treatments
Emergency department issue: Emergency department clerical error
Emergency department issue: Delay in initiating treatment plan
Delay in communicating plan of care
Physician not communicating to patient
Physician not communicating with family
Wrong test, treatment, procedure ordered
Incomplete admission assessment, hospitalization (hx)
Omission of an order
Delayed request for a consult
No consent for treatment
Delay in processing forms
Delay in initiating treatment/plan of care
Lack of coordination among interdisciplinary team about discharge plan
Patient teaching not done/completed
Inappropriate/early discharge
Physician did not prepare/inform patient of discharge
Delay in medication administration
Delay or omission in transcribing physician orders
Abnormal test results or physical findings not addressed by physician
Plan of care not acute
Incomplete plan of care
TAT to answer consult > 24 hours
Weekend or coverage issues delaying changes in treatment
Delay in implementing guideline/multidisciplinary action plan
Repeated unnecessary tests on transfer
Delay in responding to attending physician recommendations
Delay in initiating consult
  Reasons:
  - Rehabilitation
  - Psychiatry
  - Medicine
  - Surgery
  - Other

Box 8.5 (continued)   Sample List of Variances

Family-Related Variances (continued)

Delay in switching from intravenous to oral medication

Delay in ordering medication

Delay in ordering test/treatment/procedure

Order exceeds guideline recommendation: Excessive resource utilization

Plan of care inconsistent with guideline

Delay in discontinuing medication

Delay in discontinuing test/treatment/procedure

Delay in implementing guideline/multidisciplinary action plan

Appropriate guideline/multidisciplinary action plan not applied

---

should then drill down to the next level. For example, the case manager may have identified that there is a delay in a patient receiving a computed tomography (CT) scan. This would be considered a "system variance," meaning that an issue related to the organization's own internal system processes caused the delay. Once the delay has been identified as "internal system," the case manager should then categorize it as "CT scan delay." Finally, the case manager will want to determine the cause or reason for the delay. This would be the final and most detailed level.

When possible, a prospective list, such as the one in Box 8.5, should be used by all case management staff so that staff members who are identifying variances are doing so in a consistent manner. The list should reflect all potential variances and should be as specific as possible. It can be coded and automated in a database. In this way, the case manager need only identify the variance by its code number (Case Manager's Tip 8.9).

By keeping the variances as specific as possible and by creating the three-tiered system of identification, reports can be generated that will reflect any level of detail required. For example, a particular clinical department may want to know first how many total "patient-related" variances it may have had during a specific period. Then that department may want to know how many of each type. Finally, it may decide to focus on specific patient-related variances and will want to know the reasons for these variances. Automating the standard list and tracking of variances

makes these reports less time consuming and easier to generate.

During documentation of the variances, the case manager should remember that the "system" and "practitioner" variances SHOULD NEVER be documented in the medical record. These categories of variances are legally protected by being part of the "quality management" initiatives of the organization and considered confidential and privileged information. Conversely, patient and family variances should be documented in the medical record as they relate to clinical and/or psychosocial issues that will need to be clearly communicated. The case manager should always follow the policies and procedures of the organization as they relate to documenting variances in the medical record. If the variances are warehoused in a database, this too will be protected under the quality umbrella.

A variance should be documented as soon as it is identified. If the variances are being entered into a database, the database will be current and the information in it will reflect "real time" issues. If the variances require immediate intervention, the case manager should document the actions taken to correct the situation in the appropriate location as per their policies and procedures. For example, if the patient had a clinical complication such as an infection, the case manager should document this variance in the database and in the medical record. The medical record documentation should reflect the change in the plan of care (medical and transitional plan) that was made in response to the infection, as well as the expected increase in length of stay, if appropriate.

8.5. CHARTING BY EXCEPTION

Charting by exception is a system for documenting against a pre-determined, standardized set of expected outcomes. The system uses a number of tools, including standardized clinical/case management plans of care

 CASE MANAGER'S TIP 8.9

Specific Documentation of Variances

Variances should always be documented as specifically as possible so that they can be used for quality improvement projects and process redesign.

Example 1: Charting by Exception Sample When Outcome Has Been Met.
Clinical practice guideline for thoracic laminectomy.

Operative Day Interventions	Expected Outcomes	Assessment/Evaluation
Assess abdomen every 8 hours	Abdomen soft	9/1/2013
Check for bowel sounds, distension	Bowel sounds positive. No distension	10 A.M., AB

such as clinical paths or clinical practice guidelines. Fundamental to the process of charting by exception is the need to have pre-determined outcomes against which the practitioner documents. The prospectively identified outcomes are evaluated at pre-determined time intervals. The time intervals are specified in the case management plans or pathways. The practitioner assesses the patient and evaluates whether the outcome has been achieved. If the outcome has been achieved, then the practitioner needs only to time and initial the outcome. This indicates that the outcome has been met.

For a charting by exception system to be effective, the following assumptions must be made:

- The clinical practice guideline in use is appropriate to the patient.
- Outcomes are evaluated against the patient's progress at clinically appropriate intervals.
- The interdisciplinary team has agreed to the prospectively identified outcomes and their associated timeframes.
- The outcome signed against indicates that the outcome has been positively met.
- If an outcome is not met, a note in the medical record is required indicating the action plan/intervention.

When charting by exception, the expected outcome to be achieved is evaluated based on an assessment or reassessment of the patient. The assessment may include either a review of the patient's laboratory values, a physical assessment, an evaluation of educational outcomes, or direct reporting from the patient, all depending on the specific outcomes in review. If the patient has met the outcome as stated in the clinical prac-

tice guideline, the case manager initials the outcome indicating that it has been positively met and no further action is needed.

8.5.1. When Outcomes Are Not Met

Charting by exception systems require additional documentation only when an outcome has not been met. Therefore if an outcome is not met as per the patient assessment and evaluation, additional documentation is required. The unmet outcome is considered a variance. The variance is the actual outcome that was achieved by the patient. The actual outcome (variance) is then documented in the designated "variance" column in the case management plan or clinical pathway. Additional documentation of the variance in the medical record must include a description of the variance and the action plan executed to correct the situation. Sometimes variances require a complete revision of the plan of care depending on the changes in the patient's medical condition, such as intubation and use of mechanical ventilation because of respiratory arrest.

Every time case managers identify a variance, they must return to their variance documentation system (e.g., automated variance list) to log in the variance and the reason it occurred, *Example 1*. This documentation is important because such data are essential for enhancing the case management model and the system or processes of patient care delivery.

AB has placed her initials in the "Assessment/Evaluation" section of the guideline. Her initials indicate that the patient has met the outcome of "abdomen soft, no distension, bowel sounds positive." In this example, no further documentation is necessary.

Example 2: Charting by Exception Sample When Outcome Has Not Been Met.
Clinical practice guideline for thoracic laminectomy

Operative Day Interventions	Expected Outcomes	Assessment/Evaluation
Assess abdomen every 8 hours	Abdomen soft	9/1/2013 10 A.M., abdomen distended;
Check for bowel sounds, distension	Bowel sounds positive	No distension; Bowel sounds positive;
	No distension	patient experiencing some discomfort.
		MD notified, AB.

In Example 2, the expected outcome of "no distension" was not met on the operative day. Because the outcome was not met, the case manager needed to document what the actual outcome was and what his or her intervention was regarding it. If the unmet outcome resulted in an extension in the length of stay and/or a quality issue, the unmet outcome must also be documented as a variance.

8.6. TIMING AND FREQUENCY OF DOCUMENTATION

Case managers must always be visible in the medical record. Each case management department must determine its own frequency of documentation and have a policy and procedure outlining the expectations and frequency of the department's documentation. Typically, documentation is completed every 3 days or whenever there is an intervention or outcome that needs to be recorded in the medical record.

In addition, case managers and social workers must document the process of discharge planning, not just the ultimate destination. Included in this documentation should be:

- The discussion with the patient and family
- Their agreement to the discharge plan
- The physician's agreement to the discharge plan
- That the "choice list" has been given (see Chapter 6)
- That the patient and family made selections that meet their clinical needs, location of choice, and insurance coverage
- That the discharge destination is discussed multiple times throughout the course of the hospital stay
- That the patient and family understand the plan and that they have been educated about what it means to them and their clinical condition
- The duration of the home care or skilled nursing care, if appropriate

8.6.1. Admission Assessment by Registered Nurse Case Manager

Best practice for the RN case manager calls for the patient to be assessed on the day of admission. By assessing early, the initial discharge plan can be initiated. In addition, any referrals, such as to social work or home care, can be made as early in the hospitalization as possible. The process is as follows:

- *Step 1*: Review the current medical record, including all relevant diagnostic test results, such as lab values and radiology reports.
- *Step 2*: If the patient was admitted through the emergency department, review all available EMS notes.
- *Step 3*: Obtain and review prior medical records if available.
- *Step 4*: Discuss the patient with the admitting physician.
- *Step 5*: Interview the patient and/or family.

The RN case manager should use a standardized template, or mimimum data set, to guide their questions and to ensure that all relevant questions are addressed. The categories shared in Box 8.6 should be included and can be used to format the case management admission assessment form or electronic documentation. The documentation categories can be used as guidelines for case manager documentation and interactions with other members of the health care team in situations such as the following:

- Patient's admission
- Patient care rounds
- Individual case conference with members of the healthcare team
- Inquiry from patient/family/physicians/other providers
- Review of medical records
- Follow-up with external agents and vendors when needing to arrange for post-discharge services and resources (e.g., durable medical equipment, transportation)

8.6.2. Initial Assessment by Social Worker

As can be seen in the above assessment, a referral can be made to the social worker based on the triggers embedded in the standardized assessment. Once that referral has been made, the social worker can then complete a detailed and comprehensive psychosocial assessment. An example of a social work assessment is in Box 8.7.

The following are guidelines nurse case managers and social workers can use in their daily documentation. Refer to Case Manager's Tip 8.10 for an example of a daily note.

- Daily and whenever an intervention takes place
- Patient and family education provided
- Daily care progression
- Daily discharge planning activities and outcomes
- Daily discussions with interdiciplinary care team and/or physician
- Discharge delay issues
- Family concerns
- Discussion process in selecting discharge destination

Box 8.6   Categories of Documentation for an Admission Assessment

Patient Information:
- Patient demographic information

Admission Information:
- Admit date
- Admit diagnosis
- Admitting service
- Attending physician
- Admit source

Financial Information:
- Insurance
- Plan number
- Medicaid eligibility

Spoken Language(s):
- Preferred language
- Need for interpreter

Source of Admission (Admitted from Where):
- Acute rehab
- Ambulatory surgery
- Another acute care facility
- Behavioral health
- Emergency department
- Home
- Home with home care
- Long term care
- MD office or clinic
- Sub-acute

Significant Prior Medical History:
- Angioplasty
- Behavioral health
- Substance abuse
- Blindness
- CABG
- CAD
- Cancer
- Cardiomyopathy
- CHF
- COPD
- Deafness
- HIV/AIDS
- Hypertension
- Pacemaker
- Paraplegic
- Quadriplegic
- Renal failure
- Stroke
- Vent dependent
- Other
- None

Mental Status Prior to Admission:
- Alert
- Not alert
- Confused
- Oriented to time
- Oriented to time and person
- Oriented to time, person, and place

Ability to Make Needs Known:
- Able
- Unable

Living Arrangement:
- Adult home
- Apartment
- Assisted living
- Group home
- Homeless
- House
- Naturally occurring retirement community (NORC)
- Nursing home
- Shelter
- Stairs
- Elevator
- Other

Home Environment/Lives:
- With adult children
- With dependent children
- Alone
- With other family
- With spouse/significant other
- Domestic partner
- Other

Support System:
- Name
- Telephone number
- Relationship

Can Patient Return to Prior Living Arrangements:
- Yes
- No

Activities of Daily Living:
- Dependent
- Independent

Use of Assistive Device
- Yes
- No

Type of Assistive Device:
- Cane
- Oxygen
- Walker
- Other

Box 8.6 (continued)   Categories of Documentation for an Admission Assessment

Prior Resource Use:

- Children's services
- Adult services
- Adult day care
- Behavioral health services
- Dialysis center
- Home healthcare services
- Infusion therapy
- Meals on wheels
- Medication assistance program
- Nonmedical home care
- Support group
- Health Home
- Medical Home
- House calls
- Other
- None

Does Patient Have a Primary Care Provider?

- No
- Yes
- PCP Name _____
- Address _____
- Phone number _____

Social Work Referral triggers:

- Abuse–Domestic violence
- Abuse and/or neglect of a child
- Abuse and/or neglect of elder/adult
- Abuse–sexual assault
- Adjustment to illness/difficulty coping
- Behavioral management problems
- Crime victim
- Cultural and/or language issues
- Drug abuse
- Ethical concerns
- ETOH abuse
- Family concerns and/or conflicts
- Guardianship
- Homeless requesting intervention
- Hospice placement
- Inadequate social support
- Inadequate financial support
- Long term care placement
- Major illness causing lifestyle change
- Multisystem trauma
- Name of patient unknown
- Noncompliance issues
- Poor prognosis
- Shelter placement
- Uninsured
- Undocumented
- Other
- None

Referred to social work:

- No
- Yes
- Name _____
- Contact info _____

Home Care Referral Triggers

- Patients requiring assessments/education relating to:
  —New diagnosis
  —New medications or change in medications
  —New treatment
  —New equipment or devices
- Change in patient's physical environment and/or new assistive device
- Patients with unstable disease process; cardio/pulmonary, diabetes, neurological, neuromuscular, metabolic, cerebrovascular, cardiovascular, renal, cancer, pediatric/including asthma, premature infants, psychiatric
- Patients with open wounds, VAC wound care, pressure ulcers
- Patients with ostomy, tracheostomy, feeding tubes
- Patients with drainage tubes and catheters
- Patients requiring IV and injectable drug therapies
- Patients with recent change in functional status including but not limited to: falls, paralysis, fractures, amputation, or other physical impairment, change in custodial needs, orthopedic, neurology, and or deconditioned diagnosis
- Patients with pain control management
- Patients with end stage disease and palliative care needs
- Patients with new oxygen and/or nebulizer treatments
- Patients receiving any type of home care services, i.e., CHHA, LTHHCP, PCA, private care, at time of hospital admission
- Patients rehospitalized within 60 days and/or known history of repeated hospital readmissions.
- Patients requiring expedited discharges (EHD/Bridge Program)

Initial Anticipated Discharge Plan:

- Acute care–transfer
- Acute rehab
- Adult home
- Assisted living facility
- Home
- Home hospice
- Home with home care (skilled)
- Home with home care (home attendant)
- Home with home care (infusion)
- Skilled nursing facility–chronic care
- Skilled nursing facility–chronic care with hemodialysis
- Skilled nursing facility–custodial
- Skilled nursing facility–skilled
- Sub-acute rehab
- Traumatic brain injury unit
- Other
- Not known

Box 8.7 An Example of Social Work Assessment

- Date of Assessment: _____
- Consulted By: _____
- Reason for Consult: _____

Family/Social Support:

- Marital Status:
  - __Single (never been married)
  - __Married (___ years)
  - __Divorced
  - __Widowed
- Relationship(s):
- Stable & supportive
- Conflicted
- Minimal interaction
- Unsupportive
- Abusive
- Highly stressed

Support System:

- Available/helpful
- Available/occasionally
- Available with incentive
- Effective
- Limited
- None

Household Composition/Caregivers:

- Name
- Location
- Availability

Housing:

- Single story home
- Two story home
- Apartment/level _____
- Condo/townhome
- Shelter
- Hotel
- Housing authority
- Other:

Mental Health:

- Counseling/psychiatric treatment:
  - __None
  - __Past
  - __Current
- Mental health counselor/caseworker:
- Use of medications for psychiatric illness:

Substance Use:

- Nicotine
  - __Yes
  - __No
  - __Past
- Frequency: _____
- Last use: _____

- Drug use
  - __Yes
  - __No
  - __Past
- Frequency: _____
- Last use: _____
- Alcohol use
  - __Yes
  - __No
  - __Past
- Frequency: _____
- Last use: _____

Legal Issues:

- Incarceration
- Probation/length: _____
- Parole
- DWI/PI
- Comments:

Religious Affiliation:

- Active
- Nonactive
- Unaffiliated
- Comments:

Employment Status:

- Full-time
- Part-time
- Unemployed
- Retired
- Disabled

Occupation:

Employer:

- Last date of employment:
- Employer aware/supportive?
  - __Yes
  - __No

Income Status:

- Patients primary income (source/amt):
- Additional income (source/amt):

Disability Status:

- Short term disability:
- Long Term disability:
- FMLA/date:
- Social security disability:
- SSI
- Social security:

Positive Characteristics (Strengths):

- Well Informed
- Processes information well

Box 8.7 (Continued)   An Example of Social Work Assessment

- Appropriate affect
- Motivated
- Realistic
- Insightful

Negative Characteristics (Concerns):

- Stressed
- Inappropriate affect
- Evasive
- Cautious/suspicious
- Anxious
- Angry
- Hostile
- Exhibiting symptoms of depression
- Difficult to engage

Factors to Consider:

- History of family dysfunction
- Limited support system
- Current substance abuse
- Problems with transportation
- Unable to read
- Limited ability of the primary caregiver
- Limited finances
- Language/cultural barriers
- Emotional problems
- Poor coping capacity
- Hx of noncompliance
- Limited understanding
- Other:

8.6.3. Discharge Summary

Every patient should have a discharge summary. The summary is used as a tool for reviewing all the outcomes the patient has achieved in their care progression and is an indication that, based on those outcomes, the patient is safe and ready for discharge.

Summarize the stay from the case management point of view. Focus on the discharge destination and the patient's readiness for discharge. Be as specific as possible. Include the rationale for the discharge destination, the patient's agreement with the plan and the location of care or services arranged.

The discharge summary is often neglected or forgotten. It is critical that it be included on every dsicharge.

8.7. DOCUMENTING PATIENT EDUCATION

The case manager's role in patient education may be one of educator and/or coordinator. In some models the case manager may develop an educational plan of

---

 CASE MANAGER'S TIP 8.10

Example of a Good Daily Note

1/5/15 10:00 A.M.

This is day two of an expected length of stay of five days. The patient has completed diagnostic testing and an MI has been ruled in. Once stabilized, it is expected that the patient will be discharged home with home care services for medication administration and blood pressure monitoring. A referral was made to St Elsewhere Home Care today. The patient's husband will be instructed as to the patent's diet, and he has agreed to care for the patient at home. A referral has been made to nutrition for a consultation with the patient and husband.

Mary Smith, RN, Case Manager

Bager Number 1234; Mobile Phone Number is 71234

---

care, perform the educational interventions, and monitor the educational outcomes. In other models the case manager may be coordinating the educational plan and outcomes but may not be directly involved in the actual educational process with the patient.

In any case, the best way to plan, evaluate, and monitor patient education and the outcomes of a patient education plan is through a charting by exception system. As the patient's educational plan is created, expected outcomes should be developed that correlate with each educational intervention. In this way, the case manager can monitor against the achievement of the expected outcomes and update the plan or intervene as necessary.

8.6.1. Educational Outcomes Must Be Measurable

Similar to other types of patient care outcomes, all identified educational outcomes should be measurable. For example, was the patient able to "return demonstration" of what he or she was taught? Or, was the patient able to verbally repeat back the given instruction? These expected outcomes should be prospectively included in the plan, and the case manager or patient educator should chart against them. Whenever a patient is unable to meet an expected outcome, the case manager must revise the plan to reflect new interventions that address the patient's inability to meet the expected outcome and strategies to meet the outcomes at a later time. Also included should be "why" the patient was unable to meet the outcome, and the plan should reflect a change in response to the unmet outcome. In some instances it may be appropriate to refer to a family member or significant other when planning and providing patient education.

Example 3: Charting by Exception Sample of Patient Education When Outcome Has Been Met. Clinical practice guideline for asthma.

Day 1 Interventions	Expected Outcomes	Assessment/Evaluation
Instruct patient in use of metered dose inhaler (MDI) and spacer	Patient is able to return demonstration dose inhaler (MDI) and spacer	9/10/2013 2 P.M., RM

8.7.2. Patient Education and Continuum of Care

The case manager should always consider the continuum of care in any educational plan. If the patient is in the acute care setting, the case manager must ensure that the educational plan safely transitions the patient to home or to another level of care or setting. Whenever possible, the educational outcomes that have been achieved, as well as those that have not been achieved, should be communicated to the providers in the setting to which the patient is transitioning.

RM has placed her initials in the "Assessment/Evaluation" section of the guideline. Her initials indicate that the patient has met the outcome of "able to return demonstration of proper use of MDI [metered dose inhaler] and spacer." In this example, no further documentation is necessary.

In this example, the expected outcome of "able to return demonstration of proper use of MDI and spacer" was not met when RM evaluated the outcome at 2 P.M. of Day 1. Because the outcome was not met, the case manager needed to document what the actual outcome was and what her intervention was regarding it. If the unmet outcome resulted in an extension in the length of stay and/or a quality issue resulted, the unmet outcome would also need to be documented as a variance. Unmet educational outcomes may trigger a need for post-discharge services that may not have been evident at the time of the patient's admission to the hospital. Timely evaluation and documentation of educational outcomes is important because it provides evidence that justifies the need for follow-up services, ensures certification for these services, and ensures that the pa-

tient's plan of care remains appropriate throughout the care episode.

8.8. CASE PRESENTATIONS

Documentation by case managers is essential to patient care because it eliminates confusion and uncertainty from the plan of care and promotes its understanding by all of the healthcare providers involved in the delivery of care of the patient. Documentation reflects the professional responsibility and accountability of case managers toward patient care and provides concrete evidence of their role in the provision of care. To help the reader better understand the case manager's role in documentation, the rest of this chapter is a discussion around a case presentation of an elderly patient with exacerbation of heart failure who needed acute care (Case Study 8.1). Although this case presentation focuses on acute care, the concepts and skills discussed may be applied in any care setting.

Documenting the patient's care in the medical record is an important means of communication between healthcare professionals. It eliminates misunderstanding and improves awareness of the patient's condition, plan of care, and responses to treatments. Case managers' documentation is necessary to the understanding of their role in patient care. The case study and excerpts on documentation shared in Chapter 8 are only examples of case managers' documentation. Case managers are advised to review the policies and procedures related to documentation that are available in the institutions where they work and make every effort to comply with those policies and procedures.

Example 4: Charting by Exception Sample Patient Education When Outcome Has Not Been Met. Clinical practice guideline for asthma.

Day 1 Interventions	Expected Outcomes	Assessment/Evaluation
Instruct patient in use of MDI and spacer	Patient is able to return demonstration of proper use of MDI and spacer	9/10/2013; 2 P.M. Unable to return demonstration of proper use of MDI and spacer; will reinstruct later today; patient is properly using the MDI and spacer after repeated instruction and attempts. RM

CASE STUDY 8.1 ■ Elderly Patient with Exacerbation of Heart Failure

In this case study, an 86-year-old male was admitted to the coronary care unit (CCU) of a major academic medical center through the ED. Mr. D. lives by himself in an apartment building on the fourth floor. He has been admitted to the hospital four times in the past 2 months. Each time he spent 3–4 days in the hospital, of which 2 days were in the CCU. This time, he came to the ED with chest pain and shortness of breath even when resting. On physical examination, he was found to have bilateral audible crackles and 3+ edema in the lower extremities, which was worse around the ankles (pedal). No new changes were identified on the electrocardiogram when compared to the ones taken on the previous hospitalizations. According to the results of his blood tests, he was found to have a potassium serum level of 3.3 mEq, a creatinine level of 2.8 mg/dL, and a blood urea nitrogen level of 22 mg/dL.

When Mr. D. was asked about the home care services arranged before discharge during his last hospitalization, he claimed he did not get along well with the visiting nurse and the home health aide, so he asked them not to visit him again. Mr. D. also informed his case manager that he has no relatives or friends, no money, no insurance, and that he has not been taking his medications (diuretics, digoxin, potassium, and angiotensin-converting enzyme [ACE] inhibitor). He has not been compliant with his restrictive diet and has been eating whatever he could find. Mr. D. was referred to the heart failure case manager by the ED physician and later on by the primary nurse in the CCU.

The heart failure case manager, after meeting with Mr. D. and reviewing his medical history and record, wrote a screening/intake note. She assessed Mr. D. for appropriateness for case management services and wrote an acceptance note while the patient was still in the ED. The following is an excerpt from the heart failure case manager's note.

Case Management Intake (Assessment) Note

Tuesday, August 13, 2015, 10:00 A.M.

Called to see patient by Dr. Jones from the ED. An 86-year-old male with frequent hospitalizations (four times in 2 months) with same complaints of exacerbation of heart failure and noncompliance with medical regimen (medications, activity, diet, and community services). Mr. D. has no insurance coverage and no primary physician. Patient is accepted into the case management services program. Will follow up for full assessment and establishment of the plan of care in the CCU.

Jane Doe, MSN, RN, Heart Failure Case Manager

The screening and intake note written by the heart failure case manager is concise and to the point. It includes the source of referral, the reasons for acceptance for case management, and the necessary follow-up to be made. On arrival of Mr. D. to the CCU, the case manager conducted a thorough assessment of the patient, reviewed the medical record (current and previous hospitalizations), and contacted the cardiologist/heart failure team taking care of Mr. D. to discuss the plan of care. The heart failure case manager then explained to Mr. D. the reason(s) for his hospitalization, the goals of his treatment, and his plan of care (as discussed with the heart failure team). The case manager also involved Mr. D.'s primary nurse in the discussion and in the decisions made regarding his care. The heart failure case manager then proceeded to write an assessment and plan of care note in Mr. D.'s medical record. The note reads as follows:

Case Management Follow-Up Note

Tuesday, August 13, 2015, 12:00 P.M.

A thorough assessment and interview of Mr. D. regarding his past medical history and hospitalizations, medications intake, compliance with medical regimen, insurance coverage, and community services before hospitalization were completed. Medical record was reviewed, and case was discussed with the heart failure team and Mr. D.'s primary nurse.

Assessment of Needs

Mr. D.'s complex condition is related to his noncompliance with the medical regimen and the prescribed community services. His needs are summarized as the following:

1. Healthcare insurance coverage and accessibility to a primary care provider
2. Teaching regarding medical regimen and importance of compliance with the regimen
3. Discharge from the hospital into a safe environment in the community

Plan

1. Verify Mr. D.'s health insurance coverage, and contact outpatient heart failure service for follow-up on Mr. D. after discharge.
2. Teach/ensure patient teaching is done regarding medical regimen and self-care expectations after discharge.
3. Refer patient to home care services. Contact the home care intake coordinator (HCIC). Also refer patient to the nutritionist for dietary counseling.

Jane Doe, MSN, RN, Heart Failure Case Manager

CASE STUDY 8.1 ■ Elderly Patient with Exacerbation of Heart Failure

During Mr. D.'s hospitalization, the heart failure case manager continued to work with him, the heart failure team, the primary nurse, and the HCIC to facilitate Mr. D.'s care and expedite his discharge back into the community. She worked on meeting the goals of his hospitalization and the needs that were identified on admission. Every time she was able to confirm the successful completion of Mr. D.'s required care activities, she wrote a note in his medical record. The following are some examples of follow-up notes written by the heart failure case manager during Mr. D.'s stay at the hospital.

Case Management Follow-Up Note

Wednesday, August 14, 2015, 9:00 A.M.

Contacted noninvasive cardiology laboratory to expedite Mr. D.'s echocardiogram. Was able to successfully schedule the echo for today, to be done at 1:00 P.M.

12:00 P.M.

Discussed discharge planning with Mr. D. Reinforced his need for visiting nurse services and home health aide. He states, "I have been very dissatisfied with the agency, the nurse does not answer all my questions . . . always in a rush" . . . "the home health aide does not spend the 4 hours with me every day, she frequently tells me that she likes to leave early, because she's got something to do. Could you do something about this?" Reassured Mr. D. of the follow-up.

2:00 P.M.

Called for results of echo. Preliminary report to be sent to the CCU. Discussed the report with the heart failure team. No significant changes from previous echo that was done 9 months ago. Patient is stable enough to be transferred to a telemetry bed. Arranged for telemetry bed, and primary nurse will transfer Mr. D. out of the CCU by 3:00 p.m. Discussed the plan with Mr. D.; he understands the plan and is in agreement. Reassured him of case management follow-up while in the telemetry unit.

Jane Doe, MSN, RN, Heart Failure Case Manager

Case Management Follow-Up Note

Thursday, August 15, 2015, 10:00 A.M.

Home care agency was called; discussed Mr. D.'s concerns, and negotiated a change in the assignment of home care services. The agency agreed to send a different nurse and home health aide. Informed Mr. D. of the change in services; he was pleased. Also discussed the importance of compliance with the medical regimen and the home care services. Mr. D. promised to try his best. Contacted the social security and welfare offices and checked on Mr. D.'s insurance. Found out that he has Medicare and Medicaid coverage. Reactivated his coverage and requested new cards, because Mr. D. could not locate the originals. Called the outpatient heart failure services and scheduled Mr. D.'s follow-up appointments for the next 3 months. Arranged for an ambulette for transportation to the hospital for each follow-up appointment.

Jane Doe, MSN, RN, Heart Failure Case Manager

As all case managers do, the heart failure case manager reviewed Mr. D.'s medical record, particularly regarding patient teaching activities, to ensure positive patient care outcomes and to identify any variances in the care of Mr. D. that might require the case manager's interventions. It was noted that Mr. D. has good understanding of his disease process, diet restrictions, and the dosages and actions of his cardiac medications. However, he seemed to experience some problems understanding the importance of fluid restrictions, the side effects of medications, and the necessity of monitoring his weight. The heart failure case manager interviewed Mr. D. regarding teaching and reinforced the areas that still required continued teaching. The case manager then wrote the following note in the medical record.

Case Management Follow-Up Note

Thursday, August 15, 2015, 2:00 p.m.

Mr. D.'s medical record was reviewed. Mr. D. seems to still be experiencing some problems understanding the significance of fluid restrictions and daily weights, as well as the side effects of his medications.

Action

1. Provided Mr. D. with written instructions regarding his medications; reviewed with him the importance of his medications, dosage, schedule, and side effects. Assessed what he was familiar with and reinforced the areas lacking. Reinforced information regarding side effects, particularly the importance and reasons of the need for potassium supplements while on diuretics. Mr. D. was still unable to verbalize complete understanding of the side effects of medications. He was reassured that this issue will be shared with the visiting nurse for further follow-up at home after discharge.
2. Fluid restriction was also discussed with Mr. D. and

CASE STUDY 8.1 ■ Elderly Patient with Exacerbation of Heart Failure

corrected his impression that restrictions are related to water only. He was provided with instructions on how to control his fluid intake. He was able to verbalize the instructions successfully.

3. When discussed further, it was identified that Mr. D. had no problem understanding the importance of monitoring his weight. The real issue was that he did not have a scale at home. A scale was ordered for him, to be delivered to his house on discharge. He was provided with a daily log to record his weights and instructed to bring it with him every time he is back for a follow-up visit with the outpatient heart failure service.

Jane Doe, MSN, RN, Heart Failure Case Manager

It is as important for the case manager to write a discharge/disposition note in the medical record as it is to write a screening and intake note on admission. Disposition notes usually summarize the patient's progress toward recovery and whether the goals of treatment, identified on admission, are met at the time of discharge. The heart failure case manager summarized Mr. D.'s discharge as follows.

Case Management Services Discharge/Disposition Note

Friday, August 16, 2015, 3:00 P.M.

Mr. D. is scheduled for discharge on August 17, 1996. The needs identified on admission have been met. His clinical status has improved significantly: no shortness of breath while at rest; able to ambulate around the unit comfortably and without oxygen. He lost 15 pounds with the diuretics. Home care services have been reinstated with new personnel. He has better understanding of his disease and medical regimen. Mr. D.'s healthcare insurance cards will be mailed to him by social services. A scale and oxygen for emergency use at home will be delivered to his house by Saturday morning. Ambulette has been arranged for transportation back and forth on the day of his follow-up appointment. Ambulette service has also been arranged for discharge by 11:00 A.M. tomorrow. Telephone numbers of the heart failure case manager and outpatient services were provided.

Jane Doe, MSN, RN, Heart Failure Case Manager

8.9. KEY POINTS

1. Documentation by case managers is important because it is the only concrete evidence of their role in the delivery of patient care.

2. Documentation acts as a means of communication among healthcare professionals.

3. Documentation improves awareness of the patient's condition, plan of care, and responses to treatments.

4. Documentation by case managers should follow the case management process. For each step in the process, a note is expected.

5. Case managers are responsible for supervising patient education. As part of this responsibility, they should ensure that the educational needs of the patient are planned and documented.

6. Documentation of the discharge planning process is essential to the role of the case manager.

7. The case manager may be responsible for documenting variances or for designing a process for documentation.

8. Charting by exception is a system for documenting against a predetermined set of expected outcomes.

8.10. REFERENCES

American Nurses Association. (1991). Standards of clinical nursing practice, Kansas City, MO.

Bower, K.A. (1992). Case management by nurses, 2nd ed., American Nurses Association, Kansas City, MO.

Cohen, E.L. & Cesta, T.G. (1997). Case management: from concept to evaluation, 2nd ed., Mosby, St Louis. MO.

Hamilton, B. (2012). Electronic health records, 3rd ed. McGraw-Hill, New York, NY.

HealthIT.gov. August 29, 2014.

Tahan, H.A. (1993). The case manager in acute care settings: job description and function, *J Nurse Adm 23*(10):53–61.

8.11. APPENDIX 8.1

CASE MANAGER'S DOCUMENTATION RECORD

Appendix 8.1 presents an example of a case manager's documentation record. The use of a standardized record streamlines and improves documentation. The record acts as a trigger for better documentation. It also reduces the amount of time required for thorough documentation. Such records can be made flexible to fit the needs of case managers in any patient care setting. This example can also be used when developing electronic documentation, modifying existing ones, or evaluating new software applications before they are purchased and implemented for the case manager's documentation.

Important Aspects of Documentation

Effective documentation provides a written record of the following items:

- Comprehensive assessment of patient and family needs
- Actual and potential problems
- Patient and family interview on admission or during initial encounter of an episode of care (screening and intake)
- Goals of treatment and case management plan (clinical care planning)
- Case conference with health care professionals, patient and family or both
- Assessments and reassessments
- Monitoring and evaluation of outcomes
- Authorizations for services by payers and clinical care reviews
- Patient and family health knowledge assessment and health instruction/teaching
- Discharge/transitional planning (coordination of services needed post-discharge or after an episode of care)
- Referrals to other services (e.g., home care) and specialists (e.g., rehabilitation)
- Completion of patient care–related paperwork (e.g., applying for nursing home placement, Medicaid application)
- Facilitation and coordination of patient care activities (clinical care management)
- Ongoing involvement in patient care activities
- Resolving variances and delays in care activities
- Discharge summary and instructions

EXAMPLE OF A CASE MANAGER'S DOCUMENTATION RECORD

Patient's Name _____   Date of Admission/Care Encounter ___/___/___

Initial Assessment

Date_____/___/_____   Interviewed _____ Patient _____ Family/Caregiver

Review of Health Insurance Plan Availability and Type _____ No _____ Yes
Review of Medical Record _____ No _____ Yes
Review of Other Documents _____ No _____ Yes, Explain _____

Discussion with _____ Physician _____Nurse _____Other _____

Brief Medical History and Medications Intake

_____
_____
_____
_____

Diagnosis and Chief Complaint

_____
_____
_____
_____

Brief Description of Problems (e.g., Physiologic, Functional, Social, Psychological, Emotional, Financial, Coping, Self Management, Health Knowledge)

_____
_____
_____
_____

Clinical Care Planning (Goals of Care, Review and Design of the Plan of Care/Case Management Plan)

_____
_____
_____
_____
_____

Notification of Insurer (Payer) and Authorizations/Certifications of the Plan of Care and Treatments (Include Medical Necessity Review and Use of Criteria such as InterQual)

_____
_____
_____

Insurer/Payer _____ Contact Person/Case Manager_____
Authorization # _____ # of Days _____ Telephone # _____

Type of Needs as Identified by the Case Manage/Focus of Case Management Services

_____ Medical/Surgical Issues
_____ Treatments and Procedures
_____ Medications Including Use of Over the Counter Therapies
_____ Acceptance of Illness
_____ Emotional Support and Psychosocial Support System
_____ Grieving Process
_____ Nutrition/Diet
_____ Activity/Exercise/ADLs/IADLs
_____ Psychiatry/Behavioral health
_____ Parenting/Mother-Infant Bonding
_____ New Parent
_____ Health Literacy and Health Knowledge
_____ Self Management and Adherence
_____ Financial
_____ Living Situation
_____ Other

Consultations and Referrals (Include Who, Date, Time, and Reason)

_____ Physical Therapy
_____ Occupational Therapy
_____ Respiratory Therapy
_____ Nutrition
_____ Psychiatry/Psychology/Counselor
_____ Social Services
_____ Home Care
_____ Patient Representation/Advocacy
_____ Ethics
_____ Other

Meetings/Conferences/Care Management Rounds (Include Type, Date and Time, Persons in Attendance)

_____
_____
_____
_____

Outcomes of Meetings/Conferences/Care Management Rounds

_____

_____

_____

_____

Facilitation and Coordination of Care Activities, Treatments, and Services (Include Type, Reason, Date, Time)

_____

_____

_____

_____

Patient and Family/Caregiver Health Education Needs and Activities (Use the following key for outcomes of teaching: U, Verbalized Understanding; D, Return Demonstration; R, Needs Reinforcement)

_____ Signs and Symptoms of Disease
_____ Potential Complications
_____ Disease process
_____ Tests/Procedures/Treatments
_____ Equipment
_____ Assistive Devices
_____ Wound Care
_____ Medications
_____ Self Management
_____ Use of Teach-Back Method
_____ Discharge Plan
_____ Other

Transitional Planning and Discharge Planning

Level of Care Review _____ Appropriate Based on Pre-established Criteria (If No, Explain)

_____

_____

_____

_____

Certification by Insurer for Continued Stay _____ Yes _____ No Date _____/_____/_____

_____

_____

Anticipated Discharge Needs

_____ Durable Medical Equipment/Assistive Devices
_____ Supplies
_____ Monitoring Technology
_____ Home Care Evaluation
_____ Long-Term Care Facility Placement
_____ Rehabilitation (Indicate if Acute or Sub-acute)
_____ Short-Term Residence
_____ Shelter Placement
_____ Hospice Care
_____ Palliative care

_____ Transportation Home upon Discharge
_____ Transportation for Follow-up Care
_____ Home, No Needs
_____ Home with Home Health (Indicate if Home Health Aide, Home Attendant, Homemaker)
_____ Special Services, Explain
_____ Other

Required Paperwork for Discharge Planning (Include Completion Date)

_____ Personal Review Instrument
_____ Visiting Nurse Services
_____ Health Insurance Plan Authorizations/Certifications

Discharge/Transition of Care Summary (Include Summary of Care and Health Instructions)

_____
_____
_____
_____

Case Manager's Name _____

Case Manager's Signature _____

Date _____/_____/_____   Time _____ A.M./P.M.

9

Becoming a Case Manager: Training, Education, Certification, and Job Seeking

Case management has become a desired approach to patient care delivery in today's post-Patient Protection and Affordable Care Act era. Originally, in the mid-1980s during the nursing shortage, case management was a nursing care delivery model thought to enhance the effectiveness of nursing resources at a time of constraint and limitations. Today, however, almost all healthcare institutions have integrated case management into their patient care delivery. Nurses who assumed the case manager's role in the 1980s were basically prepared for the role in healthcare organizations (i.e., hospitals). Training sessions for these nurses were conducted on the premises of the institution itself, particularly at the patient's bedside and on-the-job. Since the early 1990s, however, case managers have had opportunities for training in a variety of settings. In addition to the institution-based case management training programs, today there are several programs that are college- or university-based. Despite the availability of these educational degree-granting programs, such offerings are still limited and an exception.

The Commission for Case Manager Certification (CCMC) describes case management as a professional, collaborative, and transdisciplinary practice. It also defines it as a "process which assesses, plans, implements, coordinates, monitors, and evaluates the options and services required to meet an individual's health needsin support . . . us[ing] communication and available resources to promote health, quality, and cost-effective outcomes, in support of the Triple Aim, of improving the experience of care . . . , the health of populations, and reducing per capita costs of healthcare" (CCMC, 2015). Case management programs are designed to train case managers in the case manage-

ment and patient care management processes and care delivery systems. The content of these programs is an in-depth review of the CCMC's definition of case management, the standards of practice promulgated by the Case Management Society of America (CMSA), and the perespectives of other professional associations such as the American Medical Association (AMA) and the National Association of Social Workers (NASW).

9.1. BACKGROUND OF CASE MANAGEMENT EDUCATIONAL PROGRAMS

Changes in the structure and processes of patient care delivery have resulted in the development of new educational programs and specializations or the revision of already existing ones. Case management today is considered a basic component of graduate and undergraduate nursing, social work, and other allied health curricula. In some schools it is provided as a course within a program of study or area of specialization either in the form of a post-baccalaureate certificate or a master's degree program (Haw, 1996; Spenceley, 1995; Wells et al., 1996; Scheyett & Blyler, 2002; Trieger & Fink-Samnik, 2015). Research to understand the availability of formal educational programs in case management in the United States has been lacking. A survey conducted in the mid-1990s (Haw, 1996) of 108 graduate and 98 undergraduate nursing programs regarding the inclusion of case management content in their currciula noted the following:

- Eight (7%) of the schools had a dedicated major in case management at the graduate level but none at the undergraduate level.

- Eleven (10%) of the graduate and one (1%) of the undergraduate programs had one or more required case management courses.
- Nine (8%) of the graduate and three (3%) of the undergraduate programs had one or more elective case management courses.
- Ninety-six (89%) of the graduate and 93 (95%) of the undergraduate programs had some case management-related content in required courses.
- Twenty-six (24%) of the graduate and 12 (12%) of the undergraduate programs required clinical experience.
- Forty-one (38%) of the graduate and 22 (22%) of the undergraduate programs included optional clinical experience.

Falter, Cesta, Concert and Mason (1999) conducted a survey in New York, New Jersey, and Connecticut to assess the need for developing a school-based nursing case management educational program. The study employed a sample of 69 hospitals, home care agencies, managed care organizations, and long-term care facilities. This survey guided the authors in designing a graduate level degree and a post-master's certificate program in case management that were started in the fall of 1998 at Pace University in New York City. The results of this survey showed the following:

- A master's degree was required by only five (8.6%) facilities, 45 (77.6%) facilities required a Bachelor of Science degree in nursing, and three (5.1%) hired case managers with an associate's degree.
- Thirty-one (53.4%) facilities agreed that there was a need to educate nurse case managers at the master's level, 25 (43.1%) disagreed, and two (3.4%) were uncertain.
- Fifty (86.2%) were willing to provide financial support for a case manager to attend graduate case management education.
- Fifty-eight (84%) facilities employed case managers, constituting 85%, 77%, and 57% of the facilities in New Jersey, New York, and Connecticut, respectively.
- Home care facilities were found to be in the lead of employing nurses as case managers. Next were managed care organizations, then hospitals, then long-term care. No actual frequencies or percentages were provided.
- Sixty-five percent of the facilities responded positively to hiring case managers over the next 5 years, 31% responded negatively, and 9% were uncertain.
- Clinical, home care, and utilization review experiences were the top three determining factors for hiring potential case managers. Other factors reported include (in descending order) case management experience, interpersonal skills, management experience, discharge planning knowledge, insurance knowledge, managed care, certification in case management, clinical pathways knowledge, organizational skills, and advanced degree.

In 2002, Scheyett and Blyler also conducted a survey of 100 universities to examine the state of case management education with specific focus on the inclusion of case management courses in the curricula. The researchers reviewed course descriptions in eductaional programs of helping professions including nursing, rehabilitation counseling, social work, psychology, education, and others. The study noted that these universities offered 194 case management courses of which 28% were dedicated to case management and the other 72% included case management content as part of another course. Additionally, the study found that 65% of the courses were offered at the graduate level.

Kuric and white (2005) conducted a study to identify what case management content was taught in nursing education programs and to determine the essential concepts and skills of case management relevant to nursing programs. The study included faculty of associate ($N = 29$), baccalaureate ($N = 77$), and graduate ($N = 37$) level programs as well as practicing case managers who held associate ($N = 19$) or baccalaureate ($N = 16$) educational degrees. The study found that case management content was included in the curricula but to varying degrees. The major topics addressed were client identification for case management services, planning and monitoring, collaboration, quality of care, evaluation and outcomes management, legal and ethical practice, resource management and advocacy. The study found case management content in the nursing curricula was limited, despite it being an essential function of the healthcare delivery system as a means to provide high-quality, safe, and cost-effective services and resources. It then recommended case management content which should be included in the nursing educational programs.

The lack of formal educational curricula in case management was evident in the results of the 2014 national role and function study, the CCMC conducted (Tahan et al., 2016) for the purpose of developing a blueprint for the certification examination it offers. In this study of nearly 8,000 participants, only 1.6% ($N = 117$) indicated they had learned the practice of case management by attending a formal degree granting educational program, and another 1.62% ($N = 123$) reported that they had learned case management through attending a post-graduate certificate program.

The majority learned case management through on-the-job training (89%, N = 6817), while the rest learned to practice case mangement either by attending conferences and seminars (6.35%, *N* = 486), self-directed/self-taught (0.81%, *N* = 62), or via a combination of seminars and on-the-job training (0.40%, *N* = 31).

Treiger and Fink-Samnik (2015) cited the availability of only six formal educational programs in case management today; two of which were offered online and the rest were university or college-based; however, offered primarily to nurses. Treiger and Fink-Samnick's report showed a reduction of about 60% in the number of programs offered today when compared to a study completed in follow-up to Haw's 1996 study. Toran in 1998 reported the number of schools that were offering a graduate degree in case management which at the time was about 15 programs. The programs available then offered a combination of theoretical and clinical courses (Toran, 1998). Findings from the studies reviewed suggest that the current training and education for case management roles seem to have not changed since the mid-1990s. The most common mode of learning case management practice remains the on-the-job training approach. Additionally, one may conclude that when training happens, it is limited to the institution employing case managers, excpet in the few instances where academics offer educational specialization in case management at the graduate level (degree-granting) or the undergraduate level (in the form of a special course).

When they were first implemented in the mid-1980s, case management systems were bound to healthcare practice organizations (e.g., hospitals). Education of case managers in these organizations in preparation for the emerging new roles was occurring in the practice setting as part of continuing education. Training sessions were held on the premises of the healthcare organization, both in a classroom and at the patient's bedside.

During the 1990s, case management entered the area of nursing education in the form of either lectures on case management or a 3-credit stand-alone course in a graduate and/or undergraduate nursing program. Case management programs that exist today are of three types and are classified based on the length of the program and/or the location where they are offered. These are as follows:

- Certificate programs such as those offered for continuing education (CE) credit in the form of national conferences coordinated by professional associations/societies or as formal academic credit, other than a degree, in a university or college setting.
- Noncertificate programs as those offered by health-

care organizations to their own case management staff for the purpose of orientation to the field and/or ongoing skills building.
- Degree-granting programs, such as a master's degree, offered in a university-based setting.

Regardless of the type of program provided, the case management content taught is similar to the content, context, processes, aims, and outcomes of case management discussed in this book; however, the depth of the content and the length of the training or educational offering varies dependent on the type of program. The content of case management educational programs has been described by Falter et al. (1999), Haw (1996), Sowel and Young (1997), Toran (1998), and Powell and Tahan (2007). They report the lack of clinical case management courses in schools where case manage-

---

Box 9.1 Sample Content Outline of Case Management Educational Programs

- Overview of case management
- Case management models and functional areas
- Historic perspectives of case management
- Healthcare delivery systems, care settings (continuum of health and human services), and organizations
- Diversity of the roles of the case manager
- The case management process
- Utilization management and allocation of resources
- Discharge/transitional planning process (transitions of care and hand-off communication)
- Management of clinical care and care coordination
- Health insurance plans, managed care organizations, and health insurance benefits
- Healthcare reimbursement systems and methods
- Financial systems, management, and cost-benefit analysis
- Community resources and support services
- Legal and ethical issues in case management practice
- Interdisciplinary collaboration
- Quality management and performance improvement
- Outcomes management and value-based purchasing
- Reporting on outcomes indicators and metrics: quality, safety, cost, experience of care
- Management of delays in care (variance management)
- Evidence-based practice guidelines, plans of care and clinical pathways
- Case management research and evidence-based practice
- Patient engagement, activation, and self-management
- Populations health management/management of patients with chronic illnesses
- Capacity management
- Clinical documentation improvement

ment content was incorporated into other degree programs. Box 9.1 lists common topics addressed in case management educational programs, regardless of the type.

9.2. CASE MANAGEMENT CERTIFICATE PROGRAMS

Case management certificate programs are of three types.

- The first is provided by an independent agency or a healthcare institution in the form of in-person continuing education offerings (e.g., local, regional, or national conference) which may span one to many days, usually less than a week. An example is CMSA's annual conference.
- The second is offered by organizations with educational missions, however, other than formal academic institutions. These may include professional societies, publishing companies, and elearning agencies. This type of education is usually extended using computer-assisted or web-based learning platforms with the offerings being in the form of continuing education (CE) programs while granting CE hours to the learners. An example is Kaplan University, Athena Forum, or Walters Kluwer Health.
- The third is provided by a college or university in the form of multiple credits, about 12 credits, however with no formal degree at the end.

Enrollment in the first two types (in-person or online continuing education and learning programs) are open to the diverse healthcare professionals involved in the practice of case management (e.g., case managers, nurses, social workers, pharmacists, physicians, and allied health professionals) regardless of educational background, specialty, care setting, discipline, or role (clinical, administrative, or leadership). However, the college-based certificate programs are limited to those who hold a baccalaureate degree or higher. Some colleges offer a post-baccalaureate certificate program; others offer a post-master's certificate program. Both types of programs include theoretcial (cognitive knowledge) and clinical courses (practical applications). Participants in either program are provided with a certificate in case management after they have successfully completed all of the requirements.

The University of Southern Indiana, College of Nursing and Health Professions, offers a certificate program in case management, however without academic credits. The program is web-based and given over a six-week period resulting in 40 continuing education credit hours. Participants in this program may include nurses, social workers, and other healthcare professionals. The program consists of six modules: case management concepts, case management process, coordination of services, financial aspects, disease management, and application of case management into practice. The modules are set up in an interactive way that includes reading assignments, study questions, case studies, and a comprehensive final examination. Those who successfully complete the program receive a certificate of completion also reflective of the 40 continuing education hours (University of Southern Indiana, College of Nursing and Health Professions, 2015).

Seton Hall University in New Jersey offers a certificate program with 12 post-graduate academic credits. This program was established in 1996. It is a 12-credit post-baccalaureate program in nursing case management that is offered to nurses who have just started to work in case management or are considering doing so. The program combines theory and practice and features courses in case management, financial and operations management, integrated healthcare delivery systems/networks, and legal and risk management. Admission to this program is restricted to those nurses who meet the specific criteria such as Baccalaureate degree in nursing from a National League for Nursing (NLN)-accredited program, current licensure as a registered professional nurse, and a minimum of 1 year of clinical nursing experience (Seton Hall University, 2015).

The program consists of six credits in nurse case management theory, three credits of clinical experience/practicum, and three credits in nursing resource management. The nurse case management theory courses are designed to teach participants about the role of case managers in today's healthcare environment and across various settings. They explore community resources for client support, the concepts of healthcare insurance (e.g., Medicare, Medicaid, commercial insurance health plans, managed care organizations, and other payers), utilization management, legal and ethical issues, discharge planning and transitions of care, total quality management, and case management process. Participants are developed in patient screening and selection for case management services, assessment of patient and family needs, development of the treatment plan (i.e., the case management plan), on-going case management, evaluation of patient responses to treatment, patient and family teaching, and care of the patient after discharge. Healthcare marketing strategies; financial management and healthcare cost accounting, particularly reimbursement systems;

standards of care and practice; and public policy legislation are discussed. In addition, research as a vehicle for advancing the role of the case manager is also examined (Seton Hall University, 2015).

The nurse case management practicum course provides students with the opportunity to explore, test, and expand the nurse case management theory(ies) in the organizational setting. During this course, enrollees are expected to rotate through clinical areas and be exposed to first-hand experience with case management. They are precepted by seasoned case managers. Socialization with experienced case managers permits the students the opportunity to analyze, synthesize, integrate their learning, and evaluate their effectiveness as potential/future case managers. Students are given control over their clinical experience through designing their own objectives and planning, controlling, and evaluating their learning experiences to achieve these objectives (Seton Hall University, 2015).

The nursing resource management course emphasizes healthcare organizations as "corporate entities." The business perspective of managing nursing services is a major part of this course. Complex management issues are shared and explored as they relate to managing single departments, as well as the healthcare organization as a whole. At the successful completion of the program, students are provided with a certificate of completion in nurse case management. Students have the option to enroll in the master's degree program, using the 12 credits they complete in the certificate toward the academic degree.

Another example of a certificate program in case management is a 16-credit post-matser's program offered by the University of Alabama Capstone College of Nursing. The curriculum consists of three theory courses (human relations management for case managers, financial resource management, and evidenced-based practice roles and processes) and one case management practicum (University of Alabama, 2015). This program focuses on the training and education of registered professional nurses who already hold a master's degree and either currently practice as case managers or are interested in becoming one. Similar to the certificate program offered by Seton Hall University, it combines theory and practice and prepares the case manager in roles as members of interprofessional healthcare teams, understanding the health insurance market, including reimbursement methods and utilization management procedures, and use of evidence in patient care delivery including the latest practices in care coordination, clinical care management, transitions of care, and outcomes management. Graduates of this program would have had the opportunity to practice alongside an experienced case manager to have a better understanding of the case management practice environment, including exposure to the various roles and functions case managers and their fellow healthcare professionals are involved in.

9.3. CASE MANAGEMENT NON-CERTIFICATE PROGRAMS (ORGANIZATION-BASED)

Case management noncertificate programs are those offered by healthcare institutions as part of training, orientation, and education of case managers, nurses, and non-nursing personnel in preparation for the implementation of case management systems. These programs are usually designed by individual institutions based on their policies and procedures and description, roles, and responsibilities of case managers. The design of these programs is affected by who will assume the case manager's role. In addition, the length of these programs varies from one institution to another: 2–4 weeks depending on the intensity of the program. Some institutions have been able to obtain approval for offering CE hours to the participants in these programs. This is a result of successfully completing an application for CE credits submitted to nursing continuing education credentialing boards such as the American Nurses Association's Board of Continuing Education or to the boards of the CCMC, or other allied health professional societies such as the National Association of Social Workers.

Healthcare institution–based noncertificate programs are generally taught by dedicated case management educators/professional development specialists, personnel from the nursing education department, or the institution's training and development department/office within the organizational learning area. The educators and training and development staff usually collaborate with the executive/leader of the case management department in the development of the training program and in the design of the logistics. Sometimes the organization may retain a consultant or consulting agency to train and educate the staff who are both directly or indirectly involved in case management practice, especially if a consultant is hired to oversee the design and implementation of case management systems. Topics covered in the training and education are similar to those addressed in certificate programs. The difference, however, is that the noncertificate, institution-based programs are individualized to fit the institution's policies, procedures, operations, standards of care, standards of practice, and the job description and extent of responsibilities of those who assume the case manager roles (see Case Manager's Tip 9.1 for

CASE MANAGER'S TIP 9.1

Strategies for Developing a Solid Case Management Training Program

- Involve a case management expert or consultant.
- Develop a program that is reflective of the case manager's job description, departmental functions, workflows, roles, and responsibilities of various healthcare professionals (e.g., case manager, social worker, clinical nurse, pharmacist).
- Include subject matter experts from your institution on the planning team. Have the subject matter experts teach in the program.
- Refer to what has been published in this area; limit the topics to what case managers will be involved in.
- Hold both in-person classes and on-the-job training. Assure that on-the-job training focuses on the development and assessment of role-based competencies.
- Have the main topical areas of case management include: clinical care management, utilization management and rersource allocation, continuum of care/health and human services, discharge and transitional planning, hand-off communication, customer experience and service, and value-based purchasing.
- Make sure that topics taught include those related to case management practice such as finance, reimbursement, leadership skills, conflict resolution, problem solving, communication and interdisciplinary teamwork, negotiation skills, conduct of interdisciplinary care rounds, quality/outcomes measures, and legaal and ethical practice.
- Include teaching strategies such as simulation, role play, case studies, and problem-based learning and discussions.
- Maximize the use of mentoring and coaching. Identify strong, knowledgeable and skilled case managers to act as mentors or preceptors.
- Evaluate the state of the training and education program regularly; revise the program to reflect changes in the case management department and healthcare industry as appropriate.

strategies to develop a solid case management training program).

Other noncertificate case management programs are those offered in schools of nursing as one or two courses, earning three to six credits, in baccalaureate or master's degree programs. The topical outline of these courses varies from one school to another. However, they may include the basics of case management and managed care, financial reimbursement systems, roles of case managers, case management plans, variance data collection and analysis, outcomes management, and performance and quality improvement. The con-

tent of these courses is usually approved by the state education department and/or accrediting agencies such as the NLN. Most schools that include case management courses in their programs offer such course(s) as a mandatory part of the curriculum rather than as elective courses.

Students who are enrolled in the school-based programs and nurses/case managers who attend the healthcare institution–based programs may be eligible to pursue a certification in case management. After completion of these training programs, case managers are deemed knowledgeable in case management systems and are ready for practice.

9.4. CASE MANAGEMENT ACADEMIC DEGREE-GRANTING PROGRAMS

Case management degree programs are full graduate-level programs offered in a college or university setting. They generally are a combination of traditional master's level and newly developed case management systems–related courses. At the successful completion of these programs, students earn a master's degree. An example is the Master's of Science in Nursing (MSN) program, concentration in case management for rural populations, offered by the University of Alabama, Capstone College of Nursing to graduate nursing students only. The College also offers a combined MSN/doctor in education (EdD) program with concentration in case management. The EdD program is unique in its kind in the United States. The MSN degree consists of 38–41 credit hours and the graduate of this program is able at the time of degree completion to:

- Synthesize theories and principles from the natural, behavioral, social, and applied sciences, which support specialty-nursing roles.
- Apply concepts of care coordination to culturally diverse individuals and groups emphasizing clinical prevention and population health.
- Assume accountability for ethical values, principles, and personal beliefs that acknowledge human diversity and influence professional practice decisions and nursing interventions.
- Provide organizational and system leadership in coordinating, managing, and improving health programs and community health services to promote high quality and safe patient care.
- Design cost-effective interventions/strategies collaboratively with interprofessional teams to improve population healthcare outcomes.
- Collaborate with interprofessional teams and con-

sumers in designing, implementing, and evaluating innovative health programs and community healthcare services for culturally diverse individuals and populations.

- Demonstrate initial competence in ethical translation and integration of scholarship into practice.
- Advocate for rural populations in policy formulation, organization, and financing of healthcare.
- Ethically manage data, information, knowledge, and technology to communicate and deliver safe quality healthcare within and across settings (University of Alabama, Capstone College of Nursing, graduate student handbook, 2014–2015).

The Master's of Science in Nursing program is available as a part-time or full-time study. The curriculum includes the following course topics:

- Theoretical models for advanced nursing practice with rural populations
- Advanced pharmacology
- Informatics in healthcare
- Advanced health assessment
- Advanced pathophysiology
- Basic epidemiology
- Human relations management
- Evidence-based practice roles and processes
- Research and statistics for health professionals
- Issues in community health for rural populations
- Case management practicum
- Fiscal resource management
- Thesis project (optional)

The combined degree of MSN/EdD consists of 86 credit hours and includes in addition to what is offered at the MSN level other courses that focus on qualitative and quantitative research methods, educational theories, learning methodologies, college teaching, curriculum design, health informatics, case management of rural populations, and dissertation research. Upon the completion of the EdD program, graduates are able to achieve the following in addition to the MSN-based objectives listed above:

- Create an environment in classroom, laboratory, and clinical settings that facilitates student learning and the achievement of specific cognitive, affective, and psychomotor outcomes.
- Identify individual learning styles and unique learning needs of international, adult, multicultural, educationally disadvantaged, physically challenged, at-risk, and second-degree learners.
- Employ a variety of strategies to assess and evaluate student learning in classroom, laboratory, and clinical settings.

- Formulate program outcomes that reflect contemporary healthcare trends and prepare graduates to function effectively in a variety of healthcare environments.
- Identify how social, economic, political, and institutional forces influence higher education in general and nursing education in particular.
- Apply the concepts and principles of curriculum development and revision to teaching-learning situations (University of Alabama, Capstone College of Nursing, graduate student handbook, 2014–2015).

Similar to the certificate programs, what Capstone College of Nursing offers for training and education of case managers combines theory and practice and includes courses reflective of current case management practice and the dynamics of the healthcare delievery system in the United States. Graduates of these programs are able to demonstrate a deep understanding of case management as it relates to the various settings across the continuum of health and human services, model design and strategies for success, diversity of roles and functions, measuring the impact of such models on organization- and patient-related outcomes, working in an interprofessional collaboartive environment, and maintaining ethical and legal practice.

9.5. ORGANIZATION-BASED ORIENTATION OF CASE MANAGERS

When case managers join a new healthcare organization or are new to the role within the same organization, they generally spend sometime getting to learn the new practice environment. This is referred to as a "transition period" or "orientation period" where those new case managers are paired with other experienced case managers who are responsible to familiarize those who are new with the roles and responsibilities of the case manager as designed by the organization and the structure, processes, systems, and outcomes of case management. The main goals of the transition/orientation period is to:

- Ensure that those new to a role or organizational environment (referred to as orientees) receive consistent information regarding organization's and/or department's policies, procedures, standards, and documentation to support practice.
- Familiarize the orientees with the organization's and/or department's mission, vision, objectives, strategic initiatives or goals, and organizational structure.
- Share with the orientees what is considered prac-

tice excellence and a performance expectation of everyone in the organization or department. These tend to pertain to organizational values and culture, service excellence, performance or quality improvement process, safety, and code of conduct.

Generally, orientation programs consist of three components: general organization-wide orientation, specialty orientation (department specific), and practice unit orientation (area within the department). The organization and specialty orientations are usually centralized and offered either in a classroom or online manner using a learning management system, or a combination of both approaches. The unit-based orientation tends to occur on-the-job with the support of an experienced individual in similar role. In case management, content of the specialty/department orientation is similar to that described earlier in this chapter in the section on noncertificate programs and Case Manager's Tip 9.1.

Orientation programs are improtant to enhance retention, career and job satisfaction, and engagement of staff and make them feel comfortable with the new practice environment. Effective programs are those which promote practice excellence, professional development, and a healthy environment of care. They also empower healthcare professionals, including case managers, to positively impact the patient experience of care and improve the quality and safety of the care they provide. The more innovative, evidence-based, and effective an orientation program is, the more successful the transition of those new to an organization or role becomes. Those involved are then able to feel they made the right decision to join an organization or advance their role, free to contribute to the organization, and committed to remain for years to come.

Effective case management orientation programs must at a minimum include three main content areas (Box 9.2):

1. Theoretical and technological component that focuses on a review of case management-based materials such as policies, procedures, and standards specific to the healthcare organization, structure of the case management department, technology/software applications used in the execution of roles and responsibilities, and case management knowledge for practice.

2. A unit-based (specific case manager's area of practice) orientation that facilitates an effective immersion in the environment of practice, understanding of the patient population served, building trusting relationships with various members of the interdisciplinary healthcare team, gaining familiarity with the priorities of the new environment (e.g., quality goals and performance expectations), and gaining access to work-related logistics (e.g., office, telephone, computer, and other necessary equipment). An experienced case manager usually acts as a mentor or preceptor for the new case manager and facilitates learning and the acquisition of job-related knowledg, skills, and competencies.

3. Introduction to key personnel or department heads the new case manager may come in contact with as he/she cares for patients (e.g., access center/admitting office, home care intake coordinator, risk management, patient financial services).

9.6. CASE MANAGEMENT CERTIFICATIONS

In addition to case management certificate, noncertificate, and degree programs, national certifications also exist. There are multiple certifications in case management; however, the two major ones are as follows:

■ The first is sponsored by the CCMC, which has been offered since July 1, 1995. Before then it was sponsored by the Certification of Insurance Rehabilitation Specialists Commission (CIRSC). The certification confers that the holder is a specialized person in the practice of case management (CCMC, 2015). This certification targets all professional providers such as nurses, social workers, physical therapists, and counselors who meet eligibility.

■ The second is offered by the American Nurses Credentialing Center (ANCC), Commission on Certification, since 1996. The ANA initiated a taskforce for the establishment of a credentialing examination that provides certification in nursing case management (NCM). However, this offering is limited only to nurses (ANCC, 2015).

According to Cheri Lattimer, executive director of the CMSA, there are about 250,000 case managers in the United States and in excess of 30 different certifications (personal conversation, June 2015). Over 40,000 case managers have achieved the certified case manager (CCM®) certification offered by CCMC since its inception in 1992; about 37,000 are active as of June, 2015 (CCMC, 2015). The content of the certification examinations correlates with the elements of case management: content, context, processes, aims, outcomes, and role relationships. It is also reflective of the content of the curricula in case management educational programs.

Box 9.2 Sample Case Manager's Orientation Program in Acute Care Setting

Case management orientation programs are designed to assist the new case manager receive an individualized orientation to the new role and practice environment. The following is an example only; it is not a comprehensive list of what should an orientation program consist of. It is suggested that this topical list be turned into a competency assessment orientation checklist where topics, as applicable, are stated in a competency assessment format with special notation about the mode of assessment applied. For example, "completes a clinical review with the payer representative within 24 hours of patient's admission." Mode of assessment is "observation." Modes of assessment may include for example, simulation, testing, return demonstration, presentation, peer review, and medcial record audit.

Roles and responsibilities:

1. Clinical assessment and plan of care delvelopment
   - Review of patient's medical record; history and physical completed by provider, nursing admission history/assessment including risk screens: social (e.g., home situation, prior services, etc.), functional, nutrition, etc.; records from point of entry to hospital (e.g., clinic or nursing home records, ED records)
   - Review of assessments and plans of care of other disciplines
   - Initial screening within 24 hours of admission and comprehensive assessment within 24–48 hours of admission
   - Patient and family interviewing, motivational interviewing
   - Development and documentation of plan of care with special focus on discharge needs, provider's orders, frequency of medications, tests and procedures, etc.
   - Review of clinical findings based on access area from where patient was admitted

2. Utilization review and management
   - Determining anticipated length of stay
   - Level of care and medical necessity assessment using InterQual Criteria and/or Milliman Care Guidelines
   - Mandatory utilization review requirements; clinical reviews; two-midnights rule; frequency of reviews (e.g., at the time of admission, 72 hours after admission, every 14 days thereafter for behavioral health patients)
   - Documentation of clinical reviews and outcomes
   - Identification of discharge delays; identification and documentation of avoidable delays
   - Communication regarding clinical issues, care delays, reimbursement concerns
   - Organization and presentation of review to payors
   - Gathering and maintaining knowledge of insurance/benefits
   - Verification of insurance coverage; monitoring of benefit usage throughout the patient's stay
   - Communication with physician advisor and other providers
   - Obtaining authorizations for the next level of care and post-discharge services
   - Addresses denials (concurrent, retrospective, peer to peer review)

3. Transitional/discharge planning
   - Conduct of interdisciplinary care rounds; documentation of rounds
   - Application of regulatory standards and policies for discharge/transitional planning
   - Use of criteria for screening patients for post-discharge services
   - Use of chain of command
   - Documentation of initial screening, assessments, discharge/transition/transfer note
   - Medicare important message
   - Transportation management
   - Post-discharge follow-up
   - Connections to physician organizations: who, what, where
   - Transition to ambulatory care/clinic
   - Referrals to post-acute services; dual planning
   - Refusal of discharge: HINN Letter

4. Quality and patient safety
   - Quality measures: organizational quality and patient safety
   - Use of clinical pathways, deviations from pathways
   - Value-based purchasing: tracking of measures/core measures and regulatory requirements
   - Handling ethical concerns
   - Escalation of quality of care concerns; risk management issues, significant events, reportable events
   - Readmission reviews—assessing for preventable versus nonpreventable causes
   - Case management dashboard: departmental, executive/organizational

---

Box 9.2 (continued)   Sample Case Manager's Orientation Program in Acute Care Setting

Classroom-based orientation

- Review of important skills: leadership, communciation, negotiation, conflict management, managing resitance
- Interprofessional practice and team rounding; interdisciplinary collaboration: Who is on the team? What constitutes a team?
- Electronic documentation: general, case management specific
- Event reporting system
- Personal instrument review (PRI) certification
- Use of admission/discharge/transfer (ADT) system
- Continuum of care/health and human services
- Utilization review and management: medical necessity criteria (e.g., InterQual Criteria, Milliman Care Guidelines); utilization review plan; conducting clinical reviews with payers; management of denials
- Referral procedure to social worker for complex needs assessment based on high screening criteria; activation of social work based on triggers and use of automated tasking function/notification
- Review of the role of case manager versus social worker; working as partners
- Legal tips on documentation
- Health insurance plans and contracts: Medicare/Medicaid versus commercial/managed care patients
- Peer review organizations/quality improvement organizations
- Transitions of care
- Regulatory and ethical standards related to case management
- How/when to escalate a problem to the next level (chain of command)
- Medicare important message
- Transportation management
- Dual discharge/transitional planning
- Refusal of discharge notice
- Value-based purchasing
- Quality and safety program and goals

Introduction to key personnel component

- Case management department
- Nursing
- Physician organization representative (e.g., chairmen, chiefs, medical affairs)
- Transfer/access center/admitting office/bed management
- Patient services administration
- Patient financial services
- Managed care/contracts
- Rehabilitation/therapies: physical therapy, occupational therapy, speech pathology, respiratory therapy
- Onsite vendors/services: home care, skilled care, durable medical equipment, commercial insurer/payor representative
- Revenue cycle
- Pastoral care
- Ethics
- Transportation

Certifications are offered through national testing. One must obtain a passing score on a case management certification examination to be considered certified and be able to use the designated case management credential; that is, RN-BC if offered by the ANCC, or CCM if offered by the CCMC. A nationally recognized certifying body, such as the ANCC or the CCMC, provides the testing for certification, often through a third party specialized in standardized examinations. Currently, certification for case managers is not mandatory as it is for other specialties such as midwifery, nurse anes-

thetists, and nurse practitioners. However, employers are increasingly requiring a certification in case management as a prerequisite credential for hiring case managers, especially in the health insurance/payer organizations, hospitals, occupational health, and workers' compensation areas of case management practice. Tahan et al. (2015) report based on a national survey of over 7,600 case managers that 40.4% of participants indicated that their employer requires a certification in case management and about 30% offer renumeration for certification.

Box 9.3   Definitions of Licensure, Certificate, and Certification

- *Licensure* is a mandatory and official form of validation provided by a governmental agency in any state affirming that a practitioner has acquired the basic knowledge and skill and minimum degree of competence required for safe practice in one's profession.
- *Certificate* is a document awarded to affirm the completion of, or participation/attendance in, a given educational program. It can be provided by any professional agency (private or public), university, or college. Usually a certificate is not nationally recognized in any form other than an educational credit or unit.
- *Certification* is an official form of credential that is provided by a nationally recognized governmental or nongovernmental certifying agency to a professional who meets the eligibility criteria and requirement of a particular field of practice or specialty. It usually signifies the achievement of a passing score on an examination prepared by the certifying agency for that purpose. It also denotes an advanced degree of competence.

9.6.1. Importance of the Case Manager Certification

Certification in case management is important because it affirms that the case manager possesses the knowledge and skills required to render appropriate, quality, and safe case management services to potential clients. Certifications can be used for professional growth and development or as a means for advancing one's career. They are a measure of knowledge, skills, expertise, and competence. In addition, they testify that one has achieved special/advanced competence; that is, expanded knowledge and skill in a particular area of practice, such as transitions of care, care coordination, healthcare quality, health isurance, or utilization review and management. Furthermore, they allow the public to have more trust and faith in case managers and the services they provide.

Certifications also make case managers more marketable; provide them with better job opportunities, financial rewards, and compensation; and increase their chances of recognition and celebration by their employers. Certified case managers are more likely to get promoted by their employers compared with those who are not certified. In addition, certifications in case management assist healthcare organizations in meeting the quality management and improvement standards of accreditation agencies. They also keep case managers current with their knowledge, skills, and healthcare trends.

9.6.2. Differentiating Licensure, Certificate, and Certification

It is important to differentiate certification from the terms licensure and certificate. These terms should not be used interchangeably because they mean different things. Box 9.3 contains the definitions of these terms. Licensure is a restrictive form of regulation. It is also mandatory before pursuing practice, whereas certificate and certification are voluntary. Currently, all case management certifications require a basic professional licensure as a prerequisite to certification. Both certification and licensure are obtained by achieving a passing score on an examination. Licensure recognizes basic performance, knowledge, and skill, whereas certification recognizes exceptional performance and advanced knowledge, skill, and competence. Generally, certificates do not require any form of testing and do not reflect one's level of competence but rather attest to one's participation in a particular learning experience. Licensure in nursing is achieved upon passing a standardized, nationally recognized nursing board examination. Licensure in social work, however, in some jurisdications does not require the passing of an examination.

Sometimes the term certification is also confused with accreditation. Accreditation refers to a process of reviewing an organization or program against a nationally recognized and accepted set of standards to ultimately determine whether the organization or program meets the standards and requirements of quality and excellence. The pursuit of accreditation review in case management is voluntary and conducted by nongovernmental agencies such as the The Joint Commission (TJC), URAC, and the National Committee for Quality Assurance (NCQA). Accreditation may take two forms:

- *Organization-level*: usually applies to the entire organization and entails a review of the overall systems and practices of the organization, its standards and performance, and contribution to healthcare dlivery and outcomes, including quality, safety, access, cost, and experience of care. The accreditation indicates that each of the organization's parts is contributing to the achievement of the organization's objectives, mission, philosophy, and goals and that these various parts are performing at the same level of excellence. For example, accreditation review of a health insurance plan.
- *Program within an organization*: usually applies to a review of a specialty, service, department, or center of excellence within an organization. The review focuses on same aspects as those of a whole organization, however, limited to the focus area;

for example, a case management program within a hospital or utilization management within a health insurance plan.

The ultimate goal of accreditation is for the review/accrediting agency to certify and authoritatively declare where an organization or program stands relevant to the standards of excellence. Although one may say the organization is certified (instead of accredited) to meet the standards of excellence standards, the use of the term "accredited" is more widely recognized. Certification on the other hand is primarily used to reflect that an individual has achieved specific and nationally recognized standards of excellence in performance in a certain area of practice which tend to be a decision made based on passing a certification examination in the area of specialty.

9.6.3. Choosing a Certification

As more professional organizations provide certification opportunities for case managers, certifications have gained significant meaning and recognition. They may ultimately be used for regulation and accreditation of case management programs; entry into case management practice; validation of knowledge, skills, and competence; and recognition and achievement of excellence. Today there are more than 30 different organizations which provide certification in case management. Table 9.1 lists some of the ones most commonly pursued. These organizations are mostly related to specialties such as rehabilitation and disability case management, utilization management, healthcare quality, acute care case management, nursing, managed care, gerontology, and workers' compensation and occupational health.

The decision about which case manager certification one should seek can be a confusing and frustrating undertaking. Those interested must make the decision based on the field of practice or specialty, discipline, and the requirements or criteria of the certifying body. When making the choice, case managers may want to answer the following questions first to arrive at the best decision:

- Is the certification a prerequisite for my current or potential job?
- What is the benefit of the certification for my career advancement and professional development?
- Is the certification a mandatory expectation for credentialing in my role or for accreditation of the case management department I belong to?
- What are the specific standards of care, practice,

and performance that govern my practice setting/environment (e.g., acute care, health insurance plan, managed care organization, workers' compensation)?
- What are the eligibility criteria for the different certification examinations? Which one am I able to meet?
- What is the cost of the certification?
- For how long is the certification valid?
- What are the criteria for certification renewal?
- How much information is available from the certifying bodies regarding the examinations?
- Which certification is nationally recognized?
- Is the certification more general in focus, or is it highly specialized?
- Will there be any financial compensation if I obtain a certification? Does my employer pay for certification?
- Is the certifying body a for-profit or not-for-profit organization/agency?
- Is the certifying body accredited by the National Commission for Certifying Agencies?
- Is there any published research about the validity and reliability of the certification examination? How current is such research?
- Do the certifying bodies abide by the codes of ethics?
- Does the certifying body have a clear review and appeal or grievance process?

Answering the above questions assists case managers in determining which certification is best to pursue. It is important not to make such decision arbitrarily or hastily. A well thought out decision prevents oversight, problems, and unnecessary trouble. It also allows case managers to find the certification that fits their needs, abilities, and aspirations to advance their professional identity and contribution to the field.

Often certifications are offered for a limited number of years which may range between 2 and 5 years. The certifying agency requires the certiified case manager to renew the certification then. Criteria for renewal usually include a number of continuing education hours or credits (minimum of 25 hours) and good standing and moral character (e.g., active licensure and no complaints filed within the state of jurisdiction). Fees for initial certification and renewal also vary by certifying agency; for those belonging to a professional association or society, such as the American Nurses Association, a discount may be offered for candidates who are members of the association in the form of member benefit. Fees may start at approximately $250 and may reach as high as $750.

TABLE 9.1. Certifications in Case Management.

Certification	Organization and Website
Certified Case Manager (CCM)	Commission for Case Manager Certification (www.ccmcertification.org)
Nurse Case Manager (RN, BC)	American Nurses Association Credentialing center (www.nursingworld.org)
Case Manager, Certified (CMC)	American Institute of Outcomes Case Management (www.aiocm.com)
Case Manager Administrator, Certified (CMAC)	The Center for Case Management (www.cphq-hqcb.org)
Certified Professional in Healthcare Quality (CPHQ)	National Association of Healthcare Quality (www.cfcm.com)
Continuity of Care Certification, Advanced (A-CCC)	National Board for Certification in Continuity of Care (www.nbccc.org)
Certified Disability Management Specialist (CDMS)	Certification of Disability Management Specialists Commission (www.cdms.org)
Certified Rehabilitation Registered Nurse (CRRN)	Rehabilitation Nursing Certification Board (www.rehabnurse.org)
Certified Social Work Case Manager (CSWCM)	National Association of Social Workers (www.nasw.org)
Certified Advanced Social Work Case Manager (CASWCM)	National Association of Social Workers (www.nasw.org)
Certified Managed Care Nurse (CMCN)	American Board of Managed Care Nursing (www.abmcn.org)
Certified Occupational Health Nurse/Case Manager (COHN/CM)	American Board for Occupational Health Nurses (www.abohn.org)
Care Manager Certified (CMC)	National Academy of Certified Care Managers (www.naccm.net)
Health Care Quality Management-Subspecialty in Case Management, Transitions of Care, Physician Advisor, Managed Care	American Board of Quality Assurance and Utilization Review Physicians (www.abqaur.org)
Chronic Care Professional Certification (CCPC)	Health Science Institute (www.healthsciences.org)
Accredited Case Manager (ACM)	American Case Management Association (www.acmaweb.org)
Patient Centered Medical Home Certified Content Expert (PCMHCCE)	National Committee for Quality Assurance (www.ncqa.org)

9.7. THE COMMISSION FOR CASE MANAGER CERTIFICATION

The practice of case management today is still viewed as a specialized area of practice rather than a profession. Therefore, those who pursue certification in case management are usually licensed to practice in a specific professional discipline first, such as social work and nursing. Case management experts who developed the eligibility criteria for the certification offered by CCMC agree that case management services can be provided by a variety of professionals from different health and human service professions (e.g., nursing, social work, physical therapy, pharmacy). As a result, these professionals, when certified as case managers, use the credential "CCM" in conjunction with their professional licensure (e.g., registered professional nurses use the credentials RN, CCM; clinical social workers use the credentials CSW, CCM).

The certification examination of the CCMC is accredited by the National Commission for Certifying Agencies. The examination is offered a number of times per year. The initial certification is valid for 5 years, and renewal of the case manager certification is required every 5 years. It can be achieved through re-examination or demonstration of professional development, which entails participation in approved continuing education programs. In addition, certified case managers applying for certification renewal should also provide evidence that they continue to hold the same license or certification they held at the time of the initial certification (e.g., registered professional nurse, certified social worker, certified physical therapist). More information on the certification is available at www.ccmcertification.org.

9.7.1. Eligibility Criteria for the CCMC Case Manager Certification

The CCMC has established three eligibility criteria that have to be met by all applicants at the time applications for the examination are submitted (Case Manager's Tip 9.2). One criterion is licensure; the second is employment/experience; and the third pertains to applicants being of good moral character and reputation, consistent with the CCMC's Code of Professional Conduct (CCMC, 2016).

The licensure criterion requires the applicant to have a current, active, and unrestricted licensure or certification in a health or human services discipline that within its scope of practice allows the professional to conduct an assessment independently. License must be active through the last date of test administration. The candidate may instead present confirmation to have graduated from an educational program that grants a baccalaureate or graduate degree in social work, nursing, or another health or human services field that promotes the physical, psychosocial, and/or vocational well-being of the persons being served. The degree must be

 CASE MANAGER'S TIP 9.2

Eligibility Criteria

All applicants for the Commission for Case Manager Certification examination must meet the following three eligibility criteria:

1. Licensure or education that qualifies candidates to practice in a health and human services profession.
2. Employment experience in the area of specialty indicated by the licensure.
3. Good moral character, consistent with CCMC's Code of Professional Conduct.

from an institution that is fully accredited by a nationally recognized educational accreditation organization, and the individual must have completed a supervised field experience in case management, health, or behavioral health as part of the degree requirements (CCMC, 2016). For example, registered professional nurses at the bachelor's, master's, or doctorate degree education level are eligible for participation in this certification. The CCMC only honors the educational programs that provide a license/certificate that permits the holder to legally practice without the supervision of another professional (e.g., registered professional nursing programs).

In addition to meeting the licensure or education criterion, the applicant for the case manager certification examination must provide verification of employment and experience in the area of specialty as indicated on the license or certificate. To be eligible, one must provide evidence of either (1) 12 months of full-time employment under the supervision of a certified case manager, (2) 24 months of full-time case management employment without supervision of a certified case manager, or (3) 12 months of full-time employment as a supervisor of case management services and/or case managers. Applicants should demonstrate that their employment experience entails the components of case management services as defined by the CCMC, which are assessment, planning, implementation, coordination, monitoring, evaluation, outcomes, and general. The general component refers primarily to ethical, legal, and accreditation standards (CCMC, 2016).

9.7.2. Commission for Case Manager Certification Examination Content Topics

The certification examination consists of 150 multiple-choice questions that address eight different broad activities related to the job description and roles and responsibilities of case managers and the case management process. These include, as they appear in the CCM Certification Guide (CCMC, 2016): assessment, planning, implementation, coordination, monitoring, evaluation, outcomes, and general. The examination also addresses five core components of case management knowledge. These are as follows:

1. Care delivery and reimbursement methods
2. Psychosocial concepts and support systems
3. Rehabilitation concepts and strategies
4. Quality and outcomes evaluation and measurements
5. Ethical, legal, and practice standards

CASE MANAGER'S TIP 9.3

Fifty Topics to Review for the CCMC's Certification Examination

1. Patient's bill of rights
2. Legal and ethical issues
3. Patient's privacy and confidentiality
4. Continuum of care/continuum of health and human services
5. Clinical information systems and communication of information
6. Public benefit programs
7. Patient assessment and data-gathering procedures
8. Disease processes and treatment modalities
9. Psychosocial assessment of patients and families
10. Assessment of support systems
11. Coping with and adaptation to illness
12. Evaluation of patient responses to treatments and quality of care
13. Advocacy
14. Negotiation of services
15. Commercial health insurance plans and managed care
16. Insurance principles, policy coverage, inclusions/exclusions
17. Cost/benefit analysis
18. Cost-containment strategies
19. Utilization review and management activities
20. Healthcare delivery systems
21. Screening and intake of patients for case management services
22. Coordination and facilitation of care activities
23. Patient and family education, engagement, and activation
24. Health literacy
25. Family dynamics and support systems
26. Discharge/transitional planning and levels of care; transitions of care and hand-off communication
27. Case management plans and evidence-based guidelines
28. Community resources, services, and support systems
29. Documentation of case management services
30. Role of the case manager
31. Consultation
32. Legislation and public policy related to case management
33. Liability issues/concerns of case management
34. Outcomes management; variances and variance analysis
35. Americans with Disabilities Act
36. Durable medical equipment and assistive technologies
37. Evaluating the effectiveness of case management services
38. Interpersonal communication and relationships
39. Clinical pharmacology
40. Aspects of acute and chronic illness and disability
41. Job analysis and modification
42. Work adjustment and transitions
43. Mental health and psychiatric disability management
44. Value-based purchasing; core measures, patient experience with care
45. Outcomes management; quality and performance improvement
46. Accreditation standards and requirements
47. Rehabilitation post-work-related injury or serious health condition
48. Palliative and end-of-life care
49. Data analytics (e.g., risk stratification)
50. Management of chronic illnesses and disabilities

These core components must be evident in the applicants' practices, and their focus must entail the continuum of care/health and human services, and address the ongoing needs of the individual patient being served by the case management process. Furthermore, these activities must deal with the broad spectrum of the patient's needs and must involve interactions with relevant components of the patient's healthcare team such as the physician, family members, third-party payers, employers, and other providers.

Case Manager's Tip 9.3 presents a suggested list of topics that may aid case managers in their preparation for the CCMC's certification examination.

9.8. THE AMERICAN NURSES CREDENTIALING CENTER'S NURSING CASE MANAGEMENT CERTIFICATION

The ANCC is the credentialing arm of the ANA. It offers the nursing case management certification through its certifications center. Although the ANA's certification program has been in existence since 1973, in 1991, the ANCC was incorporated as a subsidiary of the ANA and became the arm responsible for management and oversight of the specialty certifications ANA offers including some other products such as the Magnet Recognition Program. The certification in nursing case management is over a decade old. Unlike the CCMC, but similar to all the other ANCC's certifications, the case management certification is offered only to licensed nursing professionals. When certified as case managers, nurses use the credential "board certified" (BC) in conjunction with their professional licensure; that is RN, BC. The goals of the ANCC are to promote and enhance public health by certifying nurses using the ANA's scope and nationally recognized standards of nursing practice. Passing the ANCC's certification examination in case management affirms that the case manager has demonstrated knowledge, skills, and abilities within a defined area of specialty. The competency based certification examination provides a valid and reliable assessment of the entry-level clinical knowledge and skills of registered nurses in the nursing case management specialty after initial licensure as an RN (ANCC, 2015).

The ANCC case management certification is accredited by the National Commission for Certifying Agencies and the Accreditation Board for Specialty Nursing Certification (ABSNC, formerly known as the American Board of Nursing Specialties). The initial case management certification is valid for 5 years, and renewal is required every 5 years and is contingent on maintaining RN licensure in the jurisdiction of employment and meeting all recertification requirements. Renewal can be achieved through re-examination or by obtaining the specified number of contact hours of continuing education. Other options for recertification requirements are related to academic credits, publishing in refereed media, or conducting research (ANCC, 2015). More information on the certification is available at www.nursecredentialing.org.

9.8.1. Eligibility Criteria for the ANCC Case Manager Certification

The ANCC has established the nursing case management examination based on core clinical skills and standards of practice that are evident in any of the ANCC certifications or that of the American Association of Critical Care Nursing. Candidates for the case management certification must meet three criteria before they are deemed eligible to take the examination. These are as follows:

1. Hold a current, active RN license within a state or teritory of the United States or the professional, legally recognized equivalent in another country.
2. Have practiced the equivalent of 2 years full-time as a RN.
3. Have a minimum of 2,000 hours of clinical prac-

tice in nursing case management within the most recent 3 years; OR have completed 30 hours of continuing education in nursing case management within the most recent 3 years (ANCC, 2015).

9.8.2. American Nurses Credentialing Center's Case Management Certification Examination Content Topics

Content of the nursing case management certification examination is based on clinical skills and standards of nursing practice. It is provided in two forms: one with the additional core nursing specialty section (i.e., the 50 questions) and one without. Nurse case managers who elect to take this examination and do not already have a core nursing specialty certification, such as certification in gerontology, oncology, medical-surgical, or critical care nursing, are obligated to take the core specialty section as well. Those who are certified are exempted from this section. Passing the certification is dependent on passing both sections of the examination where applicable: the case management and the core specialty nursing sections. Topics addressed in the examination are based on the views and philosophies of nursing case management as defined by the ANA. Case Manager's Tip 9.4 presents a suggested list of topics that may aid case managers in their preparation for the ANCC's certification examination. These topics focus on the seven components of the framework of nursing case management certification examination and content areas based on a national study ANCC conducted in 2013 for the purpose of practice analysis. These are as follows:

1. Assessment
2. Planning and collaboration
3. Implementation, coordination, and linking
4. Education
5. Evaluation
6. Advocacy
7. Systems

9.9. THE NATIONAL ASSOCIATION OF SOCIAL WORK CASE MANAGEMENT CERTIFICATION

The National Association of Social Workers (NASW) launched its national certification program in 2000 after querying the interest of its members in offering specialty certifications which was received favorably. The certification program offers NASW members the opportunity to attain (NASW, 2015):

■ Enhanced professional and public recognition

CASE MANAGER'S TIP 9.4

Topics to Review for the ANCC's Certification Examination (ANCC, 2014)

1. Assessment
   - Client screening for case management
   - Identification of target population for case management services
   - Client consent for case management and goals
   - Validation of clinical and demographic data
   - Assessment tools
   - Motivational and adherence issues
   - Medication reconciliation
   - Review of client history and current condition
   - Health promotion and illness prevention
   - Health literacy
   - Payer sources and health insurance coverage
   - Client's level of care based on utilization review criteria

2. Planning and Collaboration
   - Client-focused case management plan and outcomes of care
   - Client engagement in care
   - Evaluation of support and social systems
   - Setting outcomes and goals
   - Identifying and selecting resources
   - Treatment options
   - Designation of appropriate levels of care, medical necessity review
   - Ascertaining appropriate providers
   - Collaboration with stakeholders (clients, employers, payers, providers)
   - Communication with stakeholders

3. Implementation, Coordination, and Linking
   - Communication with stakeholders of progress toward achieving outcomes
   - Coordination of services with stakeholders and transitions to next level of care
   - Linking clients to services and resources
   - Referrals to other providers such as complex case management or disease management
   - Cost-effective interventions
   - Compliance with regulation, standards, and legislation
   - Utilization of community resources
   - Documentation of the nursing case management process
   - Accountability for implementing the plan of care
   - Problem solving and conflict resolution
   - Negotiations with clients, payers, and providers of services
   - Barriers to availability, accessibility, and affordability of treatment
   - Documentation
   - Denial and appeal process

4. Education
   - Educational needs and patient/family teaching
   - Education regarding case mangement, disease process, treatment options, self-management, insurance benefits, transitions of care, bill of rights
   - Education of healthcare team members and payer regarding case management plan

5. Evaluation
   - Progress toward achieving goals
   - Customer satisfaction
   - Cost-benefit analysis
   - Evaluation of client's health knowledge

6. Advocacy
   - Facilitation of access to services
   - Liaison and collaboration with other disciplines and providers
   - Coordination of care to minimize delays
   - Resolution of ethical conflict
   - Client's confidentiality
   - Client's self-advocacy and autonomy
   - Brokering of services
   - Communication of client's care preferences

7. Systems
   - Outcomes data collection and tracking: utilizations, clinical
   - Outcomes measures
   - Delays in care data management
   - Change in organization and client-centered care

- Increased visibility as specialized, professional social workers
- Association with a select group of specialized, professional social workers who have attained national distinction

The specialty certifications NASW offers are not a substitute for state licensure. They are available to social workers who have graduated from accredited schools and possess academic degrees in social work. The certifications provide a vehicle for recognizing social workers who have met national standards and possess higher levels of experience and specialized knowledge, skills, and experience (NASW, 2015).

The NASW describes social work case management as a method of care where a professional social worker assesses the needs of clients and their families and provides needed services accordingly. The care addresses the individual needs of the client while considering the client's biopsychosocial status and the context of the social system in which case management operates: at the micro level which relates to interventions offered to clients and the macro level which focuses on improvement in the systems of care. The professional social work case manager "arranges, coordinates, monitors, evaluates, and advocates for a package of multiple services to meet the specific client's complex needs," (NASW, 2015). Certification is good for 2 years, after which certificants apply for renewal. Renewal is granted based on 20 contact hours of continuing education relevant to case management and adheres to the NASW's Standards for Continuing Professional Education and current valid license or certification to practice as a social worker in the state of employment.

9.9.1. Eligibility Criteria for National Association of Social Workers Case Management Specialty Certification

Membership in NASW is not required for a social worker to apply for the case management certification credential. However, if a candidate is a current NASW member, membership must be in good standing to receive the discounted rate. There are six eligibility criteria for the certified social work case manager (C-SWCM). These are:

1. *Education*: a bachelor's degree in social work (BSW) from an accredited university.
2. *Experience*: 3 years of full time work experience after completion of the bachelor's degree in social work; a total of 4,500 hours. The work experience must meet the core functions of social work case management functions. Experience must not exceed 5 years from time of application.
3. *Supervisor's evaluation*: supervisory evaluation(s) must correspond in time to the qualifying experience described in the application. The supervisor(s) must be able to evaluate the applicant's case management skills, knowledge, and abilities across the seven core functions of case management. This can be submitted from a supervisor who is specialized in social work or from another supervisor from an allied health profession.
4. *Reference from a colleague*: a confidential reference from a BSW or master's in social work (MSW) colleague. The colleague reference cannot be completed by the same person who completed the supervisory evaluation.
5. *License or credentials*: copy of current licensure or certification acquired based on passing the licen-

sure examination offered by the Academy of Certified Baccalaureate Social Workers, in the states where it is available. In the states where a BSW-level license is not available, proof of one additional year of experience and 20 additional continuing education units are accepted.
6. *Affirmation of professional standards and statement of understanding*: attestation of adherence to the NASW Code of Ethics and Standards for Continuing Professional Education (NASW, 2015).

Eligibility criteria for the certified advanced social work case manager (C-ASWCM) are similar to six criteria required for the C-SWCM, except for the following differences:

1. Education: master's degree in social work (MSW) instead of a BSW.
2. Experience: minimum of 2 years and 3,000 hours of full-time work instead of 3 years and 4,500.
3. Supervisor's evaluation: strongly preferred to be from an MSW supervisor.
4. Reference from a colleague: same as C-SWCM.
5. Licensure: current examination-based state issued MSW-level license or certification.
6. Affirmation of professional standards and statement of understanding: same as C-SWCM (NASW, 2015).

9.9.2. National Association of Social Workers Case Management Examination Content Topics

Social work case management requires the professional social worker to develop and maintain a therapeutic relationship with the client/family. This may include linking clients with needed services and resources provided in a single agency or across multiple organizations. NASW offers two specialty certifications in the area of case management practice. These are the certified social work case manager (C-SWCM) and the certified advanced social work case manager (C-ASWCM). The certification examinations cover the seven core functions of case management (Case Manager's Tip 9.5) (NASW, 2015). These are:

1. Engagement
2. Assessment
3. Planning
4. Implementation and coordination
5. Advocacy
6. Reassessment and evaluation
7. Disengagement

CASE MANAGER'S TIP 9.5

Topics to Review for the NASW Case Management Certification Examination (NASW, 2015)

Topics are based on the social work case management core functions and apply for both the C-SWCM and C-ASWCM certifications.

1. Engagement
   - Client outreach
   - Working alliance
   - Screening for needs and initial intake
   - Consent for services and release forms
   - Receiving referrals
2. Assessment
   - Needs: functional, psychosocial
   - Strengths, challenges, and opportunities
   - Biosychosocial system
   - Comprehensive intake assessment
   - Sociocultural factors
   - Financial resources
3. Planning
   - Services, interventions, treatments, and care activities
   - Care direction and goals
   - Rehabilitation services and goals
   - Crisis prevention
   - Support systems and services
4. Implementation and coordination
   - Brokering of resources and services
   - Monitoring of service delivery
   - Service provision
   - Client support
   - Crisis management
5. Advocacy
   - Systems improvement
   - Promoting client's well-being and functioning
   - Liaison
   - Mediation
6. Reassessment and evaluation
   - Monitoring
   - Efficacy, effectiveness, efficency
   - Appropriateness
   - Review and revision of plan of care
   - Data collecion and analysis
7. Disengagement
   - Terminating case management services or relationship
   - Transferring clients to another level of care or provider
   - Discharge planning

9.10. FORECASTING THE FUTURE OF CASE MANAGEMENT CREDENTIALING

Credentialing of case managers by the organization that employs them is on the rise. Healthcare organizations may use credentialing of case managers as a process to assure a professional possesses appropriate credentials to practice in the role of case manager. The current sociopolitical dynamics of the healthcare environment and the health policy work being done by professional organizations such as CMSA will make credentialing of case managers more popular. For example, CMSA continues to advocate for reimbursement for case management services in all care settings across the continuum of health and human services and not just the ambulatory care setting where reimbursement using specific current procedural terminology (CPT) codes is available. CMSA is also working on reimbursement eligibility for case managers by Medicare and Medicaid services. Such privileges will make credentialing as a normal practice for four reasons:

1. More professionals are becoming case managers, especially those with advanced degrees and education.
2. Healthcare providers and executives are pursuing practitioners with advanced preparation for the role of case manager.
3. Accreditation agencies have included credentialing in their accreditation standards and expect providers to have a process for credentialing of case managers.
4. Reimbursement for care coordination and transitions of care services, especially from the CMS.

Advanced practitioners who assume the case manager's role are licensed professionals and mostly have graduate educational degrees in a particular discipline such as nursing, healthcare management, or social work.

Credentialing is a peer review process one undergoes to provide evidence of continued competence, advanced knowledge and skills, and good standing. It is important for demonstrating that one's certification, license, and practice privileges are current and that one's performance satisfactorily meets the standards of competence. The successful completion of this process results in the endorsement of case managers for continued practice; that is, the authority, responsibility, and accountability to perform certain duties and clinical activities as designated in their job description and scope of practice. The process of credentialing must be planned and operationalized in a systematic way.

Credentialing can be implemented as an annual or bi-annual formal peer review process and may include the examination of the following:

- Professional license
- Certification/recertification status
- Educational background
- Competence
- Knowledge and skill of current practice trends
- Professional conduct—ethical and moral
- Demonstrated quality outcomes in performance/practice

Currently, credentialing is not mandatory. It is carried out by individual healthcare organizations voluntarily for ensuring public interest, consumer protection and safety, ethical practice, and professional development. Mandatory credentialing of case managers cannot occur until a nationwide standardization of the case manager's role, scope of practice, and education are established. Consumers of case management services demand the assurance that case managers are properly licensed, certified, and credentialed. Credentialing through a peer review process helps organizations meet such consumer demands.

9.11. HIRING CASE MANAGERS

Interviewing or being interviewed for a job/position is something nearly everyone has to do at one time or another during one's career. It is probably the most important, intimidating, and demanding task one will ever be involved in. The reward of interviewing well is getting hired for the job. Candidates for the case manager role face a challenging task. They need to prove to their prospective employers, on paper and in person, that they are the best candidates for the role.

The number of experienced candidates for the case manager's role has been limited while the number of available positions has been increasing because restructuring and redesigning of patient care delivery have resulted in case management systems being identified as key delivery models in most institutions. Given this demand, many schools have incorporated specific courses or content in their curricula. However, only a few programs are available today that are dedicated to the training and education for case management at the graduate or post-baccalaureate levels. Despite these efforts, finding experienced and educated candidates for the case manager role continues to be a challenge; demand outweighs the supply. This has resulted in an increased competition as recruiters and potential employers select the best candidate for the case manager's role. This section discusses the interview process of

case managers and the roles of the candidate and the interviewer. In addition, it provides some tips for success in both roles.

9.12. CANDIDATES FOR THE CASE MANAGER ROLE

Employers select their candidates for the case manager's role based on the applicant's clinical and leadership skills and knowledge in case management. The criteria considered in the potential candidate include resourcefulness, flexibility, adaptability, tolerance to stress and hard work, teamwork, dependability, truthfulness, reliability, effectiveness, perseverance, and ability to manage change and conquer challenge. Other criteria relate to clinical expertise in an area of practice (e.g., cardiology, health insurance plans, or long-term care), specialty certification, and case management certification.

To be hired for the case manager's position, potential candidates should prepare themselves to be "The Candidate." They must go beyond preparing an "attractive" resume. They need not only be able to intelligently market themselves on paper but also to sell themselves even more carefully during the job interview process. This task can be quite intimidating and requires high-level written and verbal skills.

9.12.1. Preparing the Resume and Curriculum Vitae

Today's advertisements no longer include the telephone numbers of the recruiter or recruitment office; instead a mailing address (mostly electronic) is provided. This change in advertising makes the resume and curriculum vitae (CV) extremely important. Resumes and CVs are personal marketing and sales tools and should contain accurate information reflective of the candidate's past and current experiences, skills, accomplishments, and honors. They become the only compelling source of information available to prospective employers for targeting candidates for interviews. Resumes and CVs should summarize the candidate's best attributes, including the following:

- Career objective(s) and vision
- Employment history, highlighting the most recent experience
- Education
- Licensure, certifications, awards, and honors
- Scholarship activities: previous research, public speaking activities, and citations of published materials

- Professional organizations or societies
- Volunteer work or community services
- Other skills (e.g., languages spoken, computer skills)
- Available references

Resumes and CVs require a special type of writing that may not conform to the rules of grammar or punctuation, which makes them easier to write. When preparing your resume/CV, as candidates for the case manager role you may face some challenges in articulating your previous experiences or conveying the extent of the skills you possess. To overcome this challenge, you may seek the help of professional agencies that specialize in writing resumes, or refer to books on business writing (i.e., how to write resumes and cover letters). Such books can be found in public and private libraries and in the business sections of bookstores. Today, similar information is easily found online. However, if you seek help in writing the resume, it is important that you assure the final product provides the potential employer with your comprehensive profile, stressing what contributions you potentially may offer the institution (Case Manager's Tip 9.6).

Resumes and CVs are different but also somewhat similar. They vary based on length and degree of detail. The length of the resume usually does not exceed two to three pages. However, CVs are generally longer than resumes (they may be longer than 10 pages) and include more details. Although not a standard rule, resumes tend to start with work experience first, while CVs begin with the educational background. This is why CVs are thought of as more academic than re-

CASE MANAGER'S TIP 9.6

Importance of the Resume or Curriculum Vitae

Writing a compelling resume or CV is important to guarantee an interview opportunity. Today's process for applying for a job is limited to an online approach. You may apply for a position without having a chance to speak or meet in person with a recruiter or case management leader. Therefore, preparing a resume or CV that communicates your skills, knowledge, competencies, work experience and other credentials is important to increasing your chances of being called for a job interview. Most automated systems screen candidates based on answers to specific questions and often completing a detailed application is contingent upon your answers of the screening questions. These usually include the qualifications for the job the potential employer is looking for.

sumes. The work history and experience consume most of the length (Case Manager's Tip 9.7). In both resumes and CVs, candidates may highlight their work experience and skills following either a reverse chronological format or a grouping of tasks and skills. The formats are equally appropriate. In the reverse chronological history, the work history is listed starting with the latest job held. In contrast, the grouping of tasks and skills format requires a synthesis of the categories of these tasks and skills based on all previous jobs held. The advantage of the latter format is that the candidate has the flexibility of highlighting the skills, tasks, and qualities most appropriate to the case manager's role regardless of the time they were acquired, performed, or applied. Candidates for the case manager's role who do not have case management experience are advised to prepare their resume following the grouping of tasks and skills format. This format will clearly show the qualities that make them the best candidate for the job.

Box 9.4 presents an excerpt from an ad for a case

CASE MANAGER'S TIP 9.7

Suggestions for Writing Resumes or Curriculum Vitae

- Include a summary statement about your professional background.
- Describe your work experience using factual and detailed information.
- Be specific with your educational background, credentials, licensure, and certifications.
- Include the time period of each of your past work experiences and educational background. Be accurate with dates and include the months and years.
- Organize your past experiences and educational background information in the same chronological order; reverse chronological is preferred.
- Do not include the number(s) of your license(s).
- List your accomplishments; include those that relate to your work and volunteer associations.
- Add a statement about your career vision, job objectives, and/or goals.
- Make your resume/CV reader-friendly: use a consistent format throughout, font size 12, bulleted lists, and recognizable sections.
- Be concise and to the point in your descriptions: "less is more."
- Include a list of selected publications and presentations; most recent 5 years or 10 years if not a lengthy list.
- Highlight any honors or awards you may have received.
- Highlight community service involvement.

> **Box 9.4   Excerpt from an Ad for a Case Manager's Job**
>
> In this position as a case manager you will be responsible for working with an *interdisciplinary/interprofessional team* of healthcare providers and *managing the care* of a select group of patients with complex diagnoses (chronic illnesses) and needs. You are expected to achieve *high-quality* care *outcomes* in a *safe and cost-effective* manner. You will act as a patient and family *advocate* and a *consultant* for members of the healthcare team within the institution and for health insurance plans, and for community resource agencies externally. The ideal candidate will possess a minimum of *4 years' clinical experience* and a current license as a registered professional nurse or certification as a social worker. A bachelor's degree is also required. The candidate must demonstrate strong *problem solving* skills and the ability to make *sound clinical judgments* and apply *critical thinking* in an effective manner. Excellent *verbal and written communication skills*, case management experience, and *certification* are a plus.

manager position that one might come across in a newspaper, professional nursing journal, or recruitment newsletter. Potential applicants should study the ad carefully and be able to identify the qualities, skills, and qualifications the organization is looking for in the candidate (i.e., the *italicized* areas in Box 9.4). These qualities and skills may not be clearly stated in the ad. It is the responsibility of the candidate applying for the job to synthesize the desired qualifications. The resume or CV should then be written in a way that addresses the identified characteristics of the job. Candidates must not arbitrarily submit a resume or a CV; they must stick to what is specified in the ad.

9.12.2. Cover Letter

A cover letter explaining the candidate's intent to apply for the job is important to have attached to the resume or CV before submitting an application to a potential employer. Almost all online talent acquisition software applications allow for uploading a cover letter and a resume or CV despite the use of structured features or questions. In the letter, as the candidate, you should indicate the specific ad you are responding to (i.e., specify the job title and the source of the ad). If you are applying online, this may be automatically populated as part of the process. The letter should also include your career objective(s) and highlight the acquired qualities and skills that meet the job requirements. For example, if you are responding to the ad presented in Box 9.4,

it is important that you describe your skills in communication, teamwork, negotiation, brokering, facilitation, coordination of patient care activities, and evaluation of care outcomes. It is also important to highlight your knowledge of healthcare reimbursement systems, health insurance plans, managed care organizations, and patient and family satisfaction issues. Additionally, it is beneficial to identify your clinical and leadership skills as they relate to the advertised job.

Because there will be no personal contact with the recruiter or prospective employer to discuss the job, you should put special effort into writing the best resume/CV and cover letter possible to increase your chances for an interview. You also should exercise special attention to how you answer the questions on the automated application. Your answers will determine whether you will be called for an interview; your answers will screen you in or out. The resume/CV and cover letter are your selling tools. They reflect your marketability, and they should "paint a picture" of your potential for success in the job. Review them carefully for any typographical or spelling errors, long or run-on sentences, and appropriateness of the adjectives used to describe yourself. Always remember to be concise, clear, and direct.

In the letter, candidates should indicate how their skills and previous experiences can be used in the prospective job or for the benefit of the institution. The style applied in the cover letter should appeal to the talent acquistion manager/recruiter or the prospective employer. Avoid being overly clever or too wordy. Try to be honest, warm, and sincere. Use phrases that will increase interest in you (e.g., be results oriented), and emphasize those aspects of yourself that you think will meet the case manager's role and make you look attractive. The cover letter should not be too long or boring to read. It should urge the prospective employer to review the resume/CV and call you for an interview.

9.12.3. Looking Your Best

The interview is the opportunity to prove yourself. It is an act of validating that a potential candidate is the best fit for the job. The interview process should validate for the interviewer that your description of your qualifications and skills, evidenced in the resume/CV and cover letter, is accurate. Your responses to the interview questions should strongly support what you have written in the resume/CV. You should be at your best and look your best.

One way of improving your chances of being hired for the job is by familiarizing yourself with the role or position you are interviewing for and the institution/

prospective employer. It is important for any case manager candidate to keep abreast of the latest changes occurring in the healthcare industry. Two decades ago, case management models were strange to hospitals and healthcare organizations. Training of case managers was held in the healthcare organization itself as part of the orientation to the new work environment and the role. However, because of the redesign of patient care delivery systems, today these models and roles are more popular, and formal eductaion and training in case management, although still limited, has become available in some schools of nursing or online educational agencies as certificate and degree programs. This shift into case management has increased the competition among the candidates for the case manager's role and helped prospective employers in selecting the best-prepared candidate for the job.

The healthcare-related literature contains a substantial amount of information on case management models and roles. It is important for you as potential candidates to become knowledgeable in this field before applying for the role, especially if you have not had any prior training or experience in case management.

The case manager's role varies from one institution to another. One's experience as a case manager in one institution might not be transferable. Therefore it is important for a candidate to evaluate his or her previous experience in relation to the skills and qualifications required for the job being interviewed for and to proactively determine how to maximize the benefit of this experience for the interview.

It is important for you to obtain the job description of the advertised role and the mission and philosophy statements of the institution before the interview and to study them carefully. This information is invaluable for you when you prepare for the interview and is instrumental in familiarizing yourself with the potential work environment; expectations of the role; and the institution's culture, values, and beliefs. As candidates for the role, you may ask for this information in advance through a personal letter (preferably via e-mail) addressed to the talent acquisition manager/recruiter at the address available in the ad. You may also ask for this information in the cover letter you attach to the resume/CV, either at the time you send the information to the talent acquisition manager or the prospective employer, or when you are contacted to set up a date for the interview. Either way, it is important to obtain and review this information before the interview.

Potential case managers should be able to convince their prospective employer that they are the right candidates for the job and the organization. One way to accomplish this is by conveying a sense of profession-alism. You should clearly articulate your strengths and weaknesses as they relate to the job. You should also explain your willingness to learn and improve in the areas in which you lack experience. You should be comfortable in providing evidence to the interviewer that you possess the qualities, skills, and attributes necessary for the position. Sometimes it is helpful to maximize the use of real examples related to previous experiences to convince the interviewer that you are "The Candidate." The interviewer expects a candidate to be lacking knowledge or experience in some aspects of the job, and candidates who recognize or address this issue demonstrate a clear understanding of the job requirements and willingness to learn. It is also important that you make the interviewers aware of your potential. Explain to them what it is that you are able to bring with you that is considered beneficial to the institution. Concentrate on meeting the organization's mission statement and philosophy. Make an effort to discuss your transferable skills (i.e., the skills you can carry with you to any job or organization).

The outer appearance of potential candidates for the case manager's role is important. It is the first impression you leave with the interviewer/prospective employer. The way you are dressed should create a positive and professional image. This image plays a crucial role in setting the tone for the rest of the interview. You should make an effort to look professional even if you know that the prospective employer has a relaxed dress code. You should dress for success (Case Manager's Tip 9.8).

During the interview, you should be extra careful in how you respond to the interviewer's questions. Do

CASE MANAGER'S TIP 9.8

Dress for Success

- What you wear reflects who and what you are.
- Dressing in business attire is preferred.
- Play it safe and stick to conservative colors such as navy blue, black, or gray.
- Keep jewelry and accessories to a minimum; be tasteful in your choices.
- Avoid strong cologne or perfume.
- Stand and sit erect during the interview.
- Maintain eye contact during the interview, smile, and take a pause as you articulate your answers.

Note: If the interview is done remotely using telecommunication technology such as videoconferencing it is advisable to still dress for success and follow the above recommendations.

not appear to be rigid, indifferent, or inflexible. Avoid using statements that begin with "I never . . . ," "I don't like . . . ," or "It is impossible to . . ." The following examples illustrate this point.

- *Do not say*: "In my previous job I never attempted to call the private physicians myself because it made them angry. Instead, I always asked the nurse manager to do that." It is better to say: "In my previous job I was not expected to contact the private physicians myself, but I understand the importance of discussing a particular situation with them directly. I am willing to and have no problem doing that in this position."
- *Do not say*: "In the past I found it impossible to discuss the plan of care of each patient with the various healthcare providers." It is better to say: "It is a great challenge to discuss the plan of care of each patient with the various healthcare providers, and I understand its importance in improving the quality of care. I will do the best that I can in this area."
- *Do not say*: "Why should I keep pushing for rescheduling a procedure that is cancelled? It is not my responsibility to do it. It is the responsibility of the department canceling the procedure." It is better to say: "I understand how difficult it can be to ensure that a procedure is completed as scheduled. It is important to not delay the completion of a procedure. Otherwise, the patient and the institution suffer (or the cost and quality of care are compromised)."

In your answers to interviewers' questions, use statements that convey an understanding of the case manager's role, flexibility in your opinions and attitudes, openness to change and try new methods of doing things, and willingness to learn and expand knowledge. You should avoid stating what you have always done in your previous jobs. However, you can use your previous experiences in subtle ways to support your claim of flexibility as practitioners and confirm to the interviewers that you possess the skills and qualities the interviewers seek in the potential case managers.

9.12.4. Questions That May Be Asked by Candidates

It is appropriate for candidates to ask questions during the interview process. However, questions should be asked when opportunities exist. For example, interviewers may ask candidates at some point during the interview process if they have any questions. If this does not happen, then candidates may ask their questions toward the end of the interview. Questions that are considered appropriate include the following:

- Patient population(s)
- Area of responsibility (e.g., inpatient unit, outpatient clinic, both areas)
- Expectations regarding performance, especially during first year of employment
- Expected hours of work (e.g., days, evenings, weekends, rotation)
- Reporting mechanism (i.e., the case manager's position in the table of organization; centralized team or decentralized by service lines)
- Current status (performance of the department) in relation to case management and institutional goals
- Support systems (i.e., case management assistive personnel and use of technology)
- Orientation process to the work environment and the role

The salary should not be discussed during the interview unless it is brought up by the interviewer. It is always better to negotiate the salary at the time the job is offered. Candidates may also ask the interviewer about the timeframe for filling the job or how long it will be before they are notified if they are selected. Candidates may contact the talent acquisition manager and inquire if a decision has been made if the indicated timeframe has passed. It is acceptable to ask about the reasons for not being chosen. Interviewing is a demanding skill, and one cannot improve unless if made aware of deficient areas and opportunities for further development.

9.13. CHARACTERISTICS LOOKED FOR IN POTENTIAL CANDIDATES FOR THE CASE MANAGER'S ROLE

The role of the case manager is integral to the success of the case management program. During the interview process candidates for this job should reflect potential for success in the role. There are several significant skills case management leaders look for in candidates for the case manager's role (Box 9.5). These skills are based on the job description of the case manager and are affected by the environment of work, care setting, and scope of responsibilities (i.e., the operations/systems of the organization, policies, procedures, standards of care and practice, and status and power embedded in the job as compared with other healthcare professionals on the care delivery team). The most important skills are those that make the potential candidate able to collaborate effectively with other healthcare providers within and outside the organization.

Box 9.5 Case Manager's Skills

- Clinical
- Leadership
- Teamwork, cooperation, and collaboration
- Time management and priority setting
- Decision making/problem solving
- Critical thinking and clinical judgment
- Organization
- Delegation and supervision
- Communication/open-mindedness/assertiveness
- Diplomacy/political savvy
- Tolerance
- Emotional intelligence
- Commitment and accountability
- Education/teaching
- Role modeling
- Change agent
- Motivational interviewing
- Conflict resolution
- Power
- Cultural sensitivity
- Information management and reporting
- Computer literacy
- Proficiency in case management software applications
- Flexibility and taking initiative

A person in the case manager position is expected to work with minimum direction and supervision. Because the case manager is an integral member of an interdisciplinary team of healthcare professionals, he or she is expected to demonstrate excellent decision-making and problem-solving skills. In addition, the case manager should exhibit a willingness to work with others (i.e., teamwork and collaboration). Because of the varied responsibilities of this position, the case manager should have superior organizational, priority setting, and time-management skills. This is important for increased productivity and efficiency in the role. Case managers work daily with physicians, nurses, patients and families, payer representatives, and other healthcare providers to ensure that high-quality, safe and cost-effective care and outcomes are achieved. These expectations make assertiveness, the ability to communicate well verbally and in writing, diplomacy, and open-mindedness among the many skills required for success in the role.

Case managers spend much of their time facilitating and coordinating patient care activities, advocating for their patients/families, and resolving variances or delays in care. In this role function, they are expected to demonstrate skills in leadership, clinical care activities, tolerance, emotional intelligence, communication, delegation, and negotiation. When they hold patient and family teaching sessions, they apply the adult learning theory into their practice and follow the strategies derived from the health-belief model, which means that they should be knowledgeable about the available theories on patient and family teaching and behavior change. In addition, when they are asked for help by a member of the healthcare team, they are looked at as role models and resource people. They are expected to be able to find solutions to challenging situations.

9.14. INTERVIEWER'S ROLE

During the interview process, interviewers should evaluate whether potential candidates possess the skills required for the role. If candidates are found to be lacking in any of the necessary skills or functions, interviewers should evaluate them for potential success in learning these functions and acquiring the necessary skills and competencies. The questions to be asked in an interview should cover the affective, cognitive, and behavioral aspects of the case manager's role.

The best questions to be asked are open-ended ones, referred to as behavioral interviewing questions (Table 9.2). Potential candidates should also be asked to provide practical examples that support their abilities and help demonstrate competence in their skills. As an interviewer it is your role to ask the candidate to share examples of prior experiences in a behavioral context if the candidate does not respond to interview questions in that manner. Examples are particularly important because they provide concrete evidence related to a candidate's performance in real work situations. Examples usually validate a candidate's answers because they add an objective flavor to subjective answers. When candidates are found to be struggling with giving examples, the interviewer may use hypothetical situations to help them express their opinions.

The interviewer must be careful not to ask questions that are considered against the law, as determined by the Americans with Disabilities Act, Equal Employment Opportunity Act, and Age Discrimination in Employment Act. Interviewers should avoid questions such as the following:

- How old are you?
- How many children do you have?
- How old are your children?
- Are you married?
- What religious holidays do you observe?
- What language do you speak when not at work?
- What is your ethnic background?
- What are your political beliefs?

Interviewers should take their time when conducting

TABLE 9.2. Sample Questions That May Be Asked in the Case Manager's Interview.

Questions	Behaviors/Skills Evaluated
Tell me about yourself.	<ul><li>Personality type</li><li>Energy</li><li>Optimism</li><li>Ego</li></ul>
Give me an example of when you had too many things to do at once, and tell me how you went about accomplishing the tasks.	<ul><li>Time management</li><li>Organizational skills</li><li>Prioritization</li><li>Creating a plan</li><li>Getting tasks accomplished</li></ul>
Tell me about a problem you have faced in the past with a patient/family member, co-worker, physician, or superior. How did you handle the situation?	<ul><li>Conflict resolution and problem solving</li><li>Dealing with stress</li><li>Affect/temperament</li><li>Teamwork/independence</li><li>Effectiveness</li><li>Assertiveness</li><li>Comfort level with confrontation</li></ul>
Explain to me what makes you the best candidate for the job.	<ul><li>Motivation</li><li>Self-confidence and self-esteem</li><li>Ability to discuss strengths and weaknesses</li><li>Experience</li><li>Assertiveness</li></ul>
From your past experience, tell me about a time when you had to promote change. How were you able to do it? What role did you play in it?	<ul><li>Perseverance</li><li>Change agent</li><li>Adaptability and flexibility</li><li>Openness to change and new ideas</li><li>Ability to influence others</li><li>Assertiveness</li><li>Risk taking</li><li>Creativity</li></ul>
In your opinion, what does a case manager do?	<ul><li>Knowledge and understanding</li><li>Potentials</li><li>Keeping up-to-date with changes in healthcare</li></ul>
Tell me about a time when you were able to influence the behavior of others in a positive way.	<ul><li>Encouragement of others</li><li>Teamwork/team player</li><li>Ability to provide feedback</li><li>Interpersonal skills</li><li>Creativity and paradigm shift</li><li>Willingness to try new ideas</li></ul>
Describe a situation when you were able to impact the cost of patient care.	<ul><li>Awareness of healthcare costs</li><li>Cost-containment strategies</li><li>Allocation/management of resource utilization.</li></ul>
Tell me about a time when you were faced with a problem and needed to collect some information for solving the problem. Describe to me how you analyzed the information.	<ul><li>Problem solving</li><li>Critical thinking</li><li>Use of data and evidence</li><li>Response to stressful situations/affect</li><li>Willingness to complete a project/task to come to your decision</li><li>Commitment</li></ul>

(continued)

TABLE 9.2 (Continued). Sample Questions That May Be Asked in the Case Manager's Interview.

Questions	Behaviors/Skills Evaluated
Describe to me a situation when you had to work with little or no supervision. What did you do?	• Independence • Motivation • Commitment • Productivity • Leadership
What is it that you can bring to this role/institution that will make a difference?	• Previous experience • Ability to identify one's strengths • Confidence/self-esteem • Visionary
Tell me about your career goals.	• Goal orientation • Having a vision • Future planning • Ability to be focused
Discuss the biggest mistake you ever made.	• Self-confidence • Truthfulness/authenticity • Learning • Admitting to mistakes

the interview. They should avoid making candidates feel rushed or unimportant. A reasonable interview is one that lasts an average of 1 hour. Similar to the candidates, interviewers are required to be poised, clear, direct, articulate, and skillful in the interview process. It is imperative for interviewers not to bore candidates by talking too much about the institution and the job. They should avoid unnecessary rambling. They also should begin the interview with a personal casual conversation to make the candidate feel welcome and comfortable. For example, acknowledge the candidate for his or her interest in the job and how pleased your are to meet the candidate. Also ask about the candidate's travel to the organization; was there any trouble driving, locating the organization and office? Casual conversation puts the candidate at ease.

Interviewers should prepare the interview questions in advance. As much as possible, they should use the same set of questions for interviewing all potential candidates. This pattern makes it easier to remain fair and equitable with all candidates, compare candidates and select the best one for the job. Most institutions have a standardized interviewing process in place and a predetermined set of questions that can be adapted to each specific job. If this is not the case in your institution, it is helpful to prepare interview questions beforehand.

At the end of the interview, interviewers may summarize the interview by explaining the next step(s) to candidates. This may include whether follow-up interviews are necessary and, if so, with whom, when, and where. It is also important that candidates be informed of the timeframe for filling the position and the method of notifying the selected candidate. This eliminates any confusion candidates may face while waiting to hear from the interviewer/potential employer.

9.15. FOLLOW-UP INTERVIEWS

Candidates for the case manager's role are usually interviewed more than once. They are interviewed by the talent acquisition manager and by the administrator of the case management program. Some institutions also require them to interview with a panel (i.e., representatives from the interdisciplinary team such as physicians, other case managers, directors of nursing, nurse managers, social workers, physical therapists, quality management staff, and home care coordinators). Depending on the job description and roles and responsibilities, potential candidates may be required to interview with chief physicians or chairmen of departments, or senior leaders responsible for the case management department. Candidates should prepare themselves well for impressive and successful interviews throughout the interview process an institution may have in place.

When interviewed by physicians or chairmen of departments, it is important for a candidate to convey a message of openness, collegiality, collaboration and partnership, and clinical knowledge. It is also important that he or she convey excellence in teamwork, negotiation, leadership, mentorship, problem solving, conflict resolution, and coaching skills.

Candidates are first interviewed by a talent acquisition manager, who screens them and selects those who express strong potential for success in the case manager's role. Often the screening is happening today by phone or telecommunication technology such as videoconferencing. Next they are interviewed by the administrator of the case management program. Those who are found to be impressive and show strong potential are then called for follow-up interviews. The follow-up interviews, depending on the institution, may include an interview with a physician or the chairman of the department in which the case manager will be working, and another with a panel of interviewers, including representatives from the interdisciplinary healthcare team and fellow case managers.

 CASE MANAGER'S TIP 9.9

Suggestions for the Interviewer

- Ask open-ended questions: background, behavioral, situational, conversational/nondirective, and directive.
- Establish rapport at the beginning of the interview; make the candidate feel at ease.
- Begin with "ice-breaking" questions (e.g., It is a lovely day today; how was your trip coming here?).
- Allow silence; the candidate may need to collect his or her thoughts before answering the question.
- Ask behavioral questions.
- Control the interview; you may need to redirect the conversation if the candidate starts to ramble around and is not focusing on the question.
- If you want to take notes, explain why; obtain permission from the candidate.
- Prepare the questions in advance. Questions should be based on the related job description, qualifications, and/or the candidate's resume/CV.
- Ask questions that are based on the candidate's past job experiences and the needs of the job. This allows for envisioning the future and investigating the candidate's potential.
- Ask for contrary evidence, especially when identifying an undesired or a negative skill. Contrary evidence prevents the interviewer from creating a one-sided/ subjective picture.
- Validate responses using reflective statements as needed.
- Avoid judgment, and be objective. Do not allow intuition or "gut feelings" to interfere in your decision.
- Familiarize yourself with the skills required for the job (e.g., performance, organizational, interactional).
- Apply a businesslike approach to the interview process.

 CASE MANAGER'S TIP 9.10

Suggestions for the Candidate

- Ask for the job description, the organization's mission and philosophy statements, and the case management program goals in advance. Study them well.
- Research the prospective employer and organization. This will allow you to speak with a degree of confidence and familiarity with the organization.
- Arrive for the interview on time.
- Dress for success.
- Bring your portfolio to the interview. Be prepared to share concrete evidence of your accomplishments when appropriate.
- Watch your body language/nonverbal communication. It is a part of the interview too. Sit straight and erect with your head up. Do not fidget.
- Maintain eye contact at all times.
- Do not interrupt the interviewer.
- Avoid rambling in your answers. Be poised, concise, clear, and direct.
- Support your answers with evidence (i.e., examples from previous experiences, tell a compelling story in your answers).
- Be prepared to discuss what it is that you can provide to the organization (your assets).
- Convey your self-confidence, professionalism, and self-esteem through your answers.
- Do not hesitate to explain your silence at times. The interviewer is aware that you may need a moment of silence to collect your thoughts before answering a question.
- Avoid speaking fast or stuttering. Be articulate.
- Be clear in your career goals.
- Rehearse your interview if that helps you to be better prepared.
- Apply a businesslike approach to the interview process.
- Do not downplay your achievements.
- Avoid criticizing your present or past employer or supervisor. You do not want to be perceived as a complainer.
- Be careful and guard against displaying nervous habits.

It is important to limit the follow-up interviews to only the candidates who express promising success in the role. The talent acquisition manager and the administrator of the case management program may collaborate in selecting these candidates, which usually are limited to two or three in number. Unnecessary interviews waste time and cost money. Candidates should be informed by the interviewer of the next steps, whether follow-up interviews will be conducted, and when they will be informed of such decisions.

Candidates should not forget about the interviewer after the interview is over. It is advisable to send a note (e.g., e-mail) or a card thanking the interviewer for the opportunity and the consideration. It is also appropriate for candidates to indicate in the note their continued interest in the job.

Conducting interviews and being interviewed are great challenges. One should learn how to meet these challenges. It is beneficial to read about the interview process or attend seminars to polish your interviewing skills. Another strategy to prepare for a successful interview is practicing with a colleague who is comfortable in providing authentic feedback and offer suggestions for improvement. This practice may help you get the job you desire. Case Manager's Tips 9.9 and 9.10 present some tips for the interviewer and the candidate. These tips should help both the interviewer to be better prepared for evaluating and screening the appropriate candidates for the job and the potential candidates to overcome their fear of being interviewed. The skills necessary for interviewing well are important for everyone to master because one never knows when they may be necessary. You should always remember that the written words (i.e., the resume/CV and cover letter) are the candidate's ambassador to the interviewer. They should be thought of as a glorified list of one's qualities, which when read leave a lasting impression and a desire for an in-person interview. Considering the popularity of online applications, these written words are a gateway for joining an organization and getting the dream job one desires; never compromise on the application process or underestimate its importance.

9.16. KEY POINTS

1. Case management training and education programs are of different types. They either are college/university-based, healthcare provider organization-based, or independent agency-based.
2. Case management training and education programs are available as certificate or degree granting programs.
3. Regardless of their preparation or background in case management, case managers are eligible to sit for case manager certification examination. One must be able to find the appropriate certification that advances one's professional stature.
4. Certification in case management is important because it affirms that case managers possess the knowledge, skills, and competence re-

quired for rendering case management services to their clients.
5. It is important for case managers to examine all of their certification options before they select a specific certification. Case managers must select the certification that best fits their field of practice and meets the employer's expectations.
6. The interview process for a case management position is not easy. It requires careful and thorough preparation by the candidate and the interviewer. Practice, role play, or rehearsal before the interview could be helpful.
7. Candidates for the case manager's job should always send a resume/CV with a cover letter to potential employers explaining their intent for applying for an advertised job and summarizing their qualifications for the job.
8. The resume/CV is a compelling source of information for the prospective employer. An impressive resume/CV is one that summarizes the candidate's knowledge, experiences, attributes, and skills. Most organizations use an electronic application process; make sure as a candidate to carefully and thoughtfully answer the questions on the application and convey your qualifications in an effective and powerful manner.
9. The cover letter should delineate acquired qualities and skills as a candidate, especially those that meet the requirements of the job applied for and anticipated employer's interests.
10. Avoid being rigid, indifferent, or inflexible during an interview (this is applicable for both the candidate and the interviewer).
11. If interviewing several candidates for a job, use a standardized set of questions that could be prepared based on the job description and that should reflect the skills and qualities demanded by the job. It also is helpful to apply a scoring/rating system in the process. This makes it easier to differentiate among the applicants and to select the best candidate for the job.

9.17. REFERENCES

American Nurses Credentialing Center (ANCC). (2014). 2013 Role Delineation Study: Nursing Case Management, Silver Springs, MD.

Commission for Case Manager Certification (The Commission). (2016).: CCM certification guide, Mount Laurel, NJ.

Falter, E., Cesta, T., Concert, C., & Mason, D.J. (1999). Development of a graduate nursing program in case management, *J Care Manag* 5(3):50–78.

Haw, M. (1995). State-of-the-art education for case management in long-term care, *J Case Management 4*(3):85–94.

Haw, M. (1996). Case management education in universities: A national survey, *J Care Manag 2*(6):10–23.

Kuric, J.L. & White, A.H. (2005). Case management curriculum in nursing education, *Lippincott Case Management, 10*(2), 102–107.

Latimmer, C., Executive Director of the Case Management Society of America, in personal conversation, June 24, 2015.

National Association of Social Workers (NASW). (2015). Specialty Certifications, Information Booklet with Application and Reference Forms, Certified Social Work Case Manager and Certified Advanced Social Work Case Manager, Washington, DC.

Scheyett, A. & Blyler, C. (2002). An exploration of case management courses in university curricula, *Psychiatric Rehabilitation Journal, 26*(1), 86–90.

Seton Hall University, College of Nursing. Accessed June 20, 2015. Seton Hall University's nurse case management certificate program, South Orange, NJ. Available at www.shu.edu/academics/nursing/certificate-programs.cfm

Simmons, F. (1992). Developing the trauma nurse case manager role, *Dimens Crit Care Nurs 11*(3):164–170.

Sowell, R. & Young, S. (1997). Case management in the nursing curriculum, *Nurs Case Manag 2*(4):173–176.

Tahan, H.A., Watson, A.C., & Sminkey, P.V. 2016. Informing the content and composition of the CCM® certification examination: A national study from the Commission for Case Manager Certification—Part II, *Porfessional Case Management, 21*(1): 3–21.

Toran, M. (1998). Academic case management, *Case Manager 9*(1):43–46.

Trieger, T. & Fink-Samnick, E. (2015). Collaborate for Professional Case Management: A Universal Competency Based Paradigm, Walters Kluwer, Philadelphia, PA.

University of Southern Indiana, College of Nursing and Health Professions. Accessed June 20, 2015. Case management/care coordination certificate program. Available at www.usi.edu/health/certificate-programs/case-managementcare-coordination-certificate-program

University of Alabama, Capstone College of Nursing, Graduate Student Handbook 2014–2015. http://nursing.ua.edu/student_handbook.htm.

10 Case Management Plans of Care

There is no doubt that the current healthcare delivery system in virtually every setting across the continuum of care has been experiencing massive and revolutionary changes. With the advent of the Patient Protection and Affordable Care Act of 2010 and the increased number of insured individuals, the continued popularity of commercial health insurance carries (e.g., those who have a managed care health insurance plan), managed competition and the interest of consumers in quality, safe, and cost-effective care, healthcare leaders, nursing executives in particular, are pressured to seek intelligent transformations in the way care is delivered. Most healthcare organizations, whether acute, ambulatory, rehabilitative, long term, or home care, have undergone some sort of redesign. Most importantly, case management programs have become an integral strategy of care delivery in virtually every care setting across the continuum of health and human services. Regardless of the setting, case management is viewed as the best way to assure the delivery of high-quality, efficient, safe, and cost-effective care.

Case management delivery systems have also been proven successful in caring for poulations with multiple chronic illnesses. These approaches to care use evidence-based and standardized case management plans (CMPs) that delineate the best/ideal practice and expected outcomes. Chapter 10 discusses a 10-step process for developing these plans. The process provides a template for healthcare professionals who are interested in implementing CMPs and a step-by-step guide to developing them, with practical examples to simplify the process.

Although CMPs are not new to many healthcare organizations across the continuum of care, there is a renewed insterest in their use today. What is different this time is the intentional focus on implementation of evidence-based practices with the aim of eliminating variations in care provision across providers, access to care at the right amount, by the right provider, and in the right setting, and clearly delineated expected milestones and outcomes that reflect quality and safe care. The lack of a deliberate and systematic process to develop these plans holds healthcare organizations back from creating timely and efficient results while avoiding the financial risk imposed by the current value-based purchasing program. Chapter 10 is highly beneficial for healthcare providers and case managers in particular, who are involved in the development of CMPs. They may acquire new knowledge and strategies to simplify the task of developing CMPs, or even choose to implement the proposed process if they currently do not have a formal one in place.

10.1. OVERVIEW OF CASE MANAGEMENT PLANS

Similar to case management delivery systems, CMPs are popular because of the economic and political characteristics and pressures of the healthcare environment. Some of the driving forces of CMPs are as follows:

1. Changes in reimbursement methods: prospective payment systems, case rates, capitation, bundled payments, financial risk sharing
2. The advent of managed care and managed competition
3. Consumerism and industrialization of the healthcare market

4. Standards of regulatory and accreditation agencies and their requirements of a quality, safe, collaborative, evidence-based, and seamless approach to care provision

5. Disparity in the use of resources as a result of variations in practice patterns of healthcare providers

6. Demand of consumers and consumer advocates for quality, safe, accessible, and cost-effective care

7. Demand for easy access to heathcare services and resources

8. Pressure for evidence-based decisions about best healthcare delivery strategies

9. Increase in lawsuits and healthcare litigation

10. Increasingly complex and costly innovations in healthcare technology and treatment options

Since their inception, CMPs have been used as tools to define the standards of care and practice and as guides for patient care activities that are evidence-based for all members of the healthcare team alike. Whatever they are called, they define the optimal schedule and amount of key interventions to be provided by the various professional disciplines and providers to achieve desired patient outcomes for a particular diagnosis or procedure. They are systematically developed as statements, guidelines, and strategies for patient care management. CMPs are important tools developed to assist providers in delineating the desired sequence of interventions, treatments, and services, and making decisions about appropriate and necessary interventions that effectively address particular clinical situations. They usually incorporate the best scientific evidence of effectiveness with expert opinion and recommendations of governmental, professional, or specialty organizations. Moreover, they incorporate patient preferences and values in an effort to deliver patient and family-centered care.

CMPs have been in use for over a half century; however, they have been known as practice guidelines (PGs) and were originally developed by physician groups mainly for malpractice and risk management purposes. The label case management plans has only become popular with the increased use of case management as a quality and cost-effectiveness strategy. The discipline of nursing introduced the use of clinical pathways as a strategy to address the nursing shortage of the 1980s; however they were nursing focused rather than interdisciplinary or interprofessional. With the demand for quality and safe healthcare services, the Agency for Healthcare Research and Quality (AHRQ) advocated for the development and implementation of PGs as a strategy for quality improvement and evidence-based practice. This took place in the late 1980s

and is still a focus for AHRQ today; in fact, the agency has developed and published multiple PGs and has made them available to healthcare organizations free of charge.

This development has encouraged healthcare providers of different disciplines and specialties to implement the AHRQ's guidelines in their practice. However, because of the complexity of the guidelines, it was essential for AHRQ to pursue other strategies for implementation, among which is the development of clinical pathways/CMPs. This resulted in a shift in focus of the nursing clinical pathways to interdisciplinary plans as we know them today. Because of this development, CMPs and PGs should not be used interchangeably as they are not one and the same. There exists some differences between the two and these are presented in Box 10.1.

The format of the CMPs is basically known as a "time-task" matrix that applies either an abbreviated, one-page version or a comprehensive, detailed booklet. CMPs have been developed based on the Gantt chart process and design, borrowed from the engineering industry. They can be available in either paper or electronic format; however, more commonly electronic today. Additionally, the purposes of CMPs, the way they

---

Box 10.1   Differences Between Case Management Plans and Practice Guidelines

1. CMPs focus on quality and efficiency; PGs focus on appropriateness of care.

2. CMPs are interprofessional in nature; PGs are medically focused.

3. CMPs are healthcare organization-specific; PGs are national standards.

4. CMPs may be used for documentation; PGs may not and are not written with that purpose in mind.

5. CMPs follow a specific timeline such as days or hours; PGs do not, they may apply phases of care.

6. CMPs are less costly than PGs.

7. CMPs are less complex and time-consuming to develop than PGs.

8. Variance identification and tracking is an integral part of CMPs but not PGs.

9. CMPs apply a "time-task" and "time-outcome" matrices in format; PGs follow a text or algorithm format.

10. CMPs consider the recommendations of PGs in their development; PGs are developed based on a thorough review of evidence.

11. CMPs are used by providers, payers, and consumers; PGs are limited to providers, some payers but not consumers.

are used, and the process in which they are developed are the same.

CMPs are labeled differently in different institutions. Some are copyrighted, such as Caremap®; some are not, such as interdisciplinary action plans (IDAPs). Examples of CMPs include critical path, anticipated recovery path, clinical pathway, care guide, collaborative plan, coordinated plan, integrated plan of care, action plan, or evidence-based clinical guideline. Throughout Chapter 10, these plans will be referred to by using the generic term "case management plan." Case Manager's Tip 10.1 lists the characteristics of CMPs. The use of CMPs has created a multitude of advantages. Among the most important benefits are those described in Box 10.2.

10.2. TYPES OF CASE MANAGEMENT PLANS

CMPs link the processes and outcomes of care. They are used as structured and formal plans that delineate the delivery and management of patient care services and outcomes. They also are used to identify best practices, standardize care activities, promote consistency and continuity in practice patterns across providers and levels of care, enhance interdisciplinary collaboration and a seamless approach to patient care delivery, and provide a mechanism for measuring outcomes of care and addressing variances and deviations from the standards. Healthcare organizations have designed and implemented many different types of CMPs (Box 10.3). Some of the plans include more details than others, some are multipurpose, and some may address the responsibilities of multiple disciplines and providers.

Generally, there are three main areas of focus when CMPs are developed and implemented. These are as follows:

1. To standardize new, old, or current practice; that is, to ensure consistency and continuity in care delivery and services, among providers, and across settings. CMPs are developed for this purpose when there are no other innovations, knowledge, or better ways/ideal practices for the provision of care.

2. To implement evidence-based practice or state-of-the-science care; that is, to change the current methods and strategies of care delivery and management through the use of knowledge gained from outcomes of research and clinical trials. CMPs are developed for this purpose when the latest research outcomes about new treatments and interventions have proven to be more beneficial to patients and cost-effective.

Box 10.2   Advantages of Case Management Plans

- Cost-effectiveness
- Reduction in hospital length of stay
- Elimination of avoidable readmissions to acute care settings
- Controlling number of home care visits to what is most appropriate and necessary
- Consistency and standardization in care provision (elimination of practice pattern variations)
- Implementation of best practices and evidence-based treatment options
- Improved quality of care, safety, and customer satisfaction and experience
- Better allocation of resources and coordination of services that result in eliminating redundancy, fragmentation, and duplication of care activities
- Clearly defined plans of care and delineation of responsibilities of healthcare team members
- Improved communication systems among the various disciplines and providers

Case Management Plans are known to:

- Enhance clinical outcomes and quality of care, including safety
- Integrate nationally recognized evidence-based practice guidelines into practice
- Assure the use of healthcare resources and services to the best clinical value
- Maximize use of effective communication among interdisciplinary team members
- Reduce unwanted variation in clinical practice
- Promote patient-centered care through educating family and patient about plan of care

3. To innovate and develop new practices; that is, to implement new strategies, treatments, protocols, and interventions where there are no known ideal or evidence-based practices. CMPs are developed for this purpose when experts in an organization are interested in testing different treatment options that are still considered to be controversial or have not been tested before. Such CMPs usually result in identifying ideal and evidence-based practices after the period of experimentation is concluded.

10.2.1. Issue-Specific Recommendations

Issue-specific recommendations are statements of care and decisions and are usually limited to clinical situations in their format and content. They also are clear, concise, and direct to the point. They tend not to address the total aspects of care of a patient with a specif-

---

Box 10.3   Types of Case Management Plans

1. Issue-specific recommendations
2. Algorithms
3. Protocols
4. Predetermined/standardized order sets
5. Guidelines
6. Clinical/critical pathways
7. IDAPs

---

ic diagnosis but rather an individual aspect or a related process of care, such as prescribing medications for a patient with pneumonia, or deciding the best level of care for a patient with a certain diagnosis/chief complaint (Box 10.4). In addition, they identify the role of a particular discipline, and in that regard they define the responsibility of a specific care provider to the clinical situation they address. For example, an issue-specific

recommendation regarding the discharge of patients who are receiving intravenous (IV) antibiotics while hospitalized and who are known to be IV drug users may indicate that the prescriber of care and treatments (e.g., physician, nurse practitioner) should switch an IV antibiotic to its oral form before these patients are discharged from the hospital. Another example is the need to measure the temperature of a febrile patient rectally, or to send a blood specimen for microbiology/bacteriology testing when the patient's temperature is greater than or equal to 103.5°F.

Issue-specific recommendations may stand alone as policy statements or be part of the standard of care. To elaborate, the example provided in Box 10.4 represents a standard of care or a guideline for the outpatient and ED settings. Sometimes issue-specific recommendations are incorporated in the CMPs to enhance quality and safe practice, prevent errors and medical litigation, and promote adherence to the standards of accredita-

    CASE MANAGER'S TIP 10.1

Characteristics and Benefits of Case Management Plans

- Each plan addresses a specific diagnosis, medical problem, surgical procedure, or phase in the care needed.
- The plans represent a timeline of patient care activities based on the clinical service. This could be minutes or hours in the emergency department, days in the acute care setting, weeks in the neonatal intensive care unit, months in long-term facilities, or number of visits in ambulatory or home care settings.
- The plans include well-defined milestones or trigger points that aid in expediting care and indicate an impending change in care activities (e.g., switching from intravenous to oral antibiotics when temperature is within normal range for 24 hours) or readiness of patients for different care setting (e.g., criteria for transferring a patient from an acute to a subacute or nursing home care setting). The triggers are discipline- or provider-specific.
- The length of each plan depends on a predetermined length of stay based on the diagnosis/procedure and reimbursement rules, guidelines, and mechanisms.
- The plans prospectively delineate the necessary interventions in a way that eliminates fragmentation, redundancy/duplication, and use of unnecessary resources.
- The plans clearly delineate the responsibilities of the various healthcare team members as they relate to each particular department.
- The plans identify the outcome indicators or quality measures used to evaluate the appropriateness and effectiveness of care.
- Each plan may include a specific variance tracking section to evaluate any delays in care activities/processes or outcomes.
- The plans may be used as one strategy for ensuring compliance with the standards of care of regulatory and accreditation agencies.
- The plans are interdisciplinary in nature—a mechanism that reinforces a seamless approach to the delivery of care and standardizes and ensures consistency in the care provision processes.
- The plans can be used as educational tools for housestaff, student nurses or nurses in training, and newly hired employees.
- The plans help improve performance in the areas of patient and family teaching, coordination of services, collaboration and communication among the healthcare team members, and discharge planning.
- The plans may also be developed in a "patient version," which can be given to the patient and family at the time of admission into the hospital or community care setting. This helps the patient understand what is projected to take place during the course of treatment.
- The plans may be used for negotiation of managed care contracts and reimbursement rates as they prospectively define practice and identify the critical steps in the care of patients with a specific diagnosis or procedure.

Box 10.4   Example of an Issue-Specific Recommendation: Decision to Admit a Patient Who Presents to the Emergency Department to the Acute Care Setting

Use of the CURB-65 tool to make a decision whether to admit or discharge.

- The CURB-65 is a simple scoring system easily used in the outpatient or emergency department settings to decide whether to admit a patient to the hospital.
- The CURB tool consists of five clinical factors the provider scores based on their presence. If a patient's condition meets a criterion, a score of one single point is given to the criterion.
- The criteria are:
  —C–Confusion or delirium
  —U–Blood Urea Nitrogen (BUN) > or = 20 mg/dL
  —R–Respiratory rate > or = 30 breaths/minute
  —B–Systolic blood pressue (BP) < 90 mm Hg or Diastolic BP < or = 60 mm Hg
  —65–Age 65 or older
- Decisions Criteria
  —If the cumulative score is 0 or 1 (low risk), then most likely the patient can be safely treated as an outpatient.
  —A score of 2 (moderate risk) suggests closely supervising the patient in an outpatient treatment, or observation status is appropriate.
  —A score of 3 (high risk) inidcates patient requires admission to an inpatient/hospital setting.
  —A score of 4 or 5 (very high risk) indicates the patient requires admission to an intensive care unit.

tion and regulatory agencies. Issue-specific recommendations are not as popular today; however, healthcare providers used to develop and implement them more often before the advent of other more detailed types of CMPs such as clinical pathways, algorithms, and IDAPs. Healthcare providers have used them to proactively delineate the responsibilities and practices of the various disciplines involved in patient care and in specific situations.

10.2.2. Algorithms

Algorithms are problem-based procedures of care that are developed by healthcare providers as consensus statements to delineate the process(es) of caring for a patient with a specific medical condition or health problem such as asthma or pharyngitis (Figure 10.1). They include a step-by-step guide to the care of patients and usually focus on the clinical decision-making process

regarding the patient's assessment and the required diagnostic and therapeutic interventions and treatments. Usually, algorithms are written in an "if . . . then" style; however, the use of the "if . . . then" may not always be explicit. Sometimes, arrows (indicating direction) and boxes (containing the recommended care options) are used instead of "if . . . then," such as in the example presented in Figure 10.1. Regardless of the method used, algorithms apply a stepwise format that is systematic, chronological, and outcomes driven.

Algorithms focus on the logical progression of intervention options that are driven by the patient's response to treatment and aim at resolving the patient's problem. They are rules-based and leave little room for decision making and judgment because they are prospectively developed as explicit interventions for managing specific conditions. These decisions are specified in the content of the algorithm and follow the style described above. As with CMPs, it is appropriate to deviate from the algorithm; however, the healthcare provider deviating from the plan must have a logical reason for such actions and must document the rationale of the deviation in the patient's medical record. Sometimes documentation flowsheets/tools are developed in conjunction with the algorithms to simplify the process of patient care provision and documentation, especially in a fast paced care setting such as the ED. In this case the algorithm and the documentation tool are implemented as a package; one is not used in the clinical setting without the other.

10.2.3. Protocols

Protocols are similar to algorithms in their systematic and logical progression format. They consitute a detailed, written set of instructions that provides a systematic plan for a procedure or course of treatment. They also are usually specific to a patient's problem and mainly used as integral components of clinical trials and research.

Protocols are used as formal guides to delineate all of the steps for the application of a particular procedure or intervention. They provide a standardized approach to meeting desired outcomes of care. An example is an acute coronary syndromes protocol that classifies chest pain and angina into different levels of intensity or seriousness and details the appropriate and necessary treatments/interventions for each level. In this example the protocol guides the healthcare providers in the assessment, diagnosis, and treatment of chest pain.

10.2.4. Predetermined/Standardized Order Sets

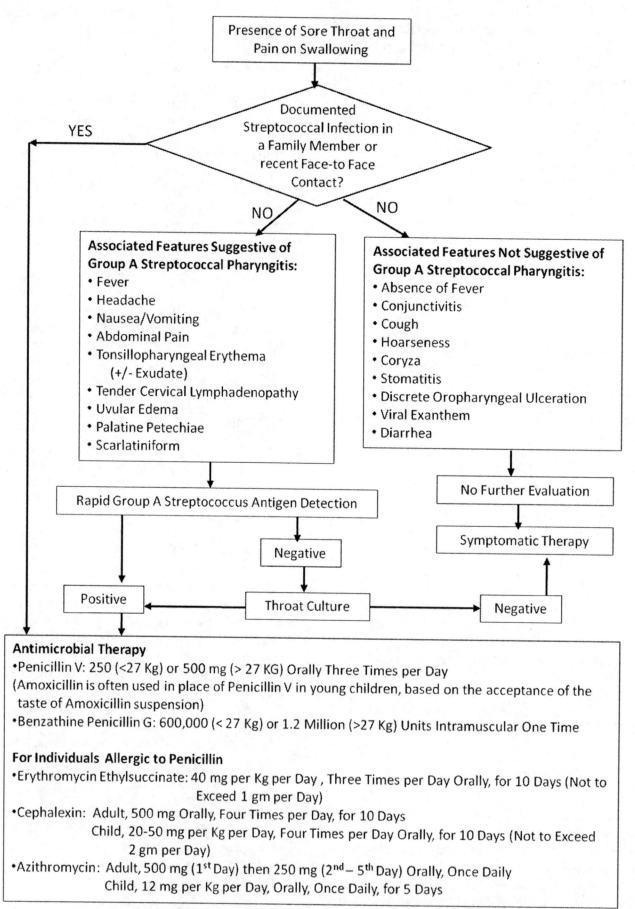

Figure 10.1 Algorithm for the care of patients with pharyngitis.

Predetermined order sets are prospectively prepared by one or more disciplines or healthcare providers to delineate a standardized process for the diagnosis and treatment of patients with particular problems. These orders focus mainly on medical/physicians' practice. However, they may also address the responsibilities and expectations of other providers, including nurses and allied health professionals (e.g., social workers, physical therapists). With the advent of electronic documentation and computerized provider order entry systems, predetermined/satandaridzed order sets have become popular in the practice of various health professionals not just physicians. These are developed based on research outcomes and the latest recommendations of professional societies such as the American Heart Association. The purposes of predetermined order sets are to standardize and expedite care, provide evidence-based treatments and interventions, and prevent variation in the practice patterns of providers. Sometimes preprinted order sets are used alone or in conjunction with CMPs. They are a positive way of increasing physician buy-in to CMPs.

10.2.5. Guidelines

Guidelines are statements of specific recommendations for the care of patients with a particular health problem such as heart failure. They are written in a narrative or outline format to provide guidance for the care and management of patients, especially in the areas of diagnostic and therapeutic tests and procedures. Unlike issue-specific recommendations, they make reference to time and may include specific timeframes for the implementation of designated actions or the achievement of certain outcomes. Guidelines have been used in anesthesia for many decades; however, they only became popular in other specialties and disciplines with the advent of case management and managed care. They are thought to reduce legal risk and are adopted by healthcare organizations and professional societies for that purpose.

Guidelines are systematically developed recommendations for care to assist healthcare providers in making decisions regarding the appropriateness and necessity of care and services. Similar to the other types of CMPs, guidelines provide practitioners with advice that is based on expert opinion, consensus statements, and research outcomes. Moreover, they intend to reduce practice variations and improve patient care outcomes (Figure 10.2). Today guidelines are developed and advocated for either internally in a healthcare organization or nationally by federal agencies such as the AHRQ and professional organizations such as the

American Medical Association. They may be broad or specific depending on their source of origin. Those developed or adopted by a healthcare organization tend to be based on the nationally acceptable guidelines and more specific in content and timeframes, taking into consideration the systems and process of care present in the particular organization.

10.2.6. Clinical/Critical Pathways

Clinical/critical pathways are specific guidelines of care developed to delineate the contributions and responsibilities of the various disciplines and specialists for the care of specific patient populations. They are problem-based and discipline-focused in content (Figure 10.3). The clinical/critical pathway format is based on the Gantt chart principles used by engineers and architects. Karen Zander was the first to use clinical pathways at the New England Medical Center in Boston, Massachusetts, in the mid-1980s. At the time, they were referred to as Caremaps, applied a one-page format, and focused almost exclusively on nursing. They were originally used as a strategy to address the nursing shortage; however, they grew to become of interdisciplinary focus and today are adopted for use by all disciplines and healthcare providers.

Similar to the other types of CMPs, clinical/critical pathways are developed based on national standards and research outcomes and are best used for evidence-based practice. However, they differ from the other types of CMPs, in that they include specific timeframes for all of the recommended activities. They also are used as cost-effective tools for the delineation of key and critical resources and activities; to specify the order, timeliness, and progression of these activities; and to provide a mechanism for the evaluation of patient care outcomes and for meeting the desired outcomes.

Clinical pathways today are embedded in the elctronic documentation and order entry systems. Often they are used as plans of care and guides for documentation. Effective ones, however, are those of the predetermined order sets for each health discipline and are embedded in the electronic order entry systems with special delineation of the day of hospital stay to communciate timeframe for execution or follow-up.

10.2.7. Interdisciplinary Action Plans

Interdisciplinary Action Plans (IDAPs) (Figure 10.4) are similar to clinical pathways in their purpose, focus, and process of development. However, they are more detailed, several pages in length (sometimes they are

Population	Adults age 50–75 years	Adults age 76–85 years	Adults older than 85 years
Recommendation	Screen with high sensitivity fecal occult blood testing (FOBT), sigmoidoscopy, or colonoscopy	Automatic screening is not recommended	No screening is recommended
Screening Tests	High sensitivity FOBT, sigmoidoscopy with FOBT, and colonoscopy are effective in decreasing colorectal cancer mortality. Risks and benefits of these screening methods vary. Colonoscopy and flexible sigmoidoscopy (to a lesser degree) entail possible serious complications.		
Frequency of Screening	Annual screening with high sensitivity FOBT Sigmoidoscopy every 5 years, with high sensitivity FOBT every 3 years Screening colonoscopy every 10 years		
Balance of Benefits and Harms	Benefits outweigh the potential harms for 50–75 years old adults	The likelihood that detection and early intervention will yield a mortality benefit declines after age 75 because of long average time between adenoma development and cancer diagnosis	
Implementation	Focus on strategies that maximize the number of individuals who get screened. Practice shared decision making; incorporate information about test quality and availability when discussing screening with patients Use a surveillance regimen for patients with a personal history of cancer or adenomatous polyps; this screening guideline does not apply to these patients		
Other Recommendations	Recommend against use of aspirin or nonsteroidal anti-inflammatory drugs for the primary prevention of colorectal cancer.		

NOTE: This guideline is used here as an example; it is not to be followed as recommendation for practice. Adapted from AHRQ, 2014.

Figure 10.2 Example of guideline, screening for colorectal cancer.

developed in a booklet format), allow room for documentation, and have medical orders embedded in them. In addition, they provide evidence of a collaborative and seamless approach to care for accreditation agencies and result in opening the lines of communication among the various providers.

IDAPs are excellent tools to standardize interdisciplinary clinical practice. IDAPs are usually developed for a specific group of primary diagnoses and to enhance practice through implementation of the latest available evidence and as a result improve

quality and optimize direct resource utilization in patient care delivery. An IDAP is an interdisciplinary, day-by-day guideline that recommends interventions, treatments, diagnostic testing, consultations, discharge/transitional planning, and patient education activities to occur at the appropriate stage of a patient's care and recovery.

IDAPs specify both the actions/interventions necessary for the care of patients and the related and expected outcomes. They detail outcomes in relation to progression toward recovery; that is, the outcomes follow a specific sequence that is temporal and allows practitioners to easily evaluate the patient's condition and progress in relation to recovery or problem resolution and to determine the appropriate next step in care. This is done by prospectively delineating the intermediate outcomes that must be met first so that the care and the patient can progress in the desired direction. The outcomes are presented in the IDAPs using specific time-

Key Elements	Admission	Day of Surgery	Post-operative Day 1	Day	Day of Discharge
Assessments	Anesthesia service Skin assessment Falls risk Neurovascular check Pain assessment Confirm operative clearance	Intake and output Check drains Neurovascular check Cardiopulmonary check Vital signs	Intake and output Check drains Neurovascular check Cardiopulmonary check Vital signs		Intake and output Discontinue drains Neurovascular check Cardiopulmonary check Vital signs
Tests	CBC Urine analysis ECG (if over 40 or based on condition) Chest x-ray (if over 60)	CBC Postoperative chest x-ray	INR (for anticoagulation)		CBC, if indicated INR (for anticoagulation)
Treatments	Physical therapy	Autoreinfusion Venodynes post surgery Intravenous fluid therapy	Physical therapy Occupational therapy if indicated Pain management Intravenous fluid therapy Respiratory inspirometer		Physical therapy Occupational therapy if indicated Pain management follow-up Discontinue intravenous Fluid therapy Respiratory inspirometer
Consults	Medicine service as indicated Cardiac or other specialty as indicated	Pain management service Physiatry service	Pain management follow-up		Pain management follow-up
Medications	Pre-op medications Additional medications	Pain medication Antibiotics: surgical prophylaxis Anticoagulation /DVT prophylaxis	Pain medication Antibiotics Anticoagulation /DVT prophylaxis		Pain medication Antibiotics Anticoagulation /DVT prophylaxis
Diet	NPO after midnight Fluid	Liquids	As tolerated Follow restrictions as per health condition		Regular diet Follow restrictions as needed
Activity/ Exercise	Bed rest	Bed rest Turn and position/posture in bed	Begin ambulation Establish activity/exercise regimen Use of assistive device as needed (e.g., walker)		Continue ambulation Use of assistive device as needed (e.g., walker)
Health Education	Orientation to unit/hospital Health instruction, procedure and other topics as needed Use teachback	Discuss post-operative care Health instruction, conditon and signs and symptoms and dressing changes Use teachback	Health instruction, conditon, signs and symptoms, and dressing changes Instruct about red flags Instruct, medications, exercise, and diet Use teachback		Health instruction, conditon and signs and symptoms and dressing changes Instruct about red flags Instruct, medications, exercise and diet Use teachback
Discharge	Assessment of post-discharge needs	Discuss post-discharge needs and services Coordinate post-discharge services	Discuss and confirm discharge plan Coordinate post-discharge services Order durable medical equipment as needed Order transportation if needed		Confirm post-discharge services Confirm durable medical equipment as needed Confirm transportation as needed

NOTE: Admission and day of surgery may be the same day for certain ti nt popula ns. Content is general for use as examples of how treatments and interventions are placed on the pl .

Figure 10.3 Example of clinical/critical pathway template.

Major Thoracic Surgery
(Thoracotomy, Lobectomy, Wedge Resection)

Clinical Service: Thoracic **Primary Nurse:**
  Physician:

Admitting Diagnosis:

Secondary Diagnoses:

Nursing Diagnoses:

#1 Knowledge Deficit	# 4 Ineffective breathing related to thoracic surgery
#2 Alteration in comfort related to pain	#5
#3 Potential for infection – surgical site	#6

Allergies: **Working DRG:**
 Working ICD-10 Codes:

ELEMENT OF CARE	Date __/__/__ Peri-Op/Day 0	Shift Check	Date __/__/__ POD # 1	Shift Check	Date __/__/__ POD # 2	Shift Check
Assessment & Monitoring	• Vital signs q4h • Telemetry • Admission height & weight • Assess pre-op site • Complete H & P and nursing admission assessment • Peri-op nursing assessment and care plan • Consent signed Outcomes: • Stable cardiac and pulmonary state		• Vital signs q1h • Telemetry • Admission height & weight • Assess surgical site • Implement PACU protocol / order set • Assess chest tube site and drainage Outcomes: • Stable cardiac and pulmonary state: heart rate, MAP WNL, & ECG • No bleeding		• Vital signs q4h • Telemetry • Intake & output q4h • Assess surgical site • Dressing change • Assess chest tube site and drainage Outcomes: • Stable cardiac and pulmonary state • Chest tube site dry, intact • Surgical site clean and intact • Balanced I & O • No bleeding	
Tests & Procedures	• Admission panel • U/A • PT/PTT/INR • CXR ☐Pulmonary Function Test		• CBC • ABGs • Chem 7 ☐Troponin X 3		☐CBC ☐Electrolytes ☐ECG ☐CXR ☐PT/INR Outcomes: • CBC, electrolytes, coagulation profile WNL/baseline	
Treatments	• Chlorhexidine shower • Pre-op lab work completed • Incentive spirometry • Intubation intraoperatively Outcomes: • Successfully demonstrate use of incentive spirometry		• Refer to PACU Critical Care Flowsheet • Evaluation for extubation • Venodyne boots • Pulse oximetry monitoring • Nasal oxygen PRN • Incentive spriometry q1h ☐Epidural pain management		• Evaluate removal of chest tube • Remove foley catheter • Nasal oxygen PRN • Incentive spirometry q1h • Venodyne boots ☐Foley catheter ☐Epidural pain management Outcomes:	

Figure 10.4 Example of an Interdisciplinary Action Plan (IDAP).

ELEMENT OF CARE	Date __/__/__ Peri-Op/Day 0	Shift Check	Date __/__/__ POD # 1	Shift Check	Date __/__/__ POD # 2	Shift Check
			Outcomes: • Extubated • Stable cardiac & pulmonary state • Transfer to Thoracic surgery unit		• Good bilateral pulmonary aeration • Oxygen oximetry WNL • Chest tube drainage < 100 cc/24 hours; no air leakage • Stable cardiac and pulmonary state	
Medications & IV	• Peripheral IV line • Fluid therapy • Antibiotic prophylaxis		• Peripheral IV line • Fluid therapy • PACU pain management protocol ☐Post-op antibiotics ☐Digitalization protocol ☐DVT prophylaxis		• Peripheral IV line • Fluid therapy • Pain management protocol ☐Post-op antibiotics ☐Digitalization protocol ☐ DVT prophylaxis **Outcomes:** • Maintained on oral medications • Adequate pain control	
Nutrition	• NPO after midnight		• Diet progression as tolerated **Outcomes:** • Tolerates diet		• Diet progression **Outcomes:** • Tolerates diet	
Activity	• OOB Ad Lib		• Bed rest, turn q2h • ROM q4h • Incentive spirometry q1h		• OOB to chair • Assist in ADL as needed • Evaluate activity progression ☐Physical therapy ☐Respiratory therapy **Outcomes:** • Tolerates OOB • Able to walk	
Consults	• Anesthesia • Medical clearance ☐Pulmonary				Evaluate for referral to ☐Home care ☐PT ☐SW ☐Pain management ☐Respiratory therapy	
Psychosocial	• Evaluate psychosocial needs and home situation • Check for any pre-op home services ☐Case management assessment **Outcomes:** • Verbalize consent to and readiness for surgery • Appropriate home		• Continue to evaluate psychosocial needs and home situation ☐Case management assessment **Outcomes:** • Primary nurse/case manager meet with patient and family, provide support and appropriate home environment		• Continue to evaluate psychosocial needs and home situation ☐Case management assessment ☐SW **Outcomes:** • Coping well • Appropriate home environment and support post-discharge	

Figure 10.4 (continued) Example of an Interdisciplinary Action Plan (IDAP).

ELEMENT OF CARE	Date __/__/__ Peri-Op/Day 0	Shift Check	Date __/__/__ POD # 1	Shift Check	Date __/__/__ POD # 2	Shift Check
	situation		confirmed			
Patient & Family Education	• Share and discuss patient/family pathway • Demonstrate incentive spirometry • Evaluate need for referrals ☐ Case management assessment **Outcomes (teach-back):** • Verbalize understanding of surgical procedure and post-operative course		• Review and discuss patient/family pathway • Evaluate understanding of incentive spirometry use ☐ Case management assessment **Outcomes (teach-back):** • Verbalize understanding of activity progression • Demonstrate appropriate use of incentive spirometry		• Coughing & deep breathing exercises • ROM/activity progression • Discuss disease process and risk factor modification • Review and discuss patient/family pathway • Discuss post-discharge care ☐ Case management assessment **Outcomes (teach-back):** • Verbalize understanding of activity progression • Verbalize understanding of disease process and healthy lifestyle behavior • Verbalize understanding of post-discharge care	
Discharge / Transitional Planning	• Review expected 4 days LOS • Evaluate ability for self-care & self-management post discharge • Evaluate appropriateness of home environment and support ☐ Case management assessment **Outcomes:** • Understand LOS expectation ○ Understand post-discharge care expectations		• Assess post-discharge care needs • Evaluate ability for self-care & self-management post discharge • Evaluate appropriateness of home environment and support ☐ Case management assessment **Outcomes:** • Identified post-discharge care needs		• Evaluate ability for self-care & self-management post discharge • Discuss discharge plan • Confirm appropriateness of home environment and support ☐ Case management assessment **Outcomes:** • On track for discharge • Post-discharge care needs identified	

Signature	Date	Signature		Date	Signature (Other)		Date
MD		RN					
MD		RN					
MD		RN					
MD		RN					

The Interdisciplinary Action Plan (IDAP) is developed as a suggested plan of care for various disciplines involved. This is only a guideline, which may be changed and individualized according to the patient condition, assessment data, and clinical judgment. This IDAP is not to be used as a substitute or replacement for clinical assessment.

Figure 10.4 (continued) Example of an Interdisciplinary Action Plan (IDAP).

ELEMENT OF CARE	Date ___/___/___ POD # 3	Shift Check	Date ___/___/___ POD #	Shift Check	Date ___/___/___ Day of Discharge	Shift Check
Assessment & Monitoring	• Vital signs q4h • Telemetry • Weight • Intake & output q4h • Assess surgical site • Dressing change • Assess chest tube site and drainage; evaluate for removal Outcomes: • Stable cardiac and pulmonary state • Chest tube site dry, intact • No signs of infection • Balanced I & O • No bleeding • Afebrile		• ☐ Outcomes: •		• Vital signs q4h • Discontinue telemetry discontinued • Write discharge orders Outcomes: • Stable cardiac and pulmonary state • Chest tube site dry, intact • Surgical site clean and intact • No signs of infection • Afebrile	
Tests & Procedures	☐CBC ☐Electrolytes ☐ECG ☐CXR ☐PT/INR Outcomes: • CBC, electrolytes, coagulation profile WNL/baseline • CXR normal – no signs of pleural effusion or pneumonia		• ☐ Outcomes: •		☐ Tests as needed Outcomes: • CBC, electrolytes, coagulation profile WNL/baseline • No signs of pleural effusion or pneumonia	
Treatments	• Remove chest tube • Nasal oxygen PRN • Venodyne boots • Pain management • Incentive spiromtery Outcomes: • Tubes removed • Good bilateral pulmonary aeration • Oxygen oximetry WNL • Chest tube drainage < 100 cc/24 hours; no air leakage • Tolerate room air • Stable cardiac and pulmonary state		• ☐ Outcomes: •		• Pain management • Incentive spirometry Outcomes: • Good bilateral pulmonary aeration • Oxygen oximetry WNL • Stable cardiac and pulmonary state • Tolerate room air	
Medications & IV	• Discontinue peripheral IV line • Oral medications ☐ Antibiotic prophylaxis ☐ DVT prophylaxis		• ☐ Outcomes:		• Peripheral IV line • PACU pain management protocol • Incentive spirometry q1h	

Figure 10.4 (continued) Example of an Interdisciplinary Action Plan (IDAP).

ELEMENT OF CARE	Date __/__/__ POD # 3	Shift Check	Date __/__/__ POD #	Shift Check	Date __/__/__ Day of Discharge	Shift Check
	Outcomes: • Maintained on oral medications • Adequate pain control		•		☐ Post-op antibiotics ☐ Digitalization protocol ☐ Digitalization protocol **Outcomes:** • Maintained on oral medications • Adequate pain control	
Nutrition	• Regular diet • Limitations as indicated by health condition		• ☐ **Outcomes:** •		• Regular diet • Limitations as indicated by health condition **Outcomes:** • Tolerates diet	
Activity	• Ambulatory • Stairs climbing • ADLs minimal to no assist ☐ Physical therapy **Outcomes:** • Tolerates ambulation • No shortness of breath upon activity • Oxygen saturation WNL upon activity		• ☐ **Outcomes:** •		• Ambulatory • Stairs climbing • ADLs no assist **Outcomes:** • Tolerates ambulation and stairs climbing • No shortness of breath upon activity • Oxygen saturation WNL upon activity and on room air • Self-care / ADL independence	
Consults	• Evaluate for referral to specialists • Follow-up on referrals made ☐ Pulmonary ☐ Oncology ☐ Pain management		• ☐ **Outcomes:** •		**Outcomes:** • Home care services in place	
Psychosocial	• Evaluate psychosocial needs • Check for any services needed at home ☐ Case management reassessment ☐ SW counseling **Outcomes:** • Coping well • Appropriate home environment • Appropriate family support • Ask appropriate questions re discharge plan		• ☐ **Outcomes:** •		• Follow-up on psychosocial needs ☐ Case management reassessment ☐ SW counseling **Outcomes:** • Coping well • Appropriate home environment • Appropriate support post-discharge	
Patient & Family	• Discuss patient/family pathway		• ☐		• Coughing & deep breathing exercises	

Figure 10.4 (continued) Example of an Interdisciplinary Action Plan (IDAP).

ELEMENT OF CARE	Date __/__/__ POD # 3	Shift Check	Date __/__/__ POD #	Shift Check	Date __/__/__ Day of Discharge	Shift Check
Education	• Demonstrate incentive spirometry • Review wound care • Review signs and symptoms of infection • Review health lifestyle behavior • Discuss engagement in own care • Begin discharge instructions (e.g., medications, red flags, follow-up care appointment) **Outcomes (teach-back):** • Verbalize understanding of activity progression • Verbalize understanding of disease process and healthy lifestyle behavior • Verbalize understanding of post-discharge care • Verbalize understanding of self-care (e.g., medications, red flags)		**Outcomes (teach-back):** •		• ROM/activity progression • Discuss disease process and risk factor modification • Review and discuss patient/family pathway • Discuss post-discharge care ☐Case management assessment **Outcomes (teach-back):** • Verbalize understanding of activity and exercise • Verbalize understanding of disease process and healthy lifestyle behavior • Verbalize understanding of post-discharge self-care (e.g., red flags, medications, wound care, dressing change, follow-up appointment)	
Discharge / Transitional Planning	• Review expected date of discharge • Implement discharge plan • Evaluate ability for self-care & self-management post discharge • Evaluate appropriateness of home environment and support • Schedule follow-up care appointment • Discuss post-discharge calls • Assure ability to obtain medications and discuss home delivery option • Assure availability of wound care supplies ☐Arrange for discharge transportation ☐Case management		• ☐ **Outcomes:** •		• Evaluate ability for self-care & self-management post discharge • Confirm availability of home care ☐Confirm discharge transportation **Outcomes:** • On track for discharge • Coordinated post-discharge care needs • Confirmed follow-up care appointment • Able to perform self-care activities • Available medications and wound care supplies	

Figure 10.4 (continued) Example of an Interdisciplinary Action Plan (IDAP).

ELEMENT OF CARE	Date __/__/__ POD # 3	Shift Check	Date __/__/__ POD #	Shift Check	Date __/__/__ Day of Discharge	Shift Check
reassessment **Outcomes:** • Understand and agree with discharge plan • Understand post-discharge care expectations including self-care and wound care • Demonstrate understanding of access to medications, care supplies, follow-up appointment and post-discharge calls						

Signature		Date	Signature		Date	Signature (Other)		Date
MD			RN					
MD			RN					
MD			RN					
MD			RN					
MD			RN					
MD			RN					

The Interdisciplinary Action Plan (IDAP) is developed as a suggested plan of care for various disciplines involved. This is only a guideline, which may be changed and individualized according to the patient condition, assessment data, and clinical judgment. This IDAP is not to be used as a substitute or replacement for clinical assessment.

Figure 10.4 (continued) Example of an Interdisciplinary Action Plan (IDAP).

frames similar to those applied for the interventions and treatments. This characteristic, as it pertains to outcomes, tends to be lacking in clinical/critical pathways. Another differentiating factor between IDAPs and clinical pathways is that IDAPs include algorithms and predetermined order sets, whereas pathways usually do not.

10.3. PROCESS OF DEVELOPING CASE MANAGEMENT PLANS

CMPs are developed best through an interdisciplinary team that is granted the authority and responsibility by a higher administrative structure in an organization, usually a steering committee charged with implementing case management systems, to develop a specific plan for a particular diagnosis or procedure. The interdisciplinary team is given the responsibility of developing the actual content of the plan. The steering committee, however, provides the team with ongoing expert and administrative support throughout the process.

Team members meet numerous times to discuss and develop the CMP. Sometimes they work individually in between meetings. The length of time needed for the development and completion of one CMP usually depends on the complexity of the diagnosis or procedure; the number of physicians and practitioners who will use the plan; the extent of the disagreements among physicians regarding the content of the plan that may arise while attempting to build consensus; the number of disciplines involved; the experience of the team members involved in the process; the availability of team members, their commitment, their productivity, and how well they can work together (i.e., group dynamics); and the presence or absence of a support person or an expert in CMP development. One CMP may take as long as 6–9 months for completion, particularly if the team is developing a CMP for the first time, or as little as a few weeks if team members are well experienced in the process and the topic of the plan is less controversial.

10.3.1. Steering Committee

The steering committee is composed of professionals who hold executive-level positions in the organization. The departments represented on the steering committee may include, depending on the sophistication of the healthcare organization, operations, finance/cost accounting, marketing, nursing/patient care services, information systems, medical records, legal and risk management, quality improvement and utilization management, managed care and case management, data management, research, and other ancillary services as deemed necessary. Members of the steering committee may be the high-ranking officers of each of these departments or their designee. It is not always necessary to have a representative from each of these departments. Some institutions may choose not to create a new stand-alone committee for this purpose. Responsibilities of a steering committee, in this case, may be added to a pre-existing committee such as a quality council or a length-of-stay or cost-reduction taskforce.

The major role of the steering committee is to put together a strategic plan for the implementation of case management systems. This plan describes the processes of training and educating those involved in the process; selecting and prioritizing the diagnoses and procedures for which CMPs are to be developed; and providing support for the teams charged with developing CMPs. Members of the steering committee provide leadership, support, and direction for the development, implementation, and evaluation of the case management system.

Most institutions have established a standardized process for the development of CMPs. The steering committee is responsible for the development of this process. Having an established formal process is important because it provides the interdisciplinary team with the foundation for successful development and implementation of CMPs, simplifies the work, and lays out the expectations. An ideal process is a simple one that clearly identifies the steps in a systematic way and makes it easier for the team to follow.

This chapter includes an example of such processes (Table 10.1) for healthcare administrators to adapt to their organizations and adjust as needed. This example follows a 10-step process that differentiates between the work and responsibilities of the steering committee and the interdisciplinary team.

The steering committee is responsible for the first four steps because they require higher administrative authority in decision making. They are related to the logistics of case management systems and plans and are part of the overall case management implementation plan put together by the steering committee and are approved by key executive personnel in the institution. The remaining six steps are the responsibility of the interdisciplinary team and address the actual work of the team and the creation of the CMP.

10.3.2. Step 1: Design the Format of the Plan

Deciding on the format is crucial, because the format guides the development of the content of the plan (Case Manager's Tip 10.2). The format should be made easy for all healthcare professionals to follow and use. This step is integral to the establishment of case management systems because it affects clinical practice and other care activities and processes (e.g., documentation, performance improvement processes, coding of the medical record, presentation of the standards of care and practice).

The CMP should be designed in such a way that includes the various elements of patient care (Box 10.5). Some of these elements are related to the medical/surgical care of the patient, whereas others are nursing in nature. In addition, there may be elements related to support or administrative services. Specific sections of the CMP should be allotted to quality indicators, outcome measures of care, variances track-

TABLE 10.1. The 10-Step Process of Developing Case Management Plans

Steering Committee	Step 1	Design the format
	Step 2	Select target population
	Step 3	Organize the interdisciplinary care team
	Step 4	Educate the team
Interdisciplinary Team	Step 5	Examine the current process of care
	Step 6	Review the relevant literature
	Step 7	Establish the length of stay for the case management plan
	Step 8	Develop the content of the case management plan
	Step 9	Conduct a pilot study/prototype test case
	Step 10	Standardize the case management plan

CASE MANAGER'S TIP 10.2

Factors That Affect Choosing a Particular Case Management Plan Format

- Whether the CMP will be used for documentation
- The number of disciplines that need to be represented in the plan
- Complexity of the diagnosis/procedure
- The clinical area or service or care setting
- Whether the plan will replace any existing preprinted physician orders or protocols
- The appropriate timeline
- Forms that must be eliminated from the patient's record on implementation of the plan
- Related risk management and legal issues
- Whether the plan will be a permanent part of the medical record
- Existing standards of regulatory and accreditation agencies
- Plans for automation of the medical record
- Whether the plan will integrate physician orders and algorithms or guidelines

---

Box 10.5 Elements of Patient Care as They May Appear on the Case Management Plan

- Patient assessment and monitoring
- Tests and procedures
- Care facilitation and coordination, including care milestones
- Consultations and referrals
- Medications
- Intravenous therapy
- Activity and exercise
- Nutrition
- Patient/family health teaching/instruction
- Treatments: medical, surgical, and nursing interventions
- Wound care
- Therapy: physical, occupational, respiratory, and speech pathology
- Pain management
- Outcome indicators and projected/desired responses to treatments (intermediate and discharge outcomes)
- Safety
- Discharge and transitional planning
- Psychosocial assessment

---

ing, and data collection. The number of the different care elements for each CMP depends on the diagnosis or surgical procedure addressed. For example, a plan for chest pain evaluation may include a pain management section but not occupational therapy. However, speech pathology and physical and occupational therapy are important when addressing a stroke CMP. A CMP to be used in a subacute care facility designated for ventilator-dependent patients should always include a respiratory care section that stresses the institution's protocol for weaning patients off mechanical ventilation.

The final format of the CMP (see Appendix 10.1 for an example) should be presented to the institutional medical records committee, legal/risk management department, and medical board for review and approval before it is made official. A decision regarding the format should be in place before authorizing any interdisciplinary team to start working on a CMP. The approved format becomes the desired CMP's template that is followed by all interdisciplinary teams to maintain consistency and uniformity of plans. The format also provides the framework based on which the team can construct the content details of the CMP. The steering committee then develops guidelines for the use of the template/final format of the CMP. The guidelines explain in detail how the template should be followed or used, the definitions of each of the care elements, and examples of the various patient care activities that

could be listed under each care element (Box 10.6). This is important because it maintains continuity and consistency of CMPs across the various interdisciplinary teams. When a team is established, a copy of the template/format and a copy of the guidelines should be presented to and discussed with the team members.

10.3.3. Step 2: Identify/Select Target Population

The mechanism for selecting target populations can be done at any time during the design phase of the CMP format. The steering committee studies the patient populations/groups served by the institution. It then selects the groups that need improvement regarding cost and quality, that present a risk for financial loss, or are a potential for increased revenue.

There are several criteria that must be considered when selecting target populations for which to develop CMPs (Case Manager's Tip 10.3). These include volume of the patient group, cost of care, complexity of care needed, institutional length of stay compared with other benchmarks, variations in practice patterns, the need for multiple services/care settings or providers, feasibility of developing the plan, potential revenue (i.e., control of resources, fragmentation, and duplication of care), opportunity for improvement in quality of care and outcomes, reports from payer groups, problem-prone/high-risk diagnoses or procedures, and

Box 10.6   Guidelines for the Placement of Patient Care Activities in the Case Management Plan

Each patient care activity should be indicated in the appropriate "care element" category. The following is a master list that should be used as a guide by interdisciplinary teams during the process of developing a case management plan.

Assessment and Monitoring

1. Physiological assessment measures (e.g., blood pressure, temperature, pulse[s], respirations, hemodynamic monitoring)
2. System assessment (e.g., cardiac, pulmonary, gastrointestinal)
3. Intake and output
4. Drainage of bodily fluids
5. Weights

Tests and Procedures

1. Laboratory tests (e.g., blood work, urine, sputum, pathology)
2. Unit-based tests (e.g., glucose fingerstick, guaiac, urine dipstick)
3. Routine diagnostic tests (e.g., electrocardiogram, chest x-ray examination, ultrasound)
4. Diagnostic/therapeutic procedures (e.g., operations, cardiac catheterization, angiogram, angioplasty, gastrostomy tube placement)

Treatments (Preventive and Therapeutic)

1. Dressing change and wound care
2. Intermittent compression device
3. Chest physiotherapy
4. Oxygen therapy and ventilator-related care
5. Central line/vascular access device site care
6. Tracheostomy care

Consults/Referrals

1. Specialty care providers
2. Home care
3. Psychiatry/Psychology
4. Child Life

Medications

1. Routine medications necessary for the particular case type (standing, as required [prn], and single dosages; premedication needs when preparing a patient for a particular procedure)

Therapy

1. Physical therapy
2. Occupational therapy
3. Respiratory therapy
4. Speech Pathology

Pain Management

1. Pain management protocol
2. Frequency of evaluating pain status and response to medications
3. Indications/recommendations for nonpharmacologic actions
4. Medications for pain management

Intravenous Therapy

1. Intravenous fluids (e.g., D5W, D5NSS)
2. Blood and blood products

Nutrition

1. Type of diet/meal
2. Instructions for diet progression
3. Fluid restrictions
4. Tube and supplemental feedings
5. Parenteral nutrition

Activity and Exercise

1. Activity limitations/ambulation
2. Safety instructions
3. Physical and occupational therapy
4. Fall risk assessment
5. Skin integrity risk assessment
6. Functional measures

Consults and Referrals

1. Routine consults (e.g., infectious disease, anesthesiology)
2. Specific consults (e.g., speech pathology for a stroke patient)

Psychosocial Assessment

1. Coping and adjustment to illness and hospitalization
2. Support system
3. Anxiety level

Patient/Family Teaching

1. Assessment for readiness to learn
2. Assessment of limitations/barriers to learning
3. Assessment of learning needs
4. Education plan, including areas of teaching (e.g., medications, disease process, activity/exercise, dietary limitations, specific medical/surgical regimen after discharge)
5. Need for particular equipment (e.g., glucometer for diabetic patients)

Box 10.6 (Continued)   Guidelines for the Placement of Patient Care Activities in the Case Management Plan

Discharge/Transitional Planning

1. Assessment of discharge needs
2. Referrals of high-risk patients to home care, social work, nutrition
3. Completion of any necessary paperwork for nursing home placement
4. Transitioning patients from one level of care to another

Outcome Indicators (Expected Outcomes of Care)

1. Intermediate outcomes
2. Discharge outcomes

Variance Tracking

1. Instructions on the use of variance section of the case management plan
2. Classifications/coding
3. Action plan
4. Date and time

Patient Problems

1. Delineate how patient problems should be stated (i.e., medical/nursing language)
2. Actual and potential problems

---

results of internal and external quality management monitoring.

It is important to evaluate the number of patients seen in a particular diagnosis-related group (DRG) when selecting a target population. The decision of which DRG should be targeted is made based on the number of patients seen in a particular DRG during a whole year. The larger the number of patients seen, the better the opportunities for improvement.

The established CMP will then be applied to a larger population, which maximizes the benefit. Because a DRG is too broad and may include several procedures that require different resources, whereas the International Classification of Diseases, Tenth Revision, Clinical Modification (ICD-10-CM) is more specific,

 CASE MANAGER'S TIP 10.3

There are many factors that assist in identifying the target population for case management plans. Case managers are best prepared to identify these opportunities based on their observation of practice and their efforts of preventing and controlling delays and variances in care. Here are some examples of these factors:

- High volume diagnoses
- Patient care quality and safety improvement opportunity
- High cost and resource utilization
- Diagnoses that involve the care of many disciplines, levels of care, and teams—opportunity to standardize care and improve communication
- Variation in care among providers that is not evidence based
- Opportunity to organize care in a more efficient manner to reduce length of stay

evaluation and analysis of patient populations for CMP opportunity should be made at the ICD-10-CM code level. Consider MS-DRG 280 (acute myocardial infarction, discharged alive with major complications and comorbiditiy) as an example. It includes several different conditions, with each designated a separate ICD-10-CM code (Table 10.2). The treatment plans for these conditions may be different; for example, patients presenting with ST elevation myocardial infarction may require an emergency procedure/intervention such as cardiac catheterization and percutaneous angioplasty or stent placement, whereas those with non ST elevation myocardial infarction may not. These variations make developing one CMP for MS-DRG 280 a great challenge. One option is developing a separate CMP for the management of patients for each of the ICD-10-CM codes. Another option may be the development of an algorithym for since presentation of patients may seem similar and then based on certain criteria different tracks for care and intervention may then be recommended; for example, a track for those who meet criteria for the procedure and anbother for those who do not.

Another example is MS-DRG 304: hypertension with major complications and comorbidity (Table 10.3). There are differences between treating hypertension related to heart disease and hypertension related to renal disease. It is best to deal with this DRG based on ICD-10-CM codes. Sometimes it is appropriate to combine two or more ICD-10-CM codes in one CMP. For example, combining renovascular hypertension (ICD-10-CM code I15.0) and hypertension secondary to other renal disorders (ICD-10-CM code I15.1) in one CMP that delineates the standard of care of hypertension related to renal disease is relevant because there may exist minimal to no variation in the treatment

TABLE 10.2. Examples of Different Procedures in MS-DRG 280.

Acute Myocardial Infarction, Discharged Alive with MCC	ICD-10-CM Codes
ST elevation myocardial infarction involving left main coronary artery	121.01
ST elevation myocardial infarction involving left anterior descending coronary artery	121.02
ST elevation myocardial infarction involving other coronary artery of anterior wall	121.09
ST elevation myocardial infarction involving right coronary artery	121.11
ST elevation myocardial infarction involving other coronary artery of inferior wall	121.19
ST elevation myocardial infarction involving left circumflex coronary artery	121.21
ST elevation myocardial infarction involving other sites	121.29
ST elevation myocardial infarction of unspecified site	121.3
Non-ST elevation myocardial infarction	121.4
Subsequent ST elevation myocardial infarction of anterior wall	122.0
Subsequent ST elevation myocardial infarction of inferior wall	122.1
Subsequent non-ST elevation myocardial infarction	122.2
Subsequent ST elevation myocardial infarction of other sites	122.8
Subsequent ST elevation myocardial infarction of unspecified site	122.9

MCC, Major Complications and Comorbidity; MS-DRG, Medicare Severity Diagnosis-Related Group.

of patients with these disorders. However, combining ICD-10-CM codes I11.9, I13.10, and I15.0 may not appropriate because treating hypertension due to heart disease versus renal disease is different, and the standard of care for both diagnoses if combined into one standard may result in confusion and ultimately may compromise patient experience and care outcomes. With the implementation of ICD-10-CM, specificity of target diagnoses for CMP development is even better compared to that of ICD-9-CM since ICD-10 applies more specificty and allows for more homgeneity among the patient population within a code.

The volume of patients seen in one DRG should not be considered in isolation from other measures, such as cost per case, cost per day, consumption of resources (e.g., the number of x-ray examinations, blood tests,

or electrocardiograms in one hospitalization or episode of care), average length of stay, outcomes, and profit and loss ratios. Patient populations that exert financial loss on the institution are considered the best target for CMP development.

Table 10.4 is an example of one administrative report that can be used to identify a target population. Examining the data presented, one can see that MS-DRGs 190, 193 and 292 have longer lengths of stay and at the same time have profit losses. Thus considering the development of CMPs for these three MS-DRGs is worthwhile because the opportunities for improvement and profit are high. To address these three MS-DRGs requires the establishment of three different teams for CMP development because the MS-DRGs are related to different services—pulmonary and cardiology.

TABLE 10.3. Example of Different ICD-10-CM Codes in MS-DRG 304.

Hypertension with Major Complications and Comorbidities	ICD-10-CM Codes
Essential (primary) hypertension	I10
Hypertensive heart disease without heart failure	I11.9
Hypertensive heart and chronic kidney disease without heart failure, with stage 1 through stage 4 chronic kidney disease, or unspecified chronic kidney disease	I13.10
Renovascular hypertension	I15.0
Hypertension secondary to other renal disorders	I15.1
Hypertension secondary to endocrine disorders	I15.2
Other secondary hypertension	I15.8
Secondary hypertension, unspecified	I15.9

MS-DRG, Medicare Severity Diagnosis-Related Group.

TABLE 10.4. Example of Administrative Report Used to Identify Target Populations.

MS-DRG	Description	Total Cases*	Average Length of Stay	Excess Days†	Profit (Loss)±
190	Chronic Obstructive Pulmonary Disease with MCC	150	6	2	($1,145.43)
193	Simple Pneumonia and Pleurisy, with MCC	165	7	3	($989.56)
195	Simple Pneumonia and Pleurisy, without CC/MCC	100	3	0	$1,120.56
292	Heart Failure and Shock with CC	200	7	3	($1,895.62)
308	Cardiac Arrhythmia and Conduction Disorder with MCC	116	4	0	$460.75

CC, Complications and Comorbidity; MCC, Major Complications and Comorbidity; MS-DRG, Medicare Severity Diagnosis-Related Group
*Total number of patients seen annually in each MS-DRG.
†Total number of days per case above or below average length of stay at comparable institutions.
±Amount per case.
Note: The figures in this table are hypothetical and are presented for clarification purposes only.

Conversely, MS-DRGs 195 and 308 are not a high priority for CMP development because the length of stay is same as comparable institutions and they are financially profitable. The institution may decide to develop CMPs for these diagnoses based on other factors and improvement efforts, such as quality of care, practice patterns, and allocation and use of resources.

Deciding which CMPs must be developed is not always the decision of the steering committee. Some healthcare organizations leave such decisions open and encourage the various departments and specialties to decide on the topics that are appropriate for them. Other organizations may purposefully leave such decisions to the clinicians and address the development of CMPs as a department-based quality improvement plan. In either case, the steering committee may institute the use of a communication tool/form so that it is kept abreast of the developments in each department (Figure 10.5). The use of this tool is beneficial to the organization. It helps keep the steering committee informed of the activities and improvements taking place at the department level. It also ensures that the departments are kept focused and on target and that their efforts are not being wasted. Furthermore, it allows the steering committee to evaluate the level of responsibility, accountability, and initiative assumed by the department.

10.3.4. Step 3: Organize an Interdisciplinary Team

Traditionally, members of the interdisciplinary team were selected by the steering committee, and recommendations from department heads were usually considered when organizing the team. Today, however, most healthcare organizations defer this responsibility to the various departments and clinical specialties. In this case, the departments and the steering committee communicate constantly. The department may also seek the advice of the steering committee when problems arise or challenging decisions need to be made. The selection of members is based on their communication skills and ability to work in a team, their clinical competence and past experiences, and their commitment to their work. Becoming a member of an interdisciplinary team and contributing to the development of processes that improve patient care can be a rewarding experience for staff members.

Based on the type of the CMP to be developed, members from the various disciplines involved in patient care are selected to serve on the team. It is important to include all disciplines so that the completed plan is thorough and well written. Every team should include representatives from various departments or disciplines such as medicine (including house staff), nursing, case management, quality improvement, patient safety, patient experience, utilization management/revenue cycle, social services, home care, and nutrition. Members from other departments may participate on a consultation basis. These departments may include pharmacy, medical records and coding, finance, patient representative, materials management, laboratory, and radiology. Some departments may be represented as needed based on the diagnosis being worked on. For example, representation from rehabilitation, occupational therapy, and speech pathology is essential for a team working on a stroke CMP, respiratory therapy for asthma, chronic obstructive pulmonary disease, or pneumonia plans.

The interdisciplinary team should be moderate in size (i.e., six to ten members). A larger team reduces its productivity, increases the risk for disagreements, and delays the process. The team is empowered by the steering committee to make independent decisions. The steering committee may designate one of its mem-

When a CMP topic is selected, please complete this form and send to the steering committee. This will allow us to maintain a database of CMPs in development and ensure that work does not commence in an area where another CMP is in development or already in existence. This also will offer an opportunity to designate an executive sponsor to the CMP development team.

Medical Service Involved: _____

Suggested CMP Title: _____

Projected Volume of Cases per Year: _____

Rationale for Development (Place a checkmark "√" for all that apply)

_____ LOS Outlier   _____ High Variance in Practice

_____ Cost Outlier   _____ High Volume

_____ Quality Concern   _____ Legal Risk

_____ Safety Concern   _____ Clincal Trial/Research

_____ Other, specify: _____

Team Members (Include Disciplines Involved and Contact Information)

Physician Co-Lead: _____

Nurse Co-Lead: _____

Case Management Co-Lead: _____

Team Members: _____
_____
_____
_____
_____
_____

Figure 10.5 Case management plan, predevelopment communication form.

bers to act as a sponsor for the team. The sponsor's role (Case Manager's Tip 10.4) includes coaching the team through the process, removing obstacles and answering unresolved questions, acting as a liaison between the team and the steering committee, and overseeing the administrative activities that keep the team functioning. In addition, it is important for the steering committee to appoint two members of the interdisciplinary team to act as the team leader and the facilitator (Case Manager's Tip 10.5). Most healthcare organizations designate a physician and a nurse to assume these roles. These two members play an important role in keeping the work of the team progressing and ensuring that the goals and objectives of the team are met within the established timeframe. Some institutions may require the team to present its recommended CMP before the steering committee when it is completed and ready for implementation.

Direct care providers should be well represented on the team as team members (Case Manager's Tip 10.6) because they are instrumental in sharing their firsthand experiences with the day-to-day patient care activities. To prevent physicians' resistance to the use of CMPs, it is recommended that they be involved in the process from the beginning and given the leader or co-leader role on the interdisciplinary team. Past experiences show that physicians who participate on a team act as champions in promoting case management systems and CMPs in their institutions and continue to be the best supporters and sellers.

10.3.5. Step 4: Educate/Train the Team in the Process

Before the team launches the development process for a CMP, members should be trained in the process.

CASE MANAGER'S TIP 10.4

Roles and Responsibilities of the Team Sponsor

1. Provides the team with administrative support and power
2. Acts as a resource
3. Answers any unanswered questions or, when unable, facilitates obtaining the answer
4. Acts as the team's liaison with the steering committee
5. Ensures that work is on track
6. Helps the team with problem solving
7. Alerts the team to not make decisions regarding issues that are beyond their realm of responsibilities or power
8. Brings feedback about the team to the steering committee

Formal training must include topics such as a general overview of case management systems and plans; the process of developing CMPs; the responsibilities of the team leader, facilitator, and member; and tools and strategies for success. Examples of the work of other teams, if they exist, should be shared. It is in this forum that the expectations from the team, the administrative support available to the team, and the role of the sponsor and the steering committee as they relate to the role of the interdisciplinary team should be discussed. The team should be given the opportunity to ask any questions or raise any concerns. It should also be informed of the ongoing support of the steering committee throughout the process. After completing the required training, the team starts its work on the plan.

One may ask who prepares the steering committee regarding case management systems and how members of the steering committee acquire their related knowledge. Most healthcare organizations hire an outside consultant (an expert in case management systems) to help and guide them through the process. The consultant plays an important role in helping the steering committee develop the best case management system for the organization. The consultant also develops an education packet specific to the institution's policies, procedures, and operations to train members of the steering committee and the interdisciplinary teams that will be developing CMPs. Sometimes organizations may prefer to hire a full-time employee (instead of a consultant) who is an expert in the area of case management to assume full responsibility for the program. The employee is usually responsible for coordinating all the activities of the program such as educating com-

CASE MANAGER'S TIP 10.5

Roles and Responsibilities of the Team Leader and Team Facilitator

Team Leader

1. Chairs the meeting
2. Prepares the agenda
3. Introduces team members and explains the charge and goals of the team
4. Guides team members through the process of developing CMPs
5. Keeps the team focused on its goals
6. Stimulates discussion regarding treatment modalities and patient care activities and seeks different opinions
7. Encourages active participation of members
8. Helps members reach a common understanding and resolutions on disagreements
9. Builds consensus of members regarding ideal/best practice to be included in the CMP
10. Guides members through problem-solving process when necessary
11. Elicits information, ideas, opinions, comments, and recommendations
12. Ensures that every member gets the opportunity to contribute
13. Obtains commitments for actions
14. Follows up on unresolved/unconcluded issues
15. Clarifies and summarizes conclusions and decisions
16. Collaborates with the facilitator of the team
17. Collaborates with the sponsor of the team

Team Facilitator

1. Coaches the team leader and the members
2. Serves as a role model
3. Ensures the participation of every member
4. Monitors group processes and relieves tension when it arises
5. Interjects as needed
6. Keeps the team focused
7. Maintains a positive and collegial atmosphere during meetings: openness, acceptance, trust, respect, support, cooperation, collaboration, listening, cohesiveness, and teamwork
8. Makes suggestions to keep the team moving forward
9. Confronts interpersonal or process problems
10. Serves as a liaison with team members between meetings
11. Offers support and training sessions as necessary
12. Clarifies ideas and decisions and makes recommendations during meetings
13. Collaborates with the team leader and the sponsor

CASE MANAGER'S TIP 10.6

Roles and Responsibilities of the Team Member

1. Participates actively in meetings
2. Attends meetings
3. Provides relevant information
4. Collects data
5. Supports the team's charge and goals
6. Cooperates in achieving consensus when needed
7. Completes assignments
8. Maintains a positive and collegial atmosphere during meetings
9. Respects the team's ground rules
10. Represents coworkers
11. Seeks guidance when needed
12. Acts as a recorder
13. Collaborates and cooperates in the team process

mittee members, interdisciplinary team members, and staff and acting in place of the consultant.

10.3.6. Step 5: Examine the Current Practice

This step represents the start of the work on the actual content of the plan. The team members usually begin with brainstorming regarding the care of a patient. Members are asked to concentrate on the routine rather than the exception (i.e., the normal recovering patient and not exceptions or extraneous situations) because exceptional patients usually represent a small number of cases. During brainstorming, members attempt to list any quality barriers regarding patient care and any experienced delays in the past. Discussing the quality barriers helps members better understand the current situation and identify the improvement efforts the CMP will address.

After brainstorming is exhausted, team members move on to developing a flow diagram for the current process. A flow diagram that highlights the most important steps in the process of caring for a patient is recommended to prevent the team from getting bogged down with the unnecessary details. The flow diagram (see Figure 1.1 in Chapter 1 for an example of a flow diagram) should reflect the projected care of the patient from admission until discharge and in some cases until after discharge or from the beginning to the end of the care episode.

There are several ways to examine current practice patterns. The two most important ones are to review medical records and to interview care providers. In medical record reviews, members concentrate on the critical elements of care presented in Box 10.7, such as assessment, tests and procedures, treatments, consultation and referrals, care facilitation and coordination, medications, IV therapy, activity level, nutrition, patient and family teaching, wound care, physical and occupational therapy, pain management, outcome indicators and projected desired responses to treatment, and discharge planning. Data collection regarding the critical elements and the associated timeframes of delivery of patient care activities is essential in the development of CMPs. Mostly, tools to simplify and standardize the process of collecting data are developed by the team members before starting the data collection process.

Particular attention is given to the care activities considered as critical milestones of care or trigger points for a change in the treatment plan. For example, it is important to collect data about when an IV antibiotic is switched to its oral form during the hospitalization of a patient with pneumonia or when an IV corticosteroid is switched to an oral form while caring for a patient with asthma. These milestones are important because they affect the length of stay and are considered outcome measures or quality indicators. It is recommended that a thorough chart review be done regarding the most significant care activities that are required for a case type, with particular evaluation of their timeframes for completion. For example, caring for a patient hospitalized for a coronary intervention procedure may require healthcare professionals (physicians, nurses, and others) to ensure the successful completion of several different care activities preprocedure, intraprocedure, post-procedure, and at the time of discharge. These activities, as specified in Box 10.5, should be the center of medical record reviews when developing a CMP for coronary interventions.

Practice patterns of individual physicians and providers should be assessed for variables such as length of stay and cost per case (Table 10.5) by examining the effect of the starting time of antibiotic therapy on the length of stay (Figure 10.6) or by reviewing the use of resources per case including the following for example:

- Volume/number of electrocardiograms (average per patient)
- Volume/number of x-ray examinations and other radiologic scans (average by type per patient)
- Blood tests and average by type by patient
- Use of medications
- Specialty consults
- Discharge and disposition (e.g., home with no services, nursing home, acute and subacute rehabilitation)
- Arranging for durable medical equiment

■ Other, such as patient demographics and route of entry to the hospital as these variables' length may affect the length of stay.

■

In the example seen in Table 10.5, physician B has the lowest average length of stay and the lowest cost per case. This physician appears to be providing care differently from the others. Medical records for this physician's patients must be reviewed and compared with other physicians' records to identify differences and to determine appropriate practice patterns for the CMP.

Using the example in Figure 10.6, one can see that the earlier the first dose of antibiotic is started in a pneumonia patient, the shorter the average length of stay will be. Based on this conclusion, the interdisciplinary team may recommend that the antibiotic to be used to treat pneumonia should be started as early

TABLE 10.5. Example of Physicians' Practice Patterns for Diagnosis-Related Group 89: Simple Pneumonia and Pleurisy, Age Greater Than 17 Years with Complications and Comorbidities.

Physician Code	Number of Cases	Average Length of Stay (Days)	Cost per Case
A	55	5.2	$9,280.56
B	50	3.0	$6,985.44
C	34	5.6	$9,986.53
D	30	6.0	$9,895.32
E	25	5.4	$9,643.50
F	18	4.8	$7,856.64

Note: The data are presented for clarification purposes only.

as the time of admission or when the patient is seen in the emergency department. This recommendation should be reflected in the timeline of the CMP for pneumonia.

After completing the medical record reviews, team members interview representatives of the healthcare team who provide care for the patient population in question. This includes physicians, house staff, nurses who provide direct patient care, and ancillary and professional staff. Similar to the medical record reviews, the interviews concentrate on the critical elements of care and their attached timeframes.

Other important documents available in the organization are also reviewed by the team and are studied carefully for their relation to and impact on the delivery of care. These may include any data reports on file in the institution (e.g., utilization, financial, quality assurance and improvement, and medical record reviews), the standards of care and practice, the preprinted physician orders, protocols, and guidelines.

As members of the CMP development team review the practice patterns of providers and a sample of the medical records, they may find that there is no consistency in treatment plans. An important strategy to address such situations and to routinely complete when developing CMP content is a review and evaluation of the related evidence literature (see step 6 below). This helps the team to decide on which plan of care to adopt.

The literature may not always provide the answer. In this case the team's next strategy is to pursue consensus building on a desirable treatment approach with key and influential providers in the organization to resolve this dilemma. Situations such as this are common, especially in areas in which treatment options are controversial, no research is available to support one type of treatment versus another, or no national stan-

---

Box 10.7 Indicators for Data Collection from Medical Records Review of Patients: Postcoronary Intervention Cases-Examples

■ Demographic data: age, sex, risk factors related to coronary artery disease, and insurance coverage (e.g., Medicaid, Medicare)

■ Comorbidities

■ Services used prior to admission/procedure (e.g., home care)

■ Resource utilization (tests): blood work, chest x-ray examination(s), electrocardiograms, angiograms, and echocardiograms

■ Medications (preprocedure and postprocedure): cardiac medications, anticoagulants

■ Length of stay (preprocedure, postprocedure, and total) and time spent in the cardiac catheterization laboratory (during procedure)

■ Length of stay in the coronary care unit, telemetry unit, and/or observation/postprocedure recovery area (as applicable)

■ Ionic/nonionic contrast use

■ Sheath: arterial, venous, or both; time spent with sheath in place; timing of sheath removal; use of vascular hemostasis device (e.g., vasoseal/collagen)

■ Ambulation: length of time on complete bed rest after sheath removal

■ Need for community services after discharge

■ Patient/family teaching regarding disease, procedure, medications, diet, prevention, and exercise

■ Complications: hematoma, pseudoaneurysm, bleeding

■ Cost per case (finance is usally able to share such data)

■ Past quality and safety concerns

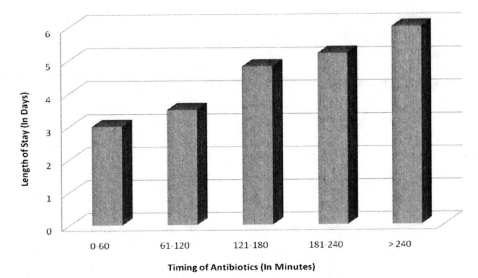

Figure 10.6 Example of physician's practice patterns: timing of first antibiotic dose and length of stay for patients in diagnosis-related group 89. Note: The data in this figure are presented for clarification purposes only.

dards/recommendations are made by professional and specialty organizations. When the CMP development team encounters such a situation, it must look at it as an opportunity for a change in practice and for innovation; that is, developing new care methods and treatment options. The team must then test the new methods and evaluate their outcomes. If the outcomes achieved are not desirable, the new methods must be altered as indicated and then retested. If found to be favorable, they should be adopted on a larger scale as the normal practice and standard of care. Such a process results in the development of new ideal/best practices in areas that otherwise might be considered controversial.

10.3.7. Step 6: Review the Available Literature

A thorough review and evaluation of the literature is essential because it raises awareness of team members to the latest trends and innovation in patient care. The available research should be studied carefully and used to validate the recommendations made in the CMP. This creates an opportunity to provide patient care that is research/evidence-based. Without consideration of the relevant outcomes of research and clinical trials, the CMP developed becomes specific to the healthcare organization and may not reflect the ideal/best practice, or the state-of-the-science care. To promote the development of a CMP that is evidence based, research utilization methodologies must be incorporated in the process of developing the content of the plan. This is achieved through a critical review, analysis, and evaluation of the literature.

The evidence literature supplies the team with the latest clinical practice evidence. However professional societies have reviewed, endorsed, and advocated for recommendations for the leatest and best care guidelines. A place to look for these guidelines is the National Guidelines Clearing House. Others are professional societies such as the American Medical Association or the Society of Hospital Medicine.

It is important to merge the processes of CMP development and research/evidence utilization. This can be achieved by applying the following actions:

- Review the research literature as it pertains to the topic of the CMP or the clinical practice problems.
- Evaluate and critique the research for its level of evidence and quality, strengths, and weaknesses.
- Evaluate the appropriateness of the research outcomes for application in practice.
- Apply the outcomes that are considered ready for implementation in practice by incorporating them as an integral part (i.e., care activities and interventions) of the content of the CMP.

Review of the literature should also include an examination of any published related quality improvement efforts, CMPs, and existing standards of care that are developed by professional organizations such as the TJC, physician groups and societies such as the American Medical Association, nursing organizations such as the American Nurses Association, or governmental agencies such as AHRQ. Other essential literature to be used in the development of CMPs is the literature on transitional planning and managed care guidelines. It is necessary to examine transitional planning to obtain information on the latest regulations about the various care settings across the continuum and their related admission and discharge criteria and associated reimbursement methods. The managed care literature relates to the Milliman Care Guidelines and InterQual Criteria. These guidelines play an essential role in ensuring that the CMPs developed adhere to the managed care reimbursement standards by including appropriate interventions and care progression activities and reinforcing the provision of quality care and services.

10.3.8. Step 7: Determine the Length of the Plan

The length of the CMP is based on several factors, including institutional administrative reports regarding the average length of stay and reports of length of stay per physician, the DRG's length of stay for Medicare and non-Medicare populations, managed care contracts and their respective organizations, variations in practice patterns as they relate to the length of stay, physician preference, reimbursement reports, benchmarks from other healthcare organizations, and improvement targets. The team should study the length of stay issue very carefully, and it should seek the steering committee's support and guidance as needed. The length of the CMP, as decided by the team, should be within the reimbursable range and lower than the institution's current average length of stay for that particular diagnosis or DRG. Also, it is crucial that improvement targets regarding length of stay, mostly decided by the steering committee, are made known to the interdisciplinary team before launching the development process of the CMP.

10.3.9. Step 8: Write the Content of the Plan

This step involves compiling all of the data collected in the previous steps. Representatives from each department are asked to write a draft of their respective part in the provision of care following the approved format of the plan and based on the results of the data collected from chart reviews, interviews, and review and evaluation of the literature and research outcomes. All drafts are then put together on one form to be discussed and finalized by the team members.

The content of the plan should reflect the state-of-the-science care and the ideal/best practice that was agreed on by the team, in realistic timeframes. For example, expecting to complete a cardiac catheterization procedure on same day of the hospitalization of a chest pain patient, knowing that the system requires a turnaround time of 24 hours from ordering to completion, may not be realistic for a nonurgent

situation. Such an unrealistic expectation will result in delays in care, compared with the plan, every time a patient with chest pain is admitted for treatment. However, the team may make a recommendation to the steering committee that the process for completing a cardiac catheterization procedure in 24 hours be evaluated so that a same day turnaround is possible. It then becomes the responsibility of the steering committee and executive sponsor to make a final decision regarding the timeframe.

When the team finishes the plan, it should be circulated for review by a group of physicians, nursing practice leaders, ancillary department heads, and support services involved in the care of the specific patient population. The CMP also must be sent to the pharmacy department to review whether the medications selected are cost-effective and to the coding division of the medical records department for a review of word choices that may enhance coding and improve reimbursement. This review must be done before concluding the content of the plan, and it could be done earlier in the process. In some organizations, the following forums may also be required to review and endorse the CMP before its implementation.

- Medical Board
- Nursing Board
- Senior leadership team
- Medical service chairs
- Nursing practice council
- Other interdisciplinary practice committees

The CMP will then undergo a final review by the team with regard to the recommendations of the reviewers. The final draft of the plan is then presented to the steering committee for approval. The steering committee may suggest the use of an approval form (Figure 10.7). In case such a form is used, the multidisciplinary development team will be required to submit the final draft of the CMP attached to the approval form for the steering committee review and approval. The use of this form is important for record keeping with regard to the review and approval process. The team clarifies any questions asked and presents the reasons a particular practice pattern was recommended. Finally, the CMP is put into practice.

10.3.10. Step 9: Conduct a Pilot Study/Test Case of the Plan

In this step the team implements the use of the CMP. Training and education regarding the CMP for all healthcare providers involved in the particular specialty

This form must be completed by the facilitator of the CMP development team. The purpose of this form is to provide the steering committee with a concise record of CMPs. The completion of this form is essential for archival of all plans, a system to expedite updates to the tools used on an annual basis, and a checklist to ensure policies, standards, and procedures for CMP development and endorsement have occurred.

Case Management Plan Title: _____

Medical Service/Department: _____

Date Completed: _____

Development Team (May Attach a List of Members with Titles and Contact Information)

Suggested Date of Implementation: _____

Standardized Order Set Developed: _____

	YES	NO
Patient/Family Version Developed:	____	____
Variance Indicators Outlined on Tracking Form:	____	____
Quality/Outcome Indicators Outlined:	____	____
Is this a Revision of an Existing CMP (If Yes, Attach Old CMP):	____	____

Reviewed by: _____

Medical/Department Chair: _____

Director of Nursing: _____

Pharmacy (Review of Suggested Drugs): _____

Medical Records/Health Information Systems: _____
(Review of Abbreviations, other Terms Used)

Figure 10.7 Case management plan communication and approval form.

or diagnosis should be completed before implementation of the plan (Box 10.8). The CMP is then evaluated for quality, feasibility of use, appropriateness of timeline and clinical activities and interventions, length of stay, any delays or variations in care, practice patterns of physicians and other care providers, and compliance. For the CMPs that include state-of-the-science care and are considered research/evidence-based, it is important for the team to evaluate the appropriateness of such content to the patient population addressed in the CMP. Therefore it is necessary for the team to evaluate the patient outcomes achieved by the CMP to ensure that they are consistent with those reported in the original research, evidence, or clinical trials. If the outcomes and other CMP features tested are found to be consistent with the intent, targets, and relevance to the current care setting and patient population, the CMP is then finalized as the standard of care.

If the outcomes are not found to be of concern, (e.g., ineffective, inappropriate to the patient population) the team must re-examine the interventions, evaluate the possible causes, determine why the outcomes are unacceptable in the current setting, and revise the content accordingly. Such process must continue until the team is pleased with the results. This evaluation may be conducted in the form of a quality improvement process or research process if the team finds it important to conduct a research study. However, this may delay finalizing the CMP and may require the use of a comparative groups—one with and one without use of the CMP.

The CMP is piloted on a group of patients. In addition to evaluating the content of the CMP, it is as

---

Box 10.8   **Education and Training of Staff and Providers on the Use of Case Management Plans**

The education and training of staff and providers must address the following objectives:

- Present an overview of CMPs
- Discuss the purpose and benefits of CMPs
- Define CMPs
- Describe the roles and responsibilities of the various professionals and providers affected by the use of CMPs
- Explain the elements of care, definition of outcomes, variances, and their classifications, and the format of the CMP
- Explain the use of the variance tracking tool
- Review an example of a CMP using a case study
- Perform documentation using a CMP
- Review the standards of care and practice, and policies and procedures pertaining to CMPs
- Discuss how CMPs integrate with electronic documentation and provider order entry systems
- Review the process to be used for evaluation of CMPs

---

important to survey the providers using the CMP for their perception and satisfaction with its use including impact on workflows and roles and responsibilities of the clinicians affected most by the CMP. Figure 10.8 presents an example of a tool that can be used for this purpose. The results of the pilot are then analyzed and discussed by the interdisciplinary team, and revisions are made accordingly. The plan is then finalized for official use.

10.3.11. Step 10: Standardize/Normalize the Plan

After completing the pilot study of the CMP and making the required changes, the interdisciplinary team meets to develop policies and procedures regarding the use of the plan. It should be made clear to all involved healthcare professionals that the CMP represents the standard of care for that particular population and should be followed when caring for the patient, except for those who meet the exclusion criteria. It should be made clear that some patients might not fit the CMP and that it is appropriate not to use the CMP in these situations (Case Manager's Tip 10.7). It is common knowledge that CMPs do not apply to every type of patient because they are developed based on the care of the average patient (i.e., for 80% of the population) and not the exceptional cases. The final plan is then added to the master manual of CMPs and circulated

 CASE MANAGER'S TIP 10.7

Implementing Case Management Plans

It is important for the interdisciplinary team developing the CMP to identify the inclusion/exclusion criteria to guide healthcare providers in the implementation of the CMP. It is also important to identify the conditions under which the CMP may be discontinued. Examples of situations when a CMP may be discontinued are as follows:

- A change in the primary diagnosis of the patient
- Significant change/worsening in the patient's condition
- Failure to meet the expected clinical outcomes within the designated timeframe, which results in a serious delay in progressing the patient as specified in the CMP

---

in the final format to key people in the institution. The plan can be shared with various healthcare providers in different forums such as grand rounds, newsletters, and administrative and departmental meetings.

Policies and procedures on the use of CMPs, particularly documentation of patient progress and variances, what to do when a patient's care needs do not fit the CMP, and why it is important to individualize the CMP, are extremely important and should be in place before implementing the use of CMPs. Such policies and procedures serve as a guide and reference for any healthcare practitioner required to use the CMPs.

10.4. PATIENT AND FAMILY CASE MANAGEMENT PLANS

The design and use of CMPs is not limited to those used by providers of care. Patient- and family-focused plans (for use by the lay public) are popular today and are viewed as essential tools for patient/family education about necessary treatments and care expectations. Patient and family CMPs have become an integral component of case management systems. They are developed as an essential progression of provider's CMPs and packaged together as a set of plans that delineate the care of patients for both providers and consumers alike.

Patient and family CMPs (Figure 10.9) are defined as tools for educating the consumers of healthcare. They are patterned after providers' CMPs and include basic information about the plan of care using lay terminology, a language that patients and their families are able

Instructions: Please Check Yes, No, or No Opinion for Each Statement	No	Yes	No Opinion	Comments
CMP Title: Date:				

1. Format
  a. Is easy to understand and follow
  b. Is easy to use for documentation
  c. Allows adequate opportunities for modification				

2. Documentation
  a. Helps improve documentation
  b. Reduces time needed for/spent on documentation
  c. Does not result in duplication (if yes, comment how)				

3. Education
  a. Prepared staff adequately for use of CMP
  b. Clearly defined each discipline's role in the use of CMP
  c. Can be used as an education tool				

4. Variance Tracking
  a. Tool is easy to use
  b. Codes are adequate for describing variances				

5. Outcomes
  a. Evaluation is easier than with a traditional plan of care
  b. Intermediate outcomes identified are appropriate
  c. Discharge outcomes identified are appropriate				

6. Collaboration
  a. CMP enhanced interdisciplinary teamwork
  b. CMP enhanced interdisciplinary team communication				

7. Patient and Family
  a. Facilitates interactions with patient and family
  b. Enhances timely completion of health instruction				

What do you like best/most about the CMP?				
What do you like least about the CMP?				
What would you like to see changed in the CMP?				

Figure 10.8 Assessment of clinician's attitudes, perceptions, and satisfaction with the use of Case Management Plans.

to understand easily. Similar to provider's CMPs, they are diagnosis, procedure, or problem specific; apply a timeline that is appropriate to the care setting they are used in; and may follow a "time-task" matrix format. Furthermore they are written in simple language (i.e., fourth to sixth grade reading level), concise, clear, and characterized by the use of graphics and clip art. The graphics are pictures and symbols used to make the plan more valuable, meaningful, attractive, and interesting to read and use for patients. This is especially important because the plans are directed to those without a medical background.

Patient and family CMPs are used to facilitate the following:

- Educate patients and their families about the normal course of treatment.
- Communicate to patients and their families realistic expectations of the care and timeline.
- Answer patients' and families' questions.
- Enhance informed and shared decision-making.
- Empower patients and enhance their ability to assume more responsibility toward their care (activation, self-management, and engagement).
- Review roles of the interdisciplinary care team members.
- Reinforce the role patients and their families play in their care as integral members of the healthcare team.

Care Providers 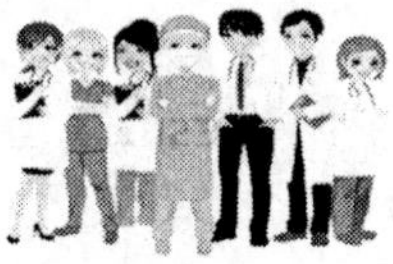	• A team of doctors, nurses, and respiratory therapists will work together to evaluate and treat your asthma.
Tests 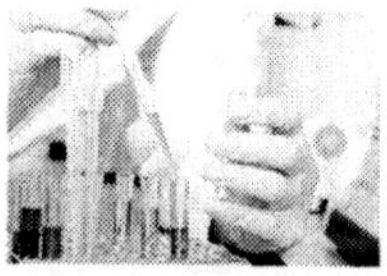	• Peak flow: You will have a simple breathing test one or more times daily. • Blood tests and x-rays (picture): These may be needed one or more times during your stay. • Oxygen measurements: Checking the level of oxygen in your system using a clip placed on your finger.
Treatments 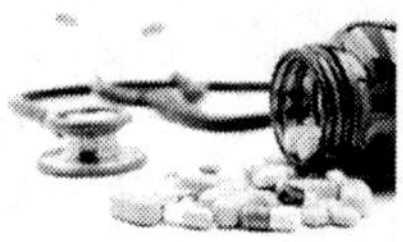	• Intravenous cortisone/steroid is usually given to you the first 24 hours, sometimes longer. • Cortisone/steroid will be changed to pills (prednisone) you take by mouth when your asthma gets better. • Bronchodilator medicine (drug that make your breathing better) will be given to you to open up your airway, more frequent at first. You will take it with a nebulizer—a breathing system that helps you inhale the medicine in the form of a vapor. As your breathing gets better, the medicine will be changed to a metered-dose-inhalor (MDI). • You may require to use oxygen at first. You will receive oxygen through a system you place close to your nose (nasal prongs) or by a face mask.
Nutrition 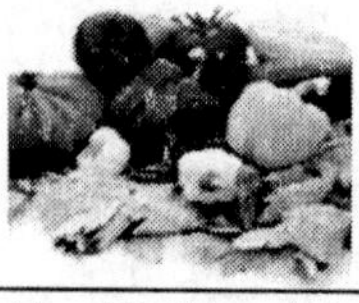	• It will be important to drink more fluids. • A nutritionist (a specialist) will visit you and discuss the foods you eat and advise you about what is best for you.
Health Teaching 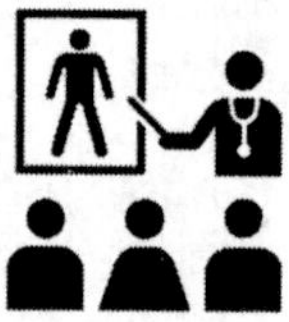	• Learning about your asthma is helpful for you to stay healthy. • Asthma is a preventable condition. By taking your medicines and following the care your health team suggests you are able to control it. • Your healthcare team and nurses will start to teach you about your asthma soon after you enter the hospital. They will teach you about how to prevent having asthma attacks, your medicines, and your inhalor (MDI). • Your health team will prepare a plan for you to use at home. • Your health team will give you information in writing when you leave to go home.
Going Home 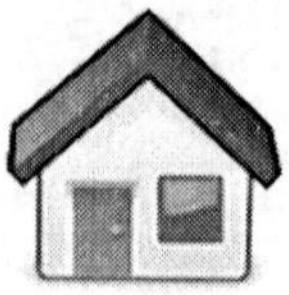	• Most people are ready to go home on the second day, sometimes the third day. • Your healthcare team will discuss with you if you need anything when you go home. • Some people may receive visits at home from visiting/home care nurses. Your healthcare team (nurse, doctor, or social worker) will discuss with you home care if they think you need it. • Your healthcare team will set up a follow-up appointment for you to see the doctor after you leave the hospital.

Figure 10.9 Example of patient and family pathway, adult asthma.

Patient care plans can also be used as a tool for contract development between a provider and a patient/family. The expected outcomes of the plan are reviewed with the patient and family and are given to them in writing as appropriate and feasible. The patient may then be asked to sign the plan, indicating that he or she agrees with it. In this way the contract is developed between patient and provider and the patient becomes an active member of the care team, participating in the development of the goals of care and the expected outcomes and timeframes for achieving the goals.

The plan is reviewed with the patient and family at the appropriate time intervals; that is, at times related to milestones of treatments, as specific outcomes are achieved, or when decisions about treatment options are needed. For example, if the plan consists of daily goals of care, then it should be reviewed with the patient on a daily basis. If the patient achieves a goal sooner than expected, then that achievement should be reviewed and the plan altered accordingly.

Patient and family CMPs are developed by an interdisciplinary team of providers that represent the various specialties and disciplines involved in the care of patients with a particular diagnosis. They are also reviewed and approved by a steering committee similar to the provider-based CMPs. The process of developing patient and family CMPs differs from that of provider's CMPs in that the development team includes a patient advocate or representative whose role is to bring the perspective of patients to the development process. The process is similar to the way patient education materials are developed. In fact, most institutions integrate the patient's CMP development team with the patient and family education committee because of their common aspects and objectives. The skills, knowledge, and expertise of members of the patient/family education committee make it easier for the team to develop patient-focused CMPs. They also enhance writing plans that are personal and conversational in nature. For example, it is common to see patient and family CMPs with phrases such as "you will need to," "you will be asked to," "your physician," "your nurse," or "your case manager." Another characteristic related to style is the use of words that are nonmedical in nature, such as "walk" instead of "ambulate," "going home" instead of "discharge," or "low blood sugar" instead of "hypoglycemia."

The type and number of care elements included in a patient and family CMP varies based on the diagnosis or procedure it addresses. Usually the number is kept to a minimum; that is, limited to those that are essential. The most common elements are tests and procedures, activity and exercise, diet, medications, pain control, teaching and instructions, and preparing to go home. The content included in these elements relates to what is predictable, essential, and standard. "Less is more" is the rule of thumb. It is important to focus on activities the patient is able to handle and control. Refraining from the use of content that patients are unable to comprehend is desirable because it may make them feel frustrated, anxious, or fearful.

10.5. STRATEGIES FOR PHYSICIAN PARTICIPATION AND BUY-IN

Physicians play a key role in the success of the interdisciplinary team charged with developing a CMP for a particular diagnosis or procedure. Physician participation in developing the plan is integral to improving consistency (i.e., eliminating variations in physician practice patterns) in the care of patients with similar diagnoses who are cared for by different physicians. Obtaining physician support is a prerequisite to achieving the identified goals of the team. Physician buy-in to the use of CMPs before their development and implementation is a key to compliance in their use afterward. Case Manager's Tip 10.8 lists some strategies that can be employed to obtain physicians' buy-in and increase their participation in the interdisciplinary teams for CMP development.

10.6. ORGANIZING THE WORK OF THE INTERDISCIPLINARY TEAM

The steering committee may provide the interdisciplinary team members with policy/guidelines that define what is expected from the team and how the work should progress in each meeting. These guidelines are used to facilitate, simplify, and expedite the process of developing and implementing CMPs (Case Manager's Tip 10.9). The steering committee assigns the team's leader and facilitator before the team's first meeting. These two members are specially trained to assume these roles. Interdisciplinary team members are also trained in the roles they play. Preparing all members of the team, including the facilitator and leader, is important because training improves the team's productivity and increases members' skills in teamwork and CMP development.

Despite the popularity of CMPs, there still exists some confusion about how to maintain an interdisciplinary focus while encouraging all disciplines to use CMPs. Selling the use of CMPs to a diverse and large group of providers is not an easy task. Obtaining buy-in from the different disciplines requires special tactics

CASE MANAGER'S TIP 10.8

Gaining Physicians' Support of Case Management Plans

Strategies and benefits that can be communicated to physicians to gain their buy-in and increase their participation in the interdisciplinary teams to develop CMPs include the following:

- Involve physicians in the process of developing CMPs from the beginning. Find a champion(s) and capitalize on his or her participation to influence others.

- Approach influential physicians who are interested in improving the quality and safety of care and reducing the related cost for participation.

- Demonstrate the benefits of CMPs to physicians' personal practice.

- Educate physicians about the use of CMPs and share with them related published materials (e.g., evaluative research, description of case management systems, physicians' opinions from other similar institutions). Also share similar information with their office staff.

- Emphasize that CMPs are recommendations for treatment rather than rigid guidelines or standing orders. Make clear to all physicians that the CMP should be individualized for each patient on initiation and that changes are possible.

- Delineate how CMPs enhance quality of care, safety, and patient experience:
  a. Clearly and proactively defined care expectations and physicians' preferences
  b. Improved continuity of patient care, especially if a patient requires care across different patient care units within the same institution
  c. Detailed patient/family education requirements
  d. Open communication patterns among various disciplines involved in the care
  e. Care-related variance data tracking; the use of variance data for continuous quality improvement efforts
  f. Clear expectations shared with patients in lay langue they understand

- Delineate how CMPs enhance cost of patient care:
  a. Predetermined patient care activities that are sequenced in a timely manner to achieve appropriate length of stay and expected outcomes
  b. Modifications of physicians' practice pattern
  c. Consistency in patient care across physicians
  d. Improvement in patient care as a result of variance tracking
  e. Benefits of the CMP in reducing risk management issues

- Communicate how CMPs improve compliance with the standards of regulatory and accreditation agencies.

- Explain how the plan could be used as an education/training tool for residents, house staff, nurses, case managers, and students.

- Emphasize that the plans may be used as marketing tools to attract more participation from managed care organizations.

- Stress opportunities for research and creativity in patient care delivery.

- Emphasize that data from tracking variances facilitate changes in hospital systems to eliminate inefficiencies in patient care.

- Share an individual physician's performance data/practice pattern and how it compares to that of other physicians in the hospital and in comparable institutions.

- Avoid a punitive approach. Reward those who are willing to participate and address the concerns of those who are hesitant.

- Use data and not emotions to gain cooperation.

- Educate physicians about the reimbursement methods, their impact on practice behaviors, and the role CMPs play in managed care contract negotiations.

and political correctness. Using interdisciplinary teams for the development, implementation, and evaluation of CMPs is a move in the right direction. However, this is not the answer to all concerns. Tahan (1998) described 14 strategies that are still applicable today for enhancing the interdisciplinary nature of CMPs and the participation of the different providers in their development. These strategies are summarized in Box 10.9.

Interdisciplinary teams need an average of six to eight meetings, 1 hour each, to complete a CMP. The following sections outline an example of how the work of the team should be planned.

10.6.1. Preparation Meeting

The steering committee assigns the team leader and facilitator based on the specific case type/CMP to be developed. A meeting is then held between representative(s) from the steering committee and the leader and facilitator, during which the goals and expectations of the interdisciplinary team are discussed. During this meeting the following issues are finalized:

- Membership of the team, including physicians
- Length of stay of the CMP
- Training and education of the team members
- Date, time, and place of the team's first meeting
- Finalizing the agenda of the first meeting
- Notifying team members of their participation on the team
- Establishing a timeline for the team's work and a target date for completion of the CMP
- Sharing of the available data (previous administrative, length of stay, and utilization review reports) related to the CMP type

10.6.2. Interdisciplinary Team's First Meeting

During the first meeting, the interdisciplinary team leader discusses the team's goals and expectations and the timeline for completion of the expected work. A list of all team members and their phone numbers is distributed. If the CMP development form is not already completed and submitted to the steering committee, it is finalized during this meeting. This meeting is geared toward educating the team members. The issues discussed include the following:

- The process of developing a CMP
- Goals for improvement
- Specific discussion regarding the responsibilities of each member in the development of the CMP

- The template of the CMP as provided by the steering committee
- The available data related to the particular case type and examples of CMPs from other institutions
- Assignments for the next meeting (plan of care related to each discipline)
- Finalizing the meeting's schedule (date, time, location, and frequency)

Box 10.9   Strategies for Enhancing the Interdisciplinary Nature of Case Management Plans

1. Every discipline is equally important regardless of the degree of its involvement in the delivery of patient care.

2. Membership in CMP development teams should be reflective of the patient population being addressed.

3. Every team member should be empowered as a champion in advocating the use of CMPs in their own discipline/department.

4. Communication to the various clinical, administrative, and support providers/staff members on all levels cannot be overemphasized.

5. Clear, concise, and crucial guidelines for the development, implementation, and evaluation of CMPs are significant factors that must not be ignored.

6. The various sources of data available in the organization are integral for making interdisciplinary decisions and building consensus and must be shared with the team.

7. Documentation in the CMP should not be limited to nursing.

8. Ensure compliance with standards of regulatory and accreditation agencies, especially a seamless approach to patient care.

9. The role of the ancillary departments (allied health and support services) is an important element of successful CMP development and must not be ignored.

10. Resource allocation and management is every department's benefit.

11. The multidisciplinary nature of CMPs increases the chances of obtaining new managed care contracts and maintaining or enhancing old ones.

12. Interdisciplinary CMPs are documented standards of care and practice for all disciplines and help reduce the risk of legal liability and malpractice litigation for all disciplines.

13. CMPs help establish an interdisciplinary outcomes- and research-based practice environment.

14. CMPs may be used as a strategy to enhance patient and family satisfaction.

CASE MANAGER'S TIP 10.9

Content of guidelines for the development of Case Management Plans

- Define a CMP using a template/example.
- Use a glossary of terms.
- Provide direction for content of the CMP using a standard set of patient care elements to be included in the plan. Define each element and include examples.
- Identify the steps to be followed by the team in the development process of a CMP (i.e., selection of the case type, how to identify opportunities for improvement [e.g., high risk, high volume, cost outlier, length of stay outlier, problem prone, quality issue, physician preference], how to identify the need for data and where to obtain them [internal and external mechanisms], and the process of consensus-building associated with defining the content of the CMP).
- Define the approval process of the CMP and the role of the steering committee.
- Define the use of a disclaimer. State an example. Clarify whether a standard statement is to be used on all CMPs. Include the statement in the guidelines and in the CMP template.
- Define the use of outcomes and their types: intermediate and discharge or process, structure, and patient-related. Include examples of each in the guidelines.
- Clarify the documentation process associated with the CMP. Review daily the process of the plan during the time it is in use/applied in patient care. State the implications for all providers and disciplines.
- Explain the use of preprinted physician orders and algorithms.
- Describe the functions of members of the CMP development team, including the roles and responsibilities of the team leader, facilitator, and member.
- Explain the process of variance (outcomes) data collection and tracking and the mechanism of reporting and feedback. Define the relationship between variance data and quality improvement initiatives.
- Identify the implementation process. Pilot the CMP before standardization and wide use.
- Define the education process: who should teach, who should attend, and how should teaching/training be conducted (e.g., area/discipline-based, centralized).
- Address the issues of patient and family confidentiality associated with the use of CMPs.
- Discuss the use of patient and family pathways. Define the reading level to be followed, the format, the use of pictures, their process of implementation, and so on.

10.6.3. Second Meeting

During the second meeting, team members conduct a medical records review and discuss the following:

- The preliminary plan of care prepared by each member of the team as it relates to the discipline he or she represents
- The timeline placement of the recommended interventions
- The assignment for the next meeting (finalize the plan of care of each discipline)

10.6.4. Third and Fourth Meetings

During the third and fourth meetings the team finalizes the recommended plan of care, compares the ideal/best practice with the review of literature available, and makes changes as needed. The team starts to discuss the expected outcomes of care and does the following:

- Finalizes the interventions and the treatment plan

- Starts discussing the intermediate and discharge outcomes of care
- Begins looking at the preprinted physician order set
- Ensures that the patient's actual and potential problems are included in the plan

10.6.5. Fifth Meeting

In the fifth meeting members of the interdisciplinary team present the intermediate and discharge outcomes of care related to their portion of the CMP. A discussion takes place on whether these outcomes are feasible within the timeline recommended. If any problems are identified, adjustments are made. The preprinted physician order set and the list of patient's problems are also confirmed. At this point the CMP is near completion. The team starts to discuss variance tracking and what types of data are to be collected.

10.6.6. Sixth Meeting

The sixth meeting is spent finalizing the significant

data for variance tracking. The team also prepares the final CMP to be shared with the chief of the department in which the CMP will be implemented. It is important to also obtain the steering committee's feedback on the recommended CMP before it is finalized. In addition, the team starts planning for pilot testing of the CMP.

10.6.7. Seventh Meeting

During the seventh meeting, the interdisciplinary team discusses the recommendations made by the chief of the department and the steering committee. The CMP is revised accordingly. The pilot-testing (prototype test case) plan is finalized, and the CMP is confirmed in its final version that is ready for testing.

10.6.8. Eighth Meeting

The last meeting is spent reviewing the pilot data. Data are analyzed, and a decision on whether the CMP is ready for wide implementation is made. Based on the data collected during the pilot period, the CMP is revised and finalized. At this point the CMP is ready to become the standard of practice. It is usually submitted to the steering committee in its final version with recommendations for implementation. The report generated by the interdisciplinary team, which is based on the pilot of the CMP, is also given to the steering committee. In this meeting the work of the interdisciplinary team is completed. The team may also decide on follow-up dates for meetings to evaluate the use of the CMP and the variance data collected to determine if any changes should be made in the CMP.

The interdisciplinary team members work on their assignments in between meetings. The actual meeting time is used for follow-up on work progress and for discussions around identified concerns or issues. Case Manager's Tip 10.10 presents strategies for holding effective meetings. These strategies can be applied by case managers when involved in running meetings, whether related to developing CMPs or not.

The use of CMPs has become more popular in virtually all patient care settings. The standardization of the process of developing these plans is extremely important. The previous discussion provides healthcare and nursing administrators and case managers with a practical, step-by-step approach to developing CMPs. It can be used as a tool to train members of interdisciplinary teams involved in developing CMPs. The method presented is flexible and can be tailored to any organization or care setting across the continuum. It can be used to develop CMPs for the care of patients in acute, ambulatory, long-term, or home care settings. The pro-

---

Box 10.10   Strategies for Running Effective Meetings

- Identify the purpose of the meeting.
- Prepare an agenda before the meeting, distribute it to the members, and allow them to add items/issues to it.
- Be sure that all agenda items are necessary and appropriate.
- Allocate in advance the time needed for discussing each agenda item.
- Start and finish the meeting on time.
- Stay on schedule during the meeting. Adhere to the allotted time for each item. If discussion is not concluded within the allotted time, follow up on the item in the next meeting.
- Assign subgroups to work on certain issues in between meetings to maximize the utility of the meeting time. Ask these subgroups to report back with the outcomes/decisions during the next meeting.
- Allow and encourage participation of all members.
- Clarify and summarize discussions/decisions before an issue is concluded.
- Ensure that the environment is conducive to the meeting: room, ventilation, temperature, seating.
- Keep interruptions to a minimum.
- Record minutes.
- Maximize the use of visual aids (e.g., handouts).
- Prevent disagreements. Use consensus building when issues arise.
- Generate a sense of team spirit.
- Ensure normal group dynamics because they are essential to accomplish the purpose.
- Limit participation in the meeting to the necessary players.
- Schedule the meeting on a date and at a time when all necessary attendees are available.
- Be sensitive to organizational politics.
- Avoid mixing business with pleasure.
- Keep conversations relevant and discussions balanced.
- Avoid editorializing.
- Promote active listening.
- Recognize individual expertise and talent.
- Do not dominate the discussion.
- Avoid value judgment statements.
- Allow for difference of opinions.
- Negotiate win-win resolutions.
- Conclude the meeting with a summary of accomplishments and follow-up work.
- Express appreciation.

cess to be followed in these settings is the same, but the content and format of the plans may vary.

The use of CMPs has successfully contained healthcare costs, reduced lengths of stay, improved quality of care, streamlined use of resources, and opened communication lines among the healthcare team members. Formalizing the process of developing CMPs is the first step toward ensuring that these benefits will be met. The proposed process is beneficial to all healthcare providers in any care setting, particularly case managers, whether they are involved in developing CMPs or are planning to get started. It can be used by interdisciplinary team members as a blueprint to develop CMPs. It serves as a guide or safety mechanism to ensure that all bases are covered during the developmental process and before the plan is concluded.

10.7. KEY POINTS

1. Case management plans in the form of evidence-based clinical guidelines or pathways are gaining renewed interest especially in the acute care setting.

2. CMPs today are thought of as tools used to ensure provision of care that applies the latest evidence, reduces practice variation, limits the overuse of unecessary resources, and reduces financial risk.

3. It is necessary for institutions interested in the implementation of CMPs to have a steering committee to oversee the development, implementation, and evaluation of CMPs.

4. It is more effective to have a formal process and structure for developing CMPs.

5. CMPs should be developed based on the literature, particularly research and evidence-based practice, expert opinion, and recommendations of professional organizations and societies.

6. It is important to seek the input of all healthcare providers involved in the care of a particular patient when developing a CMP.

7. The CMP, after it is pilot-tested and approved, should become the institution's standard of care and applied by all practitioners.

8. The interdisciplinary team charged with developing a particular CMP should be given enough guidance by the steering committee and provided with appropriate training and education regarding the process.

9. CMPs should incoproate either the Milliman Care Guidelines or InterQual Criteria into them to ensure cost-effective and quality outcomes.

10.8. REFERENCES

Agency for Healthcare Research and Quality (AHRQ). (2014). The Guide to Clinical Preventive Services-2014. AHRQ, US Preventive Services Taskforce. Available at http://epss.ahrq.gov. Pub. No. 14-05158.

Bozzuto, B. & Farrell, E. (1995). A collaborative approach to nursing care of the open heart surgical patient, *Case Manage* 6(3):47–53, 1995.

Cohen, E.L. & Cesta, T.G. (1997). *Case management: from concept to evaluation*, 2nd ed., Mosby, St Louis, MO.

Cole, L. & Houston, S. (1999). Structured care methodologies: evolution and use in patient care delivery, *Outcomes Manage Nurs Pract* 3(2):53–59.

Dykes, P. (1998). Psychiatric clinical pathways: An interdisciplinary approach, Aspen, Gaithersburg, MD.

Esler, R., Bentz, P., Sorensen, M., et al. (1994). Patient-centered pneumonia: a case management success story, *Am J Nurs* 94(11):34–38.

Ferguson, L.E. (1993). Steps to developing a clinical pathway, *Nurse Adm Q* 17(3):58–62.

Guiliano, H.H. & Poirer, C.E. (1991). Case management: Critical pathways to desirable outcomes, *Nurs Manage* 22(3):52–55.

Hampton, D.C. (1993). Implementing a managed care framework through care IDAPs, *J Nurse Adm* 23(5):21–27.

Hydo, B. (1995). Designing an effective clinical pathway for stroke, *Am J Nurse* 95(3):44–50.

Ignatavicius, D. (1995). Clinical pathways: The wave of the future, *Health Travel* 2(5):23–25, 46–47.

Ignatavicius, D.D. & Hausman, K.A. (1995). *Clinical pathways for collaborative practice*, WB Saunders, Philadelphia, PA.

InterQual, Inc. (1998). System administrators guide, InterQual, Marlborough, MA.

Janken, J., Grubbs, J., & Haldeman, K. (1999). Toward a research-based critical pathway: A case study, OJKSN document no. 1C, July 1 (clinical column). Available online at www.stti.iupui.edu/library/ojksn/cc_doc1c.pdf

Katterhagen, J.G. & Patton, M. (1993). Critical pathways in oncology: balancing the interests of hospitals and the physician, *J Oncol Manage* 2(4):20–26.

Meister, S., Rodts, B., Gothard, J., et al. (1995). Home Care Steps protocols: home care's answer to changes in reimbursement, *J Nurse Adm* 25(6): 33–42.

Parker, C. (1999). Patient pathways as a tool for empowering patients, *Nurs Case Manag* 4(2):77–79.

Schibanoff, J.M., Ed. (1999). *Health care management guidelines*, Milliman & Robertson, New York, NY.

St. Anthony Publishing. (1992). DRG: working guide, Alexandria, VA.

Tahan, H. (1998). The multidisciplinary mandate of clinical pathways enhancement, *Nurs Case Manag* 3(1):46–52.

Tahan, H.A. & Cesta, T.G. (1995). Developing case management plans using a quality improvement model, *J Nurse Adm* 24(12):49–58.

Thompson, K.S., Caddick, K., Mathie, J., et al. (1991). Building a critical pathway for ventilator dependency, *Am J Nurs* 91(7):28–31.

Zander, K. (1991). Care IDAPs: the core of cost and quality care, *New Definition* 6(3):1–3.

Zander, K. (1992). Physicians, care IDAPs, and collaboration, *New Definition* 7(1):1–4.

10.9. APPENDIX 10.1

CASE MANAGEMENT PLANS

This appendix presents a template for case management plans. Case management plans usually delineate the standards of care; identify patients' actual and potential problems, the goals of treatment, and the necessary patient care activities; and establish the projected outcomes of care. Often they are accompanied with a predetermined order set. Today there are software application packages for use of CMPs that are either stand alone or built into electronic documentation and computerized provider order entry systems. If such is available the development of the CMP must be completed with such systems in mind so that it is integrated into rather than independent of the workflows of healthcare professionals. This allows professionals to avoid duplication of activities including documentation.

Things to remember about developing interdisciplinary case management plans:

- Establish an interdisciplinary team.
- Identify team members based on the diagnosis or surgical procedure in question. Members should be chosen based on their clinical experiences, leadership skills, communication skills, tolerance to hard work, and commitment to the institution and the project.
- Identify a team leader and a facilitator.
- Provide the team with administrative and clerical support.
- Establish a project work plan (timeline of activities) before the team's first meeting.
- Train team members in the process of developing CMPs.
- Team members should prepare their work in between meetings. Meetings should be held to review the work and determine the next steps.
- Regardless of the format of the CMP, it should always include the patient care elements as identified by the organization, the patient problems, projected length of stay, and outcomes of care, a variance tracking form, and patient care activities and interventions.
- Create a timeline for the CMP as indicated by the care setting. For example, minutes to hours in emergency departments, number of visits in clinics and home care, days in acute care, weeks in areas of longer length of stay such as neonatal intensive care area, and months in nursing homes and group homes. The timeline of CMPs in subacute care and rehabilitation centers can be established based on the length of stay, goals of treatment, and intensity of activities. For the most part, it is daily or weekly.
- Pre-establish the expected (acceptable) length of stay.
- Identify the inclusion and exclusion criteria (i.e., type of patient population)
- Determine the mechanism for tracking variances and define the variance categories to be evaluated. Some must be relevant to the CMP and based on predetermined milestones of care, intermediate and discharge outcomes.
- Ensure that the CMP is the standard of care applied by all healthcare providers, including physicians.
- Include patient and family teaching and discharge planning activities in all CMPs.
- Determine whether CMPs are a permanent part of the medical record and how it interfaces with the electronic documentation systems.
- Decide on (and complete) the predetermined order set, if one is to be used in conjunction with the CMP.
- Maximize documentation on the CMP. Require all patient care services to use the CMP for documentation and incoparate it into the interdisciplinary plan of care process/workflow.
- Develop CMPs based on the latest recommendations of research evidence and professional societies.
- Avoid being rigid in recommending treatments. For example, use words like "consider" when including treatments, medications, or interventions that may not be applicable to every patient, completion may not always be possible within the indicated timeframe, or progress may be dependent on the patient's condition.
- Identify the intermediate and discharge outcomes of care in each CMP.
- Delineate the ICD-10-CM code or the DRG number of the CMP on the cover page.
- Include all disciplines involved in the care of patients as indicated by the diagnosis or surgical procedure considered.
- Stress the importance of patient care activities that historically were identified as problem areas or required improvement.
- Establish a timeframe for reviewing and revising the CMP.

Example of an Interdisciplinary Case Management Plan Template

Diagnosis: _____   Patient Name: _____

Clinical Service: _____   Location/Unit: _____

Admission Date: _____   Physician: _____

Discharge Date: _____   Case Manager: _____

Problems List: Social Worker: _____

    1.   Other: _____

    2.   _____

    3.   _____

    4.

Allergies:

_____

Care Elements	Specific Actions	Responsible Party	Expected Outcomes	Comments/Notes
Assessment & Monitoring				
Lab Work				
Problem List				
Tests & Procedures				
Treatments				
Medications				
Consults				
Activity				
Nutrition				
Intravenous Therapy				
Respiratory Therapy				
Physical Therapy				

Care Elements	Specific Actions	Responsible Party	Expected Outcomes	Comments/Notes
Occupational Therapy				
Wound Care				
Pain Management				
Patient & Family Health Education				
Psychosocial Assessment				
Discharge & Transitional Planning				
Signatures				

NOTE: The Interdisciplinary Case Management Plan was developed as a suggested interdisciplinary plan of care and based on available evidence. This is only a guideline and may be modified to meet the needs of the individual patients according to patient's condition and assessment data. This Interdisciplinary Case Management Plan is not to be used as a substitute or replacement for clinical assessment and judgment.

11 Quality and Safe Patient Care

Perhaps the most important topic in healthcare today is patient quality and safety. Although healthcare organizations have always had quality and safety at the top of their priority list and strategic plans, especially when the prospective payment systems began in the 1980s, only in recent decades has it been recognized that continuously improving and managing quality and safe patient care outcomes can make a difference. This strategic focus can be as vital as survival or providing the healthcare organization with a competitive advantage in the marketplace. Today the healthcare industry recognizes that a focus on quality and safety is the best way to ensure not only that revenues equal or exceed expenses, but most importantly that patients are safe, receive quality care, and have desirbale experience during their care encounters (Case Manager's Tip 11.1). This approach is particularly important because it prevents healthcare providers and leaders from paying more attention to cost and reimbursement than quality. It also allows them to attain an acceptable balance between the two entities while assuring patient safety is above all. Measuring and evaluating quality of care and safety, therefore, have become more imperative in today's era of value-based purchasing where an organization's quality, safety, and care experience outcomes are no longer kept secret and confidential. In addition, quality patient care and organizational outcomes have become necessary components of the process of care delivery and management.

11.1. IMPORTANCE OF QUALITY

Today's competitive healthcare environment demands constant attention to improvements in quality, safety,

and the patient's experience with care. Consumers are demanding that they receive full value for their healthcare dollar. The goal of any healthcare provider is to have consumers desire to return when necessary for their healthcare needs. If healthcare organizations fail to strive for quality and safety, they will fall behind in the highly competitive marketplace and ultimately go out of business. Focusing on quality and safety allows healthcare organizations to achieve many benefits, which may include the following:

- Efficient use of resources and services
- Meeting the demands, intesrests, preferences, and needs of consumers
- Enhancing the patient's and family's experience with care including satisfaction and engagement
- Provision of compassionate, ethical, and culturally competent patient/family-driven care
- Ensuring patient safety through timely and appropriate care, reduced risk for injury, avoidance of medical errors, prevention of healthcare acquired conditions, and safe disposition or discharge from acute care settings
- Professional and satisfactory performance by providers, including case managers
- Lowering cost of care and health services by eliminating unnecessary use of resources, duplication, and fragmentation of services while ensuring continuity and care progression

11.2. MEANING OF QUALITY

Probably the most difficult hurdle to overcome is to agree on what quality means. What are the properties,

323

CASE MANAGER'S TIP 11.1

The Healthcare Triple Aim

The IHI developed the triple aim as a framework or approach to optimizing the performance of the US healthcare system. When we examine healthcare quality and safety and the opportunity to improve in this regard, as healthcare leaders and professionals we can uuse the dimensions of the triple aim as a guide for where to focus our efforts and which quality aspects we can use to assess the impact of these efforts. Case managers must be familiar with the IHI's triple aim because they are able to influence improvements in all of its dimensions, which are (IHI, 2015):

- Improving the patient's experience of care (better individual health/better care): quality and satisfaction
- Improving the health of populations (better health)
- Reducing the per capita cost of healthcare (affordable or lower cost)

National Strategy for Quality Improvement in Healthcare

In March 2011 and after the passage of the Affordable Care Act, the IHI triple aim grew to become a national agenda and strategy for quality advocated-for and supported by the U.S. Department of Health and Human Services. The three aims of the National Quality Strategy are (USDHHS, 2013):

1. Better care: Improve the overall quality of care by making healthcare more patient-centered, reliable, accessible, and safe.
2. Healthy people and healthy communities: Improve the health of the US population by addressing the social, behavioral, and environmental determinants of health and quality healthcare.
3. Affordable care: Reduce the cost of quality healthcare for all—individuals, families, employers, and government.

---

characteristics, and attributes of care that lead us to a judgment of good or poor quality? Optimal or suboptimal care experience? Quality means different things to different people: the providers, regulators, payers, advocates, and consumers of healthcare. Historically, the providers of care have defined quality. However, since the mid-1980s consumers of care have become more involved in defining what consitiutes quality and influencing the perception of providers and payers of healthcare. Recently however, regulators are defining what quality is and are strongly influencing its focus, and how it is assessed and measured, especially by linking reimbursement to cost of care, quality of care, and perception of health by the consumer. This has recently evovlved and in a prominent way as a result of value-based purchsing—the Patient Protection and Affordable Care Act of 2010, sometimes referred to as the Affordable Care Act. This shift has also necessitated healthcare organizations and providers to show increased commitment to quality and to incorporate quality, safety, and patient experience into their strategic plans, mission, and vision.

For over a decade now the Institute of Medicine's (IOM) definition of quality has been widely accepted and used. The definition brought about an interesting focus for quality; one that is patient- rather than provider- or payer-centered, promotes the application of evidence in practice and examines the the cosnequences of care delivery using objective measures. The IOM defines quality as the degree to which healthcare services and resources provided to individuals and populations improve desired health outcomes and increase the likelihood that these desired outcomes are consistent with professional knowledge (IOM, 2001) available at the time care is provided to individuals and populations.

Consumers' definition of quality is dependent on their needs, interests, preferences, values, and equitable access to services and resources. Although these may vary from one consumer to another, what is important to them is the opportunity to be the drivers of care provision, feeling welcome, that they are important, made comfortable by healthcare providers, and being understood. In addition, consumers appreciate providers with a friendly, compassionate, and supportive attitude and with technical skills and knowledge. They also appreciate cleanliness and comfort in the physical environment of care.

Although the consumers' and providers' definitions of quality are not always the same, it is important for providers to define quality and desired outcomes of care based on the needs, values, and interests of the consumers. This match is necessary so that the individuals accessing healthcare experience the services provided to them as being of optimal quality, safe, and free of errors. It also is important for healthcare providers (both indivudal professionals and organizations) to incorporate the regulators' perspectives on quality, safety, and cost in their forcus to ensure adherence to standards, meeting expectations, and reducing or avoiding financial risks.

Quality of care may include, but is not limited to, available healthcare services, standards of providers, comprehensive assessment and documentation, shared decision making, collaborative and informed relationships with patients and families, minimal to no injuries or complications for hospitalized patients, evaluation of new technology and resources, and effective management of healthcare resources. Along with patient satisfaction and safety, the patient's view of what is important in his or her care may be seen as one aspect of quality when defining indicators and measures of quality. The overall quality of healthcare will be judged on the entire package, including health outcomes, accessibility, timeliness, efficiency of services, interdisciplinary communication, and the direct and indirect costs of illness and care (Case Manager's Tip 11.2).

11.3. CHARACTERISTICS OF QUALITY

From the consumer's point of view, there are three types of quality characteristics: "take it for granted" quality, expected quality, and exciting quality. Take it for granted quality is what a healthcare setting must offer to be acceptable (e.g., clinicans' competency). Expected quality includes those things that are necessary and are a given (e.g., food quality, cleanliness, pleasant experience with care). Exciting quality pertains to those items that are nice to have but are not necessary (e.g., environmental features and decorations). The consumers' needs and values as they relate to quality and safety are of the necessary and expected type of quality. Healthcare providers and organizations cannot ignore them, otherwise the consumer will view the services provided as being of "bad" or "poor" quality. Effective case management must work within a framework that demonstrates quality improvements while taking the patient's perceptions, values, and expectations into account to ultimately assure safe and optimal experience.

Characteristics of quality are also available based on the perception of providers. One approach to describing the characteristics of quality includes the following attributes Donabedian (1980) outlines when assessing for quality:

1. *Effectiveness*: The ability to provide care in the correct manner, given the current and available knowledge, and the ability to attain the greatest improvements in health now achievable by the best care
2. *Efficiency*: The ability to lower the cost of care and resources without diminishing attainable improvements in health
3. *Balance*: The balancing of costs against the effect of care on health so as to attain the most advantageous balance
4. *Acceptability*: Conforming to the wishes, desires, values, beliefs, and expectations of patients and their families in the care decision-making process

 CASE MANAGER'S TIP 11.2

Perception of Quality and Safety

A patient's perception of quality and safety is only as good as the last encounter and experience of care. Regardless however, during the current encounter, you as the case manager have an opportunity to shift the patient experience to being optimal and of high quality. This creates loyalty and better healthcare professional-patient/family relationship.

5. *Legitimacy*: Conformity to social preferences in care delivery as expressed in ethical principles, values, norms, laws, and regulations
6. *Equity*: Conformity to a principle that determines what is just or fair in the distribution of healthcare, its effect on health, and its benefits among the members of the population

The TJC, formerly known as the JCAHO defines other attributes of quality, some of which are similar to those of Donabedian. These attributes are as follows (JCAHO, 2001):

1. *Efficacy*: The degree to which care has been shown to accomplish the desired outcomes
2. *Availability*: The degree to which appropriate care is made accessible to meet the patient's and family's needs
3. *Optimality*: Ensuring the most advantageous balance between benefits and costs of care delivery and services
4. *Timeliness*: Ensuring that care is provided with no delay and when needed
5. *Continuity*: The degree to which care activities and services are coordinated among providers, settings, and over time
6. *Safety*: The degree to which the risk of an intervention or care environment is reduced for patients and providers
7. *Respect and caring*: Providing care with sensitivity and respect for the patient's values, beliefs, expectations, and cultural differences

Regardless of the past perspectives of Donabedian, the TJC, or any other professional organization concerning quality and safety, the current and most popular perspective is that of the IOM which describes quality using six aims. These aims have been used to articulate what quality is, and what focus one must take when assessing and improving it. They also are similar to what Donabedian and the TJC have highlighted in the past. The six aims are (IOM, 2001):

1. *Safe*: Care should be as safe for patients in healthcare organizations as in their homes.
2. *Effective*: The science and evidence behind healthcare services, resources, and care approaches should be applied practice and serve as the standard for the delivery of care.
3. *Efficient*: Care and service should be cost effective, and waste should be removed from the system.
4. *Timely*: Patients should experience no waits or delays in receiving care and services.
5. *Patient centered*: The system of care should revolve around the patient, respect patient preferences, and put the patient in control.
6. *Equitable*: Unequal treatment should be a fact of the past; disparities in care should be eradicated.

Healthcare providers historically have been concerned with the maintenance and improvement of quality of care for hospitalized patients; today however, they are concerned with all patients whether hospitalized or not. This has emerged with the recent increased focus on poulation health management, the IHI triple aim, and the National Quality Strategy. Most healthcare organizations and providers have a mission statement that tends to incorporate emphasis on quality and safety in conjunction with error free culture, set of core values and beliefs. Phrases usually include honesty, transparency, equity, fairness, non-punitive approach or just culture, commitment to patient/consumer satisfaction, and commitment to employee satisfaction in an environment that is conducive to the provision of best care and ensuring the best outcomes. The values are what the organization regards as important. They are the principles that the organization upholds and defends, the fabric that holds the organizational structure together, and the foundation on which it rests.

11.4. SETTING THE STANDARDS FOR QUALITY AND SAFETY

Everyone is interested in the quality of healthcare, including safety, how it is measured, and the results of these measurements. There are many groups that are involved in setting the standards for quality and safety (Box 11.1). Providers, payers, and consumers of healthcare services, as well as governmental and nongovernmental agencies, are all interested in quality. Each, individually, and as a group, directly or indirectly influences the national standards against which

performance is measured and evaluated. Each of these players also is interested in quality for different reasons. For example, providers' interest in quality may pertain mainly to being competitive, safe, profitable, and marketable; however, payers' interest is in ensuring cost-effectiveness and a balance between cost and quality. On the other hand, consumers may focus on the access to and delivery of appropriate and safe care, whereas governmental agencies' regard for quality may relate to keeping control of healthcare legislation and promoting what is in the public interest including safety and affordability. Moreover, nongovernmental agencies and professional associations may play a role in advocating for patients and lobbying for a change in legislation.

The motivation behind the interest of these groups in healthcare quality can be summarized in two ways. Some have pursued quality-related information to

---

Box 11.1   Examples of Groups That Set the Standards for Quality

1. Consumer advocacy groups
   - Coalition of independent groups
   - Public advocates
   - Lobbyists
2. Governmental agencies
   - The Centers for Medicare and Medicaid Services
   - US Department of Health and Human Services
   - State Departments of Health
   - Agency for Healthcare Research and Quality
3. Nongovernmental agencies
   - Institute of Medicine
   - The Joint Commission
   - Commission for Accreditation of Rehabilitation Facilities
   - National Committee on Quality Assurance
   - Institute for Healthcare Improvement
   - National Quality Forum
4. Professional associations and organizations
   - American Nurses Association
   - American Hospital Association
   - National Transitions of Care Coalition
5. Media
   - Journalists
   - Reporters
   - Television news programs
   - Magazines and newspapers
6. Healthcare providers
   - Physicians
   - Registered nurses
   - Case managers
   - Healthcare organizations

make better and more informed decisions regarding healthcare choices; whereas others have sought out such information for political reasons. Regardless of these interests, the variation in the motivation creates a healthy pursuit of, and competition for, what is best for the consumer. To survive in the healthcare market of today, healthcare executives and providers must maintain current knowledge of the interests of these groups, particularly the interests of the consumer and the changing desires of the governmental agencies, politicians, and lobbyists, and public advocates. They must also use this knowledge to ensure that their practices and care delivery systems are updated and altered to meet the expectations of these groups, and the changing dynamics of the healthcare system. If they fail to do this, they are at risk for causing consumer dissatisfaction, unsafe practices, decreased quality, increased costs, unnecessary use of resources, and lower reimbursement.

11.5. A HISTORICAL REVIEW OF QUALITY AND SAFETY

11.5.1. Quality Assurance

Until the mid-1980s, quality in healthcare was measured by concepts and processes categorized under the rubric of quality assurance (QA). This all-encompassing phrase, quality assurance, comprised the healthcare industry's breadth and depth of understanding as to what quality was about as it related to the management and treatment of individuals receiving healthcare services. The name described the underlying philosophy behind it in that quality assurance programs were designed to assure or maintain a particular predetermined level of performance, expectation, activity, process, or standard of care. QA focused on compliance, errors and problems, and most of the time it applied a retrospective process of evaluation. Therefore QA, by definition, was a mechanism for developing predetermined standards of care, implementing strategies for assuring that those standards are met, auditing the standards to examine degree of compliance, and designing an action plan to address staff/provider noncompliance, if present.

Following a QA approach to measuring quality and evaluating compliance, providers applied certain levels of expectation that were also known as thresholds. These thresholds identified a minimal level of performance that the organization would expect to accomplish. For example, the threshold for patient falls in the hospital setting might be: "less than 3% of all patients would experience a fall while hospitalized." As long as the organization did not exceed that threshold, it was satisfied and confident that quality care was being provided. Evaluation took place retrospectively.

Unfortunately, QA did not provide an effective infrastructure for improving performance or exceeding these thresholds. Organizations consistently and retrospectively measured their performance against those thresholds and did not expect to do any better if they were met. Safety was not a popular focus then and punitive approach to correcting noncompliance was more of the norm then.

11.5.2. Transforming Healthcare

As the cost of healthcare continued to rise in the 1980s, organizations began to recognize that they could no longer continue to conduct business as they always had in the past and that they had to search for mechanisms that would not only maintain quality but improve it as well. Healthcare traditionally has lagged behind other industries by 5–10 years in the area of performance improvement and quality management; changes in industry will often be indicators of changes that will eventually occur in healthcare. This was no less true for the quality initiatives undertaken by the healthcare industry in the late 1980s, early 1990s, and today in the twenty-first century. Industry began to focus on total quality improvement (QI) in the 1970s, with healthcare only following suit about a decade later. Industry such as automotive and communication technologies practiced Six Sigma in the 1980s and such approaches to quality improvement did not become a common practice in healthcare until late 1990s and early 2000s.

Other changes also had been taking place. Society and consumers of healthcare services were becoming more educated and well aware of the quality-related transformations occurring in other industries. They became less tolerant of the inefficiencies they traditionally had experienced from the healthcare industry such as lack of coordination of care, fragmentation and duplication of services, absent continuity of care or handoff communication across settings, and long waits to see physicians or receive results of diagnostic tests. This growing sophistication led to greater expectations on the part of the public/healthcare consumers, which had to be responded to by the healthcare industry.

Healthcare expenditures were also becoming a priority in the United States in both the public and private sectors. Diminishing reimbursement and the changes in its methods forced care providers to reassess how they were doing business and to begin to look for new ways to become more cost-effective and efficient. As industry had before it, healthcare began to adopt strategies such as total quality management (TQM), continuous quality improvement (CQI), and performance management as vehicles to help improve quality of care and most recently focusing on safety as well (Box 11.2).

The ability of the healthcare industry to make this shift in focus would be dependent on the extent it redefined itself, particularly in terms of how it measured its own quality and safety outcomes. One consistent theme before the 1980s was "more is better;" focus was more on volume rather than value. This related to the fact that healthcare organizations were rewarded for being bigger with lots of hospital beds, and lots of staff; for providing unlimited services to large numbers of patients; and for performing more and more tests, treatments, and procedures. But the rewards were

---

Box 11.2 Definitions of Quality Assurance, Quality Improvement, Performance Improvement, and Quality Management

Quality Assurance

- Designing a product or service and controlling its production so well that quality is inevitable, and providing assurances that quality requirements will be fulfilled.
- In healthcare, the activities and programs intended to guarantee or ensure quality of patient care and accepted care standards.

Quality Improvement

- A formal approach to the evaluation and analysis of performance and the pursuit of systematic efforts to improve it.
- Involves improving current processes and is normally accomplished with a series of projects to improve the quality of these processes.

Performance Improvement

- A systematic approach to measuring the outcomes of processes and then purposefully modifying these processes to enhance their outcomes.
- Ongoing system evaluation focused on high-risk, high-volume, and/or high-prone issues that affect the outcomes of the systems and processes such as patient expereince of healthcare services.

Quality Management

- Most common today. It is the process of integrating the improvement in quality of care, quality of service, and quality of organizational systems across a healthcare organization.
- The integration is synchronized to deliver higher standards of performance in multiple aspects of the organization's operations.

---

changing. Reimbursement structures were changing with fixed price strategies such as the inpatient prospective payment system (see Chapter 2). This kind of reimbursement scheme motivated healthcare organizations and leaders to manage fixed dollar amounts; therefore the notion of doing more and more with little concern for appropriateness was no longer financially rewarded. The new measure of success became how the organization was able to manage those dwindling returns and still come out even in the end.

Dwindling returns meant that healthcare organizations had to maintain their consumer base. Therefore it became increasingly important for the organizations to attract and retain patients. Patients needed to feel that they were receiving quality, efficient, safe, and effective care of the highest possible level.

11.5.3. Quality Improvement

It became clear that CQI had to replace QA as a process for not only maintaining quality but also constantly improving the level of quality. This is accomplished by continuously learning about the processes and outcomes of care delivery and then using this knowledge to reduce variation and to simplify these processes for both the consumer and provider of care. By reducing variation and streamlining the processes of care, the overall level of performance of the organization is improved. The organization begins to shift from a focus on individuals to a focus on systems, processes, and outcomes. In fact, outcomes become the drivers of the care delivery processes and systems. The punitive apporach to correcting quality concerns started to diminish while a focus on system issues contributing to suboptimal quality become more popular. Another significant shift in improving quality was the prospective versus retrospective approach. This meant that healthcare executives designed a process for quality improvement that focused on preventing undesired outcomes from occurring before they went on to measure the performance of the process. Additionally, safety at this time was still defined based on mortality, morbidity, and errors with limited to no financial consequences associated with quality and safety performance.

QI adds a number of dimensions to the traditional approaches of QA. It not only identifies levels of quality but also expects the organization to meet and exceed these levels. It focuses on the processes and systems that affect quality rather than on the individuals' responsible for care provision (i.e., staff or providers). It also uses data as an important tool in understanding variations in performance and seeks mechanisms to improve and reduce them. In addition, it avoids being punitive or relating the primary source (i.e., root cause) of errors and variations to staff and their actions. QI, therefore, approaches quality from a much broader perspective than that of QA and, most importantly, its work never ends. The organization does not put a stop to its strive toward continuously exceeding its own level of performance over time.

11.5.4. Performance Improvement and Quality Management

Performance improvement becomes the mechanism or infrastructure for CQI and for the purpose of management of quality and its improvement in the broader sense. It follows a logical series of steps in the process of continuous improvement with the ultimate goal of improving the outcomes or outputs of systems. Improvement is achieved by making modifications to the system in areas where it is necessary. The difference in quality mangement from quality improvement is the introduction of statistical analysis tools and process control techniques that went beyond what was known in quality assuarnce and quality improvement. These changes brought the focus on zero defects in outcomes and process variation control to the forefront of quality.

There is a large number of CQI tools and processes. Regardless of which CQI process one applies, generally it may include the following steps:

1. Identify a system, process, or outcome needing improvement
2. Determine the strategies or elements that need to be implemented to improve the problem identified or potentially may occur
3. Implement the improvement strategies
4. Monitor the effects of the improvement strategies over time
5. Change or amend the strategies as needed or maintain the improvements as standard practice

Regardless of the specific improvement plan or framework a healthcare organization may apply, the ultimate place to be is for the organization to never become stagnant, but rather to always be moving forward in its systems, processes, thinking, philosophy, and improvement approach. A primary and ongoing focus is to identify defective areas (or those that may potentially become defective) and opportunities for improvement work, and then implement an action plan for improvement applying the CQI methodology to ultimately achieve better quality and safety outcomes (Box 11.3).

11.5.5. Six Sigma and Lean

Healthcare organizations today have enhanced their performance improvement and quality management processes and efforts to focus more on eliminating de-

---

Box 11.3   Common Quality Improvement Process

The PDCA/PDSA Cycle

This process is also known as the Deming Cycle, the Deming Wheel (after W. Edwards Deming, a pioneer of quality management) or the Shew Hart Cycle. It is simple to apply and refers to the Plan-Do-Check-Act Cycle or the Plan-Do-Study-Act Cycle. Deming believed that a key source of quality is having a clearly defined, repeatable processes in place. The PDCA Cycle is an approach that has been traditionally used in healthcare organizations to assure a process produces the same outcomes repeatedly, every time it is applied. There can be any number of iterations of the "Do" and "Check" phases, as the solution is refined, retested, rerefined, and retested again until desired results are achieved. This cycle applies a prescribed sequence of its four stages with each having a set of associated tasks.

The four stages of the Plan-Do-Check-Act Cycle are as follows:

- *Plan*: Identifying, evaluating, and analyzing the problem. It may be useful to use tools such as cause and effect and map the proicess using flow charts or process flows.
- *Do*: Developing and testing a potential solution(s) for the problem. This step is about coming up with potential solutions and then testing and trying them in a specific, manageable environment and over a predetermined time period. Selecting the best of these solutions is important and then pilot-testing them on a small scale in a limited area.
- *Check*: Measuring how effective the test solution was, and analyzing whether it could be improved in any way. The evaluation usually uses measures that were specified in the plan stage. Depending on the success of the pilot test, the number of areas for improvement you have identified, and the scope of the whole initiative, repeating the "Do" and "Check" steps are sometimes necessary before wide implementation. This is the "Study" step when using the PDSA Cycle.
- *Act*: Implementing the improved solution fully after confirming it was successful and setting up controls to perpetuate the new process. However, applying the PDCA Cycle does not necessarily stop here. If the interest is continuous improvement, it is necessary to then repeat the PDCA Cycle in pursuit of further improvements.

fects and assuring that the outputs (i.e., outcomes) of a process are the same every time the process is applied. Despite the popularity of performance improvement and CQI, the focus was never on zero defects until the last decade when healthcare organizations adopted the six sigma performance improvement process and tools, similar to what has happened in the industry few decades prior.

Six Sigma emerged from the quality management and continuous quality improvement movement and tools applying frameworks such as the PDCA cycle. However, Six Sigma is an approach that focuses on measuring how far a process deviates from perfection. It is a disciplined and data driven improvement method applied to eliminating the defects in a process by assuring the absence of variation in practice. It seeks to improve the quality output of a process by identifying and removing the causes of defects (i.e., errors) and by minimizing deviations using quality management empirical and statistical techniques that inform opportunities for improvement. When done well, the Six Sigma method reduces defects to 3.4 in every one million opportunities; an opportunity is every time a process is applied and a defect is every time the process does not produce the expected outcome (American Society for Quality, 2015). Organizations which have implemented the Six Sigma method also employ the use of experts in the method and empircial techniques as part of their infrastructure; these are referred to as champions, black belts, green belts, or yellow belts.

Each Six Sigma quality management project carried out within an organization follows a defined sequence of steps and has quantified value targets, for example: reduce process cycle of turnaround time, reduce costs by eliminating inefficiencies, and increase customer satisfaction. The most common Six Sigma method is the Define-Measure-Analyze-Improve-Control framework also commonly referred to as DMAIC (Box 11.4). This is a measurement-oriented system that assures improvements that are objective and measureable. The use of DMAIC emphasizes important characteristics of quality that have become the norm in healthcare quality improvement practices such as problem definition through use of data and statistical analyses especially in the determination of impact of solutions on the problem, and using quality assurance methods to ensure the solution/interventions are sustainable (Lighter, 2013).

Lean Six Sigma is another progression of the DMAIC process attributed to Toyota before it became popular in healthcare. While Six Sigma focuses on eliminating defects, lean aims to reduce or completely remove waste from a process. Waste refers to anything that consumes resources (time, money, and personnel)

yet does not add value particularly to the consumer. An example is consumer wait time for a test or an appointment with a care provider. By eliminating waste (e.g., nonessential activities), one assures the process is streamlined and increases the likelihood of having the right thing done, by the right person, in the right amount, and at the right time.

Box 11.4   The DMAIC Six Sigma Process

Motorola championed the use of the Six Sigma proces in the 1980s primarily oustide the United States, and in the 1990s General Electric made it a core business strategy in the United States in the form of the DMAIC Six Sigma process. Healthcare organizations began to apply this process in the late 1990s, but most commonly in the early 2000s.

The American Society of Quality (2015) describes the DMAIC process as follows:

- *Define*: focus is on selecting a process to be examined and improved. Examples of questions answered at this stage are: What is the problem? Who are the customers? What are the custoemr's priorities? What are the project goals and requirements?
- *Measure*: this is when the current state of the process to be improved is examined with a focus on its current capabilities. Examples of questions answered at this stage are: How is the process performing? How is it measured? What measures reflect the customer's input or interest?
- *Analyze*: here, an understanding of the state of deficiencies or undesired outcomes is gained; cause and effect. Examples of questions answered at this stage are: What are the most important causes of the defects? What is their impact on the process? What are the outcomes saying about the process? What are the relationships between the causes and the outcomes?
- *Improve*: the focus is on potential solutions for improving the outcomes and eliminating the defects; testing the impact of the potentnial solutions on the proces capabilities. Examples of questions answered at this stage are: How do we remove the causes of the defects? What potential solutions we must attempt? What solutions may prevent defects? What improvements must be made?
- *Control*: address what needs to be done to sustain improvements made at all times of process application; future state of the process where defects are reduced to 3.4 per million opportunities or eliminated completely. Examples of questions answered at this stage are: How can we maintain the improvements? What measures should be put in place to control the process? What can we do to assure defects will not occur every time the process is applied?

When performed carefully and successfully, lean results in a process that is more efficient and effective which ultimately enhances the patient experience and expedites access to services. In case management, the use of Six Sigma and Lean results in improving the efficiency of the systems of care, eliminating delays in care (i.e., variances), and by ensuring practice patterns of providers are the same when caring for patients with the same or similar health conditions. Eliminating variation in practice patterns and preventing delays in care are part of the case manager's responsibilities (Case Manager's Tip 11.3).

11.6. USING STRUCTURE/PROCESS/ OUTCOMES TO MEASURE QUALITY

One of the biggest obstacles affecting the performance improvement and quality management strategies of any healthcare organization is the difficulty in linking structure, process(es), and outcome(s). Case management has been defined as a structure and process model because it links both of these elements to the outcomes of care. For case management to be effective, healthcare leaders have become well aware what structure elements and essential care and functional processes have to exist to produce desirable outcomes: quality, safety, cost-effectiveness, and desirable care experience.

11.6.1. The Structure of Care

The structure of the organization has to do with the characteristics of the systems of the organization and its environment of care (Box 11.5). The structure is also concerned with the characteristics of the providers of care, including case managers, and the patients themselves. Structure characteristics relate to the setting/level of care, the nature of the care delivery system/model (e.g., interdisciplinary approach, transitions of care), the credentials, competencies, and educational levels of the providers, and the health status and conditions of the patients.

 CASE MANAGER'S TIP 11.3

Six Sigma and Lean

While Six Sigma focuses on eliminating defects, lean assists in getting rid of nonvalue-adding activities. The combination of Lean Six Sigma then results in a care process that assures quality and safe outcomes while emphasizing the patient experiences the efficient provision of services and optimal healthcare encounter.

The system characteristics of any organization are complex and diverse. Those listed in Box 11.5 are just a small sample of the types, elements, or characteristics that make up the healthcare system. Each of these, either individually or in a group, has an effect on how care delivery is structured and how it ultimately affects patient and organizational outcomes.

The provider characteristics demonstrate the diversity of the care providers in any organization. It is clear from this list that each provider brings unique characteristics (i.e., skills, knowledge, competencies, and educational background including professional discipline or specialty) to the care delivery model, and based on the differences, each may approach a particular patient or clinical problem in a different way. The provider's years of experience will also affect how the group of providers may address a particular problem or patient situation. The varied experiences of the providers will ultimately impact how the interdisciplinary healthcare group, including the case manager, may problem solve a complex or challenging situation (see Chapter 7 for more on this topic).

Finally, the patients and their families/caregivers bring a unique view of themselves, of the care providers, and of what they may believe is quality and safe care. Their participation in their own care (e.g., healthy lifestyle, self-management skills) may be dependent on the providers' ability to engage the patients in ways that are relevant to them and that are consistent with their

---

Box 11.5   Elements of the Structure of Care

System Characteristics	Provider Characteristics	Patient Characteristics
Organization of services	Age	Socioeconomic status
Financial incentives such as payer mix	Gender	Educational level
The workload	Beliefs/attitudes/prejudices	Age
Specialty mix	Level of experience	Gender
Access and convenience for patients	Job satisfaction	Ethnicity
Degree of innovation in care options	Competencies	Health habits and beliefs
	Educational level	Psychosocial support system

values, beliefs, and needs. Ultimately these characteristics shape the patients' responses to care activities, their participation in the care processes, and finally the outcomes of the care interventions.

11.6.2. The Processes of Care

Healthcare is delivered using specific and predetermined processes. These processes are the procedures providers use, the methods they deploy, and the various styles and techniques they may render in the delivery of healthcare services. The processes of care (Box 11.6) are concerned with the functions and responsibilities of the healthcare providers and how they fulfill them. The processes can also be divided into two groups, the technical and interpersonal styles employed as healthcare providers care for patients and their families. These, when combined with the structural characteristics described previously, will ultimately affect the organization's ability to assist patients in their transition toward the expected outcomes of care, including meeting their goals and interests.

Members of the interdisciplinary healthcare teams apply the processes of care within the systems of care delivery, especially the structural and environmental elements such as those listed in Box 11.5 to assure the provision of quality and safe care to patients. The structure can be thought of as the skeleton, and the processes as the muscles. The processes are what gets one from point A to point B; that is, from a goal to an outcome that meets the goal such as transition from acute hospital care to a nursing home. They move patients from one destination to the next. To provide quality care, therefore, it is necessary to have both the structure and the processes well aligned.

The list in Box 11.6 is only a sample of the possible processes in any healthcare organization. Case managers will find themselves interfacing with virtually any and all kinds of processes in the course of their daily work. The providers' and case managers' technical styles may be affected by the organization they work

in and their personal (i.e., structural) characteristics as described previously. Have you ever walked onto a patient care unit and been able to feel something? You may have had an immediate sense that the environment was positive, energetic, suboptimal, or apathetic. You may not have known why you felt that way but there was something present in the environment that gave you that specific impression. What you were sensing was the interpersonal style and dynamics of the setting you were in.

11.6.3. Case Management Links Structure and Process

Case management transcends all of these structural and process variables as it attempts to move patients toward their expected outcomes of care. The case manager must consider all of the elements in the structure and in the processes while creating care plans; planning for discharge; and interacting with patients, physicians, and other healthcare providers. Case managers must consider and assess all of the variables to make cogent and appropriate plans of care for their patients. Finally, the case managers must, in conjunction with members of the interdisciplinary team, identify expected outcomes that are consistent with the characteristics within the structure of care and are compatible with the processes of care.

11.6.4. Outcomes of Care

Outcomes of care can be thought of as the measures used to examine whether the goals or objectives of the care rendered and the services provided have been met. Like structure and process, outcomes too can be categorized and thought of in various subsets or classifications. They are the end results and consequences of care delivery and processes and the effects of the structural variables/characteristics of the healthcare delivery system (Box 11.7).

A quality case management plan usually includes the structure and processes, as well as the expected outcomes of care. Each process should include an expected outcome as illustrated in Chapter 10. Each intervention should also include an expected outcome that is prospectively identified.

Typically, case managers use the clinical endpoints as indicators for when a patient has completed a particular stage in the care process and can be moved on to the next. The outcomes can be linked to those found in the InterQual criteria (McKesson, 2015) and Milliman Care Guidelines (MCG Health, 2015). For example, a drain might be removed post-operatively after the

Box 11.6	Elements of the Processes of Care
Technical Style	**Interpersonal Style**
Coordination	Manner and demeanor
Continuity	Communication
Medication administration	Patient participation
Physician ordering systems	Counseling and support
Test scheduling process	Interdisciplinary relationships
Transition of care activities	Shared decision making

Box 11.7	Examples of Categories of Outcomes		
Clinical Endpoints	**Functional Status**	**General Well-Being**	**Experience of Care**
Signs and symptoms	Physical	Health perception	Access
Laboratory values	Mental	Energy/fatigue	Convenience
Deaths	Social	Pain/comfort	Financial coverage
Health literacy level	Cognitive	Quality of life	General satisfaction
Complications	Physical function	Self management	Emotional state
Core measures	Ambulation/transfer	Engagement	Loyalty to provider

drainage has decreased to a predetermined and acceptable amount/volume per hour.

Outcomes can also be used effectively when linked with discharge/transitional planning. By moving the patient toward a predetermined set of outcomes, the time for discharge, or transition to the next level of care, is driven by the patient's achievement of those expected outcomes and is not based on arbitrary timeframes. In this way the case manager can defend the time at which a patient should be discharged if the patient, family, and/or physician are resistant. The case manager can also defend the need to extend the hospital stay in the event that a premature discharge or transition is identified based on a review of the patient's progress in achieving the expected outcomes. The case manager can also use the achievement, or lack of achievement, of the expected outcomes for clinical insurance reviews to ensure that reimbursement occurs and, when necessary, that additional hospital days are approved by a third-party payer. In these ways outcomes can be a powerful and dynamic tool that provides the case manager with objective indicators for use for a variety of purposes.

The classification of outcomes has shifted over time based on the individuals or groups defining them and also has been influenced by the changing socioeconomic and political characteristics of the healthcare environment. Traditionally, outcomes have been defined by the providers of healthcare services, particularly physicians. Physicians have always examined outcomes as measures of patient mortality, morbidity, complications to treatment, medical errors, and adverse events or side effects to treatments. These types of outcomes were driven by physician practices and reflected the interest of physicians in their own services. Not until the mid-to-late 1980s, but more so during the 1990s, did consumers of healthcare become more influential in changing the outlook of outcomes. They were successful in pressuring providers to examine the quality of care using outcome indicators that are consumer-focused rather than provider-focused. This movement resulted in defining a new set of indicators that is con-

sidered more contemporary. For example, the IOM defined outcomes based on its six aims of quality (Box 11.8). Other examples of these outcome indicators are clinical outcomes such as resolution of disease symptoms; patient's quality of life and well-being; functional ability; satisfaction with care; and financial outcomes such as cost per case/encounter, reimbursement denials, and many others. These indicators are most fit today for evaluating the impact of case management models/systems of healthcare.

Perceptions of the outcomes of care continue to evolve and shift. Today, and most importantly after the passing of the Patient Protection and Affordable Care Act of 2010, new outcomes have become popular. These are driven by the politics and economics of health, most importantly the influence of government and regulators on what outcomes of interest should be. They are referred to as core measures and value based purchasing measures. Although these core measures pertain to the quality and safety of care and the patient experience, regulators tie cost to these outcomes in an effort to examine the value of healthcare services and delivery systems. The new measures present healthcare organizations with increased financial risks when performance on these outcomes does not exceed the regional and/or national benchmarks. Examples of these outcomes are preventable readmissions to acute care settings within 30 days post-discharge and surgical site infections.

11.6.5. Using Structure/Process/Outcomes to Measure Quality

Because case management links the three elements of structure, process, and outcome (Case Manager's Tip 11.4), case managers can serve an important function in assisting their organizations in the measurement of quality of care. As case managers review the patient's achievement of the expected outcomes of care, they can also review the processes used to achieve those outcomes. The processes, as identified on the diagnosis-specific case management plan, become the standard

---

Box 11.8 Examples of Outcomes Based on the IOM Six Aims of Quality

Recognizing that aims must be accompanied by observable metrics, the IOM defined sets of measurements for each aim (IOM, 2010). For example:

- *Safe*: Overall mortality rates, medical error rates, avoidable hospital readmission rates
- *Effective*: How well evidenced-based practices are followed, such as the percentage of time diabetic patients receive all recommended care at each visit, rates of antibiotics administration intraoperatively
- *Efficient*: Analysis of the costs of care by patient, provider, organization, and community
- *Timely*: Waits and delays in receiving care, service, or results of tests
- *Patient centered*: Patient and family experience with care
- *Equitable*: Differences in quality measures by race, gender, income, and other population-based demographic and socioeconomic factors

---

of care for patients with that diagnosis. The patient's ability to reach the expected outcomes is dependent on the selection of the most appropriate processes for achieving those outcomes. It is also dependent on the organization's processes supporting the care interventions needed. For example, perhaps the case management plan calls for a particular test such as a MRI to be done on day 1 of the acute hospital stay. What are the consequences if day 1 happens to fall on a Sunday when MRIs are not routinely done? The patient's stay will most likely be prolonged, quality care will

 CASE MANAGER'S TIP 11.4

Linking the Structure and Process to Outcomes of Care

Case management has been described as a structure and process model, linking both of these to the outcomes of care.

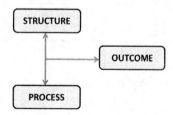

When applied effectively, it improves patient care quality and safety and reduces unnecessary cost while enhancing the patient's experience of care.

not be provided as per the case management plan, the patient's satisfaction with care will suffer, and reimbursement may be put at risk. The case manager, by collecting these delays as variances (deficiencies as per the Six Sigma process), can provide the organization with meaningful information that may assist in making organizational improvements, which in turn will result in the provision of better quality and safer care.

Another example is the switch of a patient from an IV antibiotic to its oral form as soon as it is appropriate. The case management plan may call for the switch to take place after several prerequisite clinical outcomes have been met. In the case of community-acquired pneumonia, the switch from an IV antibiotic may depend on the patient's achievement of a reduced white blood cell count, a reduction in fever, and the ability to take oral medications. What might happen if the patient achieved these outcomes but the attending physician does not write an order for the switch to take place? This may result in compromising the quality of care, prolonging the hospital length of stay unnecessarily, and increasing the cost of care or sustaining a denial in reimbursement by a commercial insurer.

11.7. QUALITY CATEGORIES OF ORGANIZATIONAL VALUES

Commonly, organizational values can be divided into five categories of quality: (1) patient/consumer focus, (2) total involvement and responsibility for quality, (3) measurement or monitoring of quality, (4) systems support, and (5) use of ongoing quality management processes and tools (e.g., DMAIC, PDCA). To differentiate the categories, it is necessary to define each more fully and to give examples of a strong versus a weak organizational commitment to quality.

11.7.1. Patient/Consumer Focus

The patient/consumer focus of quality is related to service and experience, products available, and sharing of information to both internal and external consumers of an institution (Case Manager's Tip 11.5). In this regard, customer service and experience have become common buzzwords. In fact, some organizations have developed whole departments with senior leaders dedicated for the patient experience function. Determining whether one's external consumers received the quality they valued is a powerful tool for an organization to use. In the past, most facilities believed that if they tracked the number of problems or occurrences and they remained within an acceptable level, then the organization was providing quality consumer service.

CASE MANAGER'S TIP 11.5

The Role of Customer/Consumer Service and Patient Experience in Quality

Consumer service and expereince is what defines quality in today's healthcare market and will more than likely continue to play a major role in a hospital's (or any other healthcare provider or agency) survival as we become more deeply affected by reimbursement based on patient experience.

Patient experience surveys and outcomes are currently factored into the reimbursement methods applied by the Medicare benefits program. Patient experience outcomes are also part of contractual agreements between commercial health insurance plans and providers where providers are expected to meet certain patient experience levels, otherwise agreements will not be renewed.

 CASE MANAGER'S TIP 11.6

Coleman's Care Transitions Measure

HCAHPS today includes Coleman's three-item care transitions measure. As part of the discharge instructions domain, case managers are able to improve a hospital's performance on this domain and potential reduce financial risk. The three items are as follows (Coleman, 2015):

1. The hospital staff took my preferences and those of my family or caregiver into account in deciding what my healthcare needs would be when I left the hospital.
2. When I left the hospital, I had a good understanding of the things I was responsible for in managing my health.
3. When I left the hospital, I clearly understood the purpose for taking each of my medications.

More recently, the technique of asking the consumers about their expectations of quality care was found to be much more telling and accurate rather than a hospital making random assumptions as to what the consumer needed or considered as quality care. Patient care experience surveys are now widely used in all types of settings as successful tools for quality care assessment and improvement.

As case management programs have become more visible and perceived by healthcare leaders to enhance quality and safety while assuring revenue, these programs must also now focus on their contribuition to the patient experience. Patient satisfaction surveys of the past, where they used to be a provider's choice to use, have now become a requirement that impacted reimbursement. Today's use of the Consumer Assessment of Healthcare Providers and Systems (CAHPS) surveys is one example of how voluntary patient satisfaction surveys have shifted and become required patient experience surveys by federal agaencies such as the CMS. These surveys today not only capture environmental amenities such as food and room comfort but also include the professional care received by healthcare professionals such as nurses, case managers, and physicians. The recent addition of Coleman's Care Transitions Measure (CTM) to the hospital-based CAHPS survey (HCAHPS), which consists of three items focusing on the patient's experience with transitions of care or discharge from the hospital setting, provides an aspect of the patient experience where case management can make desirable improvements (Case Manager's Tip 11.6). Focus on improving the discharge information domain of the HCAHPS survey

is essential to reducing the rate of avoidable readmissions, and therefore increasing patient safety.

It is appropriate to consider an example of an organization's commitment to quality consumer service: Patients are called after discharge to hear if their expectations were met. Their suggestions, concerns, and perhaps complaints are taken seriously, addressed, and responded to. Although it may be less likely today as a result of value-based purchasing, the organization that does not incorporate consumer service into its quality and safety program does not respond to patient complaints, and ignores suggestions made by its consumers jeopardizes its reputation, competitiveness, market share, and financial status.

11.7.2. Total Involvement

The total involvement of taking responsibility for quality relates to the fact that healthcare leaders and quality management personnel cannot be the sole personnel involved in quality and safety and QI efforts. It is everyone's responsibility to be involved in the achievement, enhancement, and maintenance of quality and safe care. Quality is the direct result of positive and desirable employee behavior. Positive employee behavior is usually the result of staff job satisfaction and engagement. Employees tend to feel ownership of their organization's values, including quality and safety, when they have been involved in the selection of those values. Productive behavior is evident when an organization's goals are clear and understood by its employees, their role in the organization is defined, and the policies and procedures governing their role are well communicated. For example, the hospital (or any other type of healthcare organization) that supports a strong case management team and empowers its members with the permission to solve problems independently and autonomously is an organization with a commitment to quality, safety and consumer experience. The hospital that shows weakness in this area of quality commitment will not address the need for a case management program and will wait for some divine intervention to solve its problems. Much at risk, at least financially, if an organization does not promote quality and safety as everyone's responsibility. Case management teams are no exception; members of these teams must be accountable for their contribution to quality of care, safe transitions, and financial returns.

11.7.3. Measurement or Monitoring of Quality

Measurement or monitoring of quality must be done to meet the goals. It is not an option, rather a mandate. Improvement is impossible without measurement. The case manager's role is to ensure that the patient is moving along in the acute, subacute, or home care level of care in a timely fashion. If any outcomes are not achieved or are delayed, it is the case manager in these settings who is responsible for determining why and for facilitating a corrective action plan. These untoward occurrences are called variances (see Chapter 12). By reviewing a patient's progress regularly and anticipating the plan, patient variances will be kept to a minimum and length of stay and transitions of care issues will be avoided. Healthcare provider variances are related to omissions, delays, or errors made by practitioners. Regulations and policies govern this area. If a healthcare provider omits a medication, this is a variance that could affect the treatment plan and outcomes. Prescribing certain medications for a patient with specific health conditions are part of the value-based purchasing program. An example is use of angiotensin-converting enzyme (ACE) inhibitors in heart failure patients.

Operational variances are those that happen within the healthcare setting and often relate to the systems, processes, and structures of care. Examples include a patient waiting for a rehabilitation bed, delays in discharge or transition, equipment failures, and test scheduling delays. Although case managers act proactively to prevent such variances from happening, and address those that occur at the time they happen, retrospective analysis and trending of variances is important from a quality management and improvement standpoint. Such analysis results in identification of those frequently occurring and their associated root causes. This analysis helps monitor quality and identify areas

for improvement. Outcomes are paramount criteria of good quality either by themselves or as related to costs if efficiency and optimality are to be determined (Donabedian, 1991).

11.7.4. Systems Support

Systems support includes planning, budgeting, scheduling, and performance management needed to support the quality management and safety efforts. If systems are well coordinated, the time it takes to accomplish the work will be reduced. Everyone should be invested in providing quality work. A team effort should be fostered to accomplish unified goals. A good example of this is the patient-focused healthcare delivery system that has become integral to many acute and nonacute care settings. This system is based on the philosophy that the patient is the center core of focus and that all disciplines involved with the patient must be able to access that patient easily and provide care that is based on the patient's culture, value system, beliefs, preferred language, interests, and preferences. Patients should not have to seek out the area needed for their treatment; it should come to them. The patient requiring physical therapy should not have to be transported to the physical rehabilitation department unless absolutely necessary; the department's physical therapist should be available in the unit in which the patient resides. This decreases the nonproductive time of transport and can ultimately have the effect of shortening the hospitalization while enhancing the patient experience of care.

11.7.5. Continuous Quality Improvement

Through continuous quality improvement and management processes, organizations foster creativity to do things better tomorrow than they did yesterday. CQI is a way of correcting flaws and making improvements. For decades now, the industrial leaders of the world realized that to remain competitive and to survive in our economy today, CQI techniques are essential. There are three individuals who stand out as pioneers in the development of QI techniques: Philip B. Crosby, W. Edwards Demming, and Joseph M. Juran. Crosby (1979) designed a 14-step approach for his quality improvement process (QIP) which is still applicable today (Box 11.9).

Demming's and Juran's work dates back to the 1920s and 1950s, respectively. They are responsible for enormous improvements in Japanese manufacturing. In 1986 Demming's approach to QI came to America. He is best known for involving the employee in the QI effort, applying a never-ending cycle of

**Box 11.9   Quality Improvement Plan:
A 14-Step Approach (Crosby, 1979)**

1. Leadership and management commitment
2. Quality improvement plan
3. Measurement of the phenomenon or area of interest (what is to be studied)
4. Cost of quality
5. Quality awareness
6. Corrective action plan (potential solutions)
7. Zero defects planning
8. Training and education of those involved and affected
9. Zero defects results
10. Goal setting
11. Error cause removal (root cause or cause and effect analysis and strategies for eliminating causes of the concerns)
12. Recognition
13. Quality councils
14. Do it all over again

Although Crosby's apporach to quality improvement still works today, it is not as popular as it used to be few decades ago. Healthcare leaders and quality management specialists use the PDCA and DMIAC cylces more often today. The PDCA sometimes is used for small test of change before wider implementation is pursued.

continuous improvement, and eliminating rework and nonvalue adding processes to reduce cost. This approach involved groups of employees coming together to discuss problem identification and problem solving. When this process is applied to healthcare, it involves strategies not only to improve quality and safety but also to reduce costs or increase revenue.

In the United States the concept of quality has matured first from the early quality control or inspection and testing effort to the middle ground of QA, in which selected specialists retrospectively monitored quality, identified errors or incidents, and kept report cards on each individual blamed for the problem. The QA specialists tend to lack the authority or clout necessary to change the way work is performed. Moreover, QA and its inspection techniques never catch the real issues affecting patient care. The fully mature quality effort later emerged in the form of continuous quality improvement or total quality management. The organizations that embrace these concepts are those advanced in the ability to empower their employees to be responsible for quality and totally own it as well as the patient experience and safe care.

In the late 1990s and early 2000s, the TJC set forth the charge to integrate QI endeavors that focus on actual performance and outcomes (JCAHO, 2001). The TJC at the time designed a model for QI and referred to it as the quality cube which is still relevant today. The quality cube depicts the focus of quality assessment for the purpose of understanding where opportunities may exist. It identified three key areas to guide quality assessment, improvement, and management (Table 11.1): dimensions of performance, patient populations, and important functions within healthcare delivery systems and services. The cube illustrates the relationship of performance and important functions to a range of patient populations and services provided. It can be used as a tool that stimulates thought related to quality assessment and identification of improvement priorities.

Healthcare professionals have successfully shifted their efforts from QA to QI and later have continued to

TABLE 11.1. Key Aspects of the
TJC Quality Cube.

Key Areas	Focus and Examples
Dimensions of Performance	• Efficiency • Appropriateness • Availability • Timeliness • Effectiveness • Continuity • Safety • Efficiency • Respect and Caring
Important Functions and Services	• Surveillance, Prevention, and Control of Infection • Management of Information • Management of Human Resources • Leadership • Improving Organization Performance • Continuum of Care • Education • Care of Patients • Assessment of Patients • Patient Rights and Organizational Ethics
Patient Population Examples	• Populations of Interest and Conditions • Adolescents • Obstetrical • Outpatients • Inpatients • Medical • Surgical

advance to such terms as CQI, TQM, and the TJC term: process improvement (PI). QA, as stated earlier, tends to focus on reduction of errors, meeting standards set up by regulatory agencies, and measuring defined outcomes. This model functions in response to problems and has a retrospective view of tracking occurrences after they have happened. QI, on the other hand, focuses on improving a process to effect improvements in the outcomes, meeting consumer needs, and measuring consumer-identified outcomes. It is a continuous and proactive process that avoids focusing on employee or punitive approaches and involves all employees at all levels. The QI approach is one in which the advantage is clear, and it assumes that most people want to do the right thing and do it well. It is common practice and philosophy today that quality in healthcare is achieved by "doing the right thing right every time," where "the right thing" is quality and safe outcomes which ultimately enhance the patient experience of care. This results from outcome management where improvements and arriving at the "right" thing is achieved by controlling the systems of care, eliminating variations and nonvalue adding processes, and proactively managing potential opportunities for failure.

We have moved from the paradigm of QA in healthcare delivery, where provider-defined outcomes (such as morbidity, mortality, and clinical endpoints) rule, to QI, which relies on consumer-defined outcomes (such as cost of care, health-related quality, and patient satisfaction), and today to quality management with special focus not only on outcomes of care of the past, but the safety of care and the patient's experience during and after an eipsode of care. QI focuses on the continued improvement of all processes rather than just those identified as a problem. This type of approach can improve quality of care for the majority of patients and also decrease statistical outliers. Outlier thresholds for some measures such those included in the value-based purchasing program are set by the CMS and are based

on regional and national rates. Length of hospital stay measures for Medicare hospitalized beneficiaries are also defined by Medicare for reimbursement purposes, the range of days a patient may stay hospitalized at the maximum reimbursement rate. Outliers are those who exceed the set range of days. In contrast, QI governs itself by the 80/20 rule (or "Pareto Principle"), which states that 80% of costs are generated by 20% of the patients. Therefore those who abide by this principle will only address a small percentage of issues. Table 11.2 provides a snapshot summary of QA versus QI activities.

11.8. CASE MANAGEMENT AND CONTINUOUS QUALITY IMPROVEMENT

How does the QI approach to healthcare fit in with a case management model? Case managers' skills, role characteristics, and context of care delivery as discussed in previous chapters, exemplify many of the descriptive elements of QI: problem solving, negotiation, mentoring, quality monitoring, consumer relations and experience, collaboration and teamwork, and outcome analysis. Usually the first function for a case manager is to select those patients who would benefit from case management. The next function is to facilitate patient treatment goals and discharge/transitional plans. In a successful case management program all patients should be monitored for quality, safety, use of resources, and length of stay. Once a patient is identified to benefit from case management, a case management plan of care is designed with his/her input. The plan is developed to optimize the treatment plan and outcomes, streamline the care to avoid delays or roadblocks, and to avoid any compromise in quality. By following these guidelines, quality issues are easily tracked and patient safety is assured. Two tools that are commonly used to track issues of quality are indicator reports and variance reports.

TABLE 11.2. Summary of Quality Assurance Versus Quality Improvement.

Topic	Quality Assurance	Quality Improvement
▪ Drivers	▪ Adherence	▪ Strategic planning
▪ Focus	▪ Errors	▪ Outcomes including defects
▪ Approach	▪ Top-down	▪ Top-down/bottom-up
▪ Process	▪ Retrospective	▪ Prospective
▪ Goals	▪ Reduce errors	▪ Satisfy the consumer
▪ Actions	▪ Track outliers	▪ Improve processes and outcomes
▪ Type of Change	▪ Incremental	▪ Incremental and continuous/ongoing
▪ Employees	▪ Not invested	▪ Participants in improvement teams
▪ Consequence	▪ Punitive	▪ Just culture/safety culture
▪ Context	▪ Inidvidual	▪ System

CASE STUDY 11.1 ■ Example of Unnecessary/Avoidable Readmission to Acute Care Hospital Setting

Mrs. Lopez is a 68-year-old woman who was admitted with a diagnosis of heart failure. She developed acute respiratory problems and was placed on a mechanical ventilator. Her family was very involved in her care and met with the case manager regularly to organize a quality-of-life discharge plan. The case manager worked diligently to provide Mrs. Lopez and her family with all the necessary tools and provisions to meet their needs for going home. The plan was to go home even if Mrs. Lopez remained on the ventilator. A respiratory company was closely involved and worked with the case manager and family to teach the necessary skills to the family and prepare the home for a ventilator. The case manager worked with Mrs. Lopez's daughter to teach her basic respiratory care and Ambu bagging techniques and to improve her confidence when dealing with her mother's ventilator. After many weeks of preparation, the doctor, case manager, patient, family, and respiratory therapy company all believed they provided a high-quality discharge plan. Within 3 days of discharge to home with home care, Mrs. Lopez was readmitted to the acute care hospital setting in respiratory distress. The family was devastated and complained that the visiting nurse from the home care agency was much delayed and did not provide the same information taught to the family in the hospital. The Ambu bag that they were using in the hospital did not work like the one provided at home; the daughter became distraught and called an ambulance. What went wrong with the quality of this care plan? Here are some questions to ponder:

- Was this the most effective discharge plan for Mrs. Lopez and her family?
- Did the case manager include all caregivers in this plan, including those involved in follow-up care?
- If the case manager had included the skilled home care agency in the discharge plan, could this outcome and readmission have been avoided?
- Was this discharge plan safe and of utmost quality?
- Were costs, patient satisfaction, and caregiver needs affected by this incomplete plan?
- What are the impacts of Mrs. Lopez retrun to the hospital on quality, safety, patient experience, and reimbursement?
- Is this the first time a readmission like Mrs. Lopez's happens? What impact this has on QI?

- Indicator reports are usually geared more to physician practice patterns and untoward occurrences as sequelae to their practice (e.g., an unplanned return to the operating room during the same hospitalization, post-operative complications, or abnormal laboratory results not addressed)—simply put, identifying anything that does not happen when it should.
- Variance reports are those that pertain to delays in care, omissions, or deviations from the expected or planned. Variance is discussed in much more detail in Chapter 12.

In general, the case manager is the driving force behind the success of quality patient care through case management. The case manager who checks on quality indicators (outcomes) and variances not only identifies problems but also must find remedies for the patient's care to continue to successfully and efficiently move through the hospital system.

A case management program has a major importance to any quality and safety effort. Case managers have the potential to reduce avoidable readmissions and the ability to evaluate the possibility of meeting a patient's healthcare needs in an alternative and probably less-costly care setting. The case manager must ensure that a patient receives adequate and appropriate care while acute and must provide adequate quality follow-up and post-discharge care. By doing this efficiently case managers reduce premature discharges/ transitions at healthcare facilities and help to guarantee that patients' discharge and transitional plans are adequate, safe, and meet their needs, with the ultimate goal of quality care, patient satisfaction, and avoiding unnecessary readmissions.

You can quickly conclude after reviewing Case Study 11.1 that had all the healthcare disciplines involved in the discharge plan of Mrs. Lopez been consulted, the undesired outcome could have been avoided. By simply and carefully reviewing Mrs. Lopez's discharge/transition plan with the home care agency, the equipment that the patient was using in the hospital versus the equipment being used at home, the undue anxiety of the patient's family would not have occurred. Had the home health nurse and case manager assessed the ventilator and related supplies that would be used in the home, the patient's well-being could have been maintained by altering the education of the caregivers in the home.

11.9. CONSUMER/PATIENT EXPERIENCE AND SATISFACTION

An important outcome of any case management program is consumer satisfaction with the care experience, including the plan of care. Patient and family satisfaction is an essential outcome to measure. Satisfaction of physicians, nurses, case managers, other healthcare team members, and other parties involved in patient care agencies, as in Mrs. Lopez example, are also key customers and stakeholders whose satisfaction is important to measure as well. Case managers must work closely with all members of the interdisciplinary healthcare team to assess, monitor, and analyze the delivery of care, the case management plan, outcomes of the care provided, and the patient/family response to the care and services. These activities are beneficial to continuously improve the organization's quality performance.

A case management plan is designed typically through an interdisciplinary and cooperative process; when executed correctly, the team's collaboration results in the designs of a single, integrated, and interdisciplinary treatment plan for a specific patient type. The plan also provides for a collection and ongoing evaluation of potential quality and safety outcome indicators and issues or concerns about care. These issues are usually identified through variances in care delivery or complications the patient experiences. The entire process enables a focus on quality and safety by continually assessing and identifying opportunities for improvement.

Case management's efforts for improvement must be accomplished case by case. Case management plays a crucial role in evaluating and monitoring a patient's case management plan and outcomes such as discharge goals and avoidable readmissions. Case managers are the professionals most aware of the patient's functional, physical, cognitive, emotional, and socioeconomic abilities and know best how these abilities may affect and determine a patient's level of functioning after discharge/transition from an acute care setting or an episode of illness. Offering the best possible discharge or transitional plan is vitally important because of the potential for reducing readmissions and providing alternative care methods for less cost—and thus the ultimate outcome of heightened patient, family, physician, and payer satisfaction.

Being able to exceed consumers' expectations for quality service must be the driving force; this central concern is a primary reason a registered nurse or social worker becomes a case manager. Quality and safe service should be a way of life for any case manager on a

CASE MANAGER'S TIP 11.7

Consumer Service Rule of Thumb

A consumer service rule of thumb case managers must remember is that a satisfied consumer will tell three people, but a dissatisfied consumer will tell 20. Consumer experience of care during and after an episode of illness or routine follow up visit to a primary care provider must be a top priority fo case managers and other healthcare professionals alike.

day-to-day basis, and it is one of the standards necessary today for healthcare to prosper and survive (Case Manager's Tip 11.7).

The CMS for several years now has implemented the use of a standardized and national survey that assesses the patient's perception of their hospital care experience. The survey is known as the Hospital Consumer Assessment of Healthcare Providers and Systems (HCAHPS). The survey consists of 32 items that encompass key topics which include communication with doctors and nurses, responsiveness of staff, medications, discharge information, cleanliness, quietness, pain management, and transitions of care (HCAHPS, 2015). Case managers without a doubt can impact a hospital's performance on this survey, especially in the areas of discharge information and transitions of care.

The survey asks a number of demographic questions that are used for risk adjustment which then allows fair comparison of performance across the participating hospitals. While many hospitals have been collecting patient satisfaction data for decades, the required use of HCAHPS in all participating hospitals allowed for standardization and ultimately benchmarking performance (HCAHPS, 2015). The HCAHPS survey is designed to address three goals:

- The standardized survey and implementation protocol produces data that allow objective and meaningful comparisons of hospitals on topics that are important to patients and consumers.
- Public reporting of HCAHPS results creates new incentives for hospitals to improve quality of care.
- Public reporting enhances accountability in healthcare by increasing transparency of the quality of hospital care provided in return for the public investment.

The CMS implemented the HCAHPS survey in October 2006, and the first public reporting of HCAHPS results occurred in March 2008. In 2013, CMS added five new items to the HCAHPS Survey: three questions about the transition to post-hospital care (care transitions measure), one about admission through the emergency room, and one about mental and emotional health. Enactment of the Deficit Reduction Act of 2005 created an additional incentive for acute care hospitals to participate in HCAHPS. Since July 2007, hospitals subject to the inpatient prospective payment system (IPPS) annual payment update provisions must collect and submit HCAHPS data in order to receive their full annual payment update. Non-IPPS hospitals, such as critical access hospitals, may voluntarily participate in the survey (HCAHPS, 2015).

Today a hospital's performance on the HCAHPS survey is part of the value-based purchasing program discussed in the next section. Use of HCAHPS in the value-based purchasing program incentivised hospitals to pay closer attention to consumer experience with care and to implement improvement strategies to increase their survey scores, thereby increasing their opportunity for an incentive payment by CMS. Hospital's performance on the HCAHPS survey is accessible on the Hospital Compare website, www.medicare.gov/hospitalcompare, where scores are posted on a quarterly basis. More detailed analyses and comparisons can also be found on the HCAJHPS website itself: www.hcahpsonline.org.

In April 2015, CMS added HCAHPS star ratings to the Hospital Compare website. HCAHPS star ratings summarize the results for each HCAHPS measure and present it in a format that is increasingly familiar to consumers, making it easier to use the information and spotlight excellence in healthcare quality. A hospital may achieve a maximum of five stars on a particular measure and the lowest being one star. There are 11 measures in the HCAHPS survey (Box 11.10) the hospital receives a star rating on each in addition to a roll-up star rating based on the hospital's performance on these various measures (HCAHPS, 2015).

11.10. HOSPITAL VALUE-BASED PURCHASING

The hospital value-based purchasing (VBP) program is a historical transformation of the way the CMS operates and reimburses acute care hospitals. This program, which went into effect in fiscal year 2013, accounts for a set of outcomes of care hospitals achieve during a specific period of time compared to performance during a preidentified period that is before the VBP program. For example, for fiscal year 2013, the time period began around October 1, 2012 where a hospital's performance is compared to a period prior to the program initiation extending between July 1, 2011 and

---

Box 11.10   HCAHPS Survey Measures and Star Ratings

There are 11 measures on the HCAHPS survey with two overall ratings:

1. Communication with nurses
2. Communication with doctors
3. Responsiveness of hospital staff
4. Pain management
5. Communication about medications
6. Discharge information
7. Care transitions
8. Cleanliness of the hospital environment
9. Quietness of the hospial environment
10. Overall hospital rating
11. Recommend the hospital

March 31, 2012. The VBP program rewards acute care hospitals with incentive payments for the quality of care they provide to Medicare beneficiaries. Although it intends to reward hospitals that provide high quality and safe care, follow best practices, keep patients healthy, and enhance the patients' experience of care during hospitalization, it penalizes those hospitals that do not (CMS, 2012).

Since the VBP program went into effect, hospitals are no longer paid solely based on the quantity or volume of the services they provide; rather, they are paid based on value: quality, safety, patient experience, and lower costs. The Patient Protection and Affordable Care Act of 2010 established the hospital VBP program. Details of this program were released in April 2011; however, a number of changes have been made since then which consist of the measures and percentage incentives. Hospitals today are able to receive incentive payments based on either how well they perform on each measure within the program or how much they improve their performance caring for Medicare patients on each measure compared to their performance during a baseline period (CMS, 2014).

11.10.1. Domains, Dimensions, and Measures of the Value Based Purchasing Program

The CMS bases hospital performance on an approved set of measures and dimensions, grouped into specific quality and safety domains. Different domains have gone into effect since the inception of this program. The 2017 domains are supposed to be stable and expected to continue to apply going forward. When the program started in 2013, it consisted of two domains,

Box 11.11   Progression of the Value-Based Purchasing Program Domains

2013 Domains
- Clinical Process of Care
- Patient Experience of Care

2014 Domains
- Clinical Process of Care
- Patient Experience of Care
- Clinical Care Outcomes

2015–2016 Domains
- Clinical Process of Care
- Patient Experience of Care
- Clinical Care Outcomes
- Efficiency

2017 Domains
- Clinical Process of Care
- Patient Experience of Care
- Clinical Care Outcomes
- Efficiency
- Safety

the clinical process of care domain which included 12 measures and the patient experience domain which contained eight dimensions. In 2016, the program has grown to include four domains compared to the initial two; and in 2017, the number of domains will increase to five. Box 11.11 shows the progression of the VPB domains since its inception in 2013.

Similar to the changing domains, measures in the VBP program have changed over time as well, where some intial measures have been eliminated while new ones added. The clinical process of care domain consists of eight measures in 2016 and three measures in 2017 comapred to 12 in 2013, while the patient experience of care domain continues to have eight dimensions since its inception in 2013. The clinical care outcomes domain went into effect in 2014 with three measures and grew to seven in 2016 and then will decline to three measures in 2017; this decline is due to reassignment of some of the measures to the safety domain. The efficiency of care domain originated in 2015 and continues to consist of one measure since. Finally the safety domain will go into effect in 2017 and will consist of six measures, two of which will be new while the other four are moved from the clinical care outcomes domain and designated as measures of the safety domain. Of note is the use of a composite measure in the safety domain referred to as the patient safety indicators (PSI) reflecting eight different safety outcomes.

Table 11.3 details the measures of the clinical process of care domain and its progression since 2013. Tables 11.4, 11.5, and 11.6 present the details of the patient experience, outcomes of care, and efficiency domains respectively (Medicare, 2015). Note that in each table the use of yes means measure is included and no means measure is excluded during that year. When a measure is listed as a yes in one year and later on as no, it means that the measure was stopped since the year where no first appears.

The Medicare spending per beneficiary (MSPB) measure assesses payments for services provided to a Medicare beneficiary during an episode of acute care. The spending per beneficiary is calculated based on care and services provided 3 days prior to the inpatient hospital admission up until 30 days after discharge. The payments included in this measure are price-standardized and risk-adjusted.

11.10.2. Hospital Performance and Incentive Payment

To determine whether a hospital is to receive incentive payment, CMS examines the hospital's performance on the various domains of the VBP program. Before a domain, dimension, or a measure goes into effect, a baseline period is identified during which the hospital's performance on the domain, dimension, or measure is examined. Often, this baseline period is about 9 months and never exceeds 12 months. For example, the baseline period for the clinical care process domain, which went into effect in fiscal year 2013, was between July 1, 2009 and March 31, 2010 while the performance period for same domain covered July 1, 2011 until March 31, 2012. Note the time lapse between the performance period a hospital is evaluated on and the actual year when a hospital may potentially receive an incentive payment, which in this case it was fiscal year 2013 (Medicare, 2015).

The baseline period changes over time as new perfromance periods go into effect. At some point a past performance period becomes a baseline period for a new performance period. For example, the baseline period for the clinical care process domain in fiscal year 2015 was January 1, 2011 through December 31, 2011 while the performance period was January 1, 2013 through December 31, 2013 (Medicare, 2015).

A hospital VBP program baseline and performance periods are a designated time span used to capture data that show how well a hospital has performed during these periods on the applicable VBP measures, dimensions, and domains. Normally, CMS expects the participating hospitals to submit their performance data on

TABLE 11.3. Clinical Process of Care Domain.

Measure	Measure Description	FY 2013	FY 2014	FY 2015	FY 2016	FY 2017
AMI-7a	Fibrinolytic Therapy Received within 30 Minutes of Hospital Arrival	Yes	Yes	Yes	Yes	Yes
AMI-8a	Primary PCI Received within 90 Minutes of Hospital Arrival	Yes	Yes	Yes	No	No
HF-1	Discharge Instructions	Yes	Yes	Yes	No	No
IMM-2	Influenza Immunization	No	No	No	Yes	Yes
PN-3b	Blood Cultures Performed in the Emergency Department Prior to Initial Antibiotic Received in Hospital	Yes	Yes	Yes	No	No
PN-6	Initial Antibiotic Selection for CAP in Immunocompetent Patient	Yes	Yes	Yes	Yes	No
SCIP-Card-2	Surgery Patients on a Beta Blocker Prior to Arrival That Received a Beta Blocker During the Perioperative Period	Yes	Yes	Yes	Yes	No
SCIP-Inf-1	Prophylactic Antibiotic Received within One Hour Prior to Surgical Incision	Yes	Yes	Yes	No	No
SCIP-Inf-2	Prophylactic Antibiotic Selection for Surgical Patients	Yes	Yes	Yes	Yes	No
SCIP-Inf-3	Prophylactic Antibiotics Discontinued within 24 Hours After Surgery End Time	Yes	Yes	Yes	Yes	No
SCIP-Inf-4	Cardiac Surgery Patients with Controlled 6 a.m. Postoperative Serum Glucose	Yes	Yes	Yes	No	No
SCIP-Inf-9	Post-operative Urinary Catheter Removal on Post-operative Day 1 or 2	No	Yes	Yes	Yes	No
SCIP-VTE-1	Surgery Patients with Recommended Venous Thromboembolism Prophylaxis Ordered	Yes	Yes	No	No	No
SCIP-VTE-2	Surgery Patients Who Received Appropriate Venous Thromboembolism Prophylaxis within 24 Hours Prior to Surgery to 24 Hours After Surgery	Yes	Yes	Yes	Yes	No
PC-01	Elective Delivery Prior to 39 Completed Weeks Gestation	No	No	No	No	Yes

Acute Myocardial Infarction, AMI; Heart Failure, HF; Immunization, IMM; Pneumonia, PN; Surgical Care Improvement Project, SCIP; Venous Thromboembolism, VTE; Process of Care, PC.

TABLE 11.4. Patient Experience of Care for the Hospital Consumer Assessment of Healthcare Providers and Systems Survey Domain.

Measure Description	FY 2013	FY 2014	FY 2015	FY 2016	FY 2017
1. Communication with Nurses	Yes	Yes	Yes	Yes	Yes
2. Communication with Doctors	Yes	Yes	Yes	Yes	Yes
3. Responsiveness of Hospital Staff	Yes	Yes	Yes	Yes	Yes
4. Pain Management	Yes	Yes	Yes	Yes	Yes
5. Communication about Medicines	Yes	Yes	Yes	Yes	Yes
6. Cleanliness and Quietness of Hospital Environment	Yes	Yes	Yes	Yes	Yes
7. Discharge Information*	Yes	Yes	Yes	Yes	Yes
8. Overall Rating of Hospital	Yes	Yes	Yes	Yes	Yes

*Coleman's Care Transitions Measure (a three-item survey) was added to the Discharge Dimension in 2015.

TABLE 11.5. Clinical Care Outcomes Domain.

Measure	Measure Description	FY 2013	FY 2014	FY 2015	FY 2016	FY 2017
MORT-30-AMI	AMI 30-Day Mortality Rate*	No	Yes	Yes	Yes	Yes
MORT-30-HF	HF 30-Day Mortality Rate*	No	Yes	Yes	Yes	Yes
MORT-30 PN	PN 30-Day Mortality Rate*	No	Yes	Yes	Yes	Yes
AHRQ Composite (PSI-90)	Complication/Patient safety for selected indicators (Composite)**	No	No	Yes	Yes	Yes
CAUTI	Catheter-Associated Urinary Tract Infection**	No	No	No	Yes	Yes
CLABSI	Central Line-Associated Blood Stream Infection**	No	No	Yes	Yes	Yes
SSI	SSI—Colon Surgery** SSI—Abdominal Hysterectomy**	No	No	No	Yes	Yes
C. Diff	Clostridium Difficile Infection**	No	No	No	No	Yes
MRSA Bacteremia	Methicillin-Resistant Staphylococcus aureus**	No	No	No	No	Yes

Outcome Mortality Measure, MORT; Agency for Healthcare Research and Quality, AHRQ; Patient Safety Indicators, PSI; Surgical Site Infection, SSI.
*Measures in 2017 make the Clinical Care Outcomes Domain.
**Measures in 2017 make the Safety Domain.
Note: PSI Composite Indicators consist of pressure ulcer, iatrogenic pneumothorax, central venous catheter-related bloodstream infection, post-operative hip fracture, post-operative pulmonary embolism or deep vein thrombosis, post-operative sepsis, post-operative wound dehiscence, and accidental puncture or laceration.

the various VBP measures during specific timeframes. CMS then compares the data collected for the performance period to data collected for each participating hospital during the relevant baseline period. CMS also assesses each hospital's total performance by comparing its achievement and improvement scores for each applicable hospital VBP measure. CMS uses a threshold which is the fiftieth percentile, and a benchmark which is the mean of the top decile hospitals to determine the number of points to be awarded to a hospital for the achievement and improvement scores. In addition, CMS compares the achievement and improvement scores and only uses whichever is greater. To determine the score in a domain with multiple measures such as the clinical process of care and outcome domains, achievement and improvement points are added across all measures (Stratis Health, 2015).

■ Achievement points are awarded by comparing a hospital's rates during the performance period with all hospitals' rates from a baseline period. Hospital rates at or above benchmark result in the award of 10 achievement points while rates below the achievement threshold results in zero achievement points. If the rate is equal to or greater than the achievement threshold and less than the benchmark, the hospital is then awarded between one to ten points (Stratis Health, 2015).

■ Improvement points are awarded by comparing a hospital's rates during the performance period to that same hospital's rates from a baseline period. Hospital rates at or above benchmark result in nine improvement points while rates at or below baseline period result in zero improvement points. If the hospital's rate is between the baseline period rate and the benchmark, it results in zero to nine improvement points (Stratis Health, 2015).

A hospital's performance of the patient experience of care domain is calculated similar to the other domains where a hospital receives both achievement and improvement scores. This domain constitutes a composite score of the hospital's perfromance on the eight dimensions of the HCAHPS survey. Dissimilar to the

TABLE 11.6. Efficiency Domain.

Measure	Measure Description	FY 2013	FY 2014	FY 2015	FY 2016	FY 2017
MSPB	Medicare Spending Per Beneficiary	No	No	Yes	Yes	Yes

TABLE 11.7. Weight of Each Domain in the Value-Based Purchasing.

Measure	FY 2013	FY 2014	FY 2015	FY 2016	FY 2017
Clinical Process of Care	70%	45%	20%	10%	5%
Patient Experience of Care	30%	30%	30%	25%	25%
Clinical Care Outcomes	N/A	25%	30%	40%	25%
Efficiency	N/A	N/A	20%	25%	25%
Safety	N/A	N/A	N/A	N/A	20%

other domains, the hospital also receives a consistency score for the patient experience of care domain. This score is calculated based on performce after the baseline period. Consistency points are awarded by comparing a hospital's patient experience of care dimensions rates during the performance period with all hospitals' patient experience of care rates from a baseline period (Stratis Health, 2015).

- If all dimension rates are at or above achievement threshold, then a hospital may receive 20 consistency points.
- If any dimension rate is at or below worst performing hospital dimension baseline period rate, the hospital then may receive zero consistency points.
- If the lowest dimension rate is greater than the worst performing hospital's rate but less than the achievement threshold, the hospital may receive 0–20 consistency points.

The CMS calculates a hospital's total performance score by combining the greater of either the hospital's achievement or improvement points for each measure to determine a score for each domain. It next multiplies each domain score by a specified "weight" (percentage) and then by adding together the weighted domain scores. The domain weights for fiscal year 2013 through 2017 are listed in Table 11.7. The weight value of each domain of the VBP changed over time since it was initiated in 2013; some have incraesed while others have decreased especially as new domains were introduced.

The hospital VBP is funded through a reduction from participating hospitals' DRG payments for the applicable fiscal year. CMS withholds a certain percentage of Medicare reimbursement dollars (e.g., 1.5% in 2015) and redistributes the amount withheld among the participating hospitals based on their total performance scores. The percentage withheld is also referred to as payment reduction. Some hospitals may end up earning more than they otherwise would have been reimbursed (i.e., earn an incentive payment), others may earn less than or nothing at all compared to what they would have reimbursed (i.e., penalized), while some others may neither earn more nor lose (i.e., receive reimbursement equal to what they would have). Table 11.8 lists the percent reductions since the inception of the program in 2013. It is anticipated that the 2017 percentage reduction rate will stay in effect in future years or at least until 2018 (Medicare, 2015).

11.11. MEANINGFUL USE

The Patient Protection and Affordable Care Act of 2010 established the Medicare Shared Savings Program to improve care coordination and to incentivize healthcare providers (i.e., individual physicians) and organizations to participate in ACOs which ultimately improve patient care outcomes, including quality, safety, and care corrdination, and reduce costs. Although participation is currently voluntary, there is no doubt that the VBP program and accountable care model will become expectations of routine healthcare delivery of the near future in both the public and private payer sectors. Indeed, commercial insurers, such as Cigna Corporation, have already launched their own versions of accountable care organizations which ultimately will reward true "meaningful use" of technology as well.

The adoption and meaningful use of certified electronic health records (EHRs) underpins the whole concept of accountable care. These systems can serve as the source of electronic data for clinical and administrative quality measures, especially those that healthcare providers are expected to report on to CMS. These mea-

TABLE 11.8. Value-Based Incentive Payment Percentage by Program Fiscal Year.

Fiscal Year	FY 2013	FY 2014	FY 2015	FY 2016	FY 2017
Percentage Reduction	1.0	1.25	1.5	1.75	2.0

sures include, for example, recording preventive health measures such as immunizations and mammography screenings, to tracking populations at risk for diabetes, hypertension, and other other chronic conditions.

The Medicare and Medicaid EHR incentive programs provide financial incentives for the meaningful use of certified EHR technology in the improvement of patient care, inclduing quality and safety (Case Manager's Tip 11.8). To receive an EHR incentive payment and to avoid financial penalties, healthcare providers and organizations have to demonstrate that they are meaningfully using their EHRs by meeting thresholds for a number of program objectives. Penalties start at reduction in payment for up to 1% and may reach over time to a maximum of 5%. The Medicare and Medicaid EHR Incentive Programs provide incentive payments to eligible professionals, hospitals, and critical access hospitals (CAHs) as they adopt, implement, upgrade or demonstrate meaningful use of certified EHR technology. Regardless however, whether a healthcare organization is a participant in a public or private ACO, it is necessary, at least from a quality and safety standpoint, that it considers ramping up meaningful use of certified EHR technology. After all, any healthcare provider interested in receiving Medicare and Medicaid EHR incentives also needs to meet value-based care measurement thresholds.

The EHR Incentive Programs have been phased-in in stages with increasing requirements which include: (1) Certified Electronic Health Records (CEHRs) adop-

 CASE MANAGER'S TIP 11.8

Benefits of Meaningful Use and Certified Electronic Health Records

1. Meaningful use employing CEHR technology may:
- Improve quality, safety, and efficiency of care delievery
- Reduce health disparities
- Engage patients and family in own care
- Improve care coordination and population and public health
- Maintain privacy and security of patient health information

2. Adherence to meaningful use and CEHR may result in:
- Better clinical outcomes
- Improved population health outcomes
- Increased transparency and efficiency
- Empowered individuals
- More robust research data on health systems

tion and data capture and sharing; (2) advanced clinical processes that allow patient information exchange and care coordination; and (3) improved patient and healthcare outcomes. Eligible professionals participate in the program on the calendar year, while eligible hospitals and CAHs participate based on the federal fiscal year (Box 11.12). Providers and hospitals must attest to demonstrating meaningful use every year to receive an incentive and to avoid a payment adjustment. They may elect to participate in either the Medicare, Medicaid, or both programs (CMS, 2015).

Over 5,000 eligible hospitals and CAHs can participate in the meaningful use incentive Programs and receive payments from both the Medicare and Medicaid Meaningful Use and CEHR Incentive Programs. Eligible hospitals and CAHs that do not successfully demonstrate meaningful use of certified EHR technology have been subjected to Medicare payment adjustments (reductions) since fiscal year 2015. For the Medicaid program, hospitals must have at least 10% Medicaid patient volume to be eligible and as of 2015, the Medicaid program did not have any payment adjustments.

The Medicare eligible healthcare professionals participating in the Meaningful Use and CEHR Incentive Program include the following providers/physicians:

- Doctor of medicine or osteopathy
- Doctor of dental surgery or dental medicine
- Doctor of podiatry
- Doctor of optometry
- Chiropractor

The Medicaid eligible professionals, however, may also include in addition to physicians (primarily doctors of medicine, doctors of osteopathy, and dentists) advanced clincian such as nurse practitioners, certified nurse midwives, and physician assistants who furnish services in a Federally Qualified Health Center or Rural Health Clinic that is led by a physician assistant. Additionally, Medicaid eligible professionals must meet one of the following criteria:

- Have a minimum 30% Medicaid patient volume
- Have a minimum 20% Medicaid patient volume, and is a pediatrician
- Practice predominantly in a Federally Qualified Health Center or Rural Health Center and have a minimum 30% patient volume attributable to needy individuals (CMS, 2015)

All eligible participants must report on the required core and menu objectives (Box 11.12) based on the number of objectives and target expectations dictated based on the Meaningful Use Stage. Measuring and reporting on clinical quality helps to ensure that the

Box 11.12   Requirements for Meaningful Use

Eligible healthcare professionals must meet the following number of objectives and related targets:

- Fifteen required core objectives
- Five menu objectives from a list of 11
- Six clinical quality measures

Eligible hospitals and CAHs must meet the following number of objectives and related targets:

- Thirteen required core objectives
- Five menu objectives from a list of 10
- Fifteen clinical quality measures

The core objectives that every eligible professional or healthcare organization must meet in order to receive an EHR Incentive Payment may include some of the following:

1. Computerized provider order entry
2. Drug-drug and drug-allergy checks
3. Maintaining an up-to-date problem list of current and active diagnoses
4. E-prescribing
5. Maintaining active medication list
6. Maintaining active medication allergy list
7. Recording patient's demographics
8. Recording and charting changes in vital signs
9. Recording smoking status for patients 13 years or older
10. Reporting ambulatory clinical quality measures to CMS/States
11. Implementing clinical decision support systems/tools to assist in improving care of patients with chronic conditions
12. Providing patients with an electronic copy of their health information, upon request
13. Providing clinical summaries for patients for each office visit
14. Capability to exchange key clinical information
15. Protecting electronic health information
16. Generating lists of patients by specific conditions to use for quality improvement, reduction of disparities, research, or outreach
17. Use of clinically relevant information to identify patients who should receive reminders for preventive/follow-up care and send these patients the reminder, per patient preference.
18. Use of clinically relevant information from CEHRT to identify patient-specific education resources and provide those resources to the patient
19. Automatically tracking medications from order to administration using assistive technologies in conjunction with an electronic medication administration record (eMAR)
20. Providing a summary of care record (transition record) when transitioning patients to another setting of care or provider or refering patients to another provider
21. Completing medication reconciliation
22. Incorporatation of clinical lab-test results into CEHRT as structured data
23. Providing patients the ability to view online, download, and transmit their health information
24. Use secure electronic messaging to communicate with patients on relevant health information
25. Capability to submit electronic syndromic surveillance data to public health agencies and actual submission according to applicable law and practice

Quality measures are defined based on the objectives and must cover at least three of the following national quality strategy domains:

- Patient and family engagement
- Patient safety
- Care coordination
- Population and public health
- Efficient use of healthcare resources
- Clinical process/effectiveness

Complied from www.cms.gov, Meaningful Use Stage 2 Grid; available at http://www.healthit.gov/sites/default/files/meaningfulusetablesseries2_110112.pdf

participating healthcare providers and organizations deliver effective, safe, efficient, patient-centered, equitable, and timely care. Therefore, the clinical quality measures (CQMs) used in the Meaningful Use CEHR Incentive Payment Program focus on measuring the quality of healthcare services provided by the eligible professionals, hospitals, and CAHs. These measures use data associated with providers' ability to deliver high-quality care or relate to long-term goals for quality and safe care (CMS, 2015). CQMs measure many aspects of patient care based on the domains of the national quality strategy and focus on the following aspects of care delivery, most of which case management has a great impact on:

- Health outcomes
- Clinical processes
- Patient safety
- Efficient use of healthcare resources
- Care coordination
- Transitions of care
- Patient engagement
- Population and public health
- Adherence to clinical guidelines

Case management departments and case managers may play an important role in meeting the Meaningful Use Incentive Program requirements. As noted in Box 11.12, most of the objectives and quality measures address key aspects of the case management functional areas and roles and responsibilities of case managers, for example, transitions of care, summaries of care with minium data elements included, patients' access to their own improtant health information, health instruction and engagement, communication among various providers of care, and use of evidence-based clinical care guidelines (i.e., standardized case management plans).

11.12. COST/QUALITY/CASE MANAGEMENT

As healthcare costs increasingly become a public issue and federally funded health insurance programs and commercial health insurance plans, including managed care organizations, spend more time examining documentation of healthcare expenses and charges, it is more apparent that quality monitoring must also include elements of not only practice patterns and patient satisfaction and experience but also cost-containment and safety strategies. With the VBP program, cost per Medicare beneficiary is under scrutiney and it behooves healthcare leaders and providers to assure cost-effective care delivery.

In healthcare organizations, problems that go undetected can have devastating effects that involve wasted time, money, and other important resources. When a problem is not fixed at the time it occurs, it will only become more costly to fix later on (Organizational Dynamics, Inc., 1991) (Figure 11.1). It is fortunate for case management that by design the role of the case manager includes a special focus on addressing variances, delays in care, or deviations from the norm at the time such undesirable events occur and sometimes even prevent such occurrence. Therefore, the case manager reduces if not compeltely eliminates the need for the healthcare organization to spend unnecessary resources on addressing a variance when it is too late and that time correcting an undesirable outcomes is perhaps too late.

It makes a difference when a problem is fixed. The 1-10-100 rule states that if a problem is not fixed when it occurs, it will only become more costly and challenging to fix later in terms of both time, personnel, and money. It may also not result in desirable outcomes compared to those would have been realized when it first occurred.

Costs usually involve the necessary expenditures and those that are avoidable. A necessary cost is one that is needed to sustain a certain standard. Avoidable costs are those that occur whenever things are done wrong, delayed, or when unnecessary steps are applied in the process. Necessary and avoidable costs can be further defined by prevention, inspection, and failure costs.

- *Prevention costs* are those intended to ensure that things will not go wrong.
- *Inspection costs* are the costs of finding an error or variance and fixing it.
- *Failure costs* are those incurred when outcomes and patient or consumer satisfaction are negatively affected.

Any institution pays a big price for a marred reputation, rework, waste, legal penalties, extra charges, or loss of business. Poor quality is costly. And since safety is the backbone of quality, we can not assess the cost of quality without factoring in the cost of safety or the lack of. To help reduce the potential costs poor quality and suboptimal safety incur, it becomes imperative that case managers facilitate QI and process improvement by making sure that they get involved and have the confidence and skills required to do their job well and assure safety at all times especially during the most vulnerable times or actions such as hand-off communication during a patient's transition to another level of care where the risk for poor quality and suboptimal experience is high. This does not mean that case managers are solely responsible for the cost of quality

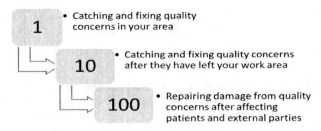

1 • Catching and fixing quality concerns in your area

10 • Catching and fixing quality concerns after they have left your work area

100 • Repairing damage from quality concerns after affecting patients and external parties

It makes a difference when a problem is fixed. The 1-10-100 rule states that if a problem is not fixed when it occurs, it will only become more costly and challenging to fix later in terms of both time, personnel, and money. It may also not result in desirable outcomes compared to those would have been realized when it first occurred.

Figure 11.1 The 1-10-100 rule (Organizational Dynamics, Inc., 1991).

and safety. They must work in concert with all of the diverse members of the interdisciplinary team, those directly or indirecelt involved in patient care.

For example, a physician writes an order for a medication that the patient has an allergy to. If the nurse notices this error as the order is picked up, it would involve a simple solution of ordering another medication that is more appropriate for the patient. However, if the order goes to the pharmacy and the allergy is not noted, and the pharmacist reviews, profiles, or fills the order, and the nurse administers the medication; it could end in a terrible tragedy. The cost of the incorrect medication is only the tip of the iceberg for this error. The dollars alone cannot fully measure the impact of such an avoidable error on the patient and the hospital. The real cost of this undetected problem shows the heightened damage as illustrated in the 1-10-100 rule. Not only has a medication occurrence added increased cost, but patient satisfaction and safety are at stake as well.

11.12.1. Prevention of Care Concerns

The obvious key to reducing costs and maintaining quality and safety is prevention. The case manager, in the daily review of patient care, works toward preventing errors, delays, ommissions, problems, and bottlenecks to care. The next best strategy after prevention is early detection and treatment of the problem. Again consider the scenario of the medication error. If the immediate physician order error goes undetected, then the first level of prevention fails unnecessarily. However, if the nurse detects the problem before administration of the dedication (referred to as a near miss event), then early detection prevents the potential full impact of the error. On the other hand, if the nurse administers the incorrect medication, then early detection is not employed. To compound this error, perhaps the patient is aware that a mistake has been made, and this is ethically necessary. Now the confidence in the physician

and hospital staff has been marred. The case manager is now involved in identifying this quality issue and must get the physician and perhaps a hospital representative in to speak with the patient and safety (referred to as disclosure) and attempt to make amends. It now becomes clearer that the cost of quality in this example could have the worst effect of all no matter how simple the issue may be—a dissatisfied patient who will never return to that healthcare facility, assuming that the effect of the error is something other than death.

11.12.2. Misuse of Resources

A second area in which cost and quality intertwine is the cost associated with misuse of personnel or equipment resources. For example, a case manager specializing in cardiac care began to notice that patients were placed on telemetry upon admission and never reassessed for continued need, nor taken off telemetry until the time of discharge, meanwhile patients awaited in the ED for telemetry beds that are not available at time of need. The case manager decided to investigate the problem of lack of telemetry beds and delays in patient admissions. By analyzing the costs of keeping patients on telemetry unnecessarily (i.e., at a higher level of care as otherwise indicated by patient's condition) and delays in admissions from the ED to the acute inpatient telemtry care unit, which sometimes results in delays in care progression. In addition, the case manager met with various physicians and the medical director to troubleshoot the rationale behind the lack of reassessment for continued need for telemtery monitoring. What was discovered by the case manager was that the cardiologists were concerned that if telemetry monitoring was discontinued a serious change in the patient's condition may go unnoticed until it was too late. One of the cardiologists recalled an incident from few years back where a patient who was not being monitored on the day of discharge sustained a cardiac arrest while about to walk out of the hospital. The case manager then set out to reassure the physicians of the indications and discontinuation including nursing assessment and close monitoring. The use of an evidence-based protocol for telemetry and review of patients for a few months showed the physicians that the quality of their patients' care had not been compromised. Because of the perseverance of this case manager, the unnecessary use of telemetry monitoring and delays in patient's admissions were diminished. By analyzing this problem the case manager identified an opportunity for QI through the most cost-effective method available to the patients.

11.12.3. Cost of Care Delays

The last area in how cost and quality inter-relate is the cost of delays. There is much at stake when quality is affected by a delayed service. All of the issues mentioned thus far come into play here. The cost associated with delays, the impact on patient satisfaction, and the misappropriation of resources and personnel will significantly affect the cost of outcomes. Delays are very costly to hospitals and can negatively influence how they are judged by regulators, accreditation agencies and payers, other physicians, consumers, and patients.

The example of the ventilator-dependent patient is useful here as well. Suppose that the patient appears to have the potential to be weaned from the ventilator. Weaning can be an arduous task, but the ultimate payoff is so exciting and cost-effective that if done successfully it can save the hospital many costly dollars. The challenge of weaning a patient from a ventilator lies with an experienced team who follows the patient very closely. This involves the efforts of case management, as well as social work, nutrition, respiratory therapy, speech therapy, physical therapy, the physician, nursing staff, the patient, and the family. The interdisciplinary approach to this complex patient's care management plan is essential to its success.

First the case manager and social worker must work with the patient and family to help them adjust to the idea that weaning their loved one may take some time and may or may not be successful. This alone is difficult and at times frustrating and disappointing for a family. Once the case manager has established that the patient and family are emotionally prepared, the next step is for the other disciplines (e.g., respiratory therapy, nutrition) to educate the family on the care required at home. The timing and availability of the other departments can make or break the length of time it takes to wean a patient. It becomes crucial for the case manager to stay on top of the whole process from start to finish so that everything is in place at the right

time. The social worker must work on applications for personal care attendants or any financial arrangements that need to be finalized before discharge. The dietitian must be closely involved with the patient, watching all food intake. The right balance of protein, fat, and carbohydrates must be monitored because weaning cannot take place without the proper caloric intake. A negative nitrogen balance from inappropriate intake can significantly delay the weaning process.

The speech therapist has the vital role of training the patient in different speech and swallowing techniques. If this is attempted with a dedicated positive approach toward the patient's progress, the odds of success are greater. Not all patients are able to meet the criteria for successful speech therapy. It is the case manager who will discuss the potential with the speech therapist and physician to see if the patient is a good candidate. Successful speech and swallow training can make the difference between a patient who will require tube feedings and the patient who can go home on oral food intake. Imagine the delays that can occur in this area alone if no one takes an aggressive risk in attempting to train the patient. Should this area not be explored or attempted with strong expertise, the patient will require tube feedings, which will surely cause a delay because of the added teaching required and post-discharge services to be needed while at home. The family will need to learn the tube feeding procedures, and the patient will have an additional psychological hurdle to get over.

This is an area in which the case manager can again be involved. A patient-teaching checklist can assist all disciplines in tracking the progress of the family and their ability to learn various tasks such as tube feeding. Without the use of such a tool, an additional delay can occur because there will be no record of the progress or lack of progress a family is making in learning the necessary skills required. Another discipline that must coordinate its intervention when weaning a patient is respiratory therapy. The therapists must monitor all of the oxygen saturation data and be willing to try the patient on and off the ventilator for periods, knowing that this is a tedious task that requires patience and perseverance. Any missed opportunities to try the patient off the ventilator could delay the ultimate weaning process and may even cause a failed weaning of the patient. Obviously if the attempts are failed the medical costs of this patient's care increase dramatically.

All interdisciplinary efforts should be to work toward keeping the cost of this patient's care as low as possible. It is very important for the physician to have a trusting relationship with all of the involved disciplines in the patient's discharge/transitional plan. If the physician becomes discouraged with the progress being made, the chances are that he or she will make the decision that the patient is not weanable. The physician must be kept well informed by other members of the healthcare team (e.g., nurses, respiratory therapist) whenever progress is being made (Case Manager's Tip 11.9).

The case manager again has the important role of assisting the physician in making educated decisions regarding whether the patient is making significant enough progress to be weaned off the ventilator. The case manager must also have the expertise to know when to call the skilled nursing agency to begin the preparations for discharge from the hospital setting. If the timing is off on this phase of the discharge/transition plan, a major delay will occur, increasing the risk for suboptimal quality of care. As in the scenario discussed earlier in Case Study 11.1, if placement of the patient in a skilled nursing facility is not included in the discharge or transition plan, the risk of an unnecessary readmission is significant. Similarly, if the outpatient home respiratory therapy company is not brought into the loop at the right time, the home may not be properly prepared for a ventilator if this patient cannot be weaned. It behooves the company to check the home electricity for the ability to accommodate the ventilator. Thus if the patient does not come off the ventilator, the potential delay of wiring the home for appropriate electricity can be avoided.

There are other tools that can assist the case manager's efforts toward a successful weaning and cost-effective quality discharge plan. The use of a clinical pathway that is specific to weaning a patient off the ventilator will serve as an excellent guideline for all disciplines involved in the case to help track areas of strengths and weaknesses. It will help to standardize the process and yet individualize it to specific patient needs. Patient teaching pathways or patient education tools can help to include the patient and family in the plan. The teaching guidelines can assist as a resource for the patient and family at times when the information being taught becomes overwhelming. The use of teach back can enhance the patient and family learning what the care entails and ultimately increases ability

for self-management. Anything that can help to reinforce teaching will be a benefit to the patient/family and lead to a timely discharge not hindered or delayed by lack of understanding on the patient's or family's part (Case Manager's Tip 11.10).

Case managers may address quality and safety concerns and ensure optimal care by being goal-oriented and intentional. For example, when an error occurs or there is delay in care, case managers may critically discuss the issue with members of the interdisciplinary healthcare team, investigate the event thoroughly including the patient's perspective, reflect on what happened, and analyze the root cause(s) of the event. Case managers assure there is no premature closure on the event investigation until all important information has been obtained and carefully examined. They then develop an improvement plan to correct the situation and assure such an event does not happen in the future. Additionally, they learn from the event and can be proactive in safe and quality care delivery. Most importantly, case managers work with the right individuals at the healthcare organization to assure complete disclosure has occurred to the patient and family. Such disclosure promotes patient-centered care and adherence to the ethical principle of truth telling.

11.13. CASE MANAGEMENT AND OUTCOMES MANAGEMENT

Outcomes management is a process that focuses on cost and quality of healthcare. It is defined as a method for the implementation of ideal and desirable patient care services that ultimately enhance patient and organizational outcomes. Case management provides the mechanism by which effective and efficient outcomes are provided, ensured, enhanced, and facilitated. Both

CASE MANAGER'S TIP 11.10

Key Elements to Help Avoid Delays in Patient Care Planning

- Make sure that family/patient education starts early.
- Maintain open physician communication.
- Include all disciplines on the team.
- Use case management plans to guide progress.
- Use patient teaching tools to assist disciplines in tracking progress.
- Include outside agencies such as home care or respiratory therapy companies early.
- To achieve your goals, be persistent, persevere, and have patience.

CASE MANAGER'S TIP 11.9

The Importance of Keeping the Physician Informed

An informed physician is better equipped to intervene appropriately and to not react to inconclusive data. Informed decision is also able to progress care in a timely manner and address care concerns as they occur to avoid unnecessary extended patient's hospitalization or costs.

outcomes management and case management processes are interested in quality, safe, and cost-effective patient care. This makes their marriage desirable and feasible. Almost all of the case management programs today include an outcomes management component whose purpose is to measure the effectiveness of the program. Other benefits of having an outcomes management program are as follows:

- Ability to identify improvement opportunities so that enhancements in patient care delivery and outcomes can be made
- Enhancing practitioner practice patterns and maximizing consistency and standardization
- Collecting pertinent and timely data for the evaluation of performance related to quality and safety
- Focusing on strategies that result in reducing readmissions to acute care setting and complications, morbidity, and mortality
- Optimizing the provision of quality healthcare that meets the interests of consumers, providers, regulators, and payers
- Determining what treatments are effective, how much they cost, and whether the results are valued by consumers
- Assisting healthcare organizations in meeting the standards of regulatory and accreditation agencies

The case manager plays an important role in monitoring and managing outcomes of care. The outcomes management process consists of a series of steps (Box 11.13) that guide the case manager toward measuring/assessing, monitoring, and managing patient outcomes over time.

Outcomes measurement is conducted by a systematic and quantitative observation and assessment of an outcome at one point in time. It is the measurement of what happens or does not happen after an action or intervention is implemented or not implemented. This is followed by the outcomes monitoring process of specific outcomes, during which repeated measures take place over time. This process allows the case manager to identify what characteristics (structure) of the patient care delivery system and processes resulted in the observed outcome; that is, making a causal inference that allows an understanding of what happened, what contributed to the outcomes, and then the design of a more effective improvement plan. Finally, the outcomes management process results in optimal outcomes through improved administrative and clinical decision making and service delivery. It takes place as the case manager and other members of the interdisciplinary healthcare team use the information and knowledge they have gained during the assessment and

---

Box 11.13 Outcomes Management Process

The outcomes management process consists of three main actions: outcomes measurement, outcomes monitoring, and outcomes evaluation and improvement. The measurement action refers to the assessment of outcomes at one point in time usually at the beginning of the outcomes management process; the outcomes monitoring action refers to assessment of the outcomes in a longitudinal manner (i.e., multiple points in time such as monthly); and the outcomes evaluation and improvement entails making sense of the outcomes and determining whether optimal or acceptable, identifying opportunities for improvement, and implementing potential solution to identified concerns.

Generally speaking, an outcomes management process may consist of the following steps:

1. Review strategic goals
2. Match goals to outcome indicators
3. Design clear, simple, attainable, measurable, relevant, time-oriented outcome indicators
4. Select appropriate outcomes measurement tools
5. Collect data
6. Analyze and evaluate data
7. Communicate findings
8. Identify, design, and implement improvements
9. Repeat the process

---

monitoring processes to improve care. Outcomes indicators measured can be classified into many categories, such as clinical, functional, and cognitive abilities (of patients); financial; knowledge; quality of life; and satisfaction with care and services (see Chapter 12 for more details).

The case management plan of care is one tool used in this process. The case management plan prospectively determines the interventions and expected outcomes or goals of care. For example, the case management plan may call for an asthma patient to be switched off IV Solu-Medrol/hydrocortisone when the peak flow reading is greater than 250 mL/min. The case manager would measure the point at which this outcome was met in the population of asthma patients and continue to monitor the achievement of this outcome over a period. The case manager might determine that on evenings and weekends a timely switch off the IV medication did not routinely take place. The interdisciplinary team would then need to identify strategies for improving this process and thereby improving the quality of the care the asthmatic patients were receiving.

By effective outcomes management, the case manager facilitates the achievement of quality patient care.

The case manager assists the interdisciplinary team in the development of the plan of care, including the identification of patient outcomes of care for specific case types. The case manager then monitors the achievement of those outcomes over time and works with the interdisciplinary team to improve processes so that the quality of patient care is continuously improving. For these reasons, it is difficult to separate out the functions of case management from those of quality/outcomes management. The two are fundamentally linked and dependent on each other for the provision of quality, safe, and cost-effective patient care.

Case management, quality improvement, and CQI are closely connected in terms of the basic philosophy and process. The asset that case management has is the ability to simultaneously consider quality, safety, and cost while delivering care and coordinating various resources and services for a patient. The tracking methods for outcomes of care used by case management help to measure the cost of good quality versus inferior quality.

The ongoing goal of any formal case management program is to identify the optimal treatment plan and most cost-effective and safe discharge/transitional plan achievable. If such plans are developed, quality is sure to follow. A case manager's quality effort takes place case by case. Case management is an organized approach to improving quality and efficiency in patient care and cost.

In the face of today's perceptions and expectations of healthcare consumers, regulators and payers, it is an ongoing challenge for case management to significantly impact quality and cost-effectiveness; the challenge must be accepted if we are to survive this tidal wave that the healthcare industry is experiencing.

11.14. MODERN VIEW OF QUALITY AND SAFETY

The modern view of quality and safe healthcare provision to patients and their families focuses on the responsibility and accountability of healthcare providers and leaders of creating an evironment of care that deals with patient safety as a top priority and of strategic focus. All members of healthcare teams (directly or indirectly involved in clinical care; both leaders and clinicians) must assure the approach care delivery in a holistic and patient centered manner at all times. Case management programs and case managers as patient advocates are best prepared to facilitate the implementation and sustaining of such approaches. Additionally because they are involved in the planning, implementation, facilitation, coordination, and evaluation of pa-

tient care, in collaboration with other members of the interdisciplinary healthcare team, they are best fit to also safeguard the safety of patients and promote quality. As such they assure care is:

- Based on the strongest clinical evidence available
- Provided in a technical and culturally competent manner
- Delivered with ongoing and transparent communication among all involved
- Planned based on shared decision making with patients and their families, especially for options and choices of care goals, treatments, interventions, and resources

Case managers also are assets healthcare organizations have the luxury to employ them in ensuring an "error-free" healthcare environments for patients and their families as well as professionals. They are able to contribute to such environments by virtue of their roles in eliminating, avoiding, and preventing delays (variances, omissions) in care and underuse, overuse, or misuse of treatments and resources. They are effective in risk reduction which ultimately improves patient safety (Case Manager's Tip 11.11).

Today's modern approach to quality improvement and patient safety focuses on managing any issues or concerns of patient care delivery that impact both clinical and operational quality (Case Manager's Tip 11.12). Case managers contribute to realizing this by sharing the data they gather while reviewing patient records, completing clinical/concurrent reviews with health insurance plans, facilitate interdisciplinary patient care management rounds, and evaluate quality indicators and outcomes of care such as the value-based purchasing core measures.

 CASE MANAGER'S TIP 11.11

Difference between Safety and Risk Reduction

- *Safety* is the prevention of accidental mistakes and/ or injuries from occuring to others (i.e., patients, the public, and fellow healthcare professionals).
- *Risk reduction* is the elimination or minimization of the possibility of injury (e.g., medical error) or loss (e.g., death) occurring because of dangerous or hazardous situations.

Case managers must be aware of the difference between these two terms and avoid using them interchangeably. They also, through their actions of advocacy and case managed care provision, must focus on both of these aspects in assuring quality and safe care.

CASE MANAGER'S TIP 11.12

Clinical and Operational Quality

Clinical quality focuses on patient care and case management outcomes that are patient health condition-related such as reduction of symptoms, mortality rate, and complications, or improvement in hemoglobin A1c in diabetic patients.

Operational quality fcuses on the systems and processes of care delivery that often are administrative in nature such as reduction of diversion hours in the emergency department, admission of a patient to an acute care bed within 60 minutes or less from time decision to admit is made, and expanding physical therapy availability over the weekend.

From a quality and performance improvement perspective, regardless of which method or process is applied, it is necessary to focus on the following four aspects of improvement for desirable transformation to happen effectively, expeditiously, and with sensitivity to the environmental factors or the cotext of patient care delivery (i.e., patient centeredness).

1. Use of technical or knowledge-based solutions to concerns of care delivery systems. This approach applies available evidence and technology to improve practice. For example, use of evidence-based practice guidelines, automated quality outcomes data collection and analysis, and patient's access to their health records.

2. Use of adaptive or behavior-based solutions to issues in care provision. This apporach capitalizes on changing attitudes, values, and beliefs of healthcare professionals. For example, adotpion of computerized provider order entry systems with standardized order sets for specific patient groups (e.g., heart failure), and implementation of clinical protocols to eliminate variation in practice patterns of clincians.

3. Understand drivers of intrinsic motivation to build momentum for improvement. These drivers come from within the healthcare professional such as energy, enthusiasm, willingness, and commitment. Upon understanding what contributes to clinicians' satisfaction in the adoption of change, we can then use these contributing factors to maximize work and behavior transformation. For example, if it is acknowledgement, implement a reward and recognition program.

4. Understand drivers of extrinsic motivation to cre-

ate urgency and business case for improvement. These drivers usually come from entities external to the clincian or the healthcare organization; often are regulatory or accreditation driven. For example, needing to change patient care activities and behaviors to meet value-based purchsing program requirements.

Finally, modern day quality and safety relies on disclosure and transparency. Unlike traditional quality assurance programs where mistakes and errors were kept as secrets and blamed and penalized clinicians, today's best practice environments that strategically focus on the delivery of safe and quality patient-centered care to ultimatey enhance the patient experience are those that have hardwired a fair and just safety culture. These have adopted nonpunitive attitudes toward proactive identification and the reporting of errors and near misses in every aspect of patient care delivery and at every level of clinicians/staff. These environments of care demonstrate quality and safety by assuring a culture of care provision that is characterized by six key components, as follows.

1. *High reliability*: organizations with systems in place that make them exceptionally consistent in accomplishing their goals and avoiding potentially catastrophic errors or unsafe situations. These organizations are specially sensitive to the operations of care delivery (whether simple or complex systems, processes and administrative transactions), reluctant to oversimplify the reasons for problems, are preoccupied with failure (acknowledge that mistakes do happen and encourage all staff to be involved in recognition of failures and contribute to change), exhibit deference to expertise and resilience.

2. *Process improvement design*: use proactive approaches to care delivcery improvements to ultimately prevent errors and enhance patient safety. For example, implement evidence-based practice guidelines, use clinical decision support systems at the point of care, and standardization of practices.

3. *Human factors integration*: use of human factor engineers to gain a better understanding of the interface of humans and available technology or systems. This is highly valuable when implementing a new process of care, EMRs, or health devices as well as when conducting a root cause analysis for an error or near miss that has already occured. This innovative approach allows a real life and practical understanding of how healthcare professionals

(humans) interact with the technology and systems (e.g., policies, procedures, standards, and organizational heirarchy) available to them in the patient care environment and at the point of care. It also assures that when investigating how an error occurred, a holistic and thorough analysis of all of the aspects in the care process that have (or potentially may have) contributed to the error, not just the human element. In addition, this approach prevents pointing fingers or blaming others (or oneself), generates more appreciation of the complexity of healthcare delivery, and how challenging it is to have a fully safe and quality care environment.

4. *Partnership with patients and their families*: seeking the voice of the customer is important especially when developing innovative systems of care or engaging in transforming exisiting care environments. Additonally, healthcare organizations who are effective in demonstrating a culture of safety (or safety first) are those that reach out to patients proactively, inquire about their care experience, and specifically seek to understand what improvement opportunities exist. Today these organizations have implemented patient and family advisory committees (PFACs) as a standard and routine structure; often these committees report up the quality and safety department or subcommittees of the board of directors/trustees which is a level high enough in the organizational governance structure.

5. *Transparency in error reporting*: this is not only having a process in place for assuring disclosure to patients and families when an error occurs, but rather having an expectation that healthcare professionals and other staff errors and near misses in an event reporting system as well. The reporting system can then provide the data necessary to identify trends and patterns of issues (factors contributing to risk for errors) which may have contributed to system and human failures, and to implement improvements as necessary. Nonpunitive culture is a prerequiste to staff transparency and report of actual or potential errors. When disclosing an error to a patient or family, it is necessary to acknowledge the failure, apologize for it, spend enough time with them, answer their questions, allow them to express themselves, and leave them feeling they have received all the information they may have wanted.

6. *Caring for the caregiver*: this characteristic is important in safe and just cultures. With transparency and disclosure comes obligation to care for the healthcare professional directly or indirectly in-

volved (or have contributed to) in the error or near miss. Caring for the caregiver allows the involved party to verbalize feelings and emotional responses to what have occurred. This focuses on providing a support mechanism for the involved party and ensure re-entry into the care environment with no blame, regret, or self-doubt.

11.15. KEY POINTS

1. Today's competitive healthcare environment demands constant attention to improvements in quality, safety, cost, and performance.

2. There are three types of quality: take it for granted quality, expected quality, and excited quality. Today's definition of quality is considered incomplete if it is not integrated with safety.

3. One can not improve quality without including a special focus on safety. Safety is the backbone of quality.

4. Organizational values consist of five categories of quality: patient/consumer focus, total involvement for taking responsibility for quality, measuring/monitoring quality, systems support, and quality improvement using CQI, DMAIC, or PDCA cycle.

5. It is everyone's responsibility to be involved in the achievement of quality and enhancement of patient safety.

6. Quality assurance focuses on reduction of errors, whereas quality improvement focuses on improving a process of care and its outcomes.

7. Six Sigma and Lean Six Sigma are common today and frequently used in quality management. They focus on elimination of defects and nonvalue-adding activities or processes. They assist systems of care to meet consumer needs and quality and safety targets.

8. The key to reducing costs and maintaining quality is prevention: prevention of errors, duplication, fragmentation, or use of unnecessary resources.

9. Case management focuses on integrating the structure, processes, and outcomes of care in effort to improve quality, assure safety, and reduce cost.

10. Hospital value-based purchasing programs have resulted in placing more emphasis on case management and increased awareness of how case management systems can improve

reimbursement by reducing financial risks and assuring the delivery of quality and safe care.

11. Creating a safe and just care environment/culture of safety relies on a number of key elements including proactively identifying risk and mitigating such risk; encouraging staff to identify and report errors and near misses; adopting the practice of transparency and disclosure; and use human factor engineers to better understand the dynamics of care delivery environments and workflows that potentially contribute to errors.

11.16. REFERENCES

American Society for Quality. Accessed June 5, 2015.What is six sigma, available at http://asq.org/learn-about-quality/six-sigma/overview/overview.html

Claflin N and Hayden CT. (1998). *Guide to quality management,* 8th ed., National Association for Healthcare Quality, Glenview, IL.

Centers for Medicare and Medicaid Cervices (CMS). (2012). Frequently asked questions, hospital value-based purchasing program. Available at http://www.cms.gov/Medicare/Quality-Initiatives-Patient-Assessment-Instruments/hospital-value-based-purchasing/Downloads/FY-2013-Program-Frequently-Asked-Questions-about-Hospital-VBP-3-9-12.pdf

Centers for Medicare and Medicaid Services (CMS). (2014). Hospital value-based purchsing, available at http://www.cms.gov/Medicare/Quality-Initiatives-Patient-Assessment-Instruments/hospital-value-based-purchasing/index.htmlospHosp

Centers for Medicare and Medicaid Services (CMS). Accessed August 22, 2015. Electronic Health Record Incentive Payment Program, Eligible hospitals; available at https://www.cms.gov/Regulations-and-Guidance/Legislation/EHRIncentivePrograms/Eligible_Hospital_Information.html

Coleman E. Accessed June 5, 2015. The Care Transitions Program, Care Transitions Measure. Division of Health Policy and Research, University of Colorado, Denver, School of Medicine. Available at http://www.caretransitions.org/ctm_main.asp

Crosby PB. 1979. Quality is free: the art of making quality certain, McGraw Hill, New York, NY.

Donabedian, A. (1980). *Exploration in quality assessment and monitoring, Vol 1: The definition of quality and approaches to its assessment,* Health Admnistration Press, Ann Arbor, MI.

Donabedian, A. (1991). The role of outcomes in quality assessment and assurance, excerpts from Annual Conference on Nursing Quality Assurance, Miami, FL.

Hospital Consumer Assessment of Healthcare Providers and Systems, Centers for Medicare and Medicaid Services. Accessed June 5, 2015. Available at http://www.hcahpsonline.org/home.aspx

Institute for Healthcare Improvement (IHI). Accessed June 2, 2015. IHI Triple Aim Initiative. Available at http://www.ihi.org/Engage/Initiatives/TripleAim/pages/default.aspx

Institute of Medicine. Crossing the quality chasm. (2001). A new health system for the 21st century. National Academy Press Washington, D.C.

Joint Commission on Accreditation of Healthcare Organizations (JCAHO). (1994). Lexicon dictionary of health care terms, organizations, and acronyms for the era of reform, Chicago, IL.

Joint Commission on Accreditation of Healthcare Organizations (JCAHO). (1996). The 1996 accreditation manual for hospitals, Oakbrook Terrace, IL.

Joint Commission on Accreditation of Healthcare Organizations (JCAHO). (2001). The 2001 accreditation manual for hospitals, Oakbrook Terrace, IL.

Lighter, D. (2013). Basics of health care performance improvement: A lean six sigma approach, Jones and Bartlett Learning, Burlington, MA.

McKesson Corporation, InterQual healthcare Guidelines. Accessed June 2, 2015. Available at http://www..mckesson.com/payers/decision-management/interqual-evidence-based-clinical-content/

MCG Health. Milliman Care Guidelines. Accessed June 2, 2015. Available at http://www.mcg.com/provider/main

Medicare, Hospital Compare. Avvessed June 5, 2015. Hospital value-based purchasing, available at http://www.medicare.gov/hospitalcompare/data/hospital-vbp.html

Newell, M. (1996). Using nurse case management to improve health outcomes, Aspen, Gaithersburg, MD.

Organizational Dynamics, Inc. (1991). Excerpts from conference presentation, Burlington, MA.

Qualis Health, Hospital value-based purchasing. Accessed June 5, 2015. Available at http://medicare.qualishealth.org/sites/default/files/medicare.qualishealth.org/Hospital_VBP_FY2017.pdf

Stratis Health. Value-based purchasing. Accessed June 5, 2015. Available at http://www.stratishealth.org/providers/vbp.html

U.S. Department of Health and Human Services (USDHHS). (2013). 2013 Annual progress report, national strategy for quality improvement in health care.

Williams, R.L. (1994). Essentials of total quality management, American Management Associates, New York, NY.

12 Measuring the Effectiveness of Case Management

As a case manager or an administrator of a case management program in your organization you may be called on to participate in the evaluation of the case management model, its effects on the organization, or its effects on patient outcomes. You may have direct responsibility for evaluating the effectiveness of the model, the outcomes of the case management plans in use, the success of the case manager's role, or the case manager's performance. Some of the evaluation criteria to be discussed in Chapter 12 may require an organizational effort in terms of data collection and/or analysis. Some you may be able to facilitate as part of your own daily job activities.

Whenever possible, it is important to have an evaluation process and a plan set up before implementation of the model. This is particularly true for those outcomes that affect the organization. Categories such as LOS, patient and staff satisfaction, clinical care outcomes, and costs of care should have baseline benchmarks against which the hospital can judge success or failure. Additional measurement points will be identified prospectively during the course of the hospital stay or course of treatment or intervention and then at the point of discharge or completion of services, depending on the care setting. Other indices, particularly those related to clinical or patient outcomes, will evolve over time.

12.1. OUTCOMES AS INDICES OF QUALITY

Broadly speaking, outcomes can be grouped by those that have an effect on the organization versus those that have an effect on patients. These indicators may be the best measures of quality because they provide an understanding of the functioning of the organization and its effects on the product of services and patient care. Outcomes are the result of actions or processes. In patient care they are defined as the goals of the healthcare process. A good outcome is one that has achieved the desired goal.

Case management, through the use of tools such as guidelines, interdisciplinary action plans, and clinical pathways, and through case management team conferencing, allows healthcare providers to prospectively identify the expected outcomes or goals of care. There are no organizational or clinical processes or tasks that are carried out that do not have an expected outcome attached to them. Therefore outcomes in their narrowest sense allow us to understand the effects on an individual patient and in their broadest sense provide us with an understanding of the functioning (i.e., efficiency and effectiveness) of an organization or the healthcare system at large. These linkages provide us with an understanding of the structure (the organization), the process (the delivery system), and the expected outcomes (goals of care).

Expected outcomes of care are of different types. Some are related to the organization's performance but are not directly related to the patient's health. Others are related to the patient's health but are not directly related to the organization's performance. Still others are solely related to the clinical processes, meaning they are purely clinical in nature.

Case management outcomes can be categorized into three groups:

- Quality
- Financial
- Productivity and regulatory compliance

357

12.2. QUALITY OUTCOME METRICS

Some outcomes directly affect the patient's clinical quality or their perception of that care, such as those listed in Box 12.1.

12.2.1. Patient Satisfaction

Understanding patients' satisfaction with the care and services we provide helps us to improve those services over time and to continuously improve patients' level of satisfaction with the care they receive. Patient satisfaction data are either collected toward the end of the hospital stay or soon after discharge. All hospitals and many other healthcare organizations collect and monitor data on patient satisfaction. Unfortunately there may not always be a mechanism for feeding that information back for the improvement of system processes or expected clinical outcomes.

In May 2005, the National Quality Forum (NQF), an organization established to standardize healthcare quality measurement and reporting, formally endorsed the Consumer Assessment of Healthcare Providers and Systems (CAHPS®) Hospital Survey. The NQF endorsement represented the consensus of many healthcare providers, consumer groups, professional associations, purchasers, federal agencies, and research and quality organizations. Commonly known as the HCAHPS—Hospital Consumer Assessment of Healthcare Providers and Systems, the tool is designed to provide a standardized survey instrument and data collection methodology for measuring patients' perspectives on hospital care.

While many hospitals had been collecting information on patient satisfaction, prior to HCAHPS there was no national standard for would enable valid comparisons to be made across all hospitals. Hospitals could choose from several instruments, purchasing them and using them as they chose to. Questions could even be modified or added. In order to remove the varation between and among instruments, it was necessary to introduce a standard instrument to be used universally.

Three broad goals have shaped the HCAHPS survey. First, the survey is designed to produce comparable data on the patient's perspective on care that allows objective and meaningful comparisons between hospitals on domains that are important to consumers. Second, public reporting of the survey results is designed to create incentives for hospitals to improve their quality of care. Third, public reporting will serve to enhance public accountability in healthcare by increasing the transparency of the quality of hospital care provided in return for the public investment (hospitalcahps@cms.hhs.gov). HCAHPS is classified as an "outcome" measure for purposes of measurement under value-based purchasing. Since July 2007, hospitals subject to the IPPS annual payment update provisions must collect and submit HCAHPS data in order to receive their full IPPS annual payment update. IPPS hospitals that fail to publicly report the required quality measures, which include the HCAHPS survey, may receive an annual payment update that is reduced by two percentage points. The Patient Protection and Affordable Care Act of 2010 included the HCAHPS survey (Box 12.2) among the measures to be used to calculate value-based incentive payments in the Hospital Value-Based Purchasing program, which began with discharges as of October 2012.

Of the nine key topics, at least three have a strong relationship to the work of case management. They are listed in Box 12.2 and include communication about medicines, discharge information, and transition of

---

Box 12.1 Quality Outcome Metrics

1. Patient satisfaction
2. Turn-around time for tests, treatments, procedures, consults
3. Readmissions
4. Discharge/disposition delays

Box 12.2 Hospital Consumer Assessment of Healthcare Providers and Systems Survey

The HCAHPS survey contains 21 patient perspectives on care and patient rating items that encompass nine key topics:

- Communication with doctors
- Communication with nurses
- Responsiveness of hospital staff
- Pain management
- Communication about medicines
- Discharge information
- Cleanliness of the hospital environment
- Quietness of the hospital environment
- Transitions of care.

The survey has a total of 32 questions.

There are four approved modes of administration for the HCAHPS:

1. Mail only
2. Telephone only
3. Mixed (mail followed by telephone)
4. Active Interactive Voice Response (IVR)

CASE MANAGER'S TIP 12.1

Improving Hospital Consumer Assessment of Healthcare Providers and Systems Scores

One strategy for improvement in the HCAHPS scores is to see the patients daily and to repeat the information about discharge planning and transitions to them multiple times. Patients need to hear information repeatedly in order to fully grasp it. Additionally, discuss the patient's medications for home use and how those prescriptions will get filled. Facilitate getting the prescriptions filled before the patient leaves the hospital if possible.

care. While case management is not the only discipline with responsibility for these key topics, case managers and social workers play a large part in the patient's experience with them.

Case management leaders should share the scores with their staff so that case managers and social workers can continuously improve their performance in these categories (Case Manager's Tip 12.1).

12.2.2. Turnaround Time for Tests, Treatments, Procedures, and Consults

Turnaround time (TAT) can be used as a measure of the organization's process improvement and efficiency after the introduction of case management. Facilitating care and managing the patient through the healthcare system should improve the TAT for completion of tests and procedures. The TAT should be measured from the time the physician places the order until the order is completed and results are recorded in the medical record. Acceptable timeframes should be decided in advance. For example, the completion time for computed tomography (CT) scans may be 24 hours from the time the order is written until the results of the CT scan are placed in the medical record.

Monitoring of these periods can be done concurrently or retrospectively through the medical record. Concurrent data collection is always preferred because it is both more accurate and timely. If any problems or delays are identified, they can be addressed immediately. Retrospective data collection, on the other hand, may be more difficult because of lapses in documentation in the patient's medical record or simply the inability to obtain the necessary information. In addition, when problems are finally identified, it is rather late to try to resolve them.

Finally, relationships should be shown between the reduction in TAT and the length of stay (LOS). As be-

fore, it may be difficult to prove sound relationships between LOS reductions and TAT because many other factors may have an effect on the LOS.

12.2.3. Readmissions

Readmissions have become a standard metric for case management. Because the Centers for Medicare and Medicaid Services (CMS) reports them on a 30 day readmission cycle, most hospitals have begun reporting them that way. However, you may want to consider expanding your reporting to include the following:

- 30 days
- 15 days
- 24 hours
- Same day

These additional timeframes allow for the identification of the root causes of readmissions that happen closer to the day of discharge. This methodology allows you to refine all readmissions into additional subsets to work on the causes and corrective actions.

Another method for reporting readmissions is by payer. Consider reporting in the following ways:

- Medicare
- Medicaid
- Managed care

Looking at all payers will help reduce your overall readmission rates as additional payers will most likely be applying penalties in the future. While not all readmissions are avoidable, some are. Understanding and tracking the hospital's performance over time will ensure that everything is being done to reduce those readmissions that are avoidable.

12.2.4. Discharge/Disposition Delays

Discharge and disposition delays are issues associated with the department's inability to transition the patient out of the hospital in a timely manner. These issues may have to do with the availability of services in the community, family issues, financial problems, or physician issues. They may also be related to the performance of the individual discharge planner. To evaluate the performance of the case management department in terms of its discharge planning processes, the department should consider monitoring and analyzing these issues on a regular basis.

Delays in service turn-around time should be tracked and trended. High volume delays should be reported to the appropriate department. Examples might include turn-around time for completion of tests, treatments, procedures, consults, as well as the reporting of same.

12.3. FINANCIAL OUTCOME METRICS

Many case management outcomes are directly related to the bottom line, or financial performance, of the organization. Examples of these include:

- Cost per day/stay
- Length of stay
- Third party denials of payment

12.3.1. Cost Per Day/Stay

Clinical cost accounting methods are being used more and more as a means of understanding not only hospital charges but also the true costs of care. This information can be used to negotiate realistic and appropriate managed care contracts because the hospital understands exactly what costs are associated with the care of a specific population of patients. Cost accounting can also be used as a way of measuring the financial impact of case management on the organization. Although understanding that reduction in LOS of a particular patient population is clearly important, it is also important to determine the amount of resources consumed in the management of that population. Organizations often focus on reducing the LOS but neglect coupling this act with an effort to improve the practice patterns related to tests, procedures, and treatments (pharmaceuticals and others) and eliminating the unnecessary activities. Sometimes they even distribute the same number of tests and procedures across the days left after reducing the LOS. This act keeps the cost of care the same even though the LOS is reduced. Reducing the LOS but consuming the same amount of resources is not as valuable and should be avoided. This will not have the same long-term benefits of shortening the LOS while reducing the amount of resources used in the care of that case type of patient (Cohen, 1991).

The two main goals of clinical cost accounting are first to identify the organization's standard use of materials for a particular diagnosis-related groups (DRG) and then to define the standard cost of each clinical service. An understanding of these costs allows the organization to assess its costs relative to the normal reimbursements, such as Medicare, Medicaid, and other payers. This information also provides a frame of reference or benchmark against which the organization can compare itself with competitors. This can be particularly useful during managed care contract negotiations when the hospital wants to make the most competitive

bid possible (Schriefer et al., 1996). Using standardized case management plans allows an organization to calculate the expected cost of care for a particular case type and facilitates the comparison of the actual cost to the expected cost. Such efforts enhance the development of an action plan for improvement.

Internally, clinical cost accounting helps the hospital measure its internal treatment patterns. This information can be linked to the medical staff to determine which physicians are rendering the most cost-effective care. Allowing the physicians to compare their cost per case with the expected cost or that of their colleagues may provide them with information they can use to improve their practice and in the revision of case management plans.

In the fictitious example in Table 12.1, physician C has the greatest LOS and the highest cost per case compared with other physicians caring for the same type of patients. This report reflects the intensity of physician C's use of resources such as medications, antibiotics, radiology, blood products, and other related supplies. This information might be used by physician C and his colleagues to develop standard protocols that address the use of resources and how it can be reduced or controlled.

Clinical cost accounting can be used by physician department heads or chiefs of services as part of staff education programs. The cost information can be used to help them gain a better understanding of the costs of clinical services and their contribution to those costs. Where differing treatment patterns exist, they can review the patient outcomes and relative costs.

On a managerial level, clinical cost accounting can be used as a component of departmental performance reports, providing administrative staff with financial information related to the efficiency of their departments. Medical staff reports such as that shown in Table 12.1 can provide clinically related information

TABLE 12.1. Example of Physicians' Cost-Per-Case Comparisons for Diagnosis-Related Group 193: Simple Pneumonia and Pleurisy with Complications and Comorbidities

Physician	Number of Patients	Average Length of Stay	Cost per Case
A	55	6.5	$9,280.56
B	50	4.5	$6,985.44
C	34	70	$9,986.53
D	30	7.0	$9,895.32
E	25	6.9	$9,643.50
F	18	5.8	$7,856.64

to guide physicians in changing their clinical practice patterns and can provide information to the finance department in terms of the cost versus volume versus profit to the organization.

12.3.2. Length of Stay

LOS is a broad umbrella term that can be interpreted in various ways to indicate the amount of time allotted to the care, treatment, or recuperation of a patient. In the inpatient setting (e.g., acute, subacute, or skilled nursing facilities/nursing homes) it can be measured by the number of bed days or the number of days the patient remains in the hospital. In the home care setting it is calculated by the number of visits to the home and the number of hours or minutes per visit or the total number of hours. In the ED the LOS may be measured in hours or parts of an hour (15 minutes). LOS statistics are most commonly used in the hospital setting. They are often used as an indicator of the success of case management in conjunction with or in the absence of a cost accounting system.

To determine success or failure of case management and case management plans and their effect on LOS, hospitals must have a clear understanding of what their LOS goals are and compare those with the current LOS statistics in the organization. Comparisons can be made between the hospital and a variety of benchmarks. The first should be the Medicare and non-Medicare DRG average LOS. Although DRGs are not the primary reimbursement system in every state, they are still used for analytical purposes. It is important to understand the history of the organization so that realistic LOS reduction goals can be set. The hospital should also benchmark against comparable hospitals. These hospitals may or may not be close geographically. National databases can be used for this purpose, such as the University Health System Consortium.

12.3.3. Third Party Payer Denials of Payment

Third-party payer denials are a commonly used financial metric. Denials can be related to actual dollars lost and are easily measured and tracked. The department of case management should keep track of initial denials received as well as those lost or recovered after appeal. Trending of the data can demonstrate significant financial returns to the hospital. The data should be routinely reconciled against the data being reported by the finance department to ensure that both departments are reporting in similar fashion.

To monitor denial data, the case management de-

> **Box 12.3   Ways of Aggregating and Monitoring Denials**
>
> - Measure reductions in initial denials
> - Measure reductions in final denials
> - Measure percent reductions on each of the above over time
> - Determine denial reversal rate
> - Measure effect of physician advisor
> - Aggregate by physician/payer

partment must keep accurate data and enter that data into a database in a timely fashion. The data should be audited periodically to ensure that it is accurate. The denials can then be correlated to actual dollars based on the hospital's specific reimbursement rates.

Box 12.3 lists the variety of ways in which denials can be aggregated and monitored.

12.4. PRODUCTIVITY AND REGULATORY METRICS

Monitoring departmental compliance with regulatory indicators is important as a measure of the compliance of the department but should be kept separately as an indicator and should not be included in your report card.

Regulatory compliance examples might include:

- Providing patients with "choice" lists for home care and nursing homes
- Appropriate documentation of discharge planning assessments
- Use of Condition Code 44
- Appropriate documentation of patient discharge disposition

Productivity measures are indicators of the volume of work performed by the department. Although they may give an indication of the amount and complexity of the work, these numbers alone don't demonstrate the organizational outcomes, but rather the volume of the work itself. If monitored, they should be used for the internal evaluation of the department and of the case management staff and should be used within the department only. The department may find, however, that it needs to evaluate the work performance of individuals in the department to demonstrate the need for more staff members. In these circumstances, productivity measures are appropriate.

Case management leadership may consider using some of the productivity measures to evaluate staff member's performance in conjunction with their annual performance review (Box 12.4).

Box 12.4   Examples of Staff Productivity Measures

- Caseloads
- Number of patients discharges with services by type of service
- Number of case management assessments completed
- Number of case management assessments completed within 24 hours of admission
- Number of insurance reviews completed
- Number of interventions on avoidable day issues
- Avoidable days capture rate

12.5. CLINICAL OUTCOMES

Each time a clinical intervention is applied in healthcare, there is an associated expected outcome (Box 12.5). Case management provides the structure for identifying those outcomes prospectively. Clinical outcomes should be interdisciplinary and should come as a result of the collective efforts of the entire clinical team.

12.5.1. Avoid Adverse Effects of Care

The hospital environment can be a dangerous place, and one goal of care is always to get the patient in and out of the hospital without doing any harm. Many of the quality indicators traditionally used in healthcare have focused on errors or problems that are associated with the way care was provided. These have included falls, nosocomial infections, medication errors, returns to the operating room, readmissions, morbidity and mortality reports, and deaths. These indicators are focused on the negative, untoward effects of the care provided to the patient and less on the identification of areas for clinical improvement that appear as patterns or trends. Nevertheless, it is important to continue to track these untoward outcomes after implementation of the case management model or case management plan.

12.5.2. Improve the Patient's Physiological Status

The next set of indicators is concerned with the pa-

Box 12.5   Expected Outcomes Directly Related to the Patient's Health

1. Avoid adverse effects of care
2. Improve the patient's physiological status
3. Reduce signs and symptoms of illness
4. Improve functional status and well-being

---

tient's clinical response to treatment. A goal of care is for the patient to be discharged in a better clinical condition than he or she was in at the time of admission or the episode of care. One measure of this is the patient's physiological status, which refers to the functioning of the various parts of the patient's organs and other body parts. The physiological status can be measured by such things as vital signs, laboratory values, and physical assessment. It is anticipated that these measures improve between the time of admission and the time of discharge.

The patient's physical abilities are assessed through a thorough review of the major body systems. These include the cardiovascular, respiratory, gastrointestinal, genitourinary, neurological, musculoskeletal, and integumentary systems.

12.5.3. Improve Signs and Symptoms

Signs and symptoms are the first stage of illness. In this stage three things generally occur: (1) the physical experience of symptoms such as pain, shortness of breath, or fever; (2) a cognitive awareness of the symptoms and a placing of meaning on them; and (3) emotional response to this awareness in the form of fear or anxiety (Ignatavicius & Bayne, 1991). At this point the person may self-treat or seek a medical opinion. In either case it is anticipated that the signs and symptoms will be reduced or eliminated. If this occurs, the patient returns to the optimal level of wellness.

It is therefore anticipated that after the clinical interventions of the case management team, the patient's signs and symptoms will be improved.

12.5.4. Improve Functional Status and Well-Being

Functional status and well-being address the patient's ability to perform in a variety of areas. These areas include physical health, quality of self-maintenance, quality of role activity, intellectual status, attitude toward the world and sense of well-being related to self, and emotional status. Functional ability refers to the patient's ability to perform activities of daily living (ADLs). ADLs include an assessment of the patient's ability to perform personal care, ability to communicate, and perception of needs (Ignatavicius & Bayne, 1991).

There are a variety of tools to measure functional status. Among these is the commonly used Functional Independence Measure (FIM), developed by Granger and Gresham (1984). The FIM helps to quantify what the patient actually can do, regardless of the clinical diagnosis. Assessment categories include self-care, sphincter control, mobility and locomotion, communication, and social cognition. The FIM helps care providers measure the level of dependence/independence of their patients in an effort to decide what kind of help they may need after discharge to the community.

When developing clinical outcomes, the previously discussed categories should all be considered. Some will be more relevant to the clinical picture than others. One approach for monitoring the expected clinical outcomes is through the identification of intermediate and discharge outcomes. These should be specific to the clinical issue at hand. Intermediate outcomes are those expected goals that occur during the course of the hospital stay. They also are triggers for change or progression in the treatment process and indicate that the patient is progressing toward meeting the discharge outcomes/criteria. Achievement of the goal or outcome should be based on the patient's expected response to treatment. These expected outcomes can occur at any point in the hospital stay and usually trigger the move to the next phase of treatment.

Discharge outcomes are those expected outcomes that the patient must achieve to be discharged from the hospital. The intermediate and discharge outcomes should be the basis for the case management plans/tools. The expected outcomes must be identified before the clinical course of events can be determined. Determination of the expected outcomes should be based on an assessment of both the appropriateness of the care (a determination of who should receive what care) and the effectiveness of care (how good the outcomes of the care are). This review of the evidence helps to relate the process of care to the expected outcomes. This review should be based on all the available evidence rather than solely on the consensus of the practitioners involved in its development (Crosson, 1995). Physicians, when presented with the factual and scientific evi-

---

> **Box 12.7   Uncomplicated Myocardial Infarction**
>
> **Intermediate Outcomes**
>
> 1. Intravenous nitroglycerin: Taper/convert to oral or topical beginning on second day
> 2. Supplemental oxygen: Discontinue once patient is hemodynamically stable (usually begins on day 2)
> 3. Ambulate on day 2 or when free of chest pain and shortness of breath
>
> **Discharge Outcomes**
>
> 1. Absence of chest pain and signs of ischemia (should occur within 48 hours)
> 2. Resolution of ischemic ECG changes
> 3. Cardiac enzymes returning to baseline
> 4. Medications converted to oral/topical
> 5. Activity progressed to preadmission level
> 6. Patient/family verbalizes understanding of the following:
>   a. Signs and symptoms of heart attack
>   b. Risk factors for heart disease
>   c. Medications
>   d. Diet restrictions
>   e. Cessation of smoking (if indicated)
>   f. Activity balanced with rest

dence behind the case management tool or guideline, are more likely to favor it and use it to guide their practice.

12.5.5. Examples of Outcomes

Boxes 12.6, 12.7, and 12.8 are examples of expected outcomes presented to help understand the differences and the relationships between intermediate and discharge clinical outcomes. Each example does not include an exhaustive list of the outcomes related to the diagnosis or procedure under which they are listed. Members of the interdisciplinary team working on developing the particular case management plan are the ones who decide on the expected clinical outcomes. They are finalized after a thorough discussion of their implications on the care of the patient, LOS, cost, and quality and are always included as an integral part of the case management plan.

12.6. PATIENT CARE VARIANCES

A variance occurs when what is supposed to happen does not take place. It is defined as a deviation from a standard or omission of an activity or a step from

---

> **Box 12.6   Lower Gastrointestinal Surgery**
>
> **Intermediate Outcomes**
>
> 1. *Ambulation*: Patient is out of bed and walking with assistance within 12 hours of surgery.
> 2. *Gastric decompression*: Nasogastric tubes to be removed 24–36 hours post-operatively for drainage under 250 mL or less than 100 mL residual; gastrostomy to be clamped using the same criteria.
> 3. *Diet*: Begin clear liquids 12–24 hours after removal of nasogastric tube or clamping of gastrostomy; advance to full liquid diet the same day; begin with full liquid diet and advance to regular diet on the following day.

Box 12.8 Inpatient Management of Mastectomy Patients

Intermediate Outcomes

1. Ambulation: ambulate when fully awake
2. Encourage ambulation within 2 hours of surgery
3. Encourage regular diet when patient is able to tolerate solids
4. Change/switch pain medication(s) to oral if pain scores are five or less for 24 hours

Discharge Outcomes

1. Patient may be discharged as soon as the following criteria have been met:
2. Proper functioning of drains
3. Site is free of signs of hemorrhage and infection
4. Pain is controlled with oral analgesics
5. Patient demonstrates ability to care for drains or home care is arranged for follow-up
6. Patient is able to ambulate independently

---

a predetermined plan, norm, rate, goal, or threshold (Strassner, 1996). Generally, variances are expectations that are not met. According to Webster's Third New International Dictionary (1986), variance is defined as "the fact, quality, or state of being variable or variant . . . a difference of what has been expected or predetermined and what actually occurs." In relation to patient care, variances are outcomes or healthcare providers' actions that do not meet the desired expectations. In relation to case management, variances are deviations from the recommended activities in any of the care elements delineated in the case management plan (Ignatavicius & Hausman, 1995; Pearson, Goulart-Fisher, & Lee, 1995; Tahan & Cesta, 1995; Cohen & Cesta, 1997). Variances often result from delays, interruptions, additions, or omissions of patient care activities and processes. They may sometimes be related to expediting patient care (e.g., performing a patient care activity before it is due is considered a variance).

In an era of increased competition in healthcare, case management plans have emerged as the most desirable tools for improving patient care quality through the elimination and/or prevention of variances, reduction in duplication and fragmentation of care elements, and the standardization of patient care activities. When followed appropriately, case management plans result in consistency in the practice patterns of physicians, nurses, and other healthcare professionals and thus reduce variations in patient care. With this comes the significance of patient care variance data collection and analysis, which are integral elements of case management. Variance data collection cannot occur until the expected outcomes of care, as they relate to the case management plan, have been identified. These expected outcomes become the benchmark against which variation in patient care can be determined.

Variance data collection is important because it provides the basis for improvement in patient care activities, processes, outcomes, and quality. The mechanism of variance data collection is usually decided on by the steering committee charged with implementing the case management model and the use of case management plans. Some institutions have delegated this responsibility to a case management department or a quality improvement committee/council. Regardless of who is responsible, the process should be made consistent across the various care settings that exist in the same institution.

There is no standardization in the method of classifying variances. Variances are classified into different categories in different institutions. Traditionally the most common broad categories used to classify variances are patient/family (Box 12.9), system (Box 12.10), and practitioner (Box 12.11).

Patient/family variances are the result of the patient's behavior or activity or the behavior/activity of a family member (family is used here in its generic sense to denote a patient's spouse, caregiver, significant other, or family member). Variances may be refusal of treatments, or they may occur as a result of changes in the patient's condition or complications of a medical or surgical procedure (e.g., refusal to sign a consent for an operative procedure, infection, fluid and electrolyte imbalance, or family unavailable to accompany the patient home on discharge). Some institutions separate patient variances from the family-related ones. They may classify changes in the patient's condition as they result from the disease process under a separate category (e.g., physiological). The family-related variances may be classified into a separate category and labeled as community variances.

Practitioner variances occur as a result of behaviors of healthcare providers. Examples of practitioner variance are omission of a treatment, test, or procedure; giving the wrong medication; incomplete follow-up and documentation of the patient's response to treatments; or a visiting nurse not showing up for a pre-scheduled home visit. These variances represent the areas that healthcare providers may have the most control over, and if prevented they can influence positive patient care outcomes, lead to timely discharge, eliminate unnecessary work, and reduce cost.

System variances are those related to the way an institution operates, and they result in delays in pa-

Box 12.9   Examples of Patient- and Family-Related Variances

Patient-Related Variances

1. Refuses tests/treatments/procedures
2. Unable to decide on treatment
3. Feels unready for discharge
4. Refuses discharge
5. Noncompliance with medical/surgical regimen, medications, treatments
6. Medical status change/complications
7. Post-operative complications
8. Unable to wean from ventilator
9. Secondary diagnosis with admission (e.g., hospitalized for asthma and diabetes)
10. Language barrier
11. Reaction to medications/allergy
12. Reaction to blood transfusion
13. Poor historian
14. Withholding pertinent information
15. Sign out against medical advice (AMA)
16. Refusing discharge because of religious beliefs, holiday, or inconvenience
17. Noncompliant with diet restrictions
18. Unable to self-administer medication (e.g., insulin)
19. Unable to learn about disease
20. Inability to care for self after discharge
21. No clothes
22. No keys for apartment/left keys at home
23. Lost glasses while in the taxi; cannot see well
24. Lost dentures before admission
25. Lost insurance card
26. Pressure ulcer present on admission

Family-Related Variances

1. Unavailable to pick up patient at time of discharge
2. Unable to provide support for care after discharge
3. Language barrier
4. Late to pick up patient on discharge
5. Inadequate level of knowledge regarding patient care
6. Difficulty with compliance
7. Unable to learn
8. Want another opinion
9. Unable to bring patient's clothes until after business hours
10. Cannot be reached
11. Cannot afford to buy necessary medical equipment or medications

Box 12.10   Examples of System Variances

Hospital/Institution-Related (Internal) Variances

1. Unavailable rehabilitation therapy program on weekends
2. Weekend medical coverage delays requiring changes in treatment (e.g., cannot switch intravenous antibiotic to an oral form)
3. Operating room overbooking
4. Cancellation of operative procedure, test, or treatment
5. Unavailable messenger/transport services
6. Machine breakdown
7. Shortage of supplies
8. Laboratory errors/delays
9. Lost requisitions for tests or procedures or treatments
10. Pending infectious disease approval of medications
11. Nonformulary medications
12. Pending results: radiology, pathology
13. Conflict in scheduling tests, treatments, procedures
14. Not enough personnel to perform tests/procedures
15. Prolonged turnaround time for tests/procedures
16. Prolonged turnaround time for referrals, consults
17. Unavailable beds in the intensive care unit
18. Unavailable beds for emergency admissions
19. Specialty patients diverted to nonspecialty beds
20. Hospital-acquired pressure ulcer
21. Hospital-acquired infection (nosocomial)
22. No pneumatic tube/carrier available

Community-Related (External) Variances

1. No nursing home bed available
2. Transfer to another institution
3. Delayed ambulette transportation
4. No home care available over the weekend
5. Inappropriate transfer from another facility
6. No bed available in a rehabilitation facility
7. Child protective services are late to come
8. Company delivered medical equipment late
9. Managed care organization disapproves home care services
10. Managed care organization did not certify patient's admission to the hospital
11. Managed care organization did not certify an extension in hospitalization (increased days)

Box 12.11   Examples of Practitioner Variances

1. Delay in communicating the plan of care
2. Miscommunication between interdisciplinary team members
3. Physician not communicating to the patient
4. Physician not communicating to the family
5. Medication error
6. Wrong test, treatment, procedure ordered
7. Incomplete documentation
8. Incomplete admission assessment/history
9. Omission of an order
10. Delayed request for a consultant
11. Delayed response by a consultant
12. No consent obtained for treatment
13. Delay in processing forms
14. Delay in initiating treatment, plan of care
15. Lack of coordination of discharge plan among the interdisciplinary team members
16. Inappropriate use of medical equipment
17. Patient teaching not done/completed
18. Delay in scheduling tests
19. Inappropriate/early discharge
20. Nurse busy with other patients
21. Failure to or delay in obtaining preapproval for treatments/interventions or community services
22. Physician did not prepare/inform patient of discharge
23. Failure to conduct financial screening

---

tient care processes. They occur because of inefficient operations and systems, and they may be called operational variances. Mostly these variances require administrative attention or intervention for resolution. System variances can also be classified as internal (i.e., within the walls of the healthcare facility [institution-based]) or external (i.e., outside the walls of the healthcare facility [community-based]). Examples of system variances are lost laboratory requisition slips or specimen, failure of an infusion pump, no nursing home bed available, payment denial, or a managed care organization not approving certain patient care services.

Variances are also classified as positive or negative (Bueno & Hwang, 1993; Hampton, 1993; Ignatavicius & Hausman, 1995; Tahan & Cesta, 1995; Mateo & Newton, 1996). A positive variance is defined as a desired outcome that occurs before it is expected (i.e., before the timeframe that is indicated/projected in the case management plan). It is also a justified type of variance. Examples of positive variance are switching

a recommended antibiotic to a different one because of a patient's allergy, changing the diet of a cardiac patient who is admitted for the management of heart failure from the salt- and fat-restricted diet recommended in the case management plan to include diabetic restrictions because the patient is also diabetic, and a patient's early discharge because all of the outcomes are met earlier than expected.

A negative variance occurs when a patient care activity is delayed and the patient does not meet the expected/desired outcomes (i.e., the recommended patient care activities in the case management plan are not achieved within the specified timeframes). For example, a patient was on anticoagulation therapy and required prothrombin time (PT) testing every 6 hours on the initial day of treatment. He was due for a PT test at 12:00 P.M., but the test was not completed until 4:00 P.M. and the result could not be retrieved from the laboratory information (automated) system until 5:30 P.M. The result of the PT test was found to be very high, and the patient required an immediate intervention, putting the anticoagulation therapy on hold temporarily. In this example, a delay in performing the prescheduled PT test was identified as a practitioner variance. This variance resulted in a delay in changing the anticoagulation therapy/plan of care, and the patient was required to stay an extra day in the hospital.

Another variance category is an add-on variance. It is defined as an unplanned or extra patient care activity or process. This type of variance occurs as an addition to what is indicated in the case management plan. An example of such variance is added laboratory tests. An add-on patient care activity is considered a variance because it may contribute to an increase in cost or a delay in discharge. Most often this type of variance results in duplication of services or performance of unnecessary patient care activities.

Because there is no standardization in classifying variances, it is difficult to share variances across care settings or institutions for the purpose of benchmarking. It is even more difficult to conduct a joint trending analysis of variance data from several healthcare institutions located in a particular community, an analysis that could sometimes be important for improving healthcare in a whole community rather than a particular hospital population. To avoid this, Hoffman (1993) recommends that the standardized critical elements of patient care included in case management plans be used as the classification system for variances (e.g., assessment and monitoring, treatments, medications, patient/family education, discharge planning). If this classification system is followed, then data become transferable within and across institutions, which is highly beneficial for improving the quality of patient care.

12.6.1. Variance Data Collection and Analysis

Designing an effective method for documenting, collecting, and analyzing variances remains a great challenge for most healthcare institutions. Whether the process of variance data collection is automated or manual, most institutions have made the case manager the one responsible for collecting variances. Variance data could be collected anytime during the patient's hospitalization. However, the best time is at the time the variance happens or when it is identified. Timely identification and resolution of variances result in the delivery of cost-effective and high-quality care and increase patient/family satisfaction. A variety of sources for variance identification can be used, such as the progress notes of physicians, nurses, and other healthcare professionals; verbal communication with other members of the interdisciplinary care team during a case conference or one-on-one; or communication with other departments.

The extent to which variance data should be collected is extremely difficult to generalize and varies from institution to institution. How to collect data and what is needed should be prospectively determined. Some institutions collect data at random or as they relate to every single patient care activity without considering their impact on the LOS and quality of care. In such situations, data might become overwhelming and unmanageable. Because of the volume, collected data can be difficult to analyze, trend, or use to efficiently generate reports that can be used for quality improvement. It is recommended that the interdisciplinary team developing the case management plan spend some time defining the significant patient care activities that need to be evaluated for variance data collection. A decision as to what should be included should be individualized to the specific diagnosis or procedure of the case management plan. In addition, variance data collection should be limited to data that affect the predetermined outcomes of each case management plan. The steering committee overseeing the process of implementing case management systems and developing case management plans is the best group to guide the interdisciplinary teams in this process. Members of the interdisciplinary team may use a set of questions (Box 12.12) as a guiding tool for better decision making when faced with the dilemma of what variance data should be collected.

Variances must be identified and corrected as soon as possible for better-quality patient care outcomes and prevention of unnecessary delays in the patient's discharge or prolongation in the LOS. Regardless of who is made responsible for variance data collection, there should be the following:

- Concurrent medical record reviews
- Immediate communication of any delays in patient care to the appropriate personnel (e.g., physicians, department chiefs, case managers, nurse managers, interdisciplinary team members)
- Immediate attempts to resolve the situation causing the variance
- Prospective plans for what, how, and when variance data should be collected

If the primary nurses are given the responsibility of collecting patient care variances, then they, rather than the case manager, are responsible for responding to the identified variance. However, the ideal way of correcting variances is for the interdisciplinary team member who has identified the variance to immediately begin to try to correct or resolve it. This approach will then result in the timeliest results and should help to avoid delays in the LOS or deterioration of quality. Members of the interdisciplinary healthcare team should be made aware of their responsibilities toward variance data collection and resolution. Open lines of communication should be established to promote effective and timely communication of variances to

---

Box 12.12   Guiding Questions to Better Decision Making Regarding Variance Data Collection

1. What are the most important patient care elements/activities that should be monitored?
2. In what format should variance data be collected?
3. Should both intermediate and discharge outcome indicators be monitored?
4. Should any type of variances be collected or only those that affect the quality of care and length of stay?
5. How easy is it to collect the suggested variance data?
6. How accessible are the desired variance data?
7. Where are the variance data located?
8. How can variance data be identified?
9. Who is responsible for variance data collection? Analysis? Reporting?
10. How will the data collected be used?
11. How will the data collected be interphased with the existing quality improvement efforts, if any?
12. What is the benefit of the variance data collected in revising the case management plan?

the appropriate administrative personnel, particularly when direct care providers such as staff nurses are made responsible for identifying and resolving variances as they occur.

12.6.2. Strategies for Handling Variances

When a patient care variance is identified, certain questions should be answered immediately to resolve the situation and improve outcomes. The answers to these questions will determine the urgency and seriousness of the situation and indicate the corrective action plan. The questions appear in Case Manager's Tip 12.2.

After careful collection of variance data, the data are analyzed. The variance analysis process (Figure 12.1) is a systematic and scientific interpretation through categorization/grouping, trending, and statistical analysis of the data collected. Variance data are usually compiled and analyzed over time to allow for better opportunities for quality and patient care process improvement.

The ideal way of dealing with variance data is to link the process to the quality improvement efforts taking place in the institution. Evaluating variances and constructing and implementing an appropriate action plan for improvement ensure better patient care outcomes and prevent the situation from happening again.

Improvement efforts should be spent addressing the

CASE MANAGER'S TIP 12.2

Questions to Help in Handling Variances and Improving Outcomes

1. What is really happening?
2. Is the situation indicative of a variance?
3. How serious is it?
4. What is causing the variance?
5. What is the effect of the variance on the patient's condition?
6. What is the category of the variance?
7. What action must be taken to correct it?
8. Who should be involved in correcting the variance?
9. How urgently should it be corrected?
10. What should be shared with the patient and the family?
11. When should follow-up take place?
12. What should be documented in the medical record?
13. What should be documented on the variance tracking tool?

recurring variances rather than the isolated, random, or single events because better patient care outcomes are affected by the extent to which the recurring variances are eliminated or prevented. The isolated variances are known to happen as a result of special causes (i.e., not directly related to the systems, operations, or processes an institution has in place). However, recurring variances are the opposite of isolated variances and take place as a result of common causes. These variances require an evaluation and analysis of the systems and processes of patient care the institution follows, as well as the policies and procedures and in some cases the standards of care and practice. It is suggested that efforts to address the isolated variances be decided based on the individual situation, particularly if these events interfere in the LOS, patient/family satisfaction, and cost and quality of care.

It is not enough to identify and resolve a variance when it occurs. It is equally important to track variances. The purpose of tracking variances is to conduct a trending analysis of each variance category. The results of such analyses are the basis for revising and improving the case management plan, reducing the incidence of variances in the future, and studying the data for necessity of quality improvement efforts, particularly those that are system/operations-related.

Variance data collection and analysis allow healthcare executives to look beyond LOS and cost of care. They are ongoing processes that are helpful in continuously improving the systems of the institution, case management plans, patient care activities, processes and outcomes, and quality of care. It is through this process that standardization of the best/ideal approach to patient care can be achieved and maintained.

Establishing variance data collection tools and formalizing/standardizing the process are integral to the accuracy and reliability of the data collected (Case Manager's Tip 12.3). Before the initiation of variance data collection, it is imperative to determine what should be measured and how and when assessment and evaluation of care are conducted. It is not uncommon that a variance tracking tool be developed as a part of the case management plan (Figure 12.2). In this case, the tool is made specific and individualized based on the diagnosis or procedure of the case management plan. An institution may elect to use a generic tool (Figure 12.3) that is applicable to any case management plan regardless of the diagnosis or procedure. In both situations, the tool is not made a permanent part of the medical record. It is dealt with as defined in the institutional policy/procedure for variance data collection and analysis.

Providing feedback regarding the effectiveness of

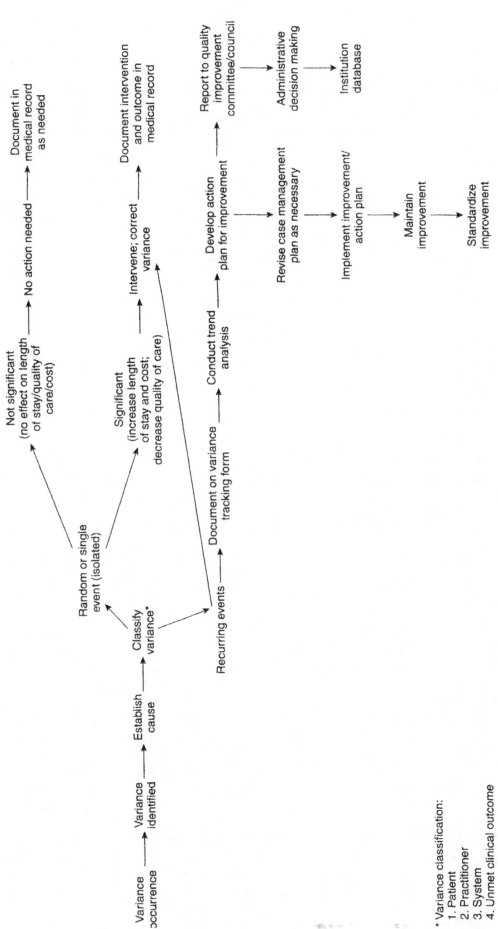

Figure 12.1 The variance analysis process. Note: Variance types may include patient, practitioner, system, community, and unmet clinical outcomes (intermediate and discharge).

CASE MANAGER'S TIP 12.3

Strategies for Making Variance Data Reporting Easy

1. If an institution decides to report variance data by source, it is useful to determine these sources (e.g., patient/family, care provider/practitioner, system), standardize them across the various care settings, and include them in the variance tracking tool. It is also helpful to include subcategories for each source. In addition, designating a code for each source and subcategory makes it easier to track, document, collate, analyze, and trend variances.

2. If an institution decides to report variance data by patient care elements applied in the case management plan (e.g., assessment and monitoring, tests and procedures, activity, medications, treatments, nutrition, patient/family teaching), it is important to determine how variances will be tracked and documented in the variance tracking tool. It is not enough to document variances as they relate to patient care elements only. Based on this method, one will only be able to report the frequency (number of occurrences) of variances in each care element. Another clarifying classification should be used in conjunction with this method. One example is the use of positive and negative classification. This way the data could be analyzed in relation to their impact on patient care processes and outcomes.

3. During the process of variance data analysis, some questions may occur that cannot be answered based solely on the data included in the variance tracking tools. In this situation, a review of medical records is suggested. The review should be conducted carefully and in a way that will answer the questions raised.

4. As much as possible, variance tracking tools should include specific places to identify the type (diagnosis, procedure) of the case management plan and the physician in charge of the care of the patient. This information is important for data analysis. It helps in analyzing the data specific to a case management plan and in identifying the physicians with minimal compliance with the plan.

5. Variance data reports should include data on the effectiveness of the case management plans, practice patterns (i.e., how well and how often the case management plan is followed by care providers), and recommendations for improvement opportunities.

6. Making recommendations for improvement opportunities may be made mandatory in each report. Areas to be addressed when recommending improvements may include the processes of care (e.g., improving the promptness of consults, developing patient education materials to be used in patient/family teaching), revisions in the case management plan (e.g., revising a timeframe for an outcome or an intervention, adding a test), and the systems of the institution (e.g., reducing the turnaround time for an echocardiography).

case management plans is important. Integral to any strategy for improving patient care is a provision for feedback to the clinicians and administrators who are involved in patient care processes and activities. A formal mechanism for communicating important and appropriate data must be in place in each institution. Reporting variance data should also be done on a regular basis with specific time intervals. Variance data reports should be distributed to members of the interdisciplinary team that was involved in the development of the case management plan and to the related administrators for initiating relevant quality improvement projects.

Patient care monitoring and timely variance identification and resolution are keys to the success of case management plans and are crucial for the delivery of cost-effective and quality care. However, establishing a standardized process for variance data analysis and management remains the best strategy for improving patient care outcomes. In addition, feedback among healthcare administrators and direct care providers is extremely important in refining the use and the effectiveness of case management plans.

12.7. OUTCOMES MANAGEMENT AND OUTCOMES CLASSIFICATION

Healthcare providers and administrators are constantly engaged in the evaluation of the outcomes of care and the care delivery system (i.e., the case management model). The interest in outcomes management is integral to case management model evaluation. One must examine both outcomes management and case management to ensure more acceptable care quality and outcomes to the patient and the healthcare organization. Some organizations have made outcomes management as one dimension of the role of the case manager. Other organizations have integrated quality management into the case management department and under the auspices of the administrator/executive responsible for the management of this department. Combining the activities of outcomes management and case management results in having the case managers accountable and responsible for outcomes measurement, monitoring, management, analysis, interpretation, and reporting and for performance improvement.

Case managers are often found to be collecting data regarding variances (e.g., delays in care), adherence to case management plans, and the outcomes of care activities of both the clinical and administrative processes. This is important for case managers because of their responsibility to "always track outcomes data for the patients in their caseload to determine the effectiveness, efficiency, and efficacy of the case management services provided. It is the ability of . . . case managers to use outcomes data intelligently to manage, plan, facilitate, expedite, advocate, coordinate, and evaluate the delivery of patient care that ultimately will result in increasing the degree of success of the case management system," (Flarey, 1998).

To facilitate the role of case managers in outcomes management and case management model evaluation, it is important for the healthcare organization to establish an outcomes classification system. Such system must aim at evaluating the case management model and must be standardized across the organization and used by all case managers. It also must identify the outcome indicators to be measured and delineate the process of data collection, aggregation, analysis, interpretation, and reporting. Moreover, such systems must adopt

---

Adult Inpatient Community Acquired Pneumonia
Place a checkmark (√) in the appropriate box
□ Less severe pneumonia □ Severe pneumonia
□ Initial antibiotics therapy did not meet guidelines for severity class
□ _____   Drug & Dosage

□ Conversion to oral antibiotics did not occur because of failure to meet:
   □ Two consecutive oral temperature readings of <100°F are obtained at least 8 hours apart in the absence of antipyretics
   □ Decrease in leukocytosis to <12,000
   □ Improved pulmonary signs and symptoms
   □ Able to tolerate oral medications
□ Orders were not written to switch antibiotics to oral form
□ Other:
   _____

□ Oral antibiotics conversion did not meet the guidelines selection
□ _____   Drug & Dosage
□ Repeat chest x-ray necessary as guideline □ Repeat chext x-ray is NOT necessary as per guidelines

□ Discharge did not occur within 24 hours of conversion to antibiotics
   □ Reason documented:
   _____
   □ Reason NOT Documented

□ Length of stay
□ Readmission within 30 days; reasons
   □ Failed outpatient management/follow-up
   □ Post-discharge services issues
   □ Other _____

NOTE: *This tool can be used as a guide to developing electronic variance tracking tools accompanying specific automated clinical pathways*

Figure 12.2 A variance tracking tool specific to a case management plan.

Variance Key:
1 – Patient
2 – Process/System
3 – Practitioner
4 – Care Planning/Discharge
5 – Community

Diagnosis:
Date Clinical Pathway Initiated: ____/____/____
Date Pathway Completed: ____/____/____
Patient Discharge Date: ____/____/____

Patient Demographics

Date	Unit	Time	Pathway Day #	Variance Description (Use Key)	Actions Taken	Case Manager

NOTE: This tool can be used as a guide to developing electronic variance tracking tools accompanying automated clinical pathways.

Codes

A. PATIENT
A1. Patient refusal/noncompliance
A2. Communication barrier
A3. Adverse effect/complication
A4. Comorbidity
A5. Altered mental status
A6. Progression ahead of pathway

B. FAMILY/LIFESTYLE
B1. Noncompliance
B2. Unavailability
B3. Environmental barrier
B4. Socioeconomic concerns
B5. Other

C. SYSTEM
C1. Interdisciplinary
C2. Transfer issues
C3. Treatment delays
C4. Delayed results reporting
C5. Other

D. PROVIDER
D1. Physician availability
D2. Response time
D3. Physician documentation
D4. Nursing delays
D5. Ancillary delays
D6. Progression ahead of Pathway
D7. Other

Physician Name: _____ Contact Information: _____

Patient Name: _____ Room Number: _____ Medical Record Number: _____

Date of Review	Day #	Code	Critical Element	Variance Explanation	Action Taken

NOTE: This tool can be used as a guide to developing electronic variance tracking tools accompanying automated clinical pathways.

Figure 12.3 Generic variance tracking tools: two examples.

the use of predetermined outcome indicators reflective of the interest of both the organization/providers of care and the patient population/consumers of care. The classification system must address the standards and requirements of accreditation and regulatory agencies and the expectations of the payers for healthcare, including managed care organizations.

One example of such classification system is shared in Figure 12.4. There is no one best system to be used. However, it is important for an organization to identify the system that works best for its providers and customers. For example, some organizations may consider the patient's functional ability as a separate classification and as independent of the clinical indicators; others may combine the two. The examples presented in Figure 12.4 do not make an exhaustive list of indicators. Others may still be added; however, it is important to define whether the indicator is a patient/family- or healthcare organization–related indicator. The examples shared here are not presented in a measurable format but rather as themes or broad classifications. A healthcare organization to be using this classification system must indicate the outcome indicators in a measurable way, for example cost per case type or an episode of care/illness or managed care reimbursement denial rate. The organization also must delineate the frequency of data collection, the sample, the formulas to be applied in the analysis, and the reporting format. Other ways of classifying outcome indicators are presented in the following sections.

12.7.1. Cost Versus Quality Outcomes

Case managers and case management departments are evaluated in multiple ways. As discussed in Chapter 12 so far, we may choose to look at outcomes in terms of those that directly affect the organization, or we may choose to look at them in terms of those that indirectly affect the organization. Another way to classify outcomes is by those that affect cost versus those that affect quality. We can further break this down to those used to evaluate the case manager versus those that are used to evaluate a department of case management (Case Manager's Tip 12.4).

12.8. ORGANIZATION-SPECIFIC OUTCOME MEASURES—EVALUATING THE DEPARTMENT OF CASE MANAGEMENT

When evaluating a department within an organization, certain measures of cost can be selected and used as they relate to the department's goals, mission, and expected outcomes. Examples may include LOS, cost per day/episode of care, cost per case, and cost associated with reimbursement denials. As each is selected, a frequency for re-evaluating each outcome should also be determined. These intervals or frequencies should be appropriate to the selected outcome and should not be too frequent as to reduce the sensitivity of the data, nor so infrequent as to lose meaning over time.

12.8.1. Length of Stay

LOS continues to be the most commonly used outcome measure in case management. If your organization or department measures LOS as an outcome indicator then the following factors should be considered:

- By DRG or International Classification of Diseases, Ninth Revision, Clinical Modification (ICD-9-CM) code
- By service line
- By physician
- By product line

12.8.2. Cost per Day/Case

Before selecting cost outcomes, consider the following question: Can you access true cost per case using a cost accounting system? If not, other strategies can be used, such as measuring specific resource utilization (e.g., tests, medications, or radiological exams). If you have access to a cost-accounting system then the following are potential measures to be used:

- Cost per physician per day
- Cost per physician per case
- Cost per diagnosis or DRG
- Cost of specific case types by department or specialty
- All of the above

12.8.3. Third-Party Payer Denials

Denial of payment by third-party payers is quantifi-

CASE MANAGER'S TIP 12.4

Outcomes based on Cost and Quality

1. Case manager:
   a. Cost at patient level
   b. Quality at patient level
2. Department/Organization:
   a. Cost at departmental and organizational levels
   b. Quality at departmental and organizational levels

able and affects the bottom line of the organization; therefore it is commonly used to measure the impact of case management on the organization. The following data elements should be considered when looking at this outcome:

- Reductions in initial denials (whole episode of care or certain hospital days)

- Reductions in final denials (that is after appealing the initial denials)
- Percent of reductions in each of these over time
- Denial reversal rate
- Impact of physician advisor in preventing and/or reversing denials
- Aggregate by physician/payer/department
- As percent of patient days

Classification	Patient/Family-Related Outcomes	Healthcare Organization-Related Outcomes
Clinical	• Improved patient care outcomes such as reduced/controlled pain, comfort, morbidity, and mortality rates • Reduction in signs and symptoms of disease and degree of progression of the disease • Prevention of adverse effects of treatments and complications of illness • Reduction in clinical practice variation	• Standardization of care processes (establishing standards of care and case management plans) • Streamlined care processes and delineation of responsibilities (reduction of practice pattern variation) • Improved turnaround time of tests, treatments, and procedures • Increased compliance with standards of regulatory and accreditation agencies
Financial	• Optimal and appropriate use of resources and services • Provision of care in appropriate setting(s)/level of care • Maximal coordination of care among providers • Streamlining of diagnostic and therapeutic tests and procedures • Reduction of zero avoidable readmissions	• Appropriate changes in staff mix/skill mix • Reduced cost (e.g., reduction in length of stay, reduction in or elimination of fragmented and duplicative care/services) • Improved reimbursement and revenue; reduction or avoidance of financial risks and penalties • Reduction in denials of claims • Improved communication among healthcare providers and payers (e.g., hospitals and managed care organizations) • Elimination of avoidable readmission
Quality of Life	• Improved/maximized physical abilities and level of independence • Improved state of well-being • Improved perception of health status • Enhanced self-care and self-management abilities and skills • Incrased engagement in care • Enhanced health knowledge and improved health literacy	• Prevention of inappropriate hospitalizations • Reduction in inappropriate utilization of emergency department services • Provision of a safe environment of care • Provision of programs that meet patient and family needs • Improved accessibility to care and services and in the right setting
Satisfaction and Experience of Care	• Increased patient and family satisfaction with and experience of care (HCAHPS) • Improved continuity of care • Enhanced communication during transitions of care • Improved patient/family-nurse/healthcare professionals relationship • Absence of medical errors	• Improved staff satisfaction • Reduced rates of staff burnout, turnover, attrition, and absenteeism • Enhanced states of communication, collaboration, and teamwork among healthcare providers and various professional disciplines (interpersonal, interdisciplinary, interdepartmental) • Enhanced just culture and transparent practice when medical errors occur

Figure 12.4 Classification of outcomes (Tahan, 1998).

12.8.4. Quality Measures

Measures of quality are as important as those of cost but may be more difficult to quantify. Measures of quality may include patient and family satisfaction, staff satisfaction, clinical outcomes, and transitional planning outcomes. Consider the following examples, knowing that without cost savings attached to them they may carry less weight.

Patient/family experience of care and staff satisfaction:

- Select a measurement tool
- Select measurement frequency
- For patients—mail-in versus on-site questionnaire
- For staff—which category of staff? What tool?
- Which role functions impact satisfaction?
- For patients—use CAHPS as required by CMS

Clinical quality outcome measures:

- Achievement of intermediate outcomes—trigger points
- Achievement of discharge outcomes
- Complication rates such as infection rates, returns to the operating room, and so on
- Transitional quality indicators system issues
- Turnaround time for completion of tests/treatments/procedures/consults
- Reporting of test result delays
- Avoidable/preventable mortalities, readmissions
- Quality improvement initiatives to reduce system delays
- Never events

Transitional planning issues:

- Delays in discharge
- Readmits within 24 hours/next day/15 days/30 days
- Returns to intensive care units
- Patient complaints regarding discharge planning
- Mortality
- Never events

12.9. REPORT CARDS

Report cards, also known as scorecards, have become a common and popular practice in quality management during the past several years. They are used as a tool for displaying outcomes data in a meaningful, concise, clear, and easy-to-read manner. Report cards can be organized applying the outcomes classification system used by the healthcare organization or the department of case management such as the one discussed earlier in this chapter. They also may include benchmark data

and/or targets, which makes the reports more meaningful and valuable (Figure 12.5). An advantage of applying an outcomes classification system to the report card is that it ensures focus on multiple elements of outcomes and not a single parameter such as cost. Adding elements such as consumer satisfaction to LOS and cost outcomes is essential.

Examples of the most common classification categories of outcome indicators are as follows:

- Demographic data and patient descriptors such as age, gender, case mix, insurance, diagnosis, type of surgery, and past medical history
- Clinical outcomes such as use of antibiotics, incision integrity, pain control, and complications
- Financial outcomes/resource utilization such as LOS, intensive care unit LOS, cost per case, and readmission rates
- Functional outcomes/physical ability and mobility such as independence status in ADLs, weight bearing status, ambulation, mental health, and social support system
- Satisfaction such as consumer satisfaction, perception of health, and quality of life

Each of these classifications may include several indicators that are measures of the activities, treatments, and outcomes of patient care practices.

Report cards provide healthcare organizations with a mechanism for data collection, aggregation, analysis and trending, benchmarking and comparing, and reporting. Standardizing the way outcomes data are displayed (by applying the above classification, for example) can be advantageous to many audiences, such as healthcare providers, administrators, payers, regulatory and accreditation agencies, and consumers. Defining the purpose of the report card and its audience is important because it influences its format, content, and level of sophistication. For example, designing a report card for a case management plan is different from designing a report card for a case management department. The case management plan's report card focuses on the topic of the plan; that is, a homogenous patient population, whereas the case management department is heterogeneous.

Report cards can be generated for a physician or other providers, such as the case manager, or for a disease entity, service or product line, case management plan, or department (i.e., case management department). Regardless of the type of audience the report card is intended for, Spath (1998) recommends that one first defines the purpose of the report card, delineates the learning opportunity intended by the card, and determines the extent of actions that need to be taken to improve outcomes and performance. It is also important

Outcome Indicators	Benchmark and Target	Actual Performance
Clinical milestone: *Initiation of intravenous antibiotics therapy for severe pneumonia*	Initiation of intravenous antibiotics therapy within 4 hours of arrival	
Clinical milestone: *Afebrile X 24 hours* *WBC decreasing to normal range*	Switch to oral antibiotics upon improvement in symptoms	
Discharge Indicators: *Afebrile* *WBC <12,000* *Tolerating oral medications*	Discharge to home or prior setting	
Complications: *Medical* *Post-operative* *Medical Errors*	None	
Variance/Deviations from Guidelines: *System* *Practitioner* *Patient/Physiologic*	None	
Length of Stay	3 Days	
Cost per Case	$6,000.00	
Readmissions within 30 Days	No avoidable readmissions	
Third-Party Payer Denials	None	
Reversal of Denials	100%	
Bad Debts	<3%	

NOTE: This tool can be used as a guide to developing electronic clinical report card tools accompanying specific automated clinical pathways

Figure 12.5 Proposed guide and format for clinical report cards.

to decide on the frequency of generating the report card and what is expected of those who receive a copy of it. Some organizations distribute the report card on a quarterly basis and as a part of their quarterly quality assurance/improvement procedures.

A report card for case management model evaluation or case management plan evaluation is necessary and it is desirable to be made available to key personnel (e.g., senior administrators, physician chairmen/chiefs, case managers, case management plan teams, and finance) in an organization on a quarterly basis. (Refer to Figure 12.6 for an example of a comprehensive case management report card). Report cards may include the elements discussed earlier in the outcomes management and classification and the national quality indicators sections of this chapter. The previous and current improvement activities must also be included as a part of such report. These activities indicate who is responsible for what and indicate the timeframe for completing an improvement activity and its expected outcome. This aspect of the report card ensures the link between the report card and the quality management department or program and communication with the various key players. Report cards that apply this format are looked on favorably by accreditation and regulatory agencies.

12.10. ORGANIZATION-SPECIFIC OUTCOME MEASURES—EVALUATING THE CASE MANAGER

In evaluating the case manager (Box 12.13), many of the outcome measures are consistent with those selected for measuring the case management department. The only difference is that the data will be aggregated in terms of the case manager; that is, based on the case manager's caseload and not the service. Included with these might be the productivity measures discussed earlier in this chapter.

12.11. NATIONAL QUALITY INDICATORS

The focus on quality and outcomes is essential for the survival of healthcare providers, payers, and agencies in today's market. The pressures of consumers of healthcare services have led to a focus on national

	Baseline	Target	Month	Month	Month	Month	Month	Month	Month	Month	YTD
LENGTH OF STAY											
Medical/Surgical											
Psychiatry/Behavioral Health High volume DRGs/CMS Geometric Mean LOS											
# Patients/% with LOS 14–20 Days											
# Patients/% with LOS >20 Days											
DENIALS BY REASON IN DAYS—PENDING ONLY											
Concurrent											
Admission											
Continued Stay											
Delay in Service											
Clinical Information not Provided											
Appropriateness of Setting											
Retrospective											
Admission											
Continued Stay											
Delay in Service											
Clinical Information not Provided											
Appropriateness of Setting											
DENIALS BY REASON IN DAYS—CLOSED/OVERTURNED ONLY											
Concurrent											

	Baseline	Target	Month	Month	Month	Month	Month	Month	Month	Month	YTD
Admission											
Continued Stay											
Delay in Service											
Clinical Information Not Provided											
Appropriateness of Setting											
Retrospective											
Admission											
Continued Stay											
Delay in Service											
Clinical Information Not Provided											
Appropriateness of Setting											

Figure 12.6 Sample comprehensive case management report card.

	Baseline	Target	Month	Month	Month	Month	Month	Month	Month	Month	YTD
DENIALS BY REASON IN DAYS—CLOSED/NO APPEAL OR UPHELD											
Concurrent											
Admission											
Continued Stay											
Delay in Service											
Clinical Information Not Provided											
Appropriateness of Setting											
Retrospective											
Admission											
Continued Stay											
Delay in Service											
Clinical Information Not Provided											
Appropriateness of Setting											
INPATIENT THROUGH-PUT											
Avoidable Days Due to No Sub-Acute Ventilator Bed Available											
Avoidable Days Due to No Sub-Acute Ventilator/Dialysis Bed Available											
Avoidable Days Reasons—Top 3 Healthcare Facility											
#1											
#2											
#3											
Avoidable Days Reasons—Top 3 Resources and Services											
#1											
#2											
#3											
Avoidable Days Reasons—Top 3 Patient/Family											
#1											
#2											
#3											
Avoidable Days Reasons—Top 3 Payer											
#1											
#2											
#3											
Avoidable Days Reasons—Top 3 Healthcare Provider											
#1											
#2											
#3											

Figure 12.6 (continued) Sample comprehensive case management report card.

DISCHARGE PLANNING													
Completion of Initial Assessment/Discharge or Transition Plan within 24 hours of Admission													
REFERRALS TO POST-ACUTE CARE													
Home with No Services (as % of Discharges)													
Home with Home Care Services (as % of discharges)													
Acute Rehabilitation (as % of discharges)													
Subacute Rehabilitation (as % of discharges)													
Subacute Medicine (as % of discharges)													
Subacute Ventilator Dependent (as % of discharges)													
Long Term Care (as % of discharges)													

NOTE: This report guide tool can be used as a guide to developing electronic reporting tools

Figure 12.6 (continued) Sample comprehensive case management report card.

Box 12.13   Case Management Outcomes Measures

Examples of Cost Measures

- Cost per case
- Length of stay
- Third-party payer denials
- Monitoring of variances
- Variance interventions and analysis
- Transitional planning efficiency and delays

Examples of Quality Measures

- Patient satisfaction scores
- Monitoring of variances
- Variance interventions and analysis
- Transitional planning efficiency and delays
- Performance evaluation
- Competencies
- Clinical outcome measures
- Documentation
- Staff's satisfaction and engagement
- Interdisciplinary relationships
- External professional activities
- Internal professional activities
- Scholarship activities

quality standards through the evaluation and measurement of certain outcome indicators of interest to consumers, payers, and providers. Different national organizations have advocated for national indicators. Although the indicators vary across the organizations, the focus is somewhat similar and to some degree the indicators are the same. The indicators basically focus on access to care and quality and cost of services. It is essential for case managers and administrators of case management programs to be knowledgeable about these national organizations so that they are better able to incorporate their recommended quality indicators in the evaluation process of the case management model.

The indicators of interest to the national organizations are usually related to performance of healthcare providers and agencies. Examples are nosocomial infection rate, fall-related injury rate, cost per episode of care, access to care, consumers' choice of services, patient satisfaction, and qualifications of healthcare providers. The national organizations most interested in quality indicators are the National Committee Of Quality Assurance (NCQA), the URAC, the CMS, The Joint Commission (TJC), and the American Nurses Association (ANA).

12.11.1. National Committee for Quality Assurance

The NCQA is a national organization comprised of healthcare quality management professionals. Originally established in 1976 to advance the profession of healthcare quality management, today its components include 48 state quality associations; an educational foundation; and an accreditation body for managed care health plans, specifically HMOs and for individual providers in healthcare quality management.

Additionally, NCQA offers a certification to healthcare professionals. Individuals certified by NCQA receive certification as a Certified Professional in Healthcare Quality. This certification recognizes professional and academic achievement through participation in this voluntary certification program (Claflin and Hayden, 1998). The national indicators and performance measures identified by NCQA and used in the accreditation standards of managed healthcare plans are known as the Health Plan Employer Data and Information Set (HEDIS). HEDIS focuses on the quality of the systems, processes, care, and services a managed care plan delivers to its clients/enrollees. Information collected by NCQA from these health plans is made accessible to both consumers and employers who subscribe to managed care plans (Box 12.14). Such information assists the consumer to choose the plan with the best quality performance. Further information about HEDIS is available at http://www.ncqa.org.

12.11.2. Utilization Review Accreditation Commission

The URAC, previously known as the American Accreditation HealthCare Commission, was established in 1990 to evaluate the methods of utilization review employed by healthcare agencies, particularly the managed healthcare plans, because at that time they were widely diverse. As a result of this examination, URAC made health utilization standards available for agencies to use in organizing their utilization review procedures. This acted as a step toward standardization in utilization review practices. In 1994 URAC developed its accreditation program for health plans that were not eligible for accreditation by NCQA, and in 1999 the program was expanded to highly integrated healthcare plans (Kongstvedt, 2001). URAC's accreditation program differs from NCQA's in that it is basically limited to utilization review programs.

URAC's accreditation program is also known today to accredit case management services. More detailed information is available at http://www.urac.org. The quality issues addressed in the accreditation standards of interest to case management are listed in Box 12.15.

12.11.3. Outcome-Based Quality Improvement

Outcome-based quality improvement (OBQI) is an approach used by homecare agencies to monitor and continuously improve their quality outcomes. The process relies on clinical, financial, and administrative outcomes data from the OASIS (see Chapter 2 for more information on OASIS) sponsored by the CMS. The goal of OASIS is to improve quality of care delivered to home healthcare patients and to provide data to CMS (Box 12.16). Uniform data must be collected on all patients, or on selected patients, in an agency. The data are compared with the same patient outcomes for the previous reporting period and against a reference sample of homecare patients. The data also are risk adjusted to control for any variable that might be affecting them. The outcomes are analyzed to determine whether they are inferior or superior to the previous

---

Box 12.14 Health Plan Employer Data and Information Set Quality Measurement Areas

- Effectiveness of care
- Access and availability to care and services
- Access to preventive services
- Consumer satisfaction
- Health plan stability
- Health plan descriptive information
- Consumer health choice
- Cost of services
- Use of services and utilization management
- Credentialing of healthcare providers

Box 12.15 Focus on Quality in Utilization Review Accreditation Commission's Accreditation Standards

- Types of consumers served
- Accessibility to services
- Delivery of case management services
- Provider's qualification and certification
- Case manager's caseload
- Consultation practices with physicians and referrals to other providers
- Quality management program
- Role of support staff
- Privacy and confidentiality practices
- Initiation and termination of services

> **Box 12.16   Outcome and Assessment Information Set Focus on Quality**
>
> - Appropriate patient selection for home care services
> - Demographics
> - Types of services required
> - Follow-up care and/or transfer to inpatient facilities
> - Resumption of care
> - Disposition status/condition

data collection period. When found to be inferior, the data are then used to spearhead further investigation in the form of a continuous quality improvement (CQI) project(s). Further information about OBQI is available at www.chspr.org/obqi3.htm.

12.11.4. ORYX—The Joint Commission

The ORYX initiative was implemented by the TJC in 1997 as a means to integrate outcomes and other performance measurement data into the TJC accreditation process. The TJC's primary mission is to continuously improve the safety and quality of care provided to the public through the provision of healthcare accreditation and related services that support performance improvement in healthcare organizations. Today the ORYX project is known as the core measures.

During the initial phase of ORYX, accredited hospitals, long-term care organizations, home care organizations with an average monthly census of 10 or more patients, and behavioral healthcare organizations select two measures from a list of core measures provided by the TJC. The measures selected must relate to at least 20% of the patient population. The healthcare organization then collects the data on the selected measures and regularly submits it to the TJC. The TJC is responsible for analyzing the data and providing performance trends and patterns to the organization in advance of a TJC survey. The organization also is responsible for explaining its rationale for selecting the specific performance measures and how the data has been used to improve performance.

12.11.5. American Nurses Association

In 1995 the ANA undertook a project (i.e., the nursing report card for acute care settings) to explore the nature of the relationships and linkages between nursing care and patient outcomes in acute care settings. This project resulted from the implementation of organizational changes that decreased the numbers of registered professional nurses providing patient care and replaced them with unlicensed personnel. Another factor that led to the demand for such a project was the increasing numbers of reports about incidents of threats to quality and safe patient care delivery. A major purpose of this project was the provision of a framework for educating nurses, consumers, and policymakers about nursing's contribution to inpatient hospital care.

The strategy used to determine the nursing indicators was based on an examination of the nursing scientific literature, consultation with experts and nurse leaders in nursing quality and outcomes research, and conduct of focus groups of nurses from all levels of practice related to the acute care setting. This project identified three categories of indicators that are still in use today (ANA, 1995). Further information is available at www.nursingworld.org. The categories are as follows:

- Patient-focused outcome indicators that include mortality rates, LOS, adverse incidents such as medication errors, complication rates such as pressure ulcers and surgical site infection, patient adherence to discharge plan, and patient/family satisfaction
- Process of care indicators that include nurse satisfaction, documentation of nursing diagnoses and the plan of care, accurate and timely delivery of nursing activities, pain management, skin integrity, patient education, discharge planning, and responsiveness to unplanned patient needs
- Structure of care indicators/nurse staffing patterns that include nurse-to-patient ratio, skill mix, nursing staff qualifications and education, nursing care hours, staff continuity, overtime, use of temporary staff, and staff injury rate

12.12. KEY POINTS

1. Outcomes can be used as indicators of quality.
2. Outcomes are the goals of healthcare delivery and can be directly or indirectly related to the patient's health.
3. Length of stay is an indicator of the success of a case management model and is often tracked to determine its effectiveness. However, it is not enough to examine it alone; it must be looked at in conjunction with other indicators such as cost of care and those shared in the report card section.
4. Clinical outcome indicators give the case manager a guide for progressing the patient from

day to day, episode to episode, or toward discharge.

5. Variance data should be collected using variance tracking tools specific to the institution. Variances should also be classified and coded for ease of tracking. The same classifications should be used across the various care settings.

6. Variance data collection may be made the responsibility of the interdisciplinary team members or the case manager only. Each institution may decide which mechanisms to be followed. Variance data should be tracked, collated, analyzed, and evaluated for improvement opportunities.

7. Results of variance data analysis should be tied into a quality improvement system. Reporting variance data and providing feedback to clinicians and administrators are important and integral to case management systems.

8. Indicators used to evaluate the case management model must be developed based on the recommendations of the national organizations interested in this area such as NCQA, URAC, CMS, ANA, and the TJC.

12.13. REFERENCES

American Nurses Association. (1995). Summary of the Lewin-VHI, Inc., report: Nursing report card for acute care settings, Washington, D.C.

Bueno, M.M. & Hwang, R.F. (1993). Understanding variances in hospital stay, *Nurs Manage 24*(14):51–57.

Claflin, N. & Hayden, C.T. (1998). *Guide to quality management*, 8th ed., National Association of Healthcare Quality, Glenview, IL.

Cohen, E.L. (1991). Case management: Does it pay? *J Nurse Adm 21*(4):20–25.

Cohen, E.L. & Cesta, T.G. (1997). *Case management: From concept to evaluation,* 2nd ed., Mosby, St Louis, MO.

Crosson, F.J. (1995). Why outcomes measurement must be the basis for the development of clinical guidelines, *Manag Care Q 3*(2):6–14.

Granger, C.V. & Gresham, G.E. (1984). *Functional assessment in rehabilitation medicine*, Williams & Wilkins, Baltimore, MD.

Hampton, D.C. (1993). Implementing a managed care framework through care maps, *J Nurse Adm 23*(5):21–27.

Hoffman, P.A. (1993). Critical path method: An important tool for coordinating clinical care, *Joint Comm J Qual Improve 19*:235–246.

Ignatavicius, D.D. & Bayne, M.V. (1991). *Medical-surgical nursing: a nursing process approach*, WB Saunders, Philadelphia, PA.

Ignatavicius, D.D. & Hausman, K.A. (1995). *Clinical pathways for collaborative practice*, WB Saunders, Philadelphia, PA.

Kongstvedt, P. (2001). *Essentials of managed health care*, 4th ed., Aspenm, Gaithersburg, MD.

Mateo, M.A. & Newton, C. (1996). Managing variances in case management, *Nurs Case Manag 1*(1):45–51.

Pearson, S.D., Goulart-Fisher, D., & Lee, T.H. (1995). Critical pathways as a strategy for improving care: problems and potential, *Ann Intern Med 123*(12):941–948.

Schriefer, J., Cali, R., Sugiyama, G., & Ryan, D. (1996). Linking process improvement, critical paths, and outcomes data to increased profitability, *Surg Serv Manage 2*(6): 46–50.

Spath, P. (1998). Nursing performance measures go public, *Outcomes Manage Nurs Pract 2*(3):124–128.

Strassner, L.F. (1996). The ABCs of case management: a review of the basics, *Nurs Case Manag 1*(1):22–30.

Tahan, H.A. (1998). Nurse case managers' responsibilities toward patient care outcomes, *Semin Nurse Manag 6(*3):100–103.

Tahan, H.A. & Cesta, T.G. (1995). Evaluating the effectiveness of case management plans, *J Nurse Adm 25*(9):58–63.

Webster's Third New International Dictionary, Vol III. 1986. Encyclopedia Britannica, Chicago, IL.

13 Application of Legal Concepts and Issues in Case Management Practice

Healthcare organizations and providers, in conjunction with the federal government, have been struggling with ways to reduce the cost of healthcare, including costs related to medical malpractice insurance and litigation. Among the efforts pursued has been the implementation of case management systems for patient care delivery and services across the healthcare continuum. When fully implemented, these systems rely heavily on the role of case managers (discussed in Chapter 4) and the use of case management plans of care. Chapter 13 discusses the legal liabilities and malpractice litigation associated with the components of case management systems. It also offers some practical tips for case managers to adhere to legal standards.

13.1. CASE MANAGEMENT SYSTEMS, THE CASE MANAGER AND THE LEGAL PROCESS

Case management has many wide-reaching effects on patients and their families. Enhanced communication with and education of patients and families allow for a better plan of care and outcomes and more fully informed decisions about the care to be rendered. Because communication is an integral strategy that assures more effective case management systems, there can be an earlier identification of patients' discharge needs, which may result in the development of improved case management plans to troubleshoot potential problem areas or barriers to quality and safe care. Case managers can identify potential problems and barriers within a desired timeframe that can be addressed proactively rather than reactively. They can prevent overlapping and overutilization of many healthcare services through

management, coordination, advocacy, and facilitation of patient care activities, thereby minimizing or eliminating delays in treatments, care, and tests required by patients. Moreover, they can facilitate changes in the provision of care, which may improve cost, timeliness of services, quality, safety, effectiveness, and efficiency of the healthcare system.

Today, case managers are found to assume responsibilities in all care settings (Box 13.1). They are obligated to actively assure that patients receive the best healthcare in the most effective, safe, and efficient manner. Their autonomy, accountability, and responsibility toward management, planning, delivery, coordination, brokering, facilitation, and evaluation of patient care practices put them at higher risk for malpractice litigation. Because of their position at the hub of the interdisciplinary care team and their role as gatekeepers of care, they find themselves increasingly involved in complex situations that require subtle decisions and present higher legal accountability, therefore increasing the chances for malpractice and liability.

Several causes of litigation appear repetitively in lawsuits, such as discourteous behavior, communication failures, lack of patient understanding, and lack of information given to the patient and family. For example, patients and/or their families may sue when common complications occur and they claim that they were not informed that such problems could occur. This concern may be a consequence of problems in the quality of the informed consent process.

If the patient is involved in a lawsuit, the case manager may encounter legal terminology that is not commonly used by the layperson. Case managers should become familiar with the legal terminology (e.g.,

---

Box 13.1   Various Settings Where Case Management Can Be Found

1. Medical and nursing practice (e.g., acute, critical, ambulatory, community, long-term care)
2. Health and wellness centers
3. Mental and behavioral health
4. Insurance-based or employee-based programs
5. Independent and private practice
6. Workers' compensation
7. Visiting nurse association and public health practices
8. Social service programs
9. Patient-centered medical homes and physician/provider group practices

---

plaintiff, defendant, malpractice suit, standard of care, and negligence) that they may come across in the case of a legal claim.

- The plaintiff is the person who brings a claim or lawsuit into court. If the case involves the death of a patient, the plaintiff is the next of kin or the appropriate legal guardian.
- The defendant in a lawsuit is the person or entity against whom a claim is brought by the plaintiff—in this case, the provider of healthcare services (e.g., the hospital, physician, case manager, registered nurse, social worker, nurse manager).
- Malpractice suits are suits filed in court against professional people (e.g., case managers or physicians) who have a level of skill and knowledge that exceed those of a lay or ordinary person. These suits are usually filed against professionals who practice healthcare below the common standards.
- The standard of care is the level at which the average prudent professional in a given situation or context would perform.
- Negligence is the failure to act as an ordinary, prudent, or "reasonable person" would under similar circumstances.

Most healthcare institutions have provided case managers with the responsibility of managing patient care in collaboration with other members of the interdisciplinary healthcare team. Such responsibility increases the risk for malpractice lawsuits against case managers.

13.2. SOURCES OF ANXIETY FOR TODAY'S CASE MANAGERS

Busy case managers can reduce the anxiety associated with the risk of legal action by gaining knowledge of the elements of malpractice lawsuits, applying the standards of care and case management in their practice, adhering to the case management ethical standards, being cognizant of the areas that have increasingly been receiving legal attention and scrutiny, and understanding the importance of accurate and timely documentation and communication, especially with the patient and family.

Case managers must "wear many hats" and instantly switch focus in their role as required by the situation at hand. By virtue of the complexity of the role, the case manager may end up being everything to everyone: a nurse, social worker, discharge or transition planner, psychologist, counselor, clergyperson, marketing specialist, communicator, translator of medical terminology, navigator of the healthcare system and insurance plans, expert in policies and coding practices, accountant, quality assurance specialist, lawyer, advocate, mediator, negotiator, health educator, financial manager, and occupational and physical therapist. Because of the diversity of this role and its functions, the case manager must possess creativity, patience, and wisdom. Once all these elements have been artfully combined, the product is then a competent case manager who can be successful in his or her role.

The new paradigm of healthcare management and delivery has grown away from the old paternalistic view of the "doctor knows best," which focused on the treatment of the symptoms, with the goal of achieving a cure. In the old paradigm the patient was passive, dependent, and his or her body, mind, and spirit were viewed as separate entities. The patient chose his or her doctor and hospital, and cost-effectiveness was not a factor in the decision making process. The new paradigm focuses on the patient as an autonomous human being, with the healthcare professional (e.g., case manager) assuming the role of therapeutic and trusted partner, counselor, guide, and navigator.

Today's emphasis is on promoting healthy lifestyles, adherence to specific health regimens, with attention paid to patterns, causes, and treatments of illnesses and reduction of their associated risk factors or the need for unplanned access to health and human services. The body, mind, and spirit are viewed as one integrated entity. Patients are approached for care as total beings rather than the focus being only on the diseased organ; for ability to adhere to the healthcare services and regimens required rather than the mere prescribing of treatment. The presence of the case manager in today's healthcare system makes it easier for the patient/family to navigate the complex care delivery systems; survive the challenges; and stay informed of the constantly changing rules, regulations, and demands.

Modern healthcare is a business whether for or not-for profit, and access to optimal care may depend on having appropriate health insurance coverage. A patient's choice of physicians or other care providers may be limited by coverage restrictions of the benefits within the patient's health insurance plan. Efficiency, cost-effectiveness, and cost-reduction are a constant focus of attention for payers, regulators, and providers alike. Quality, timely access to services, and safety are also expectations in today's healthcare marketplace. A long-term relationship with a particular physician or primary care provider is no longer the norm. Patients cannot be certain that their health insurance plan will continue to include their favorite hospital or physician. Loyalty to healthcare personnel with whom a patient has established a familiar and natural relationship is dwindling, and so is the patient's reluctance to file a lawsuit. Patients are choosing the best provider regardless of geographical limitations. They define "best" provider as someone with the highest quality star rating, someone who is safe, and who demonstrates desirable competencies in healthcare delivery including bedside manners. Finding the "best" is no longer a challenge because of the regulatory imposed transparency in reporting on outcomes and cost of care- HospitalCompare, PhysicianCompare, Health Plan Ratings, or consumer reports.

If patients feel that their rights have been violated, the care they have received is below acceptable standards, or that their provider/healthcare team has not communicated well with them and left them wondering what is going on and why undesired results have been achieved, they are most likely to sue the healthcare provider or agency involved (Box 13.2). There exists a mentality in society known today as lawsuit lottery—the chance to strike it rich by filing the right lawsuit. This is complicated by practices of some law firms who advertise aggressively on television, online, and in print media about their successful services promising potential clients they will win their case no matter what. Such law firms are sharing their past successes in headlines that shout, for example, about elderly people suing healthcare providers for exorbitant amounts of money and winning. This type of publicity increases the likelihood that patients may sue their provider if they are not satisfied with their care or feel cheated in some way. It is not surprising to learn of patients suing their healthcare provider or organization for astronomical amounts of money for suspicion of harm, even though most of the time these suspicions are unfounded.

Although an increasing number of nurses, social workers, and case managers are being named in

---

Box 13.2   Ten Common Reasons People Sue

1. Delays in diagnosing a health condition/problem or to initiate care
2. Negligent care and treatments
3. Sense of grief and loss
4. Financial gain
5. Presence of real harm/damage
6. Failure to obtain informed consent
7. Unanticipated bad results
8. Failure to consult with a specialty care provider when indicated
9. Need to punish the provider or the healthcare facility
10. Poor or unsatisfactory communication

---

lawsuits, those filed against physicians continue to dominate the trend. As patients are becoming more knowledgeable about healthcare and case management services, their expectations with regard to what type of care they may expect to receive is higher. When such expectations are not met, it is more likely that patients resort to filing lawsuits. Healthcare professionals are no longer the sole source of health-related information. It has become common for patients and their family members to show up for their appointments with information they have downloaded from the Internet or mobile devices on the signs and symptoms of a specific disease or a variety of treatment modalities that they think might be effective. This presents a challenge for healthcare professionals who are uncomfortable dealing with an increasingly educated healthcare consumer. If they leave patients' questions and concerns unanswered or incompletely or inappropriately answered, patients may feel disappointed and dissatisfied and ultimately may file complaints against their healthcare providers; some of which may be in the form of a lawsuit.

Case managers now have greater exposure to potential lawsuits because healthcare systems are increasingly reliant on them in addition to other providers and physicians, to help contain costs and provide responsible care: highest quality outcomes, desirable experience with care, and safe services. Furthermore, nurses and social workers are becoming more autonomous in their practice, especially in the area of case management. This autonomy increases the chance that they are named in a lawsuit.

Efforts to contain rising helathcare costs have led many healthcare institutions to downsize while the workloads of those remaining behind have increased, resulting in greater risk for legal action. Patient caseloads are a primary factor in the quality and safety of case management outcomes. The larger the caseload, the less likely it is for case managers to meet the expectations of delivering high-quality, safe, efficient, and cost-effective healthcare services. Reportedly, the average active monthly caseload of case managers may range from 28 to 350 cases. The wide range is due to the variation of the care settings in which case managers operate. For example, caseloads of case managers in the hospital setting are usually much smaller than the caseloads of those of health insurance plans. This diversity depends on many factors including the following (Health Intelligence Network, 2012):

- The organizational vision, mission, and values statements
- The type of organization or care setting where the case manager operates
- The systems and processes of case management services and programs, including use of technology and assistive personnel
- The goals and the definition of case management services
- The functions of case management and how they are embedded in the case manager's role: clincial care management, discharge/transitional planning, utilization management, and quality and safety outcomes management
- The acuity of the client population served
- The experience, knowledge, skills, competencies, and training of case managers
- The types of interactions between case managers, providers, and clients
- The resources available to the case manager for handling the daily workload
- Electronic versus paper documentation and records
- Regulatory environment and related standards

Many professionals have chosen to leave their practice because of increasing workloads, undesirable working conditions and pressures, confusing or vague roles and responsibilities, and high consumer demands. Most often these characteristics of the work environment put case managers in situations where they are unable to meet the needs of their patients, and ultimately at increased risk for litigation and loss of professional license and other credentials such as case management certification. The laws affecting healthcare are constantly changing, and the threat of lawsuits and disciplinary actions against the professional's license remain a silent threat to those who continue to practice.

Historically, the most common causes of legal actions against nurses have been related to negligence in care provision which may have contributed to injurious patient falls, missed care, healthcare facility acquired pressure ulcers, improper use of equipment, and medication errors (Case Manager's Tip 13.1). Malpractice payments related to lawsuits brought forth against nurses or case managers are relatively rare. This may be because most cases are settled outside the court system. Issues related to undesirable nursing practices in the areas of patient monitoring, treatment, and medication administration are the reasons behind most of the lawsuits against nurses and payments. No data bank is available yet regarding lawsuits filed directly against case managers; if any filed, it is done under the professional licensure of the case manager such as nursing, social work, and rehabilitation counseling. Regardless however, lawsuits brought against case managers have been due to patient injury as a result of inappropriate referrals for services in the community, premature discharge from the acute care hospital setting, inadequate patient assessment resulting in ineffective case management plan of care, and practicing outside one's scope or licensure.

Although the types of lawsuits filed against nurses do not relate directly to the practice of case management and the role of the case manager, they have some implications for case managers. As discussed in Chapter 4, one dimension of the role of the case manager is clinical care management. This role function focuses on the assessment, planning, coordination, facilitation, advocacy, monitoring, and evaluation of patient care delivery and outcomes. In this role function, case managers are expected to communicate with the patient and family, physician, and other members of the healthcare team regarding the patient's progress, nuances in medical and health condition, and responses to treatment. Therefore case managers can be held accountable and responsible for assuring there are no gaps in patient care and for timely communication with the healthcare team. If they fail to do so, they are at risk for litigation, especially if their lack of or delay in communication and care results in harm to the patient.

The implementation of the case manager's role is thought to reduce the risk for litigation rather than increase it. This is attributed to the fact that the case manager acts as a patient and family advocate, integrator of care and services, quality and safety coordinator, and risk manager. Furthermore, the case manager is expected to act proactively to prevent legal risk by exercising his or her established duties as defined in the scope of practice.

13.3. BASIS FOR ASSIGNING LIABILITY IN CASE MANAGEMENT

Case managers have duties that derive from the ac-

CASE MANAGER'S TIP 13.1

Charge of Negligence Against Nurses and Case Managers

A charge of negligence against nurses and case managers may arise from almost any action or inaction that results in patient injury, most often due to an unintentional failure to adhere to a standard of care or clinical practice. Such events may result in a malpractice lawsuit.

CASE MANAGER'S TIP 13.2

Conflicting Obligations of Case Managers

Liability in the case manager's role arises from the inability to integrate or broker care when conflicting obligations are present. Examples of obligations the case manager has that may be in conflict are as follows:

- Patient advocacy
- Organizational advocacy
- Quality assurance and improvement
- Cost-effectiveness or containment
- Coordination of services
- Brokerage of services
- Contractual obligations to employer
- Contractual obligations to payers
- Healthcare laws and regulations
- Ethical standards of practice

tivities in which they are involved and as defined in their job description and scope of practice. Because the law acknowledges that case management is a reasonable activity, case managers can and will be held accountable for their actions in relation to their patients. The law will hold the case manager to the reasonable standard of care for case managers. They must function within the scope of their licensure, training, and education, as well as their level of competence. They act as consultants to patients and physicians or other healthcare providers. By virtue of this role, they are able to assure efficient access to services and resources, and quality, safe outcomes, which indirectly assist in reducing litigation risk.

Although they cannot interfere with the physician-patient relationship, case managers have a fiduciary duty to communicate accurately and in a timely manner to both parties, especially in the situation of changes in the patient's condition that warrant immediate attention and potential change in the treatment/case management plan. If there is contradictory information, the case manager needs to work diligently with the patient and family or caregiver and other members of the healthcare team to determine the truth and initiate appropriate action.

Liability in case management arises from the fact that case managers are brokers and integrators of care delivery. As brokers, they are expected to arrange for the appropriate services their patients/families need and in a timely manner; as integrators, they are expected to build relationships with the patient, the payer, and the healthcare provider (i.e., the physician and/or the healthcare agency). Liability may arise from interrelating these parties (Case Manager's Tip 13.2).

13.4. THE DIFFERENCE BETWEEN NEGLIGENCE AND MALPRACTICE

Before reviewing some of the areas of litigation in case management, it is important to differentiate negligence from malpractice (Box 13.3). At first glance, negligence

and malpractice may appear as if they should belong in the same category; however, on a closer look, they are different and the distinguishing factor is "intent." Negligence is an umbrella term that is categorized based on the specific details of the individual case, which can include neglect, medical/healthcare negligence, and medical/healthcare malpractice. Negligence is an act or conduct that falls below the acceptable standard established by law for the protection of others against unreasonable risk of harm. It is an accidental departure from the conduct expected of a reasonably prudent person under similar circumstances. In contrast, malpractice is the failure to render professional services or to exercise that degree of skill and learning commonly applied under all circumstances in the community by the average reasonable and prudent, reputable member of the profession.

Claims of malpractice or negligence against case managers or healthcare providers must be brought to the court's attention within a certain period of time (statute of limitation). The statute of limitation is a specific time limit allowed for filing a lawsuit. In personal injury, medical malpractice, and breach of contract claims, state and federal laws vary. Claims should be reviewed to determine the appropriate period within which a claim can be brought against the potential defendant.

Claims of negligence or malpractice can be brought against any member of the case management team. Both usually result in harm to the client. In the case of negligence, there is no intentionality in causing harm. In contrast, an act of malpractice results from an intentional breach of trust between the healthcare

---

Box 13.3   Negligence and Malpractice

Negligence

Negligence is the failure to act as an ordinary prudent person would act in the given circumstances; applies to the acts of both laymen and professionals. It occurs when someone unintentionally or accidentally does something wrong that results in harm to another.

Malpractice

Malpractice is ignoring a standard, professional misconduct, improper discharge of duties, or failure to meet the standards of care expected of a reasonably prudent member of the profession in his or her dealings with the patient/family that causes harm to the patient.

---

professional and the client, causing harm to the client. The case manager's acts of negligence or malpractice result in injury, loss, or damage to the recipient of the case management services or to those entitled to rely on them. Negligence and malpractice may result from professional misconduct, unreasonable lack of skill or fidelity in professional or fiduciary duties, or illegal or immoral conduct.

Only those who are involved in a professional career can have a claim of malpractice brought against them. According to the law, a profession is a vocation or occupation that requires special, usually advanced, education or skill and a confidential relationship with the client. A case manager is considered a professional and is held to professional standards. A case manager may be found to have acted negligently if she/he unintentionally departed from or performed below the the expected standard of care a reasonable case manager would have followed under same circumstances, resulting in a patient's harm. The case manager may have committed malpractice when she/he neglected to perform acoording a known standard of care.

If there is an allegation of a breach of a standard based on negligence, then several areas must be evaluated. To determine a successful claim against a case manager, four elements of negligence must be evident. These elements of proof are the same for both negligence and malpractice: duty, breach, cause, injury, and damages (Box 13.4). The difference in proof is in the standard of care. One must establish the "reasonable person standard" first before an action is labeled as negligence. The standard of care for a case manager goes beyond a reasonable person standard and must be established in court so that the jury can determine whether there is liability for the case manager.

If the case manager is involved in a professional al-

Box 13.4   Elements of Proof in Negligence and Malpractice Cases (Holzer, 1999; West, 1994; Merz, 1993; Nichols, 1996)

There are four elements of proof in a case of negligence or malpractice.

1. *Duty*: establishing the presence of a duty (e.g., standard of care) the case manager owes the patient/client. For example, caring for or treating a patient in an appropriate and safe manner.

2. *Breach*: failing to act in a reasonable manner to meet the expectation of the duty owed to the patient/client-the standard of care. For example, the case manager fails to arrange for the patient's needed durable medical equipment.

3. *Proximate Causation*: the breach of the duty is the cause of the injury the patient/client suffered. The type and severity of the injury is a direct result of the failure to act in a reasonable manner. For example, a patient/client falls multiple times because the patient/client never received a needed wheelchair for ambulation and transportation.

4. *Damages*: the breach of duty resulting in the patient/client harm, personally, physically, emotionally, or financially. For example, the patient/client sustaining the multiple falls with injury requiring an acute care hospital admission and surgical hip repair.

Notes:

*Damages or injuries can include such things as loss of love and affection; pain and suffering; mental anguish; emotional distress; disfigurement; loss of consortium; past, present, and future medical expenses or lost wages; loss of guidance; loss of nurturance; loss of chance for survival; exacerbation of a pre-existing condition; and premature death.

*The proof must be provided in terms of the specific duty the case manager has toward the patient/client, the breach of that specified duty, the direct relationship between the breach and the consequences the patient suffered, and the presence of damages.

---

legation of misconduct or negligent care, then the term malpractice is used. Malpractice is defined as professional misconduct; negligent care and treatment; or failure to meet the standard of care, which results in harm to others. Let us consider the following example to understand malpractice.

A case manager fails to obtain and review pertinent patient records with the health insurance plan (i.e., payer such as a managed care organization) and as a result the patient is denied the certification for surgery or extended hospital stay, causing serious injuries (further unnecessary complications/deterioration in condition); the case manager and the managed care organization are held liable. The four elements of negligence are evident in this case. The case manager has a duty to obtain and evaluate all medical data so that the patient can receive the appropriate treatment based on needs. By failing to do so, the case manager demonstrated negligence and proximately caused additional injuries to the patient. Breach of the standard of care is also evident. The patient has a valid case.

13.5. ESTABLISHING THE STANDARD OF CARE FOR THE CASE MANAGER

In medical or healthcare-related malpractice claims, the case manager's services and treatment are judged based on the standards of care applied by other case managers with the same knowledge and experience and who are practicing under similar circumstances in a case management setting. The standard of care is then defined as a scale by which the provider's (i.e., case manager's) conduct is measured to determine if there is negligence or malpractice that has caused damage or injury to the plaintiff and if the provider acted "reasonably." To avoid malpractice litigation, case managers are advised to practice their duties in a manner consistent with their scope of practice, skills, knowledge, and competence; credentials; their job description; and the standards, policies, and procedures defined by their institution.

The sources of standards of care for case managers may include any or all of those issued by professional societies such as the following:

- National Association of Geriatric Care Managers
- Case Management Society of America
- Commission for Case Manager Certification
- National Institute on Community-Based Long-Term Care
- National Association of Social Workers
- American Nurses Association and American Nurses Credentialing Center
- Association of Rehabilitation Nurses
- American Managed Care and Review Association
- Agency for Healthcare Research and Quality
- National Institutes of Health
- The Centers for Medicare and Medicaid Services
- American Case Management Association

Case managers may also apply the evidence-based clinical practice guidelines that have been developed by national organizations and associations such as the American Medical Association, American College of Physicians, American College of Cardiology, American Diabetes Association, and Society of Hospital Medicine. If case managers receive certifications, they will be held to the standards of care of the society sponsoring the certification. Examples of these certifications are: the certified case manager (CCM), advance competency continuity of care (A-CCC), certified rehabilitation registered nurse (CRRN), certified insurance rehabilitation specialist (CIRS), occupational health nurse (OHN), certified social wrok case manager (C-SWCM), and certified rehabilitation counselor (CRC).

In situations in which the patient is involved in litigation, case managers may be called upon to testify in court, or the case management plan applied for the care of the patient and the medical record may be used to demonstrate the standard of care. Documentation (discussed in Chapter 8) that is thorough, factual, and concrete is essential to aid in the defense of the case manager and to provide a proper "picture" of the care and treatment rendered to the patient.

If there is a claim involving allegations of negligence or breaches of the standard of care, case managers will be held to the standard that was in effect at the time of the alleged incident. They will be judged by the "reasonable person's" standard, not the highest standard of care required under the same circumstances.

The standard of care measures the competence of the professional. Because a jury is not composed entirely of healthcare professionals, it is necessary to first teach the jury what a case manager does. This is done through a review of certain documents (Box 13.5) that results in establishing or clarifying the standard of care. Once the definition and role of the case manager are established in court, the jury uses this information as a template against which the follow-up information will be compared and contrasted. The jury uses the template to put the facts of the case into perspective. This enables the jury to determine if the behavior of the case manager was within or outside the standard of care for case management.

For example, the standard of care requires the case manager to inform the physician of anything significant brought to the case manager's attention by the patient, family, or staff or that the case manager personally observed or assessed. If the case manager fails to meet this expectation, he or she is committing negligence or malpractice and can be found guilty of malpractice if a lawsuit is brought forward. To illustrate, the following is an example of what can happen when the patient situation is not fully communicated to the physician or primary care provider of record. Although this case is from the 1990s, similar situations continue to happen today.

In a Georgia case, the plaintiff claimed that the nurse

Box 13.5 Sources of the Standard of Care Used in a Lawsuit

The standard of care is established by reviewing the following:

- The state nurse practice act or the practice act of other professions/disciplines if the person involved in the lawsuit is not a nurse (e.g., a social worker, vocational rehabilitation specialist, pharmacist)
- The standards of practice of case management
- Authoritative content from journal articles and books (scientific evidence for practice)
- Standards from professional organizations such as the ANA, NASW, CMSA, and Academy of Certified Case Managers
- Certification and credentialing standards
- Expert witnesses' testimony
- A review of the applicable policies and procedures from the organization for which the case manager works
- Applicable statues, laws, and regulations
- Codes of ethics and professional conduct
- Accreditation and regulatory standards
- Organizational policies, procedures, and standards of care
- Regulatory and accreditation agencies
- Equipment manuals
- Job descriptions
- Practice guidelines

was partially responsible for a baby's resulting lifelong disability because of her failure to fully communicate with the physician. A baby boy who had recently been diagnosed with a respiratory infection spiked a fever of 104°F, became limp, and began panting and moaning. His mother called the after-hours phone number of her managed care plan (health insurer) and spoke to the triage nurse. The nurse advised a cool bath while she contacted the on-call physician. The nurse told the pediatrician that she had ruled out respiratory distress in the baby but neglected to inform the physician of the baby's symptoms of panting and moaning. As a result, the pediatrician did not consider the baby's condition to be critical and directed the nurse to have the mother take her baby to a children's medical center 40 miles from home. The baby had a cardiopulmonary arrest enroute to the facility and was diverted to a nearby hospital, where he was revived. However, the color never returned to his extremities. Gangrene developed, and the baby's hands and part of each leg had to be amputated. Meningococcemia was the diagnosis. The baby's family sued the managed care plan, claiming negligence on the part of the nurse and the physician because of the delayed treatment that could have pre-

vented the gangrene. The jury awarded $45 million in this case (Sullivan, 1996).

The nurse has a duty, both to the client and physician, to relay as accurate a description of the patient as possible. If the nurse is in the role of gatekeeper, as is the case with many HMOs, triage nurses and case managers, clinics, and private practices, the physician depends solely on the input of the nurse to make his or her own medical judgment, considering the physician may not have direct contact with the patient at the time (Case Manager's Tip 13.3). This puts the nurse and the case manager in a position of responsibility and accountability not only for their practice but also for the actions taken by other providers based on their actions (Case Manager's Tip 13.4).

The case of *Darling v. Charleston Community Memorial Hospital* (33 Ill 2d 326, 211 N.E. 2d 253, 1965; cert. Denied, 383 U.S. 946, 1966) taught the nursing profession that just reporting observations to the attending physician is not enough. If the treating physician does not take action in a serious situation, the nurse has the affirmative duty to take that information up the chain of command to get help for the client. What is the chain of command for the case manager (Case Manager's Tip 13.5)? Check your organization for its chain of command policy or procedure. However, normally the chain of command starts with the immedi-

 CASE MANAGER'S TIP 13.3

Communication Strategies that Reduce Legal Risk

It is the case manager's duty to communicate to the physician or primary care provider of record any changes in the patient's condition, the plan of care, or the transitional plan. A reasonable and prudent case manager prevents communication breakdown. Examples of strategies case managers can apply to reduce legal risk associated with miscommunication are as follows:

- Convey a message using the exact words used by the patient to describe a situation or symptom(s).
- Share impressions or opinions about the situation.
- Stick to the facts.
- Be clear, accurate, and complete with the message.
- Communicate promptly.
- Communicate anyway, even if unsure.
- Repeat the information if necessary.
- Ask if the physician has any questions and provide answers as appropriate and if necessary refer back to the patient for more information.
- Assure no selective sharing of information; every piece of information is important.

CASE MANAGER'S TIP 13.4

Causation

Case managers are rarely involved in actual causation cases. Instead, they are involved in proximate causation which may result from dealing inappropriately with many different parties, factors, and/or obligations at the same time, and their actions or behaviors or inaction contribute to the harm or damage the patient experiences.

ate manager, then the department's supervisor or administrator, and may end with the department's physician advisor, department head, or the chief of medical services or chief nursing officer for the agency or facility.

13.6. STANDARDIZED CASE MANAGEMENT PLANS OF CARE

Healthcare providers have raised concerns regarding the admissibility of standardized evidence-based guidelines or case management plans as evidence in case of malpractice litigation. It has been noted by lawyers that when such plans are used for documenting the provision of care (planning, implementing, and evaluating) and are made a permanent part of the patient's medical record, it is most certain that they will be admitted into court as evidence.

A standardized case management plan is an interdisciplinary proactive set of daily prescriptions that has

CASE MANAGER'S TIP 13.5

Chain of Command

Chain of command is the order in which power and authority in the healthcare organization is distributed and delegated from top down reaching every level in the organization. As a case manager or a nurse, when you seek the attention of another healthcare provider concerning an issue you are facing with your patient/family requesting assistance or attention to the matter and you are received with no action, but you still feel the matter must be attended to; you attempt a couple of times but continue to reach no conclusion, you are obligated to pursue the chain of command as defined in your organization. This means you bring the matter to the attention of someone in a higher position than the professional you have dealt with, this professional usually is with higher authority and power and is able to address your concern to ultimately safeguard the patient's interest. Failing to follow the chain of command may result in an act of negligence or malpractice, especially if the patient sustained a preventable injury or damage.

been prepared following a particular timeline to facilitate the care of a specific patient population from preadmission to post-discharge. The plan identifies patient care activities that are thought to be effective to providing care for a specific patient population. These activities are categorized as the assessments, treatments, teaching, discharge planning, diagnostic tests, consultations, and interventions that should be completed for the patient's optimal recovery (see Chapter 10 for a detailed discussion). The plan usually holds valuable evidence because it includes information (data and evidence) about the patient's projected and actual course of treatment. It may include the following:

- Patient's actual and potential problems
- Patient's projected and actual outcomes
- Medical interventions
- Nursing and other interventions
- Projected discharge times/target times or transitional plan
- Intermediate and discharge care outcomes
- Accountabilities of various healthcare team members

Evidence-based, standardized case management plans are usually developed by professional societies, healthcare institutions, health insurance companies, or federal agencies. Sometimes they are called clinical practice guidelines or practice parameters. Professional societies and governmental agencies have developed practice guidelines to counteract or reduce the risk for liability and litigation and enhance patient's safety. They are developed and used to improve the quality of care and reduce cost through standardizing practice. They are also helpful in reducing the cost of and risk for malpractice litigation through delineating the standard of care (West, 1994).

Once a case management plan is admitted into court as evidence, it is thought to be an extremely powerful evidentiary tool used by the jury to determine the sequence of events (treatments and outcomes). If the provider was noted to have been adherent to the projections of the plan and the documentation justifies the deviation from the its recommendations, then the chances are that the provider's actions will be deemed appropriate and in accordance with the standard of care. The key in this case is appropriate documentation of variances or deviations from the plan, including rational why.

The procedure followed in the development of a case management plan affects the degree of its consideration by the jury and its reliability in the lawsuit. It is recommended that procedures be developed based on expert opinion, research, and the latest advents of treatment as recommended by professional societies

CASE MANAGER'S TIP 13.6

Points to Remember About Case Management Plans

It is the case manager's duty to communicate to the physician or primary care provdier of record any changes in the patient's condition, the plan of care, or the transitional plan. A reasonable and prudent case manager prevents communication breakdown. Examples of strategies case managers can apply to reduce legal risk associated with miscommunication are as follows:

- Can be presented as evidence if they are made part of the patient's medical record.
- Improve communication among members of the healthcare team, thus reducing the risk for liability or litigation.
- Can be determined by the injury as the standards of care.
- Should allow for deviations. However, documentation in the medical record of variances related to the plan of care, including the medical and nursing plans, is important for reducing liability.
- Helps the jury describe the sequence of events (treatments and outcomes).
- If developed by one healthcare organization, may be inappropriate for another organization.
- Will not be admitted as evidence unless proven relevant to the case in question.
- Should be flexible prescriptions and allow for deviations as long as they are justified.
- Should be developed following a scientific method.
- Standardize the care provided by multiple providers.

---

and governmental agencies (Case Manager's Tip 13.6 contains a list of suggestions for case management plans). However, if a case management plan is developed poorly and arbitrarily, it will hold no power in court and the standards of care will be judged as inappropriate. As a result the care provider will not be able to defend the case.

13.7. INFORMED CONSENT

Case managers are often involved in some way in the process of informed consent. Informed consent is consent given for a kind of intervention or service by a patient or the next of kin, legal guardian, or designated person in the medical durable power of attorney after the provision of sufficient information by the provider. The elements of disclosure (Box 13.6) are those items that must be discussed with the patient by the healthcare provider performing the treatment, procedure, or surgery.

There are several exceptions to obtaining informed

> **Box 13.6 Five Elements of Disclosure**
>
> The standard of care is established by reviewing the following:
>
> 1. The type of procedure(s) to be performed (e.g., debridement of knee wound)
> 2. The material benefits (e.g., reversal of symptoms, delay in disease progression) and risks or hazards inherent in the procedure (e.g., infection, bleeding)
> 3. The projected/desired outcome(s) hoped for (e.g., elimination of infected tissue and revitalization of new tissue)
> 4. Available alternatives, if any (e.g., medication)
> 5. Consequences of no treatment (e.g., continuation of pain, necrosis, sepsis, or possible amputation)

consent and discussing all of the elements of disclosure with the patient. The first exception is if there is an emergency situation and/or a situation in which the client is unconscious or incompetent (e.g., the patient is in a life-threatening situation and there is no time to have a discussion). Second, a therapeutic privilege may be invoked if it is medically contraindicated to disclose the risk and hazards to the patient or if it may result in illness, emotional distress, serious psychological damage, or failure on the part of the patient to receive life-saving treatment. Third, the patient may waive the right to informed consent. Finally, the patient may have had the procedure performed once before and waives the right of informed consent because he or she has already received the information. This information must be documented appropriately in the medical record to protect healthcare providers against malpractice litigation.

13.8. PATIENT CONFIDENTIALITY

As is any healthcare provider, case managers are obligated to safeguard the patient's privacy and confidentiality. Unauthorized disclosure of information is considered breach of confidentiality and may result in litigation. It is important for case managers to seek the guidance of a legal counsel before disclosing any information. In spite of confidentiality laws, reporting of certain events such as elder or child abuse, certain contagious diseases, death, birth, and animal bites is mandatory and protected by federal laws. Some information requires the patient's permission for release of information (written and signed release). The release should delineate the name(s) of the party the information is to be released to. Examples of such information include the following:

- Substance use; drug or alcohol abuse treatment
- Mental and behavioral health/psychiatric care
- Sexually transmitted diseases
- HIV or AIDS status
- Abortion
- Specific medical or surgical history

It is important for case managers to remember and respect patients' rights every time they face a legal or ethical dilemma or any challenges related to the provision of care. The patient has several rights that must not be forgotten (Box 13.7).

The case manager can play an important role in advocating on behalf of the patient and family. During such situations, the case manager should always remain aware of the patient's legal and ethical rights, as well as issues of confidentiality pertaining to patient care. Case management plans can serve an important function in protecting the rights of both the patient and the healthcare provider. Special attention should be paid to the process of their development, their use, and the way documentation is incorporated into them.

13.9. CASE MANAGEMENT "HOT SPOTS" THAT HAVE ALREADY RECEIVED LEGAL REVIEW

Case managers are at increasing risk for legal action because of the nature of their role. As the scope of their practice and accountability increases, so does their risk (Case Manager's Tip 13.7). This section reviews some of the areas in case management practice that have been noticed to receive legal attention more than others (Box 13.8). One area that presents increased legal risk is negligent referral, which is a claim that is usually brought about when there is a large network of providers. Getting the patient into the appropriate case manager's caseload is the best starting point. For

 CASE MANAGER'S TIP 13.7

Be Aware of the Law in Your Locality

Healthcare laws and regulations may vary from one state to another. Case managers are advised to remain aware of their state laws and statutes and the latest related changes. Information about the laws and regulations are available and easily accessible on the Internet, on governmental and state-based websites. Consultation with superiors/supervisors, the risk management, and/or legal departments is recommended if the case manager is unsure about a situation or has any concerns.

example, if a patient is admitted to the hospital and is diagnosed with new onset diabetes, the patient may be placed on a diabetes clinical pathway/plan of care while hospitalized. The inpatient case manager may follow the patient. A referral to the appropriate disease state case manager may then be placed so that he or she can follow the patient after discharge from the acute care setting. The patient is also screened for his or her risk level at the primary care site to determine the frequency of needed interactions and follow-up care with the disease state case manager. If a patient has a poor outcome, all parties involved in the patient's care will come under scrutiny, including perhaps those who made a referral to the contracted provider involved in the patient's case.

13.10. NONADHERENCE/MISMANAGEMENT

If it can be proven that there has been nonadherence to the case management plan of care agreed on by the family, case manager, and members of the interdisci-

---

Box 13.7   Patient Rights

- Right to access needed health and social services
- Right to treatment with dignity and respect
- Right to confidentiality
- Right to privacy
- Right to know cost of services
- Right to self-determination and choice
- Right to comprehensive and fair assessment
- Right to notification of discharge, transition to another level of care, termination, or change of service
- Right to withdraw from a case management program
- Right to a grievance procedure
- Right to choose a particular community service agency or long-term care provider

---

Box 13.8   Areas of Increased Litigation in Case Management

1. Negligent referral or act
2. Failure to investigate a claim
3. Failure to communicate or document
4. Inadequate or premature patient discharge/transition to another level of care
5. Fraud and abuse
6. End-of-life decisions and surrogate decision making
7. Denial of services
8. Breach of confidentiality
9. Failure to assess and monitor patient's condition or secure necessary durable medical equipment
10. Failure to act as a patient advocate

plinary team, then there may be a claim of mismanagement. It is important for providers, including case managers, to explain to the patient and family that certain complications or undesired outcomes may occur regardless of the efforts made to prevent them. Sometimes it is the natural progression of the patient's health condition (i.e., disease). It is also helpful to avoid providing false guarantees regarding outcomes of care and prognosis, particularly when the situation at hand is considered to be high risk and life threatening. False guarantees of this kind may be viewed as nonadherence to the plan or mismanagement of the standards of care and practice. When guarantees are provided but not met, and the patient and/or family are able to prove that the guarantees were not met, the situation results in potential breach.

Case managers must practice within the realm of the responsibilities and scope of practice defined by the professional license that they hold and must not infer in any way that they are developing medical treatment plans for their patients. Any evident nonadherent with the regulations governing the practice of nursing (or the discipline the case manager belongs to, such as social work) may present potential problems, which may result in medical malpractice litigation. It may also be a potential problem wherein the case manager is viewed as practicing medicine. This can result in a disciplinary action and an impingement on the license (e.g., revocation, suspension, or probation).

13.11. DOCUMENTATION

A case manager must act as the patient's advocate and look out for what is in the patient's best interest. If it is determined that the physician and/or facility that the patient has been referred to is not properly performing or providing the services needed, then action to change the situation must be taken and should be documented so as to protect the provider and patient. Documentation should occur when reviewing and evaluating credentials and performance of practitioners and facilities that patients have been referred to so that the case manager can determine if they are providing the appropriate levels of care needed by patients and families. In addition, follow-up documentation regarding actions taken to correct any identified problems must be evident, along with subsequent documentation of the outcomes of these corrective measures. Moreover, documentation must also include actions the case managers perform in addition to the referrals mentioned previously (e.g., patient/family teaching and counseling) and their related outcomes. Case Manager's Tip 13.8 presents some areas in which accurate and thorough

 CASE MANAGER'S TIP 13.8

Areas in Which Documentation is Critical

- Plan of care agreed on with patient and family
- Medical stability of patient within 24 hours of discharge
- Safety precautions
- Falls prevention
- Restraints management
- Third-party (insurance) reimbursement
- The TJC accreditation of facility
- Discharge planning and patient's readiness for discharge, including post-discharge services
- Patient/family health teaching
- Informed consent
- Disclosure of information
- Advance directives
- Living wills
- Medical durable power of attorney
- Reportable events (e.g., violent injuries, communicable diseases, abuse)
- Do not resuscitate orders

documentation is considered critical in reducing malpractice litigation.

Documentation serves multiple purposes, including the following:

- Evidence of the provision of care
- Justification of the need for referrals to specific providers
- Evaluation of the patient's condition in light of treatment
- Evidence that proper investigation of the qualifications, credentials, and competencies of healthcare providers is completed
- Communicating the plan of care of individual patients to the various members of the interdisciplinary healthcare team
- Protection against litigation
- Assistance in determining whether the resources are being used appropriately
- Clarification of continuity of care after the hospital stay, including post-discharge or transition services
- Summary of nursing and medical history for use in future admissions
- Reporting of data for quality of care review and risk management
- Reporting of data for continuing education and research
- Review of data for billing and reimbursement purposes

- Recording care that forms the basis of evaluation by accreditation agencies (e.g., the TJC, NCQA, URAC), and regulatory bodies (e.g., state department of health and human srvices, CMS)
- Legal evidence for use by the hospital, other healthcare providers, the patient and/or family, and members of the judicial system

13.12. LEGAL AND ETHICAL DILEMMAS FOR THE CASE MANAGER

Common legal and ethical issues that are potential areas of exposure and litigation in the area of case management may or may not involve case managers directly. Examples of such issues include the following:

- Third-party payers and healthcare facilities can be held legally accountable when inappropriate decisions regarding medical services result from defects in design or implementation of cost-containment mechanisms instituted by the facility or insurance company.
- Physicians and other providers can be held liable if they comply with the limitations imposed by third-party payers and do not protest when the patient can be harmed by these decisions. Physicians are ultimately responsible.
- Breach of contract, bad faith, and refusal to provide services and pay benefits or claims are also issues that may be litigated. A contract is an agreement consisting of one or more legally enforceable promises between two or more parties. The elements of a contract are offer, acceptance, consideration, and breach.
- If there is a breach of implied covenant or good faith and fair dealing, legal actions may be taken.
- Clients may also allege a failure to exercise due care in the discharge of the contractual duties.
- A failure to properly investigate an insider's claim is a potential litigation.
- If standards of medical necessity that are significantly at variance with community standards are applied, there may be legal exposure.
- Failure to properly document care activities and/or outcomes.
- An allegation of good faith violation of duty may be alleged when a subscriber's claim for hospital benefits is denied and the subscriber (an enrollee of a managed care organization) is not informed of his or her contractual right to impartial review and arbitration of the disputed claim.
- Failure to obtain all of the necessary documents/

medical records can result in the denial of care needed, which then exerts potential liability.
- Allegations of negligent referral claims may be filed if there is evidence of failure to properly investigate the qualifications and competencies of the providers and/or facilities to which case managers refer patients for treatment. In addition, if it can be shown that case managers were not reasonable in making a referral to that particular facility or provider, the allegation of negligent referral can be made.
- Failure of case managers to act as patient advocates or in the patients' best interest.
- Failure to apply the "reasonable" standard to the care of patients.
- Any type of "kickback" or "incentive" program with a provider/payer and the case manager. Such practices are considered illegal (conflict of interest). They also are unethical behaviors that may result in the patient not receiving the best possible care by the most appropriate provider.

A list of suggestions to help prevent or minimize malpractice litigation appears in Case Manager's Tip 13.9.

Healthcare organizations and case managers should be aware of the reputation and operations of other providers to whom patients are referred for further treatment. Decisions should be made in the best interest of patients and their families. Several considerations should be reviewed to determine if the providers to whom patients are referred are appropriate and meet the interests and needs of patients. Examples of these considerations include the following:

- Types of services provided and current practices
- Reports of patient and staff satisfaction scores
- Resource utilization practices
- Practices of quality assurance, assessment, monitoring, and improvement
- Timeliness of delivery of services
- Billing practices (e.g., how they bill, what types of insurance they accept)
- Insurance coverage (i.e., are they properly and adequately insured?)
- Records of any settlements and/or judgments against the facility or healthcare provider (check the courthouse records; do a computer search)
- The allegations of the breaches of the standard of care found in the medical malpractice settlements or judgments (do the allegations pertain to the type of care that would be rendered to the patients to be referred for services?)
- Current licensure (check with the state boards)

- Current accreditation (check with the appropriate agencies)
- Reports on outcomes of care of patients with similar problems to the ones to be referred

As a patient advocate, the case manager must always act in the best interest of the patient. The case manager must document that a reasonable evaluation

 CASE MANAGER'S TIP 13.9

Suggestions for Preventing Malpractice Litigation

To prevent malpractice litigation, the healthcare organization and the case manager may do the following:

- Delineate a referral process for community services, post-discharge service coordination and care provision that is in the best interest of the patient and family. The referral process should be accessible in writing to all those involved (i.e., healthcare providers). It should be clear and concise.
- Ensure that corrective measures are taken and action plans are developed immediately if a healthcare issue arises or if care is questionable. Evaluation and follow-up on such plans should be reflected in the patient's medical record or the hospital's administrative reports as needed.
- Develop and implement policies and procedures regarding the process of developing case management plans that are easily understood and applied. They should reflect the best interest of the patient and family. In addition, the procedure for documentation of care activities and variance identification and collection should be made easy and explicit.

To minimize malpractice litigation, the case manager may do the following:

- On admission, and in collaboration with the patient and family and the interdisciplinary healthcare team, individualize the standardized, evidence-based case management plan to meet the patient's and family's needs.
- Always consult the treating physician.
- Review the patient's medical record thoroughly before contacting the payer representative (e.g., health insurance plan including managed care organizations).
- Ensure that precertifications or preauthorizations for treatments have been obtained in a timely manner.
- Adhere to the law (e.g., patient privacy and confidentiality procedures).
- Make certain that the patient and family consent to the indicated treatment plan and procedures.
- Advocate for the patient and family.

was completed to determine the need for a referral, if one is being made. To protect the case manager and the employer from liability related to the provider offering the referred services, the healthcare organization must have a method in place to review the credentials, certifications, and documented complaints of all providers used in the referral process. The organization must also make sure that the client and family are given several options so that they make the choice that is best for them. An effective strategy is to have a resource manual of providers (e.g., provider panel) available for use by patients and their families or caregivers when a referral is warranted.

13.12.1. Failure to Investigate a Claim

This usually arises out of contract law. The client has received a denial of service and claims that the case manager did not act in good faith when reviewing the medical record. Two cases, *Taylor v. Prudential Insurance Company* and *Aetna Life Insurance Company v. Lovoie*, have been reported (Sturgeon, 1997) in this type of lawsuit. In both cases the jury based its decisions on the case of "incomplete information": sharing of incomplete information with the health insurance plan/MCO and the plan/MCO's failing to examine the claim thoroughly. Both insurers were found liable, and the juries ruled in favor of the clients. To avoid similar lawsuits, an MCO must have a formal process in place for claims review. It also must gather all of the pertinent data before a decision is made (i.e., denial of services) and be able to clearly show the basis of the decision to the client. Applying these strategies diligently assists the case manager and the insurer in the defense against this kind of claim.

13.12.2. Failure to Communicate and/or Document

This is an accusation that should never have to occur. Case managers do so much for their patients and their families, but sometimes they fail to reflect their efforts in the patient's medical record. The medical record must always reflect all of the interventions made on behalf of, or for, the patient. However, case managers must be careful in their documentation and focus only on the facts (Case Manager's Tip 13.10). An easy way to remember what to document is to apply the ABCs of documentation: accurate, brief, and complete. This way of documentation includes the following:

- Identity/role of those involved in the patient's care
- Consultations, consultants, and referrals

- How care decisions are made and incorporated in the case management plan of care
- Clarifications about certain conflicting or confusing situations
- Follow-up on issues, especially those related to changes in the patient's condition and progression of care
- Consent to or refusal of treatment
- Agreements on and share decision making regarding treatment options and services

 CASE MANAGER'S TIP 13.10

Strategies for Better Documentation

- Document legibly. If the information is in the medical record but it cannot be deciphered, it is worthless and may even be the source of an error. Use of electronic medical records prevents this issue.
- Record information in the medical record promptly. The lapse of time will increase the margin of error.
- Make sure that the medical record reflects the fact that the physician is driving the care and heading up the team.
- The medical record should reflect every transaction that occurs over the course of case management and the patient's healthcare encounter.
- Be specific, factual, complete, timely, accurate, and free of judgmental statements.
- Use descriptive terms for behaviors rather than generalizations.
- Document the plan of care and the transitional plan, including the post-discharge services arranged for.
- Document the patient's responses to treatments and actions implemented to progress care.
- Use quotations (exact words used by the patient/ family) when appropriate.
- Document refusals of treatments and options.
- Document consents to treatments.
- Record patient and family education activities.
- Be clear when recording the goals of treatment and the plan for meeting them.
- If using electronic and structured documentation, assure that the record is telling the patient's story and reflects only what is applicable to the indviudal patient.
- Assure documentations of various healthcare professionals involved in the patient's care are not conflicted.
- Be objective in your documentation; refarin from subjectivity, interpretation of what the patient/family says, inference, or improsing judgment.
- Never go back and change the documentation after the fact. Maintain honesty at all time; when you find you have committed a documentation error, amend your documentation in a timely manner and include a special note explaining the error made.

13.12.3. Inadequate or Premature Discharge/Transition

This may result in negligent act. When planning transitional care, make sure that the patient is stable for discharge or transition to the next level of care and as indicated by the patient's condition. It is customary in the acute care hospital setting to assess a patient for discharge and assure that certain criteria are met indicating the patient's stability for discharge within 24 hours before discharge or transfer from the hospital. If any of these criteria is present at the time of discharge, the discharge is considered inappropriate or premature. Examples of these criteria are as follows (refer to your hospital's specific standard for patient's discharge or transfer to next less acute level of care):

1. Parameters for temperature: > 101°F orally or 102°F rectally
2. Parameters for pulse: > 120 beats/min or < 45 beats/min with or < 50 beats/min without beta blockers
3. Parameters for blood pressure: systolic < 85 or > 180 mm Hg; diastolic < 50 or > 110 mm Hg
4. IV fluids and medications after midnight or on the day of discharge
5. Presence of a wound that has bloody or purulent discharge
6. Abnormal test results that have not already been addressed

Another example of discharge criteria from the hospital setting is advocated for by the American Thoracic Society (ATS) which states that as a general rule, patients hospitalized for an acute change in condition (i.e., exacerbation) can be deemed ready for discharge once the reasons for admission is resolved. The ATS identified the following criteria for discharge of patients with chronic obstructive pulmonary disease (COPD) based on consensus (ATS, 2015).

1. Symptoms are returning to baseline, including eating and sleeping
2. Hemodynamic stability
3. Oxygenation returning to baseline (maintaining arterial oxygen saturation at >90%)
4. Inhaled beta-agonist therapy is required less frequently
5. Patient able to resume ambulation (if patient was able to ambulate prior to current condition)
6. Patient able to eat and sleep without frequent awakening by dyspnea
7. Patient is off parenteral therapy for a minimum of 12 hours

8. Patient or home caregiver understands correct use of medications

9. Follow-up and homecare arrangements have been completed (e.g., visiting nurse service, oxygen therapy, and meal provisions

To prevent the legal risk associated with inappropriate or premature discharge, the case manager must notify the physician in the event that the patient's vital signs fall out of the criteria ranges, test results are abnormal, or there is the presence of discharge from wounds or surgical sites. If the physician still approves of the patient's discharge, documentation of such should be present in the medical record. In this case, the case manager must ensure that plans for follow-up care and post-discharge services are arranged for. The case manager must also educate the patient and family about the need for follow-up care and document these interventions and the physician's response in the medical record.

In reviewing the transitional care plan, consider whether the plan is appropriate to the patient and that it meets the patient's physical, emotional, social, functional, mental health, and safety needs. Documentation of the discharge or transition plan must include the following:

- Patient/family/caregiver's consent to the plan and communications with patient and family
- Patient responses to interventions and progress toward discharge including meeting criteria for discharge or transition to next level of care
- Contacts with other providers and agencies, as well as names, dates, times, and agreements with them, including purpose for the contact

- Patient limitations and refusals of care
- Any changes in the plan of care
- Arrangements made for post-discharge services and the use of durable medical equipment in the home setting
- Educational needs and instructions provided about medications and other treatments: what to watch for and what symptoms to report immediately to the physician or nurse; also include outcomes such as patient understanding of teaching and responsibilities for self-management
- Hand-off communication to the healthcare team or provider at the next level of care

A thorough patient assessment at discharge is critical because it prevents a premature discharge from inadvertently occurring. If significant issues or recent changes in the patient's condition were identified which warrant a change in the plan, the case manager could then stop the discharge or transition and address them with the physician and the interdisciplinary healthcare team.

Close to the claim of premature discharge would be a claim of negligence due to the delay in patient transfer. In the case *Henry v. Felici*, (758 S.W. 2d 836 Texas, 1988) a 3-year-old child died as a result of delay in transfer to another facility for CT scan and surgery. The court found that the nurses who are given the responsibility to implement a transfer have a duty to see to it that the transfer is made in accordance with the physician's order and as required by the patient's condition. If for any reason beyond the control of the nurses a complication or delay in implementing an order is anticipated, the nurses have the clear and unequivocal responsibility to immediately inform the attending physician so that he or she may take whatever action is deemed appropriate under the circumstances. In this case, the nurses failed to inform the physician. Often case managers are involved in a patient's transfer from one care setting or level of care to another. Case managers must assure the safe and timely transition and implement strategies to prevent quality or safety concerns such as delay in transfer or avoidable deterioration in patient's condition due to untimely treatment.

13.12.4. Fraud and Abuse

These are claims that can carry severe penalties for the perpetrators. Case managers can prevent fraud and abuse practices by appropriately exercising their responsibility and accountability toward patient care planning, delivery, coordination, documentation, and management. Considering that in some hospital organizations case management departments also include oversight for documentation improvement, coding of patient's medical records in preparation for claims submission for reimbursement, tends to be a case management responsibility. Therefore, manipulation of coding (e.g., upcoding or unbundling) for the purpose of increasing revenue must be avoided. Fraud is intentional deception or misrepresentation that could result in some unauthorized benefit. The most common type of fraud arises from a false statement or misrepresentation that is material to entitlement or payment under the Medicare program. The violator may be a provider, a supplier of DME, a beneficiary, or some other person or business entity (Case Manager's Tip 13.11).

The term abuse is used to describe incidents or practices of providers that are inconsistent with accepted sound medical, business, ethical, or fiscal practices. These practices may directly or indirectly result in unnecessary costs to the services provided, improper payment, or payment for services that fail to meet professionally recognized standards of care or that are medically unnecessary. Examples of abuse include overutilization of medical and healthcare services, unbundled or exploded charges, excessive charges for DME, claims for services not medically necessary or not medically necessary to the extent furnished (Case Manager's Tip 13.11).

 CASE MANAGER'S TIP 13.11

Differentiating Medicare's Fraud and Abuse (USDHHS, 2014)

Fraud: intentional schemes, ranging from individual acts to broad-based operations by an institution or group of people, that result in unfair or unjustified revenue.

Examples are:

- Knowingly submitting false statements or making misrepresentations of facts to obtain a federal healthcare payment for which no entitlement would otherwise exist (e.g., billing for unprovided services, manipulating coding to receive higher payments)
- Knowingly soliciting, paying, and/or accepting remuneration to induce or reward referrals for items or services reimbursed by federal healthcare programs (e.g., receiving kickbacks, bribes, rebates)
- Making prohibited referrals for certain designated health services
- Knowingly billing for services not furnished, supplies not provided, or both, including falsifying records to show delivery of such items or billing Medicare for appointments that the patient failed to keep
- Knowingly billing for services at a level of complexity higher than the service actually provided or documented in the file (e.g., altering claim forms to obtain a higher payment amount; deliberately applying for duplicate payments)
- Use of another person's Medicare card in obtaining medical care

Abuse: practices that are inconsistent with the goals of providing patients with services that are medically necessary, meet professionally recognized standards, and are priced fairly. They may directly or indirectly result in unnecessary costs to the Medicare program. Examples are:

- Billing for services that were not medically necessary (e.g., misrepresenting the diagnosis of the patient to justify the services or the equipment furnished)
- Charging excessively for services or supplies
- Misusing codes on a claim, such as upcoding or unbundling codes

Federal laws governing fraud and abuse include the following (USDHHS, 2014):

- False Claims Act (FCA)
- Anti-Kickback Statute (AKS)
- Physician Self-Referral Law (Stark Law)
- Social Security Act
- United States Criminal Code

The Healthcare Integrity and Protection Data Bank (HIPDB) is the electronic data bank created by the Health Insurance Portability and Accountability Act of 1996 to combat fraud and abuse in health insurance and healthcare delivery. It is a national data collection program for the reporting of and the disclosure of certain final adverse actions (e.g., civil judgment, criminal convictions) by federal or state licensing agencies taken against healthcare providers, suppliers, and practitioners, including physicians and nurses, related to the delivery of a healthcare item or services. The HIPDB is a nationwide flagging system that serves primarily as an alert to users indicating that a comprehensive review of the provider's, supplier's, or practitioner's past actions may be prudent. The HIPDB became part of the National Practitioner Data Bank (NPDB) in May 2013. Information previously collected and disclosed through the HIPDB is now collected and disclosed through the NPDB (USDHHS, Health Resources and Services Administration, 2015).

It is important for the case manager to understand fraud and abuse to then be able to prevent such acts or recognize them when they occur, and refer them for investigation by the compliance office of the healthcare organization where the case manager works. It is also as important for the case manager not to confuse an innocent mistake for an act of fraud or abuse. Here is a simple description of the differences:

- *Error*: a mistake such as inaccurate coding
- *Waste*: inefficiencies in the systems of care resulting in medically unnecessary service
- *Abuse*: bending the rules and upcoding a record for increased revenue
- *Fraud*: intentional deception such as billing for unprovided services (USDHHS, 2014)

A New York judge allowed to proceed with a class action suit that claimed that an HMO health insurance plan committed fraud and breach of contract by allowing nonphysicians to make decisions about lengths of hospital stay. Two plaintiffs brought the lawsuit on behalf of themselves and other subscribers to the HMO or its subsidiary. The lead plaintiff alleged that while she was in the hospital being treated for Crohn's disease, her physician recommended that she remain in the hospital for additional tests. However, the HMO denied coverage for the extra hospital stay, and she was discharged. One month later, the plaintiff was hospitalized again for a ruptured intestine. She contended that this condition would not have occurred had she been allowed to remain in the hospital for further tests. The plaintiff claimed that this decision was not made by a physician but by a "concurrent review nurse," or clinical reviewer, based on actuarial guidelines. The plaintiff argued that the HMO's promotional materials had represented that decisions of medical necessity were made by trained physicians (*Batas v. Prudential Insurance Company of America*, No. 107881/97, NY, Sup. Ct. NY City, May 20). The plaintiff won this lawsuit. In a case such as this the case manager can prevent such legal risk by applying good and responsible utilization review and management practices (Case Manager's Tip 13.12).

13.12.5. Elderly Abuse

The National Center on Elder Abuse (NCEA) estimates that nearly 2.2 million elder Americans encounter abuse each year and about 9.5% of the elderly population experience some form of abuse. NCEA also reports that over two-thirds of those suffer abuse are women (67%); 66.7% are White, and the median age of those abused is 77.9 years. As for the form of abuse, NCEA reports neglect (55.8%) as the most reported form, followed by physical abuse (15.7%), finaical ex-

CASE MANAGER'S TIP 13.12

Strategies for Better Utilization Review and Management

- Follow the policies and procedures of your organization consistently.
- Apply the criteria of utilization review and transitional planning adequately and in all cases.
- Apply the stipulations of the managed care contract that relate to the case in review.
- Be timely in your review and communications with appropriate parties (e.g., managed care case manager, provider-based case manager, physician, administrators, patient and family).
- Document all transactions.
- When unsure, always ask for clarification or help.
- If you disagree with a denial of service, appeal to review it with the responsible party in a supervisory role.
- Always apply the ethical and legal principles in your practice.

ploitation (12.3%), and emotional abuse (7.3%). Additionally, 66% of the reported abuse cases are perpetrated by adult children or spouses (US Department of Justice, Bureau of Justice Statistics, 2014).

Case managers have an affirmative duty to report known or suspected cases of elder abuse to the local investigating agency. Many times, because of their experience in patient assessment, care and transitional planning, and coordination of services, case managers may be able to identify a potentially stressful situation that could lead to abuse and intervene to change the outcome. Healthcare organizations should have policies and procedures to guide case managers in reporting and assisting in the investigation of suspected abuse. Protective reporting laws exist to protect the professional against defamation claims when reporting abuse or neglect.

13.12.6. End-of-life Decisions and Surrogate Decision Making

These are two topics that have the potential for legal entanglements, especially when the patient's wishes are not followed or when the patient and family wishes are conflicting or at odds. The Patient Self-Determination Act of 1991 (Sections 4206 and 4751 of the Omnibus Reconciliation Act of 1990, Public Law 101-508, November 1990) requires that hospitals, nursing homes, HMOs, home healthcare agencies, and other healthcare facilities receiving Medicare and Medicaid funds have policies and procedures in place with regard to advance directives. It also requires healthcare providers and agencies to inform their patients of their rights under state law to make decisions concerning treatment or nontreatment. Advance directives are legal documents that are drawn up by patients for use in case they become incompetent or incapacitated. The information included in advance directives refers to decisions regarding the execution, withholding, or withdrawing of medical treatment.

An advance directive can be a living will, a medical healthcare power of attorney, or a document that combines the two. To prevent legal risk, information received from the patient about the existence of the advance directive must be present in the medical record at all times. In addition, all members of the healthcare team must be aware of its presence and act by it as they make decisions regarding the patient's care and treatment options. Healthcare providers, including case managers, are expected to not discriminate against a patient who does or does not have an advance directive.

Some states recognize another document known as

a prehospital advance directive that directs prehospital caregivers regarding the patient's wishes for resuscitation outside of the acute care setting. In many states, the statutes identify the persons able to act as surrogate decision-makers in the absence of the written directives and when the patient is incompetent or unable to do so himself or herself. Problems arise when there is disagreement with the patient's directives and the patient is deemed incompetent, unconscious and failing, when the document cannot be located, or when the surrogate decision-maker is at odds with other family members. Knowing the state law and the institutional policies and procedures about advance directives and surrogate decision making are the case manager's best defenses against these types of legal entanglements. Knowing the client's status regarding resuscitation is another.

When advance directives or other legally binding documents reflective of patients' wishes are unavailable and patients lack capacity to speak for themseleves, controversies about end-of-life care decisions may arise potentially leading to ethical or legal concerns (Case Manager's Tip 13.13). In such cases, pursuing surrogate decision making is advised. However, conflict among the patient's family members or between family members and healthcare provider may also occur. The stories of some cases have made national news in the past such as a family seeking a court order to remove life support from a patient who, medical experts say, is in a vegetative state with no hope of recovery and no legal documents available to protect the healthcare provider wishing to terminate care. For example, the most recent Schiavo case in 2005, the Cruzan case in 1990, and the Quinlan case in 1976.

In the absence of such written documents, supporting the patient's wishes by honoring verbal statements made by the patient to a another close person (e.g., a family member or friend) prior to losing capacity allows healthcare providers to respect the patients wishes. However, there are situations where the patient's wishes are unknown; for example, when patients have not made their decisions about medical/healthcare known to others including family, friends, or healthcare team. The ethical and legal procedures then focus on implementing the patient's presumed wishes through what is knows as "substituted judgment." This means that a patient's surrogate must make the decisions for the patient. If the patient has not appointed a surrogate in an advance directive, healthcare proxy, or any other legal form, the patient's close family members are ethically and legally empowered to make decisions for the patient. The trend is the past when such situations first arose, has been to override refusals of treatment. Since the 1980s however, the trend has shifted to honoring them, even when doing so may cause the patient's death and may run counter to the interests of the patient, family, community, society, and/or healthcare professionals.

In one case, *Allore v. Flower Hospital* (121 Ohio App3d 229, 1997), the client had signed a living will and then went into respiratory distress during the night. The nurse was unaware of the living will and there was no copy on record; therefore the nurse initiated lifesaving measures while trying to reach the patient's doctor. The patient died in the ICU later that day, but the patient's estate sued claiming medical malpractice and medical battery arising from wrongful administration of life-prolonging treatment. The court held that the nurse complied with applicable standards of care regarding emergency care in the absence of knowledge of existing directives and that there was no battery because the patient had signed a consent for treatment when he entered the hospital. As a result the estate could not recover any damages. Educating clients on the value of advance directives and making their wishes clear to those involved in their care is an important job of the case manager.

Some states have specific laws about palliative and end-of-life care, such as in the state of New York which has passed a law that went into effect in February 2011 (Palliative Care Information Act of 2010). This law requires physicians and nurse practitioners to offer terminally-ill patients information and counseling concerning palliative and end-of-life care options. The law applies only to patients with a condition that is reasonably expected to cause death within six months. It assures that patients are fully informed of the options available to them when they are faced with a terminal illness or condition, so that they are empowered to

CASE MANAGER'S TIP 13.13

End-of-Life Care Concerns

Traditionally, the ethical and legal concerns with end-of-life care have focused on the interest of patients based on autonomy and self-determination, especially for those who have capacity to make such decisions. Going against a patient's wishes is an inexcusable invasion to autonomy and right to choice. When a patient is deemed incompetent or becomes unconscious and no longer can make wishes known, honoring his/her wishes and interests expressed in available advance directive, healthcare proxy, living will, or power of attorney is a way of maintaining the person's right to choice and autonomy.

make choices consistent with their goals for care, and their wishes and beliefs, and to optimize their quality of life.

13.12.7. Denial of Service

This is never received well by patients and their families. Often the case manager acts as a mediator when dealing with denials of services by an MCO. To mediate successfully and effectively, case managers must be knowledgeable about the denials and appeals processes, the patient's bill of rights, and state laws that govern the operations of MCOs. In *Payton v. Aetna US Healthcare*, attorney Robert Payton sought coverage from his Aetna US Healthcare HMO for inpatient rehabilitation for substance abuse in January 1998 while hospitalized for a first-time drug overdose (*Payton v. Aetna US Healthcare*, 100440/99). When the company did not respond, he repeatedly requested coverage and reimbursement, as did his treatment facilities. The requests were denied. In June 1998 he filed a formal complaint with the state attorney general. Within 6 weeks the state attorney general notified Aetna that Payton's individual policy "plainly" covered inpatient substance abuse rehabilitation. Payton also filed a grievance with Aetna. An internal appeals hearing decided that he was entitled to coverage. However, by that time Payton had been deceased for 8 days after a second drug overdose. Payton's estate sued Aetna, charging that the HMO was responsible for his death as a result of negligently delaying coverage (Riccardi, 2000).

Some of the decisions case managers make may result in professional liability, depending on the outcomes of these decisions and their effect on the patient (Case Manager's Tip 13.14). To avoid legal action related to professional liability similar to the cases discussed, case managers, whether they work for a health insurance plan, an MCO, or a healthcare provider, have

an obligation to act as a patient advocate, especially in negotiating decisions regarding services and financial coverage. If a conflict arises, case managers should refer the situation to their superiors so that it can be dealt with appropriately. They may refer the situation to the risk management department or the lawyer as a potential litigation situation so that legal risk is avoided or prevented. A proactive approach such as this usually works in favor of both the patient and the healthcare organization.

A judge ordered $120.5 million in the case of *Teresa Goodrich v. Aetna US Healthcare of California* (Robbins, 1999). This is the largest award against a managed care company to date. The case dealt with denying payment for treatment that was deemed experimental. No mention or explanation of this term was given in the 20-page handbook that Aetna members were given, even though this was the justification of the denial. *Nelene Fox v. Healthnet* (Thomasma and Marshall, 1997) is another case that involved "experimental procedures" that resulted in an award of $89.3 million to the plaintiff. The final outcome in both cases was the death of the patient. A rule of thumb for preventing such cases of litigation is that case managers must always advocate for their patients. The healthcare community can no longer maximize financial concerns at the expense of patient concerns.

Payers, health insurance plans, and MCOs have a duty to inform patients of their right to appeal insurance denials. Many times it is the case manager who informs the patient of the appeal and grievance processes. It is not uncommon for a request for service to be denied because of a lack of some important information. Case managers must communicate clearly, thoroughly, and in a timely fashion with regard to the patient's condition and the medical necessity of the service or equipment.

Sometimes a letter from the physician or a conference call with the payer's representative (e.g., physician-to-physician review) successfully clarifies a point of conflict. In other instances, the sharing of pictures or consumer letters may be needed. Case managers must remember that they cannot resolve every conflict or denial. Sometimes no amount of information is enough to reverse or prevent a denial, and a full appeal process becomes the only option for the patient. In situations where denial of a service is unavoidable and the case manager feels that the patient truly needs the service, the case manager may try to obtain charitable contributions from agencies that provide the needed service. It is advisable that case managers keep information on such resources available for use when needed.

 CASE MANAGER'S TIP 13.14

Case Manager's Professional Obligations and Liability

A case manager is obligated to participate actively in the patient's medical management and care decisions to ensure quality healthcare in the most cost-efficient manner. If the case manager's decisions result in harm to the patient, denial of an essential service (i.e., diagnostic or therapeutic procedure or test), or interference with or corruption of acceptable medical judgment, there may be grounds for professional liability.

13.12.8. Breach of Confidentiality

This is a claim that can sometimes bring severe consequences for the claimant. A former patient of a reputable hospital claimed that the medical institution ruined his life by giving information about his psychiatric troubles to a disgruntled former friend without his permission/consent. He sued the institution for $12 million. The former patient said that the hospital released his medical records to a former friend and business partner who claimed to be him. The former colleague then shared the information about his drug abuse problems with his other friends, family, business associates, and clients (Graham, 2001).

The claim in this case according to the court documents was that the plaintiff had suffered, and continued to suffer, severe injury to his personal and professional reputation and standing in the community, loss of business, physical stress, mental and emotional anguish, and humiliation. This claim was made based on the argument that the plaintiff's suffering is a direct and proximate result of the hospital's unauthorized disclosure of medical records. However, the hospital stated that it acted in good faith and that the request for the medical records had all the requisite information. They believed that the signature on the request was a forgery. This trial is currently pending (Graham, 2001). Case managers can safeguard a patient's confidentiality by reinforcing compliance with the law and regulations regarding disclosure of information and the patient's bill of rights (Case Manager's Tips 13.15 and 13.16).

Healthcare is one of the most personal services rendered in our society, yet to deliver this care, scores of personnel must have access to intimate patient information. In return, the healthcare provider, including the case manager, must safeguard the patient's confidentiality and right to privacy at all times. In the

 CASE MANAGER'S TIP 13.15

Confidential Information

Information shared by the patient or family with the case manager or any other member of the healthcare team is considered confidential and privileged and must not be shared with an unauthorized party without the patient's consent/knowledge. This information is usually shared under circumstances of trust and confidence. Examples of such information are medical history; medications intake; results of the medical/physical examination; information gathered by assessment, observation, and monitoring; and treatments and procedures.

 CASE MANAGER'S TIP 13.16

Safeguarding the Patient's Privacy and Confidentiality (Bernzweig, 1990)

- Abide by the law at all times.
- Have the patient/family/caregiver sign a release of information before any information is shared with other parties.
- Ensure moral and ethical conduct at all times.
- Exercise the duty to treat patients with decency, respect, and utmost privacy.

Exceptions to the privacy rule are as follows:

- When the patient is a public figure whose actions are considered to be of legitimate interest to the public.
- Duty to communicate communicable diseases, child or elder abuse cases, domestic violence cases, and/ or bioterrorism to appropriate law enforcement authorities.

case of *Hobbs v. Lopez* (645 N.E. 2d 261 OH, 1994), a 21-year-old woman was seen by a physician who diagnosed her pregnancy, discussed options available to her, then sent her home to think over her decision regarding the continuation of the pregnancy. A few days after the visit, the doctor asked the nurse to contact the young woman and find out about her decision. The nurse unwittingly released sensitive information to the young woman's family regarding her pregnancy. She made the parents aware of the girl's consideration of abortion as an option. The young woman later sued based on invasion of privacy, breach of privileged information, and breach of contract.

The Nightingale Pledge states, ". . . I will do all in my power to maintain and elevate the standard of my profession and will hold in confidence all personal matters committed to my keeping and family affairs coming to my knowledge in the practice of my calling. . . ." The American Nurses Association Code of Ethics for Nurses states that "the nurses safeguard the right to privacy for individuals, families, and communities. . . . The nurse has a duty to maintain confidentiality of all patient information, both personal and clinical in the work setting and off duty in all venues including social media or any other means of communication," (ANA, 2015). Judiciously protecting information of a confidential nature and maintaining patient confidentiality is not an easy task. Healthcare providers have a strong tradition of safeguarding private health information. However, in today's world the old system of protecting paper records in locked file cabinets no longer applies and the use of social media makes it more challenging to assure privacy and confidentiality at all times.

The automation of medical information permits the collection, analysis, storage, and retrieval of vast amounts of medical information that may not only be used but also may be shared with other providers at remote locations. The Health Insurance Portability and Accountability Act of 1996 (HIPAA) came about because of the advent of EMRs. The portability aspect of this regulation ensures that individuals moving from one health plan to another will have continuity of coverage and will not be denied coverage under pre-existing condition clauses.

The Privacy Rule for the first time creates national standards to protect individuals' medical records and other personal health information. It gives patients more control over their health information and sets boundaries on the use and release of health records. To protect the privacy of health information, the Privacy Rule also establishes appropriate safeguards that healthcare providers and others are required to adhere to. In addition, it holds violators accountable with civil and criminal penalties that can be imposed if they violate the patient's right to privacy.

HIPAA enables patients to find out how their information may be used and what disclosures of their information have been or are to be made. It generally limits the release of information to the minimum reasonably needed for the purpose of the disclosure, and it gives patients the right to examine and obtain a copy of their own health record and to request corrections if they choose to. For the average healthcare provider or health plan, the Privacy Rule requires activities such as the following:

- Providing information to patients about their privacy rights and how their information is used
- Adopting clear and appropriately communicated privacy procedures in their practice
- Training employees so that they understand the privacy procedures
- Designating an individual to be responsible for seeing that the privacy procedures are adopted and maintained at all times
- Securing patient records containing individually identifiable health information so that they are not readily available to those who do not need them (45 CFR Parts 160 and 164)
- Civil penalties for noncompliance with the security standards of HIPAA may range from $100 to $50,000 per person, violation, or record with a maximum penalty of $1.5 million per year for violations of identical nature per calendar year. Violations can also result in criminal charges and jail time (USDHHS, 2015)

- HIPAA violation categories and associated penalties per violation are as follows:
  - Did not know: $100–$50,000; $25,000 for repeat violations with a maximum of $50,000
  - Reasonable cause: $1,000–$50,000
  - Willful neglect—corrected: $10,000–$50,000
  - Willful neglect—uncorrected: $50,000 and/or imprisonment for up to 1 year if a person knowingly obtains or discloses individually identifiable health information
  - An indiviudal involved in a violation may also face, in addition to the fine, an imprisonment up to a year. For violations committed under false pretenses may result in penalties up to $100,000 with also up to 5 years of imprisonment. Violations of the intent to sell, transfer, or use individually identifiable information for commercial advantage, personal gain, or malicious harm may result in fines of $250,000 and up to 10 years of imprisonment (USDHHS, 2015).

Case managers are advised to assure that HIPAA expectations are adhered to and to remain abreast of the latest practices and changes in the law.

13.13. ROLE OF THE MEDICAL RECORD REVIEW IN A LAWSUIT

What happens when a patient sees an attorney about a complaint? Usually the medical record is requested for review by the patient and/or his or her legal representative. For "discovery," the attorney or the attorney's appointee will review the record for evidence of negligence, violation of the standard of care, or any other type of violation; for example, patient's rights. Discov-

CASE MANAGER'S TIP 13.17

Who Can Be Named in a Lawsuits

Any member of the interdisciplinary healthcare team directly or indirectly involved in the care of the patient can be named in a lawsuit, dependent on the the concerns the patient is suing for. This may include the following:

- Physician of record/primary care provider
- Specialty care provider
- Case manager
- Clinical nurses
- Social worker
- Physical therapy (other therapists)
- Pharmacist
- Employer of the providers
- Healthcare facility where care is provided

ery is defined as finding legal merit in a case through the collection of evidence and putting the evidence together in the form of elements of the theory that make the case for legal pursuit.

If it is determined that the case has merit and it does go to court, the record is copied and reviewed again right before the court date. The second review of the medical record aims at identifying any additions or changes made to the record that were not there before the action was taken. If there were new entries, this would give the appearance of tampering with the record and would not bode well for the healthcare provider or facility named in the lawsuit (Case Manager's Tip 13.17).

A similar review process takes place by the attorney representing the healthcare provider or the facility named in the lawsuit. Case managers may be involved in a lawsuit if they had anything to do with the care of the patient suing. If the patient has been discharged or transitioned from the healthcare facility to another and care is no longer being provided, case management and other treatments or services should have been terminated and the medical record should be considered closed. Termination of services and closure of the patient's medical record refer to the episode of care (e.g., the acute care hospital stay). Any additional documentation in the record will be considered falsification and will serve against the healthcare provider(s) named in the lawsuit. Case managers can review the medical record for completeness before it is shared with the patient's attorney. However, sometimes they may not have the privilege to conduct a final review because of time constraints and attorney or court pressures.

13.14. PROFESSIONAL MISCONDUCT

When a nurse is accused of professional misconduct,

 CASE MANAGER'S TIP 13.18

Case Managers Under Investigation Due to Lawsuit

When a case manager is being investigated or reviewed for professional misconduct due to a patient/family complaint or a lawsuit, not only the state licensing board of the jurisdiction governing the region where the case manager operates gets involved in the investiogation or review, other credentialing agencies such as a certifying body (e.g., Commission for Case Manager Certification, American Nurses Credentialing Center/ANA) also gets involved if the case manager possesses a certification from such agencies.

the state board of nursing usually investigates the claim by conducting an administrative review. This is a separate appearance from a civil action in court. The state board of nursing can take disciplinary action against a nurse for any violation of the state's nurse practice act. In all states and provinces, the board of nursing has the authority to discipline a nurse if he or she endangers the patient's health, safety, or welfare. Furthermore, the nurse could find herself listed with the NPDB if a violation is confirmed.

When case managers are accused of professional misconduct, depending on the professional background of the case manager, the state board governing the professional background also gets involved. For example, for nurse case manager, the nursing state board, and licensing agency get involved in the investigation; for social work case managers, the social work licensing board gets involved. In the states where there is no licensing board for social work, the state agency responsible for credentialing social workers and granting work permission gets involved instead (Case Manager Tip 13.18).

The NPDB was created by the Health Care Quality Improvement Act of 1986 and became operational in 1990 (USDHHS, 2000). The NPDB collects information about practitioners who may endanger the public welfare. The data is available to employers in an effort to restrict the ability of incompetent practitioners to move from state to state. Information reported about nurses to the NPDB includes the following:

- Malpractice payments made by a healthcare professional (a case manager, nurse, or social worker), including judgments, arbitration decisions, and out-of-court settlements
- Actions taken against a healthcare professional's clinical privileges
- Adverse licensure actions, including revocations, suspensions, reprimands, censure, or probation
- A healthcare professional can dispute a report, even if it requires taking his or her claim to the Secretary of Health and Human Services. It is important to note that the NPDB is the repository of information about professionals licensed by states to work in medicine, nursing, pharmacy, physical therapy, occupational therapy, and social work. Case managers are subsumed under the profession reflective of the background such as nursing or social work.

13.15. RISK MANAGEMENT

Risk management refers to the process of identifying issues of concern in patient care such as delays in ser-

CASE MANAGER'S TIP 13.19

Prevention of Risk Management Concerns

It is necessary for case managers to adopt a risk management style in daily practice to prevent issues of risk and ultimately malpractice and litigation. A guide for such style is constant focus on communication, compassion, competence, and documentation.

- *Communication*: honesty; discretion; respect; open, accurate, timely, and responsible communication help prevent miscommunication, conflict, misaligned expectations, issues or concerns.
- *Compassion*: express sympathy toward the patient and family, be supportive and available/accessible to them. Assist the patient and family in all ways possible during care provision; provide emotional support and counseling to alleviate their concerns and apprehensions.
- *Competence*: it is important to maintain current knowledge, skills and competencies in the practice of case management and in healthcare delivery.
- *Documentation*: document what is important and necessary in the patient's medical record. Be accurate, factual, transparent, and timely in your documentation. Assure the patient's medical record tells the patient's story and the documentation is free of judgment, subjectivity, or information that is conflicting with the documentation of other healthcare professionals involved in the patient's care.

vices, omissions of treatments, or significant medical errors. Case managers are able to identify actual or potential risk management concerns either during a patient's medical record review or from interdisciplinary patient care management rounds and communication with those involved in the care. No matter the degree of seriousness of such events, a thorough review/investigation is necessary whether independently or in collaboration with a member of the quality, safety, or risk management department. When not addressed effectively, these events may result in potential lawsuits by the patient/family against healthcare providers including the facility and the case manager. Box 13.9 describes an approach for the prevention of lawsuits as a result of risk management concerns.

13.16. PROTECTING THE CASE MANAGER IN A LITIGIOUS SOCIETY

Education should be one of the most important values of the professional case manager. Therefore the first piece of advice for case managers to protect them-

selves from litigation is to never stop learning! Other recommendations are as follows:

- Make it a point to stay abreast of the legislation that impacts healthcare and case management practice both at the federal and state level.
- Always review the state professional practice act just to bring to mind what the statutes describe as case management practice.
- It is not necessary to subscribe to every journal of nursing or other fields, but case managers should review pertinent journal articles that address their clinical area of practice. This can be accomplished relatively painlessly by covering current articles in an executive summary format at department meetings. Several members may review different journals and report to the group.
- Maintain membership in professional associations. This helps case managers to stay current in their field and gives them a voice in government and in the eye of the public.
- Network with professional colleagues. This may help the case manager with problem solving and may strengthen the case management profession.
- Maintain rapport with patients and their families or caregivers. This is one of the simplest and most important things case managers can do to stay out of the courtroom and away from disciplinary action.
- See and care for the patient as a whole person. The importance of this aspect of care cannot be overstated.
- Tailor care to meet the specific needs of the individual patient.
- Follow up on issues with sincere concern—become a touchstone for the patient in a world that has become increasingly impersonal.
- Establish a connection or a bond with the patient and the family. This will go a long way toward protecting the case manager from litigation.
- Be transparent with the patient and family; disclose care events as they occur and support the patient and family through tough times. Consult with risk management, patient representative/advocacy department, or patient safety officer as necessary before you disclose.
- Engage the patient and family in shared decision-making about care options, especially post-discharge services and setting.
- Assure appropriate procedure of informed consent. Ensure that consent includes discussion of risks and benefits.

We do not live in a perfect world, and sometimes, despite everyone's guidance and care, unfortunate things happen to a patient. Reviewing a chart that has carefully and thoroughly documented the case management process will often cause a case to be dismissed during the discovery phase. Remember that the chart is a potential witness in the courtroom—one that the case manager can influence by ensuring that all of the significant information is accurately recorded. The patient's record must reflect communication between the case manager and the following:

- Patient, family, or caregiver
- Physician of record, consultants, and specialty care providers
- Case management team (i.e., other healthcare providers involved in the patient's care)
- Health insurance plan and sources of authorization for care/services

Case management is not a job for the faint of heart. An understanding and appreciation of the legal process, areas of potential liability, and the critical importance of communication support the case manager in giving sound and legitimate care to clients. Those who endure are the crusaders who are leading the nursing, case management, and other professions forward into the challenge of modern healthcare and who are paving the road for their colleagues with their dedication, creativity, and devotion to the patient.

13.17. KEY POINTS

1. Consumers of healthcare services are most likely to sue providers (including case managers) and/or payers if they feel that their rights have been violated or their care was substandard.

2. Case managers are becoming increasingly exposed to potential lawsuits because of the increased autonomy and independence of their roles.

3. Case management is considered a reasonable activity. It may increase or curtail the likelihood of a lawsuit.

4. Failure to communicate or document an inadequate or premature patient's discharge or transition to another care setting is more likely today than ever before to result in litigation against case managers.

5. Denials of services may result in lawsuits if these decisions were not made based on na-

tionally recognized and evidence-based standards in utilization management.

6. Applying a formal approach to shared-decision making prevents patient's lawsuits. Such an approach assures informed consent and protects patient's right to choice, autonomy, and self-determination.

7. Education, knowledge, skills, and level of competence are the case manager's best defense against legal risk.

8. Case managers can be held liable. They should be aware of the legal process and the legal terminology used.

9. Standardized, evidence-based case management plans are admissible in court. They can be reviewed by the jury to determine the standard of care followed at the time care was provided. These plans should be developed following a scientific and evidence-based process.

10. Thorough documentation in the medical record is extremely important. The patient's medical record can be admissible in court as evidence.

11. Case managers can curtail legal risk by being proactive in their role (e.g., by anticipating and preventing variances or delays in care delivery and outcomes) and act as patient advocates above all.

13.18. REFERENCES

American Nurses Association. (2015). Code of ethics: the center of ethics and human rights, Silver Springs, MD.

American Thoracic Society. Accessed June 10, 2015. Chronic obstructive pulmonary disease guidelines: criteria for hospital discharge. Available at www.thoracic.org/copd-guidelines/for-health-professionals/exacerbation/definition-evaluation-and-treatment/inpatient/criteria-for-hospital-discharge.php

Bernzweig, E.P. (1990). *The nurse's liability for malpractice: a programmed course*, 5th ed., Mosby, St. Louis, MO.

Graham, S. (2001). Hopkins sued for $12M, hospital released man's medical files, *Baltimore Business J 19*(13):24–30.

Health Intelligence Network, Healthcare Performance Benchmarks. (2012). Healthcare Case Management, Wall Township, NJ.

Holzer, J.F. (1990). The advent of clinical standards for professional liability, *Qual Rev Bull 16*(2):71–79.

Merz, S.M. (1993). Clinical practice guidelines: policy issues and legal implications, *J Qual Improve 19*(8):306–311.

National Practitioner Data Bank, Healthcare Integrity and Protection Data Bank. Accessed December 19, 2001. Fact sheet on the healthcare integrity and pro- tection data bank. Available online at www.npdb-hipdb.com/pubs/fs/nh017fs.pdf

Nichols, D.J. (1996). Legal liabilities in case management. In Flarey, D.L., Smith-Blancett. S.: *Handbook of case management,* Aspen, Gaithersburg, MD.

Nolin, C.E. & Lang, C.G. (1992). *An analysis of the use and effect of caremap tools in medical malpractice litigation,* The Center for Case Management, Inc., South Natick, MA.

Riccardi, M. (2000). Negligence claim against HMO stands, *New York Law J 223*(57):1.

Robbins, D.A. (1999). Putting care above profit, *Continuing Care 18*(4):18.

Sturgeon, S. (1997). Legal issues in the operation of referral and utilization review systems, *Manag Care Interface 10*(12):66-70.

U.S. Department of Health and Human Services, Health Resources and Services Administration, Bureau of Health Professions. Accessed December 19, 2001. National Practitioner Data Bank, 2000, annual report. Available online at www.npdb-hipdb.com/pubs/stats/00annrpt.pdf

U.S. Department of Health and Human Services, Health Resources and Services Administration. Accessed June 10, 2015. National Practitioner Data Bank, available at www.npdb.hrsa.gov/resources/hipdbArchive.jsp

U.S. Department of Health and Human Services. Accessed June 10, 2015. Improving the health, safety and well-being of America, Understanding health information privacy, available at www.hhs.gov/ocr/privacy/hipaa/understanding/index.html

U.S. Department of Health and Human Services, Centers for Medicare and Medcaid Services, Medicare Learning Network. 2014. Medicare Fraud and Abuse: prevention, detection and reporting, August 2014, ICN 006827.

U.S. Department of Justice, Office of Justice Programs, Bureau of Justice Statistics. 2014. Elderly abuse statistics.

West, J.C. (1994). The legal implications of medical practice guidelines, *J Health Hosp Law 27*(4):97–103.

Zweig, F.M. & Witte, H.A. (1993). Assisting judges in screening medical practice guidelines for health care litigation, *J Qual Improve 19*(8):342–353.

14

Ethical Issues and Standards in Case Management

In recent years, Americans have witnessed well-documented and widely discussed changes in their healthcare system. Unlike an earlier era of "unmanaged" health insurance, millions of Americans today are covered by health insurance plans that employ various techniques to curtail rising healthcare costs. These techniques have shifted a considerable amount of decision-making authority from physicians and patients to health insurance plans including the Centers for Medicare and Medicaid Services (CMS) and managed care organizations (MCOs). This shift has also given rise to skepticism concerning the quality and safety of healthcare patients can expect under a tightly controlled system of health insurance.

The changes in the American healthcare system also present a number of ethical problems and challenges for healthcare professionals, and case managers are no exception. Professional ethics has to do with standards of "right" and "wrong" conduct as they apply to members of a particular profession. Ethical dilemmas commonly arise when the professional is faced with a situation where two conflicting duties may apply and it is unclear which one is most appropriate resulting in moral distress. When this happens, the professional must decide which duty takes precedence over the other and on what grounds. Case managers sometimes are required to work through these dilemmas alone, without the support or counsel of other members of the organization for which they work. Over time, the stress of making these decisions without organizational and expert support can result in reduced job satisfaction, resentment, or burnout.

Chapter 14 discusses the types of ethical problems that case managers may face in their everyday practice. Case managers confront many of the same ethical problems as other healthcare professionals working in provider settings, governmental healthcare agencies, and health insurance plans including MCOs. Nonetheless, these problems are particularly challenging for case managers because nurses and social workers have long defined themselves as patient advocates (Jansen, 2001). By understanding the underlying causes of the ethical problems in some detail, a framework for resolving them can be identified. This framework, known as the deliberative framework, is one that case managers are well suited for given their education, training, and experience.

14.1. COMMERCIAL HEALTH INSURANCE, MANAGED CARE, AND PATIENT ADVOCACY

Many who have written about ethics in the era of increased scrutiny by commercial health insurance plans and managed care have assumed, either explicitly or implicitly, that the traditional ethics of the profession can and should be simply applied to the new circumstances. It is true that case managers need to be familiar with the code of ethics for their profession and health discipline. However, it is a mistake to think that the traditional principles of ethics can be easily applied within the context of tightly regimented health insurance plans. Although the traditional principles of justice, autonomy, and beneficence are important, the meaning of these principles in the context of health insurance plans and managed care organizations must be substantially rethought. Moreover, new principles and new ideals need to be articulated and defended for nurses, case managers, social workers and other healthcare professionals who work in this context.

To understand why this is the case, we need to begin by considering the traditional ideal of the nurse or social worker as a patient advocate. This ideal has a strong claim to be the foundation on which traditional nursing and social work ethics rests (Jansen, 2001) and therefore, case management ethics. As this ideal has been commonly understood, the nurse, social worker, and other professionals involved in the practice of case management are expected to look out for and promote what is in the patient's best interest, irrespective of the patient's race, sex, age, value system, socioeconomic class, health insurance status, and cultural background.

14.1.1. Patient Advocacy and Beneficence

Patient advocacy relates to the ethical principle of beneficence (Case Manager's Tip 14.1). According to this principle, the case manager works with the physician and other members of the interdisciplinary healthcare team to advance the best interests of the patient and family. This ethical principle basically focuses on "promoting the interests of others;" where one may translate it to the act of preventing harm or improving the situation for the patient/family. Due to the nature of the relationship case managers have with their patients, they are obliged to weigh and balance the possible benefits against potential risks of an action, intervention, or treatment; even decisions, especially concerning care options. They also are expected to protect and defend the rights of their patients/families, help those unable to speak or assist themselves, especially during unsafe or potentially dangerous situations. For example, encouraging patients to engage in healthy lifestyle behavior, adhere to follow-up care appointments, and assure safe transitions of care advance the patient's interests and prevent the unnatural progression of health condition or disease state.

The principle of beneficence should be distinguished from the virtue of benevolence. The benevolent person is well disposed toward others. He or she cares about the others' well-being. By contrast, beneficence is an ethical principle that directs the healthcare professional to take action to promote the safety and well-being of his or her patients. The terms benevolence and beneficence should be distinguished because it is possible for case managers to promote the good of others without being well disposed toward them, and it is possible to be well disposed toward others and yet fail to promote their interests.

The principle of beneficence, at least as it has been

CASE MANAGER'S TIP 14.1

The Case Manager as Patient Advocate

An essential role of the case manager is patient/family advocate. An advocate is someone who is able to plead the cause of another (i.e., beneficence). In this role the case manager may be presented with conflicting choices. Using the principle of beneficence, the case manager should always select the choice that will advance the best interests of the patient and family. As a rule of thumb, everything a case manager or healthcare professional does should be subordinate to the patient's interest. As a patient advocate, the case manager must provide patients and their families with the information necessary to help them make better informed decisions concering their healthcare services and must support the decisions they make.

understood in medicine and healthcare, is not general, but rather specific. It directs the healthcare professional to promote the interests of his or her patients rather than the interests of all patients or of all potential patients (Beauchamp & Childress, 1994). For example, it is sometimes said that a special relationship exists between healthcare professionals and their particular patients and that this relationship grounds the requirement of beneficence (Beauchamp & Childress, 1994).

Finally, the principle of beneficence in medicine and healthcare delivery has traditionally been understood to be an "interest-maximizing" principle. This means that it requires healthcare professionals to not just promote their patient's best interests, but rather to do all that can be done to advance these interests.

14.1.2. Beneficence and Nonmaleficence

Case managers must understand the difference between beneficence and nonmaleficence. While beneficence concerns doing what is in the best interest of others, nonmaleficence is doing no harm to others. From the perspective of the ethical principle of nonmaleficence, case managers must assure that the healthcare interventions, services, and case management plans provide effective treatments and care for their patients, which means provision of quality, safe, efficient, and cost-conscious care. This presents a challenge because some treatment options or interventions may come with certain levels of risk or may be viewed as burdensome by patients or their families. For example, when case managers transition some patients from the acute to the subacute or skilled care setting, despite their effective hand-off communication and carefully designed transition of care plans, continuity of care when the patient is at the next care setting may still turn out to be suboptimal, medical errors may occur, and some patients may return to the acute care hospital setting. These outcomes are not ususally directly linked to case managers' actions of intentionally "doing harm" to their patients. Regardless however, case managers must assure the patient's transition is safe, free of concerns, and that the healthcare team at the next level of care is ready, knowledgeable of the plan of care, and comfortable to safely care for the patient post-transition.

Case managers should balance the risks with benefits when deciding on the plans of care for their patients. They also must educate patients and their families about an intervention's potential undesired effects before implementing the intervention, or ensure they are educated by another member of the interdisciplinary healthcare team. Because some treatments and interventions may cause harm while at the same time present patients with certain benefits, the principle of nonmaleficence alone provides little concrete guidance in deciding about the care of patients. Case managers must consider this principle together with the principle of beneficence and balance against it. In such cases, the risk for harm potentially inflicted by the treatment must be examined carefully against the potential benefits. Case managers in these situations can counsel and educate their patients about the treatment options and assure the patients understand the risks and benefits and are able to make informed decisions while considering these potential benfits and harms.

A common ethical dilemma arises from the action of balancing benefits (i.e., beneficence) and risks or harm (i.e., nonmaleficence). Such situations may potentially be present in nearly every dscision a patient or family must make; for example, which skilled or subacute care facility is best for the patient who must transition to from the acute care hospital setting? Case managers also face such dilemmas when offering patients and their families with a list of choices about potential facilities. Some may have better safety and quality outcomes than others. By assisting patients with making informed decisions, case managers assure that patients understand the potential risks and benefits and decide on the option where the benefits outweigh the risks for the decision to then be considered ethical or has met ethical standards.

Accordingly, the traditional ethical ideal of the case manager as a patient advocate is an ideal that directs the case manager to act in ways that will maximize the best interests of his or her own patients and their families. There is little doubt that this ideal is inspiring. It has given, and continues to give, content to the ideal that nursing, social work, case management, and other healthcare-related professions are moral professions. Yet, notwithstanding its strong appeal, in recent years many have begun to challenge the principle of beneficence that forms this ideal. Experts have argued that this principle is actually socially irresponsible and that it has contributed to the accelerating costs of healthcare. These doubts have become all the more pronounced as we have moved into a healthcare delivery environment and system that places a provider at financial risk based on patient care quality outcomes, safety, and experience of care.

Given its importance, let us look at this criticism in a little more detail. According to the critics, the traditional principle of beneficence, which forms the traditional ideal of the nurse (social worker or any healthcare professional) as a patient advocate, rests on an outdated model of the clinician/patient relationship. This model inaccurately characterizes the clinician/patient relationship if applied in a health insurance plan context including MCOs. This is true for a number of reasons, among which are the following:

1. The principle of beneficence assumes and takes as its paradigm an overly individualistic relationship between the healthcare provider and patient (Buchanan, 2000).
2. The principle of beneficence assumes that the healthcare provider is unconstrained by his or her role in an organization or by organizational policies (Buchanan, 2000).
3. The principle of beneficence characterizes the healthcare provider's obligation to his or her patient in interest-maximizing terms, which is socially irresponsible given the scarcity of healthcare resources and the need to contain healthcare costs (Daniels & Sabin, 1997).

These criticisms are compelling. Whatever one thinks of healthcare insurance plans and MCOs, it is clear that it has transformed the clinician/patient relationship. Through their decisions regarding insurance coverage, health insurance plans, especially MCOs, have assumed the authority to decide effectively when, where, and how to limit access to a range of medically beneficial services. These coverage decisions are crucial to the cost-containment techniques characteristic of health insurance plans and MCOs.

This transfer of decision-making authority to the health insurance plan (i.e., the payer) has in turn transformed the relationship between healthcare professionals, case managers, and their patients/families. Physicians are no longer in a position to provide their patients with all of the care that might reasonably be expected to benefit them and in any setting of their choosing. During the fee-for-service era of healthcare delivery, care providers could act as if their patients were the only patients there were and they could proceed, at least in many cases, with no concern for costs. In so doing, it was commonly thought they discharged their duty of beneficence. But with the current healthcare reimbursement system where the provider is at an increased financial risk whether due to utilization management practices of MCOs and payers or value-based purchasing programs—with strong emphasis on cost-containment, delivery of safe and quality care—the fee-for-service approach is no longer a viable option.

For the same reasons, the traditional ideal of the case manager as a patient advocate is not a viable option in the context of increased focus on cost reduction. It is an ideal that has a place when the clinician/patient relationship is conceived in individualistic terms and when the need to contain healthcare costs is not pressing. Still, it would be a mistake to conclude from this that case managers working in strict health insurance and managed care environments should cease to think of themselves as patient advocates (Case Manager's Tip 14.2). If nursing and social work are to remain as moral professions, then case managers should not abandon the ideal of patient advocacy when they case manage patients in today's healthcare environment that is challenged with cost reduction, value-based purchasing, hospital readmission reduction programs, and transparency in reporting outcomes of care including patient experience during an episode of care. Instead, they must rethink the content of this ideal for these new circumstances.

14.1.3. Rethinking Ethics

Case managers must adjust their ethical self-understanding to fit today's competitive and challenging healthcare environment in which they practice. Like the traditional physician/patient relationship, the traditional nurse/patient and social worker/patient relationship is transformed once cost containment becomes a pressing issue. Under health insurance plans, nurses—and case managers in particular—have conflicting loyalties. They have obligations both to their patients and to the payer organization for which they work. Balancing these obligations in an ethically appropriate way requires that they cease thinking in terms of maximizing the interests of their patients. Recognition of this important point is the first step in reformulating the traditional ideal of the case manager as patient advocate.

Often case managers are found to advocate for the patients they serve and execute on case management plans that are intended to safeguard what is in the best interest of patients. Simultaneously however, case managers work with representatives of the health insurance plans and managed care organziations (i.e., the payer) to assure effective utilization of healthcare resources and adherence to the insurer's utilization management procedures such as provision of a treatment after it has been authorized by the health insurance plan. In such situations, waiting for authorization may result in delaying treatment which may ultimately contribute to suboptimal outcomes. The case manager in these situations ends up struggling between safeguarding the patient while at the same time meeting the expectations of the health insuarnce plan; therefore experiencing moral distress (Case Manager's Tip 14.3).

14.2. CASE MANAGEMENT AND NEW ETHICAL CHALLENGES

The emergence of the health insurance market has brought with it an increased need for case management. HMOs, PPOs, and MCOs have found it necessary to enlist the services of case managers in their efforts to contain costs and maintain quality. According to the ANA, case managers focus on care coordination, financial management, and resource utilization to yield cost-effective outcomes that are patient-centric and safe, while assuring that care is provided in the least restrictive setting. They also consider patients, families, and other stakeholders as essential members of the interdisciplinary healthcare team (Leonard and Miller, 2012). The goals of case management are mainly the provision of quality healthcare that enhances the client's quality of life, efficient utilization of patient care resources, and cost containment. These are all important goals in today's healthcare environment that rewards quality, safety, and lower costs. Done well, case management can reduce the tension between providing quality and safe healthcare while containing healthcare costs. However, it would be a mistake to think that

 CASE MANAGER'S TIP 14.2

Rethinking Clinical Care Decisions

In the past, clinical decisions were made between the patient and the physician. Health insurance plans of today and MCOs have introduced a third party in the clinical decision making process: the insurer/payer. Case managers should always assist patients and families with disputing any decisions made that seem unethical, unfair, or dangerous to the well-being and best interest of the patient.

CASE MANAGER'S TIP 14.3

Moral Distress

In virtue of their roles, case managers assume multiple responsibilities and are accountable to various stakeholders. Often they are found to be accountable to stakeholders with competing demands such as patients and payers. In such circumstnaces, case managers are faced with the conflicting demands of doing what is in the best interest of the patient while at the same time assuring effective resource utilization with special focus on cost reduction. Sometimes, the payer denies a patient a treatment option whether because the payer sees it as unindicated or inappropriate for the care setting the patient is at. The case manager may appeal the payer's decision to deny the treatment or service and the payer may still uphold its decision that the treatment is not indicated. The case manager is put in the situation of advising the patient of the payer's decision, resulting in the case manager feeling moral distress.

Moral distress is a human response to situations of conflict when an indivdiual, such as the case manager in the above example, knows what is ethically appropriate to do but feels unable to take action, leaving the individual feeling loss of integrity.

CASE MANAGER'S TIP 14.4

Balancing Cost and Quality and Safety

When balancing issues of cost versus quality and safety, case managers should always err on the side of quality, safety, and/or the best interest of the patient. Reimbursement should always be a secondary consideration. Assuring the provision of efficient, quality, and safe care reduces financial and reimbursement risks.

---

this tension can ever be fully overcome. Accordingly, the ethical challenges confronting case managers who work in the health insurance plan/payer settings center on how to manage this tension and what to do when the tension becomes too great.

14.2.1. Balancing Cost and Quality

To understand the nature of this tension, we must clarify the competing goals that can come into conflict. The goal of providing quality healthcare must not be identified with the interest-maximizing principle of beneficence discussed previously. Given the scarcity of healthcare resources, case managers should not view themselves as under an obligation to provide maximal care to their patients. Instead, the goal of providing quality and safe healthcare must be understood to refer to a "reasonable" level of care.

The second goal is cost containment. Managing care with limited resources requires case managers to oversee their patients' journey through the healthcare system with an eye toward eliminating inefficiency and unnecessary expense, especially that which results from duplication and fragmentation of services. Moreover, in organizations with a capitated payment system, case managers must balance the needs and in-

terests of different patients to stay within a fixed budget. Additionally, those who work for an organization that is a participant in the Medicare's value-based purchasing program must assure the provision of efficient, safe, and quality services which assure optimal patient experience of care while keeping a close eye on the cost of these services.

The goal of providing quality healthcare grounds obligations to specific patients. The goal of containing costs grounds obligations to third-party payers, provider systems, and society at large (Case Manager's Tip 14.4). This last point is important. Cost containment is often disparaged as a financial rather than a medical and quality goal. This is only partly true because cost-containment techniques are essential to provide members of society—all of whom are either patients or potential patients—with affordable healthcare. When case managers function within a legitimate health insurance and managed care environment to limit costs, they are not merely serving the interests of insurance companies but are serving the interests of society as well.

But what is a legitimate health insurance and managed care obligation? And when are decisions to limit care "reasonable?" These questions must be squarely confronted if we are to understand the ethical challenges facing case managers under the payers pressure of cost-reduction and financial or reimbursement risks. Unfortunately, these questions are not easily answered. Not only are there no socially accepted standards of reasonable medical care, but also experts disagree among themselves as to what should count as a just healthcare entitlement (Buchanan, 2000). In the face of this uncertainty and disagreement, any decision to limit healthcare to contain costs is in danger of appearing ad hoc and arbitrary. A number of writers have proposed procedural standards that must be satisfied if cost-cutting decisions are to be legitimate (Buchanan, 2000). These procedural standards can be grouped under the following three principles:

1. The principle of impartiality

2. The principle of publicity
3. The principle of contestability

Case managers need to understand these principles because adhering to them is crucial. It assures that case managers respond ethically to the tension between providing quality and safe healthcare and containing costs.

14.2.2. The Principle of Impartiality

The principle of impartiality requires that similar cases be treated alike. At the minimum, this means that case managers should not make cost-cutting decisions that discriminate against groups on the basis of irrelevant differences such as ethnicity, race, age, gender, or socioeconomic class. The principle also demands that healthcare workers do not provide differential treatment to friends, family members, or those who they deem to be socially or professionally more important. When consistently adhered to, the principle of impartiality mitigates the worry that cost-reduction decisions made by case managers will be arbitrary (Donagrandi and Eddy, 2000).

14.2.3. The Principle of Publicity

As important as the principle of impartiality is, it is not sufficient for legitimate healthcare decision making. Decisions to limit healthcare must not only be fair, but they must also be viewed as fair. This brings us to the principle of publicity (Buchanan, 2000). Cost-cutting decisions, whether made by case managers or others who work with health insurance plans such as HMOs and PPOs to contain costs, must be made on the basis of standards and rules that are both publicly known and publicly justified (Buchanan, 2000). This means that these rules and standards must be accessible to healthcare professionals and their patients alike. Without this kind of openness, it will be difficult to quell the suspicion that coverage decisions are being made on an arbitrary basis.

In addition to being public, these rules and decisions also should be publicly justified. This means two things. First, it means that the reasons or considerations that justify the rules and standards are themselves made public. Second, it means that these reasons and considerations must be based, as far as it is possible to do so, on needs and values that are widely shared. Norman Daniels and James Sabin have expressed the importance of this last point well. What they stated almost two decades ago still applies today:

If the [healthcare] organization shows through the pattern of reasoning (the "case law") reflected in its public reason-giving that its decisions rest on the kinds of reasons all can consider relevant to deciding how to meet varied patient needs under reasonable resource constraints, then even those who disagree with the specific decisions made should acknowledge they are reasonable decisions that are arguably aimed at producing fair outcomes: safe, quality, efficent, and lower cost care (Daniels and Sabin, 1997).

In other words, although adherence to the principle of publicity cannot eliminate disagreement, it may be able to ensure that those who "lose out" in a decision at least will be able to view the decision as one made on grounds that they can recognize it to be appropriate.

14.2.4. The Principle of Contestability

The principle of contestability supplements the other two principles. Decisions made by case managers, as well as others in the health insurance plans or managed care environments (i.e., payers), should be contestable. Physicians, case managers, and other healthcare providers should be encouraging their patients and families to participate in the informed decision-making process and to offer constructive public criticism. One way in which this can be accomplished is for decision-making bodies within payers, MCOs, and PPOs to establish formal dispute resolution procedures such as the process for appealing denials of services. These would allow those who believed that they had been treated unfairly or improperly to make an appeal for redress without resorting to legal action. Case managers can assist widely in facilitating such processes by teaching and guiding patients and their families as to how to go about filing such appeals.

This is important for at least two reasons. First, in the dispute resolution process, new information or new considerations might come to light. This in turn could result in the formulation of better standards for making coverage decisions in the future. Second, by encouraging criticism of their decisions, case managers and others who must make coverage decisions would ensure that they remain accountable to those who are affected by their decisions. This accountability, and the public recognition of it, is crucial to the legitimacy of the decision-making process (Buchanan, 2000).

Legitimate decisions by health insurance plans including MCOs must, accordingly, be impartial, publicly justifiable, and contestable. This is particularly true for decisions to limit care on the basis of cost. Earlier in this chapter it was discussed that the traditional understanding of medical and healthcare beneficence as a duty to maximize the best interests of one's patient—and the ideal of patient advocacy premised on this understanding—must be rethought in the context of managed care and the need for authorizations for certain services, interventions, and treatments. Medical and healthcare beneficence and patient advocacy should be understood in terms of providing one's patient with a reasonable, not a maximal, level of care, and timely care interventions necessary based on the patient's health condition not because of convenience. This suggestion can now be made more concrete. A reasonable level of care can now be understood to be a level of care that is determined by the patient's health insurance plan that makes legitimate coverage decisions despite the case manager's review of medical necessity, where legitimacy is understood in terms of the principles of impartiality, publicity, and contestability.

Accordingly, when case managers act as patient advocates in the context of health insurance plan or payer coverage, they must attempt to provide their patients with the best possible care that is efficient and consistent with legitimate cost-lowering and coverage decisions. By doing so, they will be able to balance their obligation to promote the interests of their patients with their financial and societal obligation to contain healthcare costs and maintain or improve quality and safety.

14.3. MAINTAINING ETHICAL INTEGRITY

The three principles discussed in the previous section ameliorate the tension between providing quality healthcare and containing healthcare costs. However, it is doubtful that the tension can ever be completely overcome. This means that even when payers or health insurance plans make legitimate decisions, healthcare professionals may sometimes find themselves in situations in which they cannot support these decisions in good conscience. When this occurs, how they ought to respond is an important ethical question. For example, consider the case study presented below.

14.3.1. The Problem

A 54-year-old male patient, Mr. Jameson, was being treated with beta-blockers for hypertension. He went to his primary care physician complaining of a dry cough. Mr. Jameson was diagnosed with nasal polyps, and the cough was attributed to postnasal drip. Both Mr. Jameson's physician and case manager responsible for his care believed that he ought to undergo a total systems review. However, limits set by the health insurance plan (an MCO) or payer precluded this. As a result, Mr. Jameson's symptoms were addressed from a cost-only approach, and a specialist denied him care.

14.3.2. Ethical Decision-Making Process to Resolve the Problem

In this case, both Mr. Jameson's physician and his case manager confronted a conflict between their obligation to promote his best interests and their obligation to work within the cost-containment guidelines established by the health insurance plan. To determine how they should have responded to this conflict, we first need to distinguish between two scenarios. In the first scenario, the health insurance plan/MCO does not make legitimate coverage decisions. In other words, it fails to adhere to the principles of impartiality, publicity, and contestability. By contrast, in the second scenario the health insurance plan/MCO does make legitimate coverage decisions.

What should Mr. Jameson's physician and his case manager do in the first scenario? One option is for them to adopt the role of the "saboteur," to use a phrase coined by Allen Buchanan (Buchanan, 2000). Saboteurs seek to circumvent the coverage limits imposed by the health insurance plan or payer. They do this by falsifying diagnoses to get the insurer to cover the services for their patient that they think he or she needs or deserves. In general, this type of response is ethically unacceptable. It requires healthcare professionals to engage in deception, and it does nothing to improve the decision-making processes of the health insurance plan.

A better response in this scenario is for Mr. Jameson's physician and his case manager to press for changes in the way in which their health insurance plan makes coverage decisions. For example, they may advise Mr. Jameson to take legal action against the insurer as a way of putting external pressure on the insurer to make changes. They also may consider lobbying the insurer to establish public appeals procedures that would allow patients like Mr. Jameson the opportunity to challenge the coverage decisions that affect him. Finally, if the insurer is sufficiently unresponsive to making changes that would make it legitimate, they should consider limiting their involvement with the insurer as much as possible.

Most insurers are not as illegitimate as the one envisioned in this first scenario of the case under discussion. Let us turn then to the second scenario of the case. Here the health insurance plan makes impartial and publicly justifiable coverage decisions. When it limits coverage, it does so for reasons that all can accept as valid. Moreover, it permits and even encourages physicians and case managers to contest its decisions in public appeals procedures.

Still, even legitimate health insurance plans or payers can make coverage decisions that strike healthcare professionals as misguided. In the case we are considering, Mr. Jameson's physician and his case manager may still believe that the coverage decision made by the insurer was incorrect. How then should they respond? Clearly, in this scenario they should be not engaged in sabotage. The role of the saboteur is ethically questionable even when the coverage decisions are illegitimate, and when these decisions are legitimate, it is plainly an ethical mistake to falsify a diagnosis. Doing so is deceptive, and it frustrates the legitimate financial and societal goal of containing healthcare costs.

Mr. Jameson's physician and case manager believed that a total systems review was necessary in his case. After this was denied, they should not attempt to circumvent the legitimate decision-making procedures of the health insurance plan. Instead, they should serve as Mr. Jameson's advocate in the appeals process for denial of service. Here they should not argue that Mr. Jameson has a claim to all possible medical care that might reasonably be expected to benefit him. They should rather argue either that the cost-containing policies that affect him ought to be revised or that an exception should be made to these policies in Mr. Jameson's case. If they are unsuccessful, then they should explain to Mr. Jameson that they have done all they could do, given the policies of the organization in which they function. They should also explain to him that although they disagree with the decision of his health insurance plan, they recognize that the organization has a legitimate interest in containing healthcare costs and provision of healthcare services in most appropriate level of care or setting. Finally, if they are aware that a total systems review for Mr. Jameson would have been provided by an alternative insurer, then they should inform him of this fact.

14.3.3. Acting Responsibly

As this case illustrates, the ethics of cost-containment involves in large measure an ability to function responsibly in an organizational setting. This requires a shift in perspective from that of an "individualist" who strives to do all he or she can do for his or her patients to that of a "cooperator" who strives to perform his or her role well within a larger organization (Buchanan, 2000). In turn, this shift in perspective suggests that many ethical problems that arise under utilization management procedures of health insurance plans cannot be resolved by individualistic or "monological" reasoning. Rather

they are problems of "organizational ethics," which require case managers to engage in shared-decision making, not just between the physician and patient, but also between patient care representatives, discharge planners, social workers, other providers, and hospital administrators. This highlights an important ethical role for the case manager under commercial health insurance plans or payers in general. As the person responsible for coordinating the delivery of care to patients, case managers must also assume responsibility for initiating shared decision making to resolve ethical problems that may arise.

14.4. THE DELIBERATIVE FRAMEWORK

It was suggested previously that the traditional ideal of the case manager as a patient advocate must be seriously rethought in the context of health insurance plans and appropriate utilization of resources. We now have seen why this is true. The maximizing ethic of beneficence that supported this traditional ideal has no place in health insurance plans that are aggressive in their cost cutting measures, and the individualistic character of the ideal does not sit well with the need for organizational decision making within the restrictions imposed by health insurance plans: utilization management procedures. The procedural principles of legitimate decision making that we have discussed, as well as the illustrative case of Mr. Jameson, suggest that we need to develop a new framework for understanding the ethical responsibilities of case management professionals, including nurses and social workers, who work under health insurance plans and MCOs.

The framework used to address these types of dilemmas, known as the deliberative framework, consists of two main components:

1. A commitment to shared decision making
2. An account of the nature and purpose of deliberation

14.4.1. Shared Decision Making

Shared decision making has become an important ideal in medicine and healthcare delivery. However, for the most part it has been proposed as an ideal for specific types of interactions (Case Manager's Tip 14.5). For example, shared decision making has been proposed as a model for the physician/patient relationship, case manager/patient relationship, and any healthcare professional/patient relationship. It has much less often been proposed as a model for healthcare decision making in general (Jansen, 2001; Elwyn et al., 2013; Elwyn

CASE MANAGER'S TIP 14.5

Shared Decision Making

For shared decision making to be effective, the parties involved must work in a collaborative and cooperative manner. They also must put the team's agenda over personal interests, be transparent in sharing information, and have a clear understanding of the common purpose or goals. Additionally, options must be clear to everyone involved for the process to result in desirable decision(s).

CASE MANAGER'S TIP 14.6

Deliberation

It is important for everyone involved in the deliberative process, including the case manager, is to stay patient-centered and always remember that you are advocating for the patient and not for personal gain. For deliberation to be effective, you must know your patient/family well including the patient's health condition, values, beliefs, preferences, and interests.

et al., 2012). With the advent of managed care, value-based purchasing, and hospital readmissions reduction programs, this needs to change. Physicians and nurses must work with case managers to come up with comprehensive guidelines for providing care. These guidelines should be the product of joint decision making in which physicians, nurses, health insurance representatives, and administrators in managed care organizations all are encouraged to participate actively.

This type of shared decision making is not only necessary to arrive at better guidelines and healthcare decisions, but also it is crucial to the legitimacy of utilization management and cost reduction procedures of both health insurance plans and providers. As has already been pointed out, legitimate cost-limiting decisions must adhere to the principles of impartiality, publicity, and contestability. Shared decision making, in which all affected parties are given the opportunity to participate, will make it much more likely that these principles will be satisfied. This is particularly true of the principle of contestability, which requires that patients and their physicians and case managers have public opportunities to challenge the decisions made under utilization management proccedures of health insurance plans.

14.4.2. The Nature and Purpose of Deliberation

The second component of the deliberative framework concerns the nature and purpose of the deliberation that should take place among those engaged in shared decision making. The purpose of this deliberation is to arrive at decisions that are both legitimate and seen to be legitimate. For this to be possible, all participants must be open to rational discussion and transparent in sharing relevant information. At the very least this means that participants must consider it a genuine possibility that they will learn something from the deliberative discussion and that they might change their minds about the issues before them (Case Manager's Tip 14.6).

In addition, participants in the discussion must view one another as equal deliberative partners. This does not mean that they cannot bring their particular expertise, whether it be medical, administrative, or patient representation/advocacy to bear on the discussion. However, it does mean that they must not think in hierarchical terms. For example, administrators should not think that physicians must always defer to them and physicians must not think that nurses or case managers must always defer to them. In genuinely deliberative discussion, hierarchical relations and attitudes have no place. They obstruct, rather than facilitate, the process of rational discussion.

These conditions for deliberative discussion are fairly demanding. In practice, most of the time they will not be fully realized. However, they can serve as an ideal toward which healthcare workers under managed care should strive. The deliberative framework, then, is an ideal to be approximated; however, it is the main argument of Chapter 14 that this ideal must be realized to a substantial extent if healthcare professionals, and in particular case managers, are to make ethically responsible decisions given the restrictions imposed by health insurance plans and value-based purchasing programs which potentially may present financial risk on the healthcare organization, leader, or provider.

14.4.3. Clinical Ethics Consults

To illustrate this last point, consider the role and function of the ethics consult. Before the advent of managed care organizations, capitated insurance plans and requirement of specific utilization management procedures such as preauthorization for services, an ethics consult would be necessary only when a relatively well-defined ethical problem presented itself—clinical care concerns. Most of the time physicians and nurses could proceed as patient advocates, providing all of the care to their patients that could reasonably be expected to benefit them. However, if it is true that the traditional understanding of the ideal of patient advocate must be given up under managed care, then physicians and case managers will often confront a whole new range of challenging ethical questions about what level of care, the quantity of services, and the timing of care their patients are legitimately entitled to receive. These are not questions they will be able to answer on their own. They will need to consult others about what the health insurance and managed care cost containment guidelines require and permit and when exceptions can legitimately be made to these guidelines. Often these questions will not have determinate answers until after deliberative discussion has resolved them. Accordingly, under health insurance and managed care utilization management procedures there is an increased need for ethics consults, and these consults, at least when they function well, are instances of deliberative shared decision making.

14.5. ORGANIZATIONAL ETHICS

The type of ethics consult that a case manager is likely to call differs in significant respects from the traditional "clinical ethics consult." In large measure the clinical ethics consult centers on how individual practitioners can best resolve ethical conflicts that arise when they are treating their patients; for example, deciding whether to terminate care/treatment. However, the conflicts that arise in the context of case management and health insurance and managed care utilization management procedures and decisions are more organizational in nature (Case Manager's Tips 14.7 and 14.8). In some respects these conflicts can better be grouped under a category of "organizational ethics"

 CASE MANAGER'S TIP 14.7

Organizational Ethics

As a case manager, if your organization does not have an organizational ethics committee, you should advocate for the development of one to assist you in solving ethical dilemmas that you may come across, such as those related to utilization management procedures, resource allocation and utilization, and discharge/transitional planning. Having a utilization management committee is not enough because such committee is not the best forum to address ethical concerns of organizational nature. Also remember that organizational ethics committees must have participants who are not traditionally present in clinical ethics committees. These include experts in health insurance plans and agreements, administrative processes, and systems of care.

 CASE MANAGER'S TIP 14.8

Reporting Structure of Organizational Ethics

Organizational ethics committees should be subcommittees of the organization-wide ethics committee and should report their issues and decisions back to the ethics committee on a regular basis.

rather than the traditional category of "clinical ethics." Organizational ethics deliberation requires the participation of those who understand systems of care, utilization management procedures, and health insurance plans rather than clinical care.

Organizational ethics deals with an organization's behaviors as they relate to the individuals represented by that organization (including patients, care providers, and other employees), the community served by that organization, and other organizations with whom that organization may interact. There are a number of different categories of organizational ethics (Box 14.1). However, the types of organizational ethics conflicts that case managers must address will be limited to the unique roles that they play inside the healthcare organization. For example, the roles that case managers play give rise to the types of conflicts for which an ethics consultation would be appropriate:

1. Resolving care-related conflicts
2. Preventing delays in treatments
3. Increasing and facilitating access to care and resources
4. Brokering services within and outside the healthcare organization
5. Obtaining authorizations for treatments from health insurance plans and MCOs
6. Advocating for patients while working with health insurance plans and MCOs

To illustrate, consider the following case.

14.5.1. Organizational Ethics Consult Case Study

Mr. Gaynor was found unconscious. He was admitted out of network (a healthcare facility that is not a participating provider in the health insurance plan Mr. Gaynor has) to the ICU at a nearby inner city hospital. He remained in the hospital for 6 months before being discharged to his home in another state. Two weeks after his discharge, Mr. Gaynor experienced another syncopal episode. His wife requested that the ambulance bring him back to the original hospital where he had spent the past 6 months. Because he had full understanding of the patient's condition, had treated him in the past, and had developed a professional rapport with him, the physician from the inner city hospital agreed that this would best serve the patient's medical and health interests. However, because the patient was "out of network," the case manager was called on to make a decision as to whether the admission was appropriate.

Cases such as this have become more common in an era of health insurance plans and managed care restrictions. In this type of case, case managers best discharge their ethical responsibilities by deliberating with others to determine what response is appropriate. However, the types of people whom the case manager would most likely need to consult will differ from those whom a physician or nurse would consult in a dilemma of clinical ethics. In addition to the patient's family and physician and a trained ethicist, the case manager will also want to deliberate with a member of the managed care department, legal department, patient relations, and social work.

Given their training and institutional role in today's healthcare system, case managers must develop skills for collaborating with physicians, nurses, social workers, patients, and family members of patients on developing comprehensive and integrated healthcare delivery plans for their patients. These collaborative skills are the types of skills that are needed to engage effectively in deliberative decision making to resolve problems of organizational ethics likely to arise under managed care health insurance plans and the utilization management restrictions imposed.

With these points in mind, we can finally return to the traditional ideal of the case manager as patient advocate. This ideal can now be understood not to be an individualistic ideal (Case Manager's Tip 14.9) in which the case manager acts to maximize the interests of the patient but rather a collaborative ideal in which the case manager deliberates with others to determine the appropriate type of services and level of care for the patient.

Like other healthcare workers, case managers need to adjust to the changing circumstances brought on by managed care. This will require them to rethink some of the traditional ethical ideals that have formed the profession. In particular, an ethic appropriate to today's health insurance plans and managed care organizations must be one that is responsive to the legitimate societal need to contain healthcare spending.

Rather than providing guidance as to how to resolve specific ethical problems, Chapter 14 provides case managers with strategies that can be used when they are presented with any ethical dilemma whether clinical or organizational in nature. These strategies focus on a certain type of process for resolving ethical problems that are likely to arise in the context of utilizational management restrictions and expectations imposed on healthcare providers by health insurance plans and managed care organizations (Case Manager's Tip

---

Box 14.1   Examples of Categories of Organizational Ethics

Healthcare Business

- Cost shifting
- Billing practices
- Financial incentives
- Resource allocation
- Conflicts of interest

Societal and Public Health Considerations

- Serving the medically underserved
- Antidumping issues (Emergency Medical Treatment and Active Labor Act [EMTALA])
- Discrimination against patients
- Public disclosure of clinical errors
- Guardianship

Healthcare Advertising

- Making unrealistic promises
- Endorsing specific medical products
- Marketing of healthcare institutions

Scientific and Educational Issues

- Education of future healthcare providers
- Performing research and clinical trials

General Business Practices such as Relationships with:

- Employees
- Vendors
- Payers
- Outside agencies
- The public at large

 CASE MANAGER'S TIP 14.9

Ethics Consults

Case managers can function as patient advocates in the following two ways:

1. They can ensure that ethics consults are called when they need to be called.
2. They can ensure that their patients' interests are fully represented and protected in these consults.

CASE MANAGER'S TIP 14.10

Strategies for Approaching an Ethical Dilemma

- Enforce and promote mutual trust among all parties involved.
- Maintain the patient's confidentiality, privacy, right to choice, and self-determination.
- Affirm the dignity and worth of each party involved.
- Project commitment to truthfulness.
- Respect diversity of values and difference of opinion, including right of refusal of care.
- Ensure congruence between verbal and nonverbal communication messages.
- Avoid task orientation—be person- and goal-oriented instead.
- Allow sufficient time for each ethical issue.
- Spend enough time with the patient, family, and other healthcare providers, as indicated, for each dilemma faced.
- Interview/meet with patients and families in private rooms and comfortable settings.
- Believe that good communication results in good and desirable outcomes.
- Assume and project a sense of responsibility and accountability for own actions.
- Always involve others in shared decision making regarding the issue at hand.
- Deliberate in accord with a relatively consistent set of values and goals.
- Distinguish ethical problems from other general patient care management issues.
- Seek the assistance of others, especially experts, when unable to address the issue independently.
- Be thorough and timely in gathering information. Value uncertainty over confidence. Such attitude allows you to be comprehensive in information gathering rather than biased to your preconceived notions.
- Always apply the institutional policies and procedures; they are intended to support and guide practice.
- Document pertinent information in the patient's medical record.
- Remember to always be patient-centered and allow patient-driven care planning. Keep benefits patient-focused rather than healthcare team-focused.
- Avoid premature closure on issues; such practice prevents you from confirmation bias and deciding on the issue before all the facts have been gathered and carefully examined.
- Be mindful, reflect on what you have done; ask yourself if you could have done anything differently; go back and check whether you have missed anything of importance.
- Promote disclosure and transparency, especially when an error occurs or when you need to share bad news. Be honest, compassionate, and empathetic; tell the truth; and build trust through effective and respectful communication.

14.10). The process is deliberative and involves shared decision making between a wide range of professionals. However, to facilitate this process, case managers should also have knowledge of the specific code of ethics for their profession as case managers and professional discipline (e.g., nursing, social work), as well as with the mission, vision, and value statements of the organization in which they work. Boxes 14.2 through 14.6 include a number of professional codes of ethics specific to the field of case management.

14.6. ETHICAL FRAMEWORK FOR SHARED DECISION MAKING

Case managers may use an ethical shared decision making approach with their patients/families to assure informed decisions about care options and adherence to ethical principles and standards. This approach (Case Manager's Tip 14.11) is not limited to concerns with health insurance plans and ethical dilemmas; it rather is a part of every step of the case

CASE MANAGER'S TIP 14.11

Shared Decision Making

Case managers often work with the patient and family to ensure informed decision making especially to arrive at choosing a care option that is in the best interest of the patient. They also work with health insurance plan respresentatives to assure authorizations for the services the patient requires to address the health condition at hand. It is important for case managers to be aware of what effective shared decision making is.

Shared decision making is a two-way approach (i.e., discussion) case managers use to identify the patient's needs, preferences, interests, values, and goals, and to discuss uncertainties, experiences, and costs to ultimately support patients in making informed decisions about their care options. Case managers also apply the same approach when communicating with representatives from health insurance plans in attempts to obtain authorizations for services and treatments to be offered to patients. Applying such approaches promotes ethical practice and ethical decision making.

Box 14.2   American Nurses Association's Code of Ethics (ANA, 2015)

The ANA's code of ethics is a statement of ethical values, obligations, duties, ideals, nonnegotiable standards, and understanding of commitment to society. The code describes eight provisions, as follows.

1. The nurse, in all professional relationships, practices with compassion and respect for the inherent dignity, worth, and uniqueness of every individual, unrestricted by considerations of social or economic status, personal attributes, or the nature of health problems.
2. The nurse's primary commitment is to the patient, whether an individual, family, group, or community.
3. The nurse promotes, advocates for, and strives to protect the health, safety, and rights of the patient.
4. The nurse is responsible and accountable for individual nursing practice and determines the appropriate delegation of tasks consistent with the nurse's obligation to provide optimum patient care.
5. The nurse owes the same duties to self as to others, including the responsibility to preserve integrity and safety, to maintain competence, and to continue personal and professional growth.
6. The nurse participates in establishing, maintaining, and improving healthcare environments and conditions of employment conducive to the provision of quality healthcare and consistent with the values of the profession through individual and collective action.
7. The nurse participates in the advancement of the profession through contributions to practice, education, administration, and knowledge development.
8. The nurse collaborates with other health professionals and the public in promoting community, national, and international efforts to meet health needs.
9. The profession of nursing, as represented by associations and their members, is responsible for articulating nursing values, for maintaining the integrity of the profession and its practice, and for shaping social policy.

Box 14.3   National Association of Social Workers Code of Ethics (NASW, 2008)

The following broad principles are based on social work's core values of service, social justice, dignity and worth of the person, importance of human relationships, integrity, and competence. These principles set forth ideals to which all social workers should aspire.

1. *Value*: Service
   Ethical principle: Social workers' primary goal is to help people in need and to address social problems and placing people's interests over self-interest.

2. *Value*: Social justice
   Ethical principle: Social workers challenge social injustice; pursue social change, particularly with and on behalf of vulnerable and oppressed individuals or groups of people.

3. *Value*: Dignity and worth of the person
   Ethical principle: Social workers respect the inherent dignity and worth of the person; treat each person in a caring and respectful manner, mindful of individual differences, and cultural and ethnic diversity.

4. *Value*: Importance of human relationships
   Ethical principle: Social workers recognize the central importance of human relationships; engage people as partners in the healing process and that relationships are important vehicles of change.

5. *Value*: Integrity
   Ethical principle: Social workers behave in a trustworthy manner and act honestly and responsibly and promote the ethical principles in the organizations they are affiliated with.

6. *Value*: Competence
   Ethical principle: Social workers practice within their areas of competence and develop and enhance their professional expertise; strive to increase their knowledge and skills and apply them in practice.

The NASW also highlights a number of standards of ethical social wrok practices including responsibilities toward the client, colleagues, practice settings, as professionals, the social work profession, and to the broader society.

Box 14.4   National Association of Social Workers Standards of Social Work Case Management (NASW, 2013)

The NASW developed specific standards for social work case management. One of the standards addresses case management ethics and values. It states that the social work case manager shall adhere to and promote the ethics and values of the social work profession, using the NASW Code of Ethics as a guide to ethical decision making in case management practice. In another standard, NASW also states that the social work case manager shall advocate for the rights, decisions, strengths, and needs of clients and shall promote clients' access to resources, supports, and services. NASW refers to the individuals cared for as clients and not patients.

The NASW Standards of Social Work Case Management states that the social work case manager:

- Prioritizes service to clients above professional or personal self-interest.
- Provides services in a culturally and linguistically appropriate manner.
- Acts on individual and systemic levels to ensure clients' access to needed information, services, and resources.
- Facilitates clients' maximal participation in decision making.
- Treats clients in a caring manner, respecting their self-determination and valuing their strengths.
- Enhances clients' capacity to improve their circumstances and achieve their goals.
- Promotes the role of human relationships in the change process and cultivates a therapeutic relationship with each client and engages the client as a partner in care.
- Undertakes all actions with respect for clients' goals, exercising judicious use of self, avoiding conflicts of interest, and applying professional judgment in the provision of services to clients.
- Recognizes that self-care is essential to being present for clients and attends to self-care accordingly.
- Promotes client self-determination while helping clients navigate complex service delivery systems. When a client's decision-making capacity is limited, the social work case manager collaborates with the individual who is legally authorized to represent the client.
- Informs the client of the full range of existing choices so the client may decide which services will best meet her or his needs.
- Uses peer review, ethics committees, or external consultation, or advocates for internal change to resolve the ethical dilemma or other concerns.
- Ensures the client has the requisite information to provide informed consent in all aspects of the case management process.
- Terminates a service when it is no longer helpful to the client or is detrimental to the client's well-being and growth; promptly notifies the client that a service will be interrupted or terminated by a service provider.
- Makes the necessary transfer or referral if the client needs specific services to ensure continuity of care post current episode of care.

---

management process. It is also present during every interaction between case managers and their patients or their patient's families. When used proactively, the chances of ethical conflicts and dilemmas are redcued if not completely disappear. Shared decision making promotes the building of a trusting and respectful relationship between healthcare professions/case managers and patients/families. At its core, shared decision making accepts that the patient's self-determination and right to choice including refusal of care is an essential goal and that case managers must support their patients in achieving this goal. It also recognizes the need to support patient's autonomy while establishing these relationships (Elwyn et al., 2012).

Self-determination and autonomy are important for protecting the patient's well being and interests. Despite the tendency for interdependence when patients and case managers are involved in interpersonal relationships, informed decision making extends beyond

the transfer of information from case managers to their patients/families; rather case managers facilitate the making of decisions about care options while assuring they are in the best interest of the patients, balancing benfits and risks, and promoting independence and freedom of choice. These tactics adhere to the ethical principles of advocacy and beneficence. Box 14.7 describes a framework for ethical shared decision making case managers may use when working with patients and their families (Elwyn et al., 2012).

The shared decision making framework described in Box 14.7 is most productive when it takes the form of face-to-face deliberation. If face-to-face is not feasible, a telephone conversation may be appropriate depending on the seriousness of the situation and decision to be made. Electornic communications are not advised for deliberation, nor to address any other ethical concern. Deliberation allows case managers to work collaboratively with their patients/families and other members of the interdisciplinary healthcare team. It involves a discussion of the benefits and risks of various relevant care options, assessment of the implications of these options, and addressing any emotional concerns the patients/families may exhibit. It also respects and protects the patient's self-determination, autonomy, and right to choice.

Case managers may use the shared decision making framework to ensure that the case management plan of care meets the patient's needs, preferences, value and belief system, and personal health goals. They also may apply this framework when planning and executing the transitional plans of their patients. For example, if a patient's condition requires the transfer from an acute care hospital to a subacute or acute rehabilitation level of care, the case manager initiates the choice talk with the patient and family informing them about the need for transition emphasizing that they have a choice in the matter and their preferences are important

to share for consideration in the decision making process and ultimately the final decision to be made. The case manager may follow the following steps in his/her conversation with the patient and family regarding the transition:

1. Assess the patient and family's understanding of the patient's condition, the case management plan, and need for rehabilitation before transitioning to the home setting.
2. Inform patient and family that a decision needs to be made and that they have choices in dealing with the situation. Need to indentify the preferred rehabilitation facility the patient likes to transfer to; perhaps more than one facility is to be identified such as choices number one and number two.
3. Take the time to gather and understand the patient and family's preferences and explain that these preferences matter. Acknowledge and discuss dif-

---

Box 14.5   Code of Professional Conduct for Case Managers, Commission for Case Manager Certification (Commission for Case Manager Certification, 2015)

The CCMC identifies several values of case management practice and rules of conduct expected from certified case managers who hold the credential offered by CCMC. Although these apply for those certified by CCMC, the code has applicability and use for the larger body of case management.

The underlying values are as follows:

1. Belief that case management is a means for improving the client's health, wellness, and autonomy through advocacy, communication, education, identification of service resources, and service facilitation.
2. Recognition of the dignity, worth, and rights of all people.
3. Understanding and commitment to quality outcomes for clients, appropriate use of resources, and the empowerment of clients in a manner that is supportive and objective.
4. Embracing the underlying premise that when the individual reaches the optimal level of wellness and functional capability, everyone benefits: the individual being served, the individual's support system, the healthcare delivery system, and the various reimbursement systems.
5. Understanding that case management is guided by the ethical principles of autonomy, beneficence, nonmaleficence, justice, and fidelity.

Rules of conduct are as follows:

The rules are listed in terms of unethical practices and as violation statements that may result in denial or sanctions on the part of CCMC up to and including revocation of the individual's certification. Those certified through CCMC are expected to always abide by these rules.

- Rule 1: Intentionally falsifying an application or other documents
- Rule 2: Conviction of a felony
- Rule 3: Violation of the code of ethics governing the profession on which the individual's eligibility for the certified case manager (CCM) credential is based
- Rule 4: Loss of the primary professional credential on which eligibility for the CCM designation is based
- Rule 5: Violation or breach of the standards for professional conduct (i.e., professional misconduct)
- Rule 6: Violation of the rules and regulations governing the taking of the certification examination

The CCMC code also describes several standards for ethical case management practice which include client advocacy, professional responsibility, case manager/client relationships, confidentiality, privacy, security and recordkeeping, and professional relationships.

Box 14.6   Case Management Society of America (CMSA, 2010)

In its 2010 Standards of Practice for Case Management, the CMSA emphasizes ethics as one of its standards of practice and highlights advocacy as another. It states that case managers should:

1. Practice and behave in an ethical manner. Case managers can demonstrate adherence to this standard if they abide by the tenents of the ethical codes that underlie their professional backgrounds and credentials (e.g., nursing, social work, rehabilitation counseling). Case managers may demonstrate ethical behaviors by:

   a. Being aware of five ethical principles and their application: beneficience (to do good), nonmalficence (to do no harm), autonomy (to respect individual's rights to make own decisions), justice (to treat others fairly), and fidelity (to follow-through and to keep promises).

   b. Recognizing that the primary obligation is to the patient/client.

   c. Maintaining respectful relationships with peers, employers, and other professionals.

   d. Recognizing the laws, rules, policies, insurance benefits, and regulations are sometimes in conflict with ethical principles. In these situations, case managers must address the conflicts to the best of their abilities and seek consultation as necessary.

2. Advocate for the client/patient at the point of healthcare service delivery, administration of health insurance benefits, and policy makers level. Case managers may exhibit advocacy behaviors through documentation that demonstrate:

   a. Promotion of client's self determination, informed and shared decision making, autonomy, growth, and self advocacy.

   b. Education of other healthcare professionals about respecting the needs, strengths, and goals of the client/patient.

   c. Facilitating client/patient access to healthcare services and educating the client and support system about service availability within the care setting.

   d. Recognition, prevention, and elimination of disparity in accessing high quality care and outcomes.

   e. Expansion or establishment of services and for client/patient-centered changes in policy.

   f. Upholding client advocacy, as possible, whenever a conflict arises regarding cost-constraints and limited resources.

Box 14.7   A Framework for Ethical Shared Decision Making

When case managers engage in a conversation with their patients/families which aims to arrive at important decisions, following a formal model or framework that assures shared decision making is necessary. The following is an example of a model which consists of four main steps case managers may engage in the context of deliberation with their patients/families.

Step 1: Choice Talk conveys awareness to the patient/family that a choice exists. Assuring the patient/family are well aware of the presence of choice is important so that they do not misunderstand the conversation as if it were for the purpose of information transfer only or that no decision is needed on their part. This step presents the case manager with the opportunity to check the patient and family's preferences and reactions.

Step 2: Option Talk presents the various available and relevant options for care, treatments, or services. This allows the patient/family to examine if those shared meet their own desires, preferences, and goals and to ask questions if none seemed to meet their interests. To assure this step is effective, case managers may first check the patient's existing knowledge before they engage in health education activities, use of health instruction aids such as health videos and counseling, and encourage the patient/family to share own personal preferences. Education and counseling allow the sharing of benefits and potential harms, important for ethical decision making and adherence to the principle of beneficence.

Step 3: Decision Talk supports the patient and family in deciding about what matters most to them, especially that they are at this stage well informed based on the content of the previous steps. It is important at this step for the case manager to avoid premature closure; but rather to allow the patient/family to carefully consider the options and ask any questions they may have.

Step 4: Decision Making facilitates the choosing of the preferred care option after careful deliberation and consideration of risks and benefits. To ensure that the patient/family make an informed decision and they are confident with the choice made, case managers review the choice and offer to address anything that may have been unclear or still questionable.

ferences if any between what the patient and family preferences are and what the situation at hand requires. This is necessary to eliminate any unrealistic expectations and to address any gaps. It is likely that the patient and family may not be aware of the rationale for a transfer to a rehabilitation facility, or what rehabilitation means. In such situations, spending some time in counseling and health education is important for informed decisions.

4. Assure the patient and family you will support them throughout the process and are available to answer their questions.
5. Ascertain who is going to make the decision. For example, is it the patient, a family member, or both?
6. Present the patient and family with their options. For example, you may provide them with a list of potential rehabilitation facilities that accept the patient's health insurance plan and that is within a certain geographical area from their residence.
7. Check the patient and family's understanding of the options; clarify misunderstandings and answer their questions. Offer to give more information if necessary; encourage the family to visit the potential rehabilitation facilities before finalizing the decision.
8. Inquire if the patient and family are ready to make a decision. If not ready, agree on a date or time for follow up while clarifying when the decision has to be made. In the mean time continue to support them as they consider their options.

Sometimes the decision is made in one meeting with the patient and family; other times it may require multiple meetings. If it is a challenging situation and the patient and family are confused or have conflicting opinions, a case conference may be helpful to resolve the concerns. In such case, you may need the participation of the physician and certain members of the interdisciplinary healthcare team, in addition to the patient and family. In some situations where ethical conflicts or concerns are present, having a patient advocate/representative and an ethicist may be beneficial. When decisions are not made in a timely fashion, be aware of the health insurance plan's utilization management procedures and make every effort to adhere to them to avoid denials of services or reimbursement for extended hospital stay.

14.6.1. Advocacy

Case managers may not be effective when they engage in shared decision making activities with their clients without respecting the ethical principle of advocacy. Regardless of which case management professional organization one may refer to, to understand the nature of case management advocacy, one will find it to focus on doing what is in the best interest of the patient and family, protecting their rights to choice, informed decision making, and safeguarding their autonomy, self-determination, and independence. The Commission for Case Manager Certification (CCMC), for example, expects case managers to serve as patient/client advocates. It explains that case managers can meet this expectation by conducting comprehensive assessments of their patients/families to identify their needs and interests, providing them with options for healthcare services so that patients are able to choose based on their preferences, and assuring access to services and resources that meet their needs (CCMC, 2015) (Case Manager's Tip, 14.12). The Case Management Society of America (CMSA) describes advocacy as the "act of recommending, pleading the cause of another; to speak or write in favor of" another (CMSA, 2010). CMSA also explains that case managers have the obligation to engage in advocacy at three levels:

- The point of delivery of healthcare services to patients and their families or caregivers
- Administration of the patient's health insurance benefits
- Policy making at the organizational and healthcare system or governmental levels

Case managers according to the ANA's Code of Ethics for Nurses with Interpretive Statements are expected to promote, advocate for, and strive to protect the health, quality, safety, and rights of patients. The ANA explains this role with a focus on safeguarding the patient right to privacy and confidentiality. It also emphasizes the expectation of protecting patients engaged in research studies (rights as subjects of or

 CASE MANAGER'S TIP 14.12

Advocacy

The CCMC describes advocacy in case management as a process that promotes beneficence, justice, autonomy, self-determination, and independence for clients/patients and their families or caregivers. It involves educating clients about their rights, benefits, and healthcare and human services, facilitating informed decision making, and considerations for the client's values, beliefs, interests, and culture (CCMC, 2015).

participants in research) and addressing questionable healthcare and impaired practices (ANA, 2015).

Other case management related professional organizations also describe case managers as patient advocates and are explicit about how they demonstrate such role expectation. For example:

■ NASW, in its standard on advocacy and leadership for social work case managers, states that case managers shall advocate for the rights, decisions, strengths, and needs of their clients (patients) and shall promote clients' access to healthcare resources, supports, and services (NASW, 2013).

■ The American Case Management Association (ACMA), which focuses primarily on hospital-based case managers, includes advocacy as one of its standards of practice and scope of services. It states that "advocacy is the act of supporting or recommending on behalf of patients/family/caregivers and the hospital for service access or creation, and for the protection of the patient's health, safety, and rights," (ACMA, 2013). To enhance the role of advocacy and to meet ethical expectations in practice, the ACMA offers several actions case managers may engage in while caring for patients and their families. These are:

—Knowing who the legal decision maker is, the patient or a surrogate.

—Sharing information on benefits, risks, costs, and treatment alternatives including option of no treatment.

—Protecting the patient's self-determination and respecting the care choices and wishes including advanced directives and informed decisions.

—Promoting culturally competent care.

—Working with the payer/health insurance plan to ensure the patient accesses his/her full benefits and negotiating exceptions when needed.

—Balance resources with patient preferences and seeking the assistance of experts (e.g., ethics committee) to resolve conflicts and ethical dilemmas.

—Addressing suspected cases of abuse, neglect, or exploitation; for example, referring such cases to appropriate agencies or personnel (ACMA, 2013).

14.6.2. Informed Decision and Consent

Other aspects of successful shared decision making are informed decision and informed consent (Case Manager's Tip 14.13). One of the most beneficial ways to assure the provision of safe and high quality patient-centered healthcare services is having fully informed patients and families. Such allows them the ability to participate fully in shared decision making including arriving at informed decisions and informed consent where appropriate. In this regard, case managers educate their patients and families about various options for healthcare services, explain their health insurance benefits, and answer their questions so that they are able to decide on what is best for them. This is done in concert with advocacy; and therefore, protecting the patient's autonomy, independence, self-determination, and right to choice.

The CMSA explains in its standards for case management, that case managers educate "the client[/patient], the family or caregiver, and members of the healthcare delivery team about treatment options, community resources, insurance benefits, psychosocial concerns, case management [services], etc., so that timely and informed decisions can be made," (CMSA, 2010). In addition, CMSA emphasizes the importance of empowering the patient and family to solve problems and explore alternate care options to enhance the achievement of desired outcomes. These activities must be incorporated into the shared decision making framework, esepcially when the case manager explains

 CASE MANAGER'S TIP 14.13

Informed Decision and Informed Consent

Informed decision making is a two-way dialogue between the patient/family and the healthcare provider (e.g., case manager), about care options and their benefits, risks, and future consequences, while considering the patient's personal situation, culture, preferences, interests, and priorities. Such interaction is free of judgment and maintains respect for the patient's right to choice.

Informed consent is the end point of the informed decision-making process where the patient (or when appropriate, a family member, caregiver, or healthcare proxy) documents the agreement to a plan of care and/or a specific treatment option. Ususally at this point the patient has received appropriate information about the risks and benefits of the plan or treatment. Documentation of such consent is a traditional risk management and legal practice, completed to meet regulatory and accreditation standards.

Effective informed decisions and informed consents are those that conform to ethical and legal principles and standards. It is important for case managers to assure that processes of informed decision and informed consent adhere to these standards to prevent ethical concerns, risk management issues, or malpractice.

to the patient and family they have a choice (choice talk step), and discuss options for care during the option talk step.

Effective informed decisions are made when case managers, and other healthcare professionals, take the time to ensure the patient and family have clear appreciation and understanding of the relevant facts, care options, and future implications and consequences of the decision(s) they make or the service option they choose. Rushing such processes may result in premature closure and ineffective shared decision making. Respecting the patient's right to choice means allowing the patient to exercise his/her right to self-determination, which includes the right to have information necessary to make decisions in a confident, safe, and comfortable manner; void of coercion, judgment, or manipulation. Ultimately, respecting and understanding the patient's right to both consent or refuse care (sometimes to withdraw already established consent), service, treatment, intervention, or resource. Examples of information case managers may share with their patients during informed decisions are, but not limited to the following:

- Expert and reliable information or health instructions.
- Answering the questions patients and families may raise.
- Discussing the pros and cons, or the risks and benefits, of different care options.
- Briefing the patient and family about the potential plan of care and the recommendations of the interdisciplinary healthcare team.
- Presenting the various discharge options and post-discharge services.
- Explaining who is who on the interdisciplinary healthcare team and why each party is involved in the care.

Informed consent is a legal term that denotes a patient has given permission or authorization to receive care and services from healthcare providers, including case managers. Often it is used by healthcare providers in two general contexts: (1) to obtain a generic authorization for care provision and (2) to obtain permission to perform a specific procedure on the patient. The reality, however, informed consents should not be limited to a signature on a document, nor a single event; rather they should entail a process of ongoing dialogue between the healthcare provider and the patient/family throughout the course of an episode of care. During the legal informed consent process, healthcare providers share specific types of information with the patient and family or caregiver which result in the informed decision to grant a consent. These include the following:

- The nature of the proposed treatment.
- The known benefits and risks or side-effects of the treatment.
- Any alternative treatments or courses of action.
- What may happen if the proposed treatment does not occur.
- Questions and answers regarding the treatment.

Informed consents do not always result in having written documents as proof in a patient's medical record. They may take one of two forms as appropriate: implied and explicit.

- *Implied consent*: agreement through actions demonstrative of adherence to care instructions.
- *Explicit or express consent*: clearly stating agreement. It may be done either verbally or in writing.
  —*Verbal consent*: express agreement where a patient verbalizes permission or authrozization.
  —*Written consent*: authorization or permission provided in writing including the patient's signature as evidence.

Informed decision making honors the healthcare provider's expert knowledge and the patient's right to have the necessary information. In this collaborative process, the provider (e.g., case manager) shares what is known about the treatment or intervention of interest including the available scientific evidence while allowing the patient to ask questions and express his/her concerns, ensuring appropriate considerations for the patient's values and preferences. Formal or comprehensive documentation of the patient's active involvement in informed decisions does not always occur; however, healthcare providers usually document patient/family teaching and health instructions. In contrast, documentation of informed consent is a legal requirement. It is usually made available as evidence in the patient's medical record. It is advisable to use written informed consents, instead of implied or verbal, especially in the case when risks outweigh the benefits.

14.6.3. Manipulation

One of the risks case managers may face when engaged in shared decision making with their patients/families or fellow healthcare professionals is being perceived as coercive, self-serving, or having a hidden agenda. Such misperception may result from case managers acting passionately about something (e.g., a specific treatment option), rushing a decision (e.g., premature closure-finalizing a decision despite not all of the facts have been considered), or strongly advocating for the use of a specific healthcare agency or vendor. Case managers may also be perceived in these situations as "manipulative." There is a fine line between being self-serving and being selfless; case managers must be careful not to be perceived as manipulative.

Manipulation is a type of influence where the person being influenced is unaware that he/she is being influenced. Despite the fact that case managers' first and foremost responsibility is patient advocacy, they may be easily misperceived as being manipulative despite their selfless intention; especially because they are relentless at addressing care concerns. For example, they are pressured to implement cost-effective care strategies and to resolve challenging situations such as delays in care, timely rescheduling of tests, bringing a patient/family to agree or decide on the plan of care, or negotiating authorizations of services from the payer. Such perceptions may potentially result in an ethical concern for the case manager.

Case managers may prevent being perceived as manipulative by applying the following strategies while caring for their patients/families or dealing with fellow colleagues:

- Share all available information with the patient and family as well as other healthcare professionals and avoid incomplete or selective discolsure, distortion of the facts, obscuring a situation, decision, or bias.
- Take the time in the deliberation process with others, including the patient and family, so that all parties involved carefully and thoughfully arrive at a comfortable decision and therefore avoiding being perceived as persuasive, deceptive, or self-serving.
- Be transparent, explicit and open about the issues, no matter what they are, to avoid being viewed as having a hidden agenda or covering something up.
- Respect the patient's right to autonomy, self-determination and choice, especially during care planning and resolving problems. Seek the input, assistance, and feedback of others.
- Behave in a fair manner, consistently show concern for others, and maintain integrity during all encounters.

14.7. GENERAL ETHICAL PRINCIPLES APPLICABLE TO CASE MANAGEMENT

There is a number of general ethical principles in healthcare practice that also apply to case management. In addition to advocacy, beneficence, and nonmaleficence, ethical principles such as autonomy, objectivity, fidelity, justice, distributive justice, and veracity

are important for case managers to be aware of and to adhere to while caring for patients and their families (Box 14.8). When case managers execute their actions in a way that adheres to ethical standards, they are able to aid clients/support systems in achieving care objectives in a timely and efficient manner and assuring the patient and family have an optimal experience of care. On the other hand, when case managers remain inactive, they directly or indirectly hinder the patient's progress toward achieving desired goals. Such inaction is considered unethical and improfessional. Applying relevant ethical principles in practice, such as those in Box 14.8, assists case managers in their efforts to maintain professional credibility and good standing; ultimately they are safeguarding the public's interest not just the interests of their patients/families.

At some point patients may no longer need or benefit from case management services and case managers must terminate the services and their relationships with their patients/families. In such situations, they

---

Box 14.8   Ethical Principles Most Commonly Applied in Case Management Practice

- *Advocacy*: The act of pleading the cause of another; recommending and protecting what is in the best interest of others.
- *Autonomy*: A form of personal liberty of action in which the patient holds the right and freedom to select and initiate his or her own treatment and course of action and to take control of his or her health (i.e., fostering the patient's independence and self-determination).
- *Beneficence*: The obligation and duty to promote good, to further and support a patient's legitimate interests and decisions, and to actively prevent or remove harm (i.e., to share with the patient the risks associated with a particular treatment option).
- *Fidelity*: Keeping promises and commitments.
- *Justice*: Maintaining what is right and fair and making decisions that are good for the patient.
- *Distributive justice*: Deals with the moral basis for dissemination of goods and evils, burdens and benefits, especially when making decisions regarding the allocation of healthcare resources.
- *Nonmaleficence*: Refraining from doing harm to others (i.e., emphasizing quality and safe care outcomes).
- *Objectivity*: Refraining from imposing one's values on others including patients and their families. Also objectivity implies accepting the patient and family as they are including respecting their values, beliefs, culture, choices, and priorities.
- *Veracity*: The act of telling the truth which requires communicating honestly and objectively and sharing relevant, accurate, and understandable information.

CASE MANAGER'S TIP 14.14

Termination of Case Management Services

When terminating case management services, consider all the various aspects of the patient's situation (e.g., health, physical, financial, psychosocial) and the impact of service termination such as adverse or unintended consequences. You must first assure that your patient/family will no longer benefit from the services and they are ready for and in agreement with terminating these services.

---

must take necessary and reasonable steps to avoid the patients' feeling abandoned, concerned, or dissatisfied (Case Manager's Tip 14.14).

Careful termination of case management services and assuring that the patient and family are ready minimize the potential for suboptimal care, unsafe situations, and poor experience of care. The following are examples of strategies to enhance a desirable termination of services experience.

- Notify the patient/family before service termination and assure they are able to assume responsibility for self-management.
- Decide to terminate services based on the patient's condition, status of the case management plan and related goals, health insurance plan's utilization management procedures, and agreement of the interdisciplinary healthcare team.
- Refer the patient/family to other services as needed to assure continuity of care and the availability of ongoing support; for example, meals on wheels, charitable care.
- Discuss the patient's condition and status of the plan of care with the representative of the patient's health insurance plan.
- Provide the patient/family with a summary of care and detailed instructions about follow-up care.
- Offer the patient/family contact information and explain the procedure of calling for assistance or to obtain answers for questions which may arise post-termination of services.

 14.8. KEY POINTS

1. The traditional ethical principles of justice, autonomy, and beneficence must be rethought in the context of case management and health insurance plans including managed care; in most cases, new principles will need to be articulat-

ed, especially those pertaining to cost-cutting or lowering measures and utilizations management procedures.

2. When case managers function within a legitimate health insurance and managed care environment to limit costs, they are not only serving the interests of payers of healthcare services but the interests of consumers as well.

3. Applying the ethical principles of impartiality, publicity, and contestability is crucial to responding ethically to the tension of maintaining a balance between access, cost, safety, and quality of healthcare.

4. The case manager as a consumer advocate applies a collaborative idea (collaborates with consumers, providers, and payers) to determine the appropriate type, quantity, level, cost, and quality of care/services for the patient and family.

5. Case managers must be familiar with the codes of ethics of case management and their professional discipline (e.g., nursing). They also must apply the code(s) in their daily function.

6. Applying the ethical framework of shared decision making in all interactions with patients and families and colleagues allow case managers to adhere to ethical principles and standards and promotes effective decision making.

7. Informed decisions and informed consents are not exchangeable terms. The case manager must understand the similarities and differences of these terms, their relationship with ethical and legal standards, and protect the patient's right to agree to or refuse certain care options, and remain free of coercion and judgment.

8. It is important for case managers to identify and differentiate clinical and organizational ethical concerns and address them in collaboration with the right individuals and experts. The process of managing clinical ethical issues is somewhat different from that of organizational ethics nature.

14.9. REFERENCES

American Case Management Association. (2013). Standards of Practice and Scope of Services for Health Care Delivery System Case Management and Transitions of Care Professionals, Little Rock, AR, 2013.

American Nurses Association. (2015). Code of ethics: The center of ethics and human rights, Silver Springs, MD.

Beauchamp, T.L. & Childress, J.F. (1994). *Principles of biomedical ethics*, 4th ed., Oxford University Press, New York, NY.

Buchanan, A. (2000). Trust in managed care organizations, *Kennedy Institute Ethics J 10*(3):189–212.

Case Management Society of America. (2010). Standards of Practice for Case Management, Little Rock, AR.

Commission for Case Manager Certification. (2015). Code of Professional Conduct for Case Managers, Mount Laurel, NJ.

Daniels, M. & Sabin, J. (1997). Limits to healthcare: fair procedures, democratic deliberations, and the legitimacy problem for insurers. *Philos Public Aff 26*(4):303–350.

Donagrandi, M.A. & Eddy, M. (2000). Ethics of case management: implications for advanced practice nursing, *Clin Nurs Spec 14*(5):241–249.

Elwyn, G., Lloyd, A., Joseph-Williams, N., Cording, E., Thomson, R., Durand, M. & Edwards, A. (2013). Option grids: Shared decision making made easier. *Patient Education and Counseling, 90*; 2017–212.

Elwyn, G., Frosch, D., Thomson, R., Joseph-Williams, N., Lloyd, A., Kinnersley, P., Cording, E., Thomson, D., Dodd, C., Rolnick, S., Edwards, A., & Barry, M. (2012). Shared decision making: A model for clinical practice. *Journal of General Internal Medicine, 27*(10): 1361–1367.

Jansen, L.A. (2000). Deliberative decision making and the treatment of pain, *J Palliat Med 4*(1):23–30.

Jansen LA. (2001). The role of the nurse in clinical genetics. In Mahowald M, McKusick V, Scheurle A, et al. (Eds.), *Genetics in the clinic: Clinical, ethical, and social implications for primary care*. Mosby, St Louis, MO.

Leonard, M. & Miller, E. (2012). *Nursing case management: review and resouce manual*, 4th ed. American Nurses Credentialing Center, Silver Springs, MD.

National Association of Social Workers. (2008). Code of Ethics of the NASW, Washington, DC.

National Association of Social Workers. (2013). NASW Standards for Social Work Case Management. Washington, DC.

15 Accreditation in Case Management

Agencies involved in the accreditation of healthcare organizations, and case management programs are usually private enterprises. They, in addition to regulatory agencies, set industry standards for quality, safety, and credible healthcare services and delivery systems. Among these standards are usually based on current acceptable practices within the healthcare system, they still convey a direction toward future industry objectives and innovations. Accreditation agencies are comprehensive and cutting edge in their approaches to the assessment of healthcare organizations' quality, safety, focus on the consumer, and performance improvement practices. They also base their requirements on the healthcare industry trends, regulatory must haves, expert opinions of healthcare provdiers and organizations, and interests of consumers and their advocates. Pursuing accreditation is usually voluntary where accreditation agencies hold no direct authority over the interested healthcare organizations. However, achieving accreditation indicates recognition to reimbursement intermediaries, consumers, regulators, and the healthcare industry that acceptable quality standards are maintained, are safe, and quality patient care is delivered to the likings of consumers.

Accreditation agencies conduct nationwide assessments of many types of healthcare organizations and facilities such as the following:

- Acute care
- Long-term care
- Ambulatory care and patient centred medical homes
- Home care and visiting nurse services
- Subacute care
- Acute and subacute rehabilitation
- Specialized programs within an organization
- Behavioral health
- Health insurance plans

Each accreditation survey incorporates specialty requirements into the the general standards to enable the most complete review of a specific healthcare facility or program within a facility. Regardless of the accreditation agency and its specializations, the approach for the review includes not only the structure and processes of care delivery, but also pays special attention to outcomes as well. The standards may measure and evaluate an organization's practices (or program within an organization such as case management or utilization management) in the following four general areas of focus:

- *Individual*: patient and practitioner
- *Structure*: facility and environment of care
- *Process*: delivery of service and systems of care
- *Outcomes*: performance assessment and improvement

The intent of the accreditation review is to broadly assess the overall organizational performance, in meeting quality, safety, and patient experience with care standards. When the purpose of accreditation is a program or center of excellence within an organization, then the assessment is limited to the performance of the program or center. By weaving the review throughout the many facets of the healthcare organization (or program), accreditation agencies take the opportunity to survey if and how well the organization manages itself and its performance including care outcomes.

Almost all accreditation agencies center themselves around the measurement of quality and safety in an organization. They have defined for healthcare appropriate indications of quality by establishing standards reflective of the best possible practice and by providing guidelines to indicate the acceptable safety and compliance measures. The Joint Commission (TJC) standards, for example, require a healthcare organization to assess and evaluate its performance on all levels. This may begin with the organization's vision, mission, objectives, and structure, and it encompasses its actual day-to-day operations, functions, and departmental roles. The review continues with communication at and between all levels of personnel and departments within the organization, with careful examination of adequate and planned use of resources and the inspection of the general physical plant facilities. URAC and the National Committee for Quality Assurance (NCQA) follow similar processes as the TJC, however, they do not focus on physical plant and facilities operations.

Accreditation agencies have generally organized their standards into broad categories dealing with specific healthcare delivery components including evaluation of outcomes: quality, safety, and access to services. Generally speaking, accreditation standards can be divided into three categories as described in Box 15.1. However, this list is more comprehensive than what an individual accreditation agency may require or focus on.

15.1. PATIENT-FOCUSED STANDARDS

Patient-focused standards reflect the appropriate care and treatment phases for the patient rather than the provider. The standards tend to cross all departments or divisions within an organization. Accreditation agencies may judge them based on the information the organization shares with other disciplines, the patient, and family, and the appropriateness of improvement actions taken based on the data collected (i.e., performances or needs).

Accreditation agencies urge healthcare organizations and professionals to reduce the amount of duplication present within the healthcare system and improve patients' access to care and services. In an effort to promote both efficient use of resources (staff and time) and customer satisfaction, accreditation agencies encourage the use of interdisciplinary communication and documentation tools. What is most important is that accurate, validated data be used to plan, implement and evaluate care. Collection and reporting of data may be delegated to the most appropriate healthcare personnel (e.g., case managers) and used by other disciplines once validated (Case Manager's Tip 15.1).

Box 15.1 Standards and Functions

Standards of care (clinical care delivery and focus on the patient/client)
- Patient-centered care
- Patient rights
- Organizational and clinical ethics
- Assessment of patients
- Provision of care for patients
- Transitional and discharge planning
- Education and health instruction/patient engagement
- Continuum of care/health and human services
- Patient safety

Organization functions (administrative or operational and focus on organizational systems and processes)
- Improvement of organization performance
- Management of the environment of care inlcuding life safety and emergency/disaster management
- Management of human resources
- Management of information including health information technology
- Infection surveillance, prevention, and control
- Quality and safety
- Reporting of outcomes data to accreditation and/or regulatory agencies

Structures with Functions (personnel and departments and focus on the organization)
- Governance and board of directors/trustees
- Leadership and management of staff
- Medical professionals
- Nursing professionals
- Allied health professionals

The patient-focused standards guide the patient through an episode of illness back to the most appropriate care setting or level of care. The intent is to efficiently move the patient through the healthcare system and continuum of care while meeting the needs of the patient and family or caregiver. Past ideas of only seeing the patient through an episode of illness are no longer appropriate. The healthcare industry has recognized the need to employ a comprehensive approach to care and treatment. The introduction of cost containment by reimbursement parties with payment denials and finaical risk programs (e.g., value based purchasing) has cautioned the industry to plan appropriately and well but within reason.

Cognizant of these trends, accreditation agencies have enhanced the focus on and importance of developing efficient, effective, and safe care management plans for patients/families/caregivers which span the continuum of care. Point of entry into the healthcare

CASE MANAGER'S TIP 15.1

Promoting Efficient Resource Use and Customer Satisfaction

Use of interdisciplinary communication and documentation tools and structures (e.g., interdisciplinary plan of care and daily patient care management rounds) enhances outcomes (e.g., clinical quality, safety, and cost-effectiveness) and assures desirable patient care experience.

system, whether hospital, primary care center, or physician's office, is the point of initiation of discharge/transitional planning and the patient's return or transfer to the most appropriate care setting. Fundamental in this approach is strong, timely communication of information between and among the various entry points and providers. Meeting the patient-focused accreditation standards means putting the patient and family/caregiver in the center and allowing the established healthcare organization's processes and systems to flow around the patient.

Case managers are able to enhance the patient experience of care and improve associated care outcomes. They assure that:

- Patients experience hospitalization or an episode of illness in the most seamless way possible.
- Hospital rules, policies, and procedures smoothly facilitate the flow of patients across the continuum of care (within and outside of a healthcare organization).
- Patients' return to the community care setting is timely and well planned.
- Health education and care follow-up are clearly outlined, appropriate, and occur in a timely manner to ultimately improve patients' ability to manage needed lifestyle adjustments.
- Necessary considerations for the cultural diversity of the patients, families, and caregivers are addressed. For example, each patient participates in planning care and treatments and in addressing specific needs, which may include cultural, ethnic, and spiritual considerations.

15.2. ORGANIZATIONAL FUNCTIONS

The patient-focused standards do place the patient, family, and caregiver at the heart of the delivery of services. They clearly delineate the need to adopt a holistic approach in providing care and meeting institutional objectives. In the "organization functions" standards,

accreditation agencies may establish requirements to ensure that the healthcare organization engages in a number of functions such as those described in Box 15.2.

This group of standards focuses on the institution's development of working relationships and systems that allow it to provide patient-centered care. The intent in the measurement of these standards is usually to see strong interdisciplinary teams that are knowledgeable of their individual departmental requirements and those institutional objectives that guide the operations of the facility, always with the patient at the center of the team.

15.3. STRUCTURES WITH FUNCTIONS

This set of standards governs "structures with functions" in the healthcare organization. The five main areas (i.e., governance, leadership/management, medical staff, nursing personnel, and allied health professionals) set the tone for the direction, guidance, and operation of the healthcare organization. Accreditation agencies may require the organization to clearly define and communicate the following to its healthcare personnel and the consumers it serves.

- The mission, vision, and ethical code of operations
- The scope of services provided and the type of populations served

---

Box 15.2   Examples of Healthcare Organizational Functions

- Design efficient processes and systems for safe and quality care delivery
- Examine practice in an organized, planned, and ongoing manner
- Identify opportunities for performance improvements
- Implement cost-effective measures to ensure smooth operations
- Establish job requirements and measurable criteria for staff performance and competence
- Maintain a safe, clean, and appropriate environment of care for all: patients, families, healthcare professionals and other personnel, and visitors
- Develop effective methods to facilitate the communication of information among all involved
- Proactively examine practice and institute process changes to reduce medical errors, prevent harm, and promote patient safety
- Report publically on performance and outcomes such as the value-based purchasing program measures and patient experience of care

- The requirements of the practitioners and leaders of the organization, including education, experience, competence, and clinical privileges
- The involvement of each leader in planning future services and developing operating budgets
- The relationship of the governing board in strategic planning, day-to-day operations, and the flow of information within the organization

It is easy to see how accreditation agencies have focused and developed their standards to guide healthcare organizations toward quality and safety endeavors. They present their manuals of standards in a way that emphasizes such focus and to guide healthcare organizations in this regard.

15.4. CONTINUOUS SELF-EVALUATION AND IMPROVEMENT

In addition to defining the quality and safety standards, accreditation agencies may set an expectation for the healthcare organization to continuously evaluate itself and implement measures to improve the delivery of services and related outcomes. A healthcare organization is expected to select a systematic process of quality/performance improvement and apply it across the board to all areas to ensure a consistent approach. An example of the quality assessment and performance improvement methodology is design, measure, assess, improve, control, and redesign. This process is one way to actualize continuous quality improvement (CQI) and to guide projects/teams through the steps needed to effect sound prioritized change. It asks that each component be examined and defined in relation to the type and amount of services provided, the type of customers served, and the most important components of the services delivered and their associated outcomes. Once the components of service have been outlined, consideration can then be given to assessing and establishing expected performance measures.

Moving through the process, data are collected, aggregated, displayed, and analyzed to determine whether performance is satisfactory or it needs improvement. If improvement is warranted, a plan is developed, implemented, measured, and evaluated for success. All of this work is then shared within the organization/department to document improvement strides.

Accreditation agencies may also require the healthcare organization to examine the many facets or dimensions of performance inherent in "doing the right thing" and "doing the right thing well, every time." The dimensions include appropriateness, efficacy, timeliness, availability, effectiveness, continuity, safe-ty, efficiency, patient-centeredness, respect, and caring. Additionally, accreditation agencies ask that the personnel with the most knowledge and those with the ability to implement changes work together in interdisciplinary teams to improve performance and effect better outcomes. Certainly this indicates a most comprehensive approach to reviewing and determining how well an organization meets quality and safety industry standards.

Accreditation agencies usually invest resources in developing standards that are future oriented. They strive to incorporate the very best of current practice while anticipating the needs of tomorrow. They also are careful to balance the requirements of the future with the abilities of today. Before revisions of existing standards or the addition of new ones go into effect, they pursue public comments to ensure that the expectations are realistic, relevant, appropriate, and manageable by those to adhere to them. Moreover, accreditation agencies may expect to see evidence of current best practices, society guidelines, and recommendations used in consideration with adopting organizational change and setting priorities. This expectation crosses all standards and reinforces the commitment of accreditation agencies to the promotion of appropriate, safe, and quality care and outcomes.

The industry's concern with patient safety and medical error reduction has prompted accreditation agencies to require healthcare organizations to conduct intense analysis of events (i.e., root cause analysis [RCA]) that cause or expose a patient to actual or potential harm. They also encourage healthcare organizations to proactively examine their processes and systems of care to identify opportunities to reduce risk to patients. Continuous change, evolution of responsibility and accountability, and integration of clinical practice with administrative direction have become the new constants of the accreditation standards. As standards are adopted and refined, clear emphasis is placed on the relationship, integration, and interdependence of these standards. Selection of care issues (e.g., pain management, transitions of care, continuity) and linkage of the issues to all applicable standards define for all members of the healthcare team the quality and optimal outcomes to be achieved when providing care. This concept parallels the intent of practice guidelines, interdisciplinary case management plans and clinical pathways used in case management models of patient care delivery.

Examining the requirements to meet standards awakens a realization that systems, processes, manuals, policies, and medical records are not enough to position the healthcare organization and providers to achieve the quality outcomes they desire. What is needed is a well-developed, cohesive, and interactive approach by the organization and its personnel to accomplishing its stated goals, objectives, and mission. Adoption of a model and commitment to that model are the first steps in realizing success. Support and encouragement of the model and education regarding the need for change are the next logical steps. Finally, allowing change to occur by empowering those individuals (e.g., case managers) who need to champion the change with the ability to do so establishes the model as a working concept. Continually evaluating and improving the model maintains its original intent—to improve care, services, and their related outcomes.

Accreditation standards direct healthcare organizations, providers, and other professionals to consider their primary focus first—the patient, family, and caregiver. They proceed with the organizational functions needed to achieve the goal of quality and safe patient care and end with the requirements for knowledgeable, progressive leaders who demonstrate the ability to encourage and produce change within the organization. However, this is certainly easier to describe than to achieve.

15.5. RELATIONSHIP OF CASE MANAGEMENT TO ACCREDITATION STANDARDS

The case management model or program in an organization embodies the same principles as those of accreditation standards. It uses the patient-focused care standards as its base and builds on them with the addition of the organization functions. The model is enforced by the commitment and acknowledgment of the structures with functions as to its appropriateness, timeliness, effectiveness, efficiency, continuity, efficacy, availability, safety, patient-centerdness, and attention to respect and caring. The model complements the intents of accreditation standards and introduces a practical working approach to ensuring quality in a cost-conscious and safe environment of care.

Case management reinforces the commitment to doing the right thing and doing the right thing well, every time, all the time. Careful assessment and evaluation of patient needs allow appropriate selection of those patients requiring special attention to move through the healthcare system. Determining complexity of needs allows healthcare providers to tailor plans of care to meet customer, institutional, and regulatory expectations.

Case management focuses on getting the patient, family, and caregiver through the healthcare system in the most efficient and safest way possible. An expectation of this is to begin the process upon entry into the system. By beginning with a careful needs assess-

ment on admission/access, potential patients needing case management and post-discharge (or post episode of care) services can be identified. Point of entry may be the physician's office, hospitalization, ambulatory care, or health insurance plan enrollment. Taking a proactive approach to identifying care and post-discharge/post episode of care needs and to the allocation of appropriate resources allows provisions to be made for a smooth experience through an episode of illness.

By design, case management sets care and outcomes expectations for patient populations with particular diagnoses or procedures for a specific timeframe. It establishes the norm based on industry standards to treat approximately 80% of those patients with the same diagnosis (Case Manager's Tip 15.2). By defining the norm and establishing sound care paths/clinical practice guidelines with delineated outcomes, efficient, safe, and appropriate management of patient care is outlined and can thus be measured. Establishing structure allows providers to maintain control and prepare the patient for the anticipated experience. It makes provisions to begin post-discharge education early during the hospital stay or during an ambulatory care encounter. Allowing for time to evaluate and reinforce critical health instructions ensures sound preparation in returning the patient to the appropriate care setting.

One of the intents of case management programs is to move the patient through the healthcare system and necessary levels of service/care (acute care, ambulatory care, or home care) with minimal effort, reduced cost, and maximum efficiency and safety. These programs are able to accomplish well-defined outcomes (Box 15.3) and to assist the healthcare organization meet its goals and mission in patient care delievry.

 CASE MANAGER'S TIP 15.2

Standardized Care Practices Using Interdisciplinary Case Management Plans of Care

Case managers are astute at identifying how a standardized interdisciplinary case management plan, clinical pathway, or clinical practice guideline applies to the care of an individual patient. They are well aware that these plans are for the 80% of the patients suffering a particular health condition. The other 20% tend to suffer other issues which make the standardized plans inappropriate to meet their needs. This is the 80-20 rule. For these 20% of patients, case managers know not to automatically apply the standardized plans, rather dvelop, in collaboration with the interdisciplinary healthcare team, case management plans of care specific to meet their care goals and needs.

Box 15.3 Contribution of Case Management Programs—Special Focus on Care Delivery and Outcomes

- Provide caregivers an objective determination mark to move the patient to the next most appropriate level of care
- Allow objective measures for performance, quality, safety, cost and variance evaluation
- Address the overall care needs of the patient while allowing for individualization
- The patient remains the focus, the center of case management services. Patient care objectives may include the following:
  —Smooth transition of the patient from one phase of care to the next
  —Providing needed care and treatments in a timely, efficient, and effective manner
  —Appropriate resource utilization and management: time, staff, supplies, tests and procedures, costs, and length of stay
  —Appropriate, timely, and safe discharge/transitional planning and preparation
  —Ensuring that patient, family, and caregiver have the right tools (durable medical equipment, health education, supplies, health regimen) to manage lifestyle adjustments while in the community
  —Addressing a holistic approach in the delivery of care by involving the necessary members of the interdisciplinary team

---

Looking at the standards of accreditation agencies and case management objectives, it is apparent how well the use of one satisfies the requirements of the other. Accreditation standards have strongly urged healthcare organizations (and case management programs) to take a hard look at themselves and to examine both how they provide services and their outcomes. The overall objective is to outline current processes and systems and to assess how well they function. Implicit in the intents of accreditation agencies is the review of these functions from the patient's and family's perspectives. Healthcare organizations are asked to place themselves in the patient's shoes and walk through the process of hospitalization, experiencing it from the consumer's viewpoint. Many hospitals choose to diagram the steps and find that many steps have been added over time to meet departmental needs. Often these additions make the process a little longer, unnecessarily complex, and more confusing to the patient/family. A commitment to improving services and the quality of care delivered leads organizations to perhaps ask the following questions:

- Why are things done this way?
- How can the processes of care be streamlined to improve efficiency, quality, and safety?
- Which nonvalue-adding processes can be eliminated, and which ones are necessary to keep?

The basic goal is smooth transition of the patient from one phase of care to the next, each step along the way. Other goals are improved customer satisfaction and experience of care, a decrease in duplication of services (or complete elimination), timely delivery of appropriate, safe, and continuum-based services, improved efficiency, reduced cost, a seamless approach to patient care delivery and transitional planning, and an improved overall healthcare organization's image or reputation.

Examining the development of case management, the same principles are seen. A review of current practice outlines the various steps of treatment and care for the patient. Looking at current practice for a specific diagnosis, outlined by day of hospital stay (or visit in case of home care, long-term plans of care in case of ambulatory care settings), allows healthcare providers to review and decide if services could be scheduled sooner or less frequently. It ensures that providers plan needed care efficiently, with attention to cost-effective and safe solutions. It further enables these providers to develop standards of practice that address patient care needs and ensure the delivery of services in a timely manner. This also allows each healthcare discipline the time to interact with the patient, family, and caregiver, and to meet specific outcomes.

The flow of hospitalization from one phase/day to the next and from one discipline to the other must be seamless to the patient and family. For example, the TJC emphasizes this expectation through its continuum of care/discharge planning accreditation standard (Box 15.4). The continuum of care is defined as an integrated system of settings, services, healthcare providers, and care levels along which case managers match patients' needs with appropriate levels and types of care and resources. (See Chapter 6 for more information about the continuum of care and transitional planning).

If the goal of the case management model is to place the patient at the center of care delivery, then the work, care, and treatments must flow around the patient. Use of the case management model to facilitate the process of hospitalization or the management of an episode of care ensures that a plan of care is mapped out and that the care and services are delivered to the patient rather than the patient being brought to the care and services; that is for the convenience of the patient not the healthcare organization. The communication and planning

---

Box 15.4   The Continuum of Care and Case Management (TJC, 2015a)

The goal of the continuum of care/discharge planning standard is to maximize the coordination of care activities provided by the various healthcare providers and across the different settings/levels of care. Case managers can enhance meeting this standard by facilitating and ensuring the following activities:

Before admission:

- Assess the patient and family care needs
- Screen the patient and family for the need for post-discharge services and community resources
- Make the information about community resources available and easily accessible to the patients and healthcare team
- Ensure open lines of communication and networks across providers, settings, and facilities

During admission:

- Provide services that are consistent with the healthcare organization's mission and philosophy and that meet the needs of the patient population served
- Provide care and services based on the complexity of the patient's medical and social condition, risk, and staffing levels
- Facilitate the patient's admission and transfer from one level of care to another
- Consult with other healthcare providers and facilities for patient transfers or for meeting patient needs

During hospital stay:

- Ensure continuity and consistency in care planning and provision of care
- Facilitate care coordination among all providers and across settings
- Engage the patient and family in deciding about the next level of care and obtain their agreement on the transitional plan and services

Before discharge:

- Coordinate post-discharge services based on the patient's assessed needs
- Provide patient and family education in preparation of discharge or transfer to another facility
- Ensure the appropriateness of patients' transfers to other facilities

At discharge:

- Refer patients to other providers and for post-discharge services to ensure that the continuing care needs are met
- Share relevant and necessary information with providers or other facilities to be responsible for the post-discharge care and services

Case managers must coordinate and facilitate patient care throughout all of the phases of care provision; during the patient's entry into the system (e.g., admission to the hospital); and while assessing the patient's needs, diagnosing the problems, planning the treatment and discharge plans, implementing the care, and transferring the patient to other facilities or discharging back into the community.

- Discharge/transitional planning must focus on the patient's continuing physical, emotional, symptom management (e.g., pain, nausea, shortness of breath, fatigue), housekeeping, transportation, psychosocial, and other needs
- Discharge/transitional planning must assure quality and safety at all times and improve communication, handoffs, and continuity of care across healthcare provider and care settings

---

processes developed by a healthcare organization are the necessary investments in transitioning from an adopted model to a working plan. This model is a perfect illustration of how to implement or adhere to accreditation standards. The case management model then is an operational approach to meeting the following demands:

- Customer expectations by providing a well-planned, seamless approach to care management and across the continuum of care
- Institutional needs by addressing cost-effective and safe solutions to the management of care

- Healthcare provider needs by allowing timely interventions for the delivery of care within a structured framework
- Regulatory needs by encompassing the principles and standards of the accreditation and regulatory agency and in outlining the management of care
- Patient care safety expectations (Box 15.5) by preventing delays in and variances of care delivery processes

The case manager is responsible for moving patients with a range of needs through the system and along the continuum of care in a seamless, continu-

---

Box 15.5   Patient Care Safety and Case Management

Accreditation agencies focus on patient care safety and medical/healthcare errors reduction as part of the environment of care and leadership standards. Case managers can facilitate meeting this requirement because of their role in, or contribution to, risk management, variance management, and delays in care activities and error prevention. Often accreditation agencies require the healthcare organization's leadership staff to be responsible for implementing an organization-wide safety program, including activities such as performance improvement, environmental safety, and risk management. The safety program must focus on patients, visitors, and staff. Case managers may facilitate the implementation of the safety program by doing the following:

- Fostering a culture of safety
- Encouraging recognition and awareness of risks and hazards to patient safety
- Acknowledging medical/healthcare errors
- Initiating actions to reduce variances, delays, errors, and risks
- Encouraging voluntary reporting of errors and near misses and promoting a "blame-free" environment of care
- Supporting effective responses to occurrences
- Effecting a proactive approach to errors reduction
- Participating as members of error reduction committees and taskforces
- Participating in performance improvement teams and activities that enhance patient safety and improve quality
- Collecting, tracking, aggregating, and analyzing data on quality and patient safety
- Facilitating communication among members of the interdisciplinary healthcare team to promote a seamless, safe, and effective patient care delivery process

---

Box 15.6   Clinical Pathways/Practice Guidelines and Case Management

Accreditation agencies do not mandate but rather recommend the use of clinical practice guidelines for patient care planning and management. They advocate that the guidelines be evidence-based, outcome oriented, and interdisciplinary in nature. Case managers can facilitate the development, implementation, and evaluation of these guidelines. To meet the requirements of accreditation standards, healthcare organizations can ensure that clinical practice guidelines do the following:

- Are developed in an interdisciplinary forum
- Prospectively address the care of patients with particular diagnoses or procedures during hospitalization and across the continuum of care and settings
- Reduce variation in practice by establishing uniform standards
- Anticipate and capture variances and deviation from the plan
- Identify expected outcomes of care and clinical decision points
- Are used for evaluating performance and outcomes
- Ensure appropriate use and allocation of resources
- Assist clinicians in making decisions on the prevention, diagnosis, treatment, and management of selected medical and surgical conditions
- Are used to identify opportunities for improvement and systems redesign

---

ous, safe, and consistent manner. Standardized interdisciplinary case management plans (see Chapter 10 for more details), proactively developed as baseline tools or standards of care, facilitate and arrange for an array of care, treatment, and services required in caring for complex patients. The use of clinical practice guidelines for this purpose (Box 15.6). The benefit of the case management model is the provision of an individual practitioner (e.g., a case manager) to do this.

Generally, accreditation agencies do not set different standards for different types of patient populations. Rather, they outline high-quality and safety standards for all. The ability to meet the standards for the group of patients with complex needs is chal-

lenging. The case management model recognizes this challenge and meets it by placing the care of complex patient populations in the hands of a dedicated healthcare professional. The case manager is an additional investment by the organization to meet the increasing demands of today's complex and chronically ill patient populations.

Using all of the creativity and know-how necessary to maintain patients "on track" toward discharge from a hospital or safe at home and in the community, the case manager must plan and intervene as necessary to meet the unique needs of these complex patients. The case management plan/clinical practice guideline provides the necessary vehicle to accomplish this task. Its ability to organize care and treatments, coupled with its outlined progression to outcome achievement, makes it a natural approach for managing care for the patient holistically while meeting regulatory standards. The ability of case managers to facilitate the process of care for those patients with complex needs is crucial to meeting the needs of the patient, healthcare provider, organization, payer, and accreditation agency standards.

15.6. CASE MANAGEMENT AND ROOT CAUSE ANALYSIS

One function of case management models is the prevention of untoward events or medical errors to ultimately enhance patient care safety. This takes place under the umbrella of quality management and the delivery of quality, safe patient care services and outcomes. This focus has gained increased attention because of the public interest in medical error reduction and the consumer's right for a safe healthcare environment and services. Case managers, by virtue of their involvement in risk management, play an essential role in the prevention, investigation, and evaluation of medical errors and sentinel/significant events. RCA is the process used in the effective and comprehensive review and analysis of events patients may encounter during an episode of care (Case Manager's Tip 15.3).

A sentinel event is an occurrence that has resulted in an unanticipated death or major permanent loss of function, not related to the natural course of the patient's illness or underlying condition (TJC, 2015a). Examples of sentinel events are as follows:

- Suicide of a patient while under the supervision of a healthcare provider (i.e., while in a facility such as a hospital or crisis stabilization center)
- Infant abduction or mix-up
- Administration of wrong blood transfusion (i.e., wrong blood group type)
- Surgery on the wrong patient or body part
- Elopement-related death
- Restraint-related death
- Fall-related death
- Assault/rape while under the supervision of a healthcare provider or while institutionalized

The use of clinical practice guidelines or standardized interdisciplinary plans of care improves the processes of patient care delivery and enhances safety. Accreditation agencies encourage healthcare organizations and providers to have a standard and formal process for the development, implementation, evaluation, approval, and revision of their clinical practice guidelines and care plans where both clinical and leadership staff are involved and are representative of the various departments and disciplines. In addition, effective plans are those which apply specific criteria for the selection and implementation of practice guidelines. Without a doubt, case managers are able to monitor, evaluate, facilitate, and enforce these activities.

Accreditation agencies do not require the mandatory reporting of sentinel events; however, the state health departments usually do. Case managers, depending on the organization where they practice and established job descriptions, may be required to facilitate the RCA process, evaluation, and reporting of sentinel events. In such cases, they must be knowledgeable and skilled in the effective conduct of an RCA process. An RCA is considered acceptable if it does the following:

- Focuses on the system and care processes and not just the provider(s)
- Answers the "why" questions
- Includes human factors engineering analysis
- Identifies changes that could be implemented to reduce risk and prevent similar incidents in the future
- Is conducted in an interdisciplinary, collaborative manner
- Includes participation by leadership staff, risk management staff, and others as appropriate
- Provides an action plan for implementation, monitoring, and evaluation of the necessary changes, including an identification of the personnel responsible for implementing the changes

15.7. DOCUMENTATION STANDARDS

Accreditation standards including documentation challenge healthcare providers and organizations to accomplish the following tasks:

- Design and implement efficient patient journeys through the continuum of care
- Decrease duplication through interdisciplinary team work
- Manage information and communication across providers and settings
- Be cognizant of resource utilization, fiscal responsibilities, and length of stay issues
- Provide quality and safe care based on sound current principles and national standards
- Use documentation standards and systems to reflect the above tasks

Taken at face value, it is easy to see how case man-

 CASE MANAGER'S TIP 15.3

Root Cause Analysis

RCA is a process used by healthcare providers and administrators to identify the basic or causal factors that contribute to variation in performance and outcomes or underlie the occurrence of a sentinel or significant event which undermines patient safety and may result in death or long-term injury and disability.

agement tools and documentation fit into the overall scheme of accreditation standards. Examining each charge separately reinforces the importance and necessity of carefully developing interdisciplinary plans (clinical pathways or practice guidelines) to outline specific outcomes to be achieved within specific timeframes and the documentation in patient's records (see Box 15.6).

After reviewing the intent of accreditation and seeing the relationship between the standards and case management, it is necessary to look at the documentation tools and their relationship to these standards. This provides further evidence of the efficacy of case management in meeting the accreditation requirements.

The familiar saying, "if it's not documented, it's not done," holds true when fiscal intermediaries, accreditation and regulatory agencies review patient medical records. Any type of retrospective review that is used to evaluate the quality and safety of care and services provided to patients relies heavily on the evaluation of documentation. Appearances count. Little can be said to give credence to sloppy, illegible, contradictory entries in a patient record. One of the assumptions made when records are not neat, consistent, or complete is that the care rendered is less than adequate, inconsistent, and lacking (Case Manager's Tip 15.4). Thankfully, electronic documentation systems have assisted in addressing this concern.

One should always remember that during an accreditation survey the accreditation agency often reviews both concurrent (open) medical records and retrospec-

CASE MANAGER'S TIP 15.4

Documentation

With the advent of electronic documentation, computerized provider order entry systems, and electronic medical records (EMRs), healthcare professionals, including case managers, have been able to overcome the concerns of illegible documentation. However, other unintended consequences resulted from implementation of electronic documentation. Healthcare professionals must be aware of and address. For example, unnecessarily length of medical records, fragmented documentation, and use of structured documentation tools that impact the ability to individualize care for a specific patient. Often electronic medical records have resulted in concerns related to complexity of navigation and retrieval of important information especially during an accreditation survey or a visit from a regulatory agency giving the impression that key information is missing or an important care activity was not completed for a patient.

CASE MANAGER'S TIP 15.5

Evaluating the Quality of Documentation: Review of Records

Keep in mind that the accreditation agency reviews both concurrent (i.e., open) and retrospective (i.e., closed) medical records during its survey. The objective is to compare the care and treatment currently rendered and documented with past completed documentation and to established standards, policies, and procedures.

tive (closed) records. Its objective is to see the care and treatment currently rendered and documented and to compare this to past completed documentation (Case Manager's Tip 15.5). Specific diagnoses are chosen for review. The diagnoses chosen usually have high-risk, high-volume, and problem-prone issues or concerns surrounding them and require added interventions—physical, emotional, ethical, psychosocial, or spiritual. This part of the accreditation survey evaluates the quality of the documentation reflecting the holistic and seamless approach to needed care and treatments for the patient, family, and significant other.

Accreditation agencies may use a comparison to describe the closed medical record review. They liken the completed record to a book that details a story of patient care. The aim is to see a beginning (assessment and planning for patient care), a middle (interventions, outcomes, and patient responses to the care rendered), and an end (evaluation of services and goals and evidence of a thoughtful and safe discharge plan and preparation). Each phase is necessary in assessing the overall patient outcomes of a hospitalization or an encounter of care.

Accreditation agencies have provided structure to assist healthcare organizations and professionals in resolving issues/concerns related to documentation. They require professionals to base clinical practice on standards of care. These may take many forms, including policy, procedure, and protocol or guideline. The key is that they are based on established and nationally accepted practice. Accreditation agencies also require periodic review and update of care standards to reflect current practice and latest evidence. Changes made must be substantiated with sound reasoning (e.g., regulatory changes, new scientific research outcomes, patient safety, error reduction).

Once standards have been developed and accepted, all involved or affected must be educated to expected practice, and the documents must be accessible as reference guides for healthcare professionals. Use of the standard becomes the established norm, and variations in practice must be documented and explained. When the standard is established and applied in the clinical setting, accountability for individual practice may be enforced and evaluation must demonstrate adherence to the new expectations.

The documentation tools (e.g., interdisciplinary case management plans) developed for the case management model are formulated applying the same principles of quality, safety, access to care, and cost-effectiveness. They serve several purposes (Case Manager's Tip 15.6) and are developed with input from all healthcare providers who use them. Representation is usually from the various professional disciplines. They outline current practice for the practitioner based on actual retrospective medical record review and current published evidence-based standards and guidelines. They are designed to facilitate communication by condensing each discipline's plan of care into one document, thereby decreasing duplication and improving timely communication. By outlining care and treatments in an organized manner, an immediate flag is activated when patient care progression deviates from the predetermined actions or interventions already included in the case management plans. These variations may lead to the following:

- Increased cost
- Prolonged length of stay
- Potential for medical errors, unsafe situation or quality issues
- Indication of a need to revise the plan to reflect changes in practice

 CASE MANAGER'S TIP 15.6

Purposes Served by Documentation Tools

A key point to remember is that the documentation tool (e.g., case management plan) does more than just meet documentation requirements of accreditation and/or regulatory agencies. It serves several purposes, and it acts as the following:

1. The patient map of care through the system and service delivery
2. The practitioner guide to staying on track when providing necessary care and treatments
3. The communication tool for the interdisciplinary team and across levels of care and settings
4. An evaluation tool for quality management to ascertain variations in practice and project fiscal and quality of care implications
5. A standard of care and practice for regulatory and accreditation agencies

The basic premise of outlining the case management plan or clinical pathway and scheduling interventions correlated to length of stay supports the seamless and consistent approach to care. Using the outline, services can be activated for the patient as needed and when required. This type of preplanning allows the work to flow around the patient and enhances the patient/family's view of appropriate holistic care. This approach also creates a positive perception of the healthcare team and contributes to improved customer satisfaction or experience of care.

Another contribution toward improving satisfaction with the delivery of care is the charge to decrease paperwork and duplication of data collection. Case management documentation tools support this charge. Objective documentation on the case management plan lets each healthcare professional discipline review what has been done for and accomplished by the patient. Healthcare providers can then validate required information and patient responses rather than asking redundant questions. Several providers all performing the same assessment and data collection suggests to the patient that nobody is talking to each other and that each discipline must have to complete its work separately from the rest. Certainly this is neither the intent nor the objective of an interdisciplinary and collaborative team effort. It is, however, a distinct impression imparted to the patient, family, and caregiver.

To meet the documentation requirement of accreditation agencies (e.g., decreasing duplication and fragmentation), documentation tools may be developed for the various disciplines to build on data collected by the team. Initial assessments may be gathered by one care team member, then reviewed and added to by the next. The purpose is to accomplish the following:

- Reduce duplication, fragmentation, or redundancy
- Organize data logically to support collaboration and access to information for the interdisciplinary healthcare team members
- Delegate to the appropriate healthcare provider the most appropriate function
- Prepare providers for the computerization of clinical data
- Ensure an interdisciplinary approach to care

Building and refining old principles of documentation standards have led healthcare providers to creative solutions for complex issues. Case management is one of these creative solutions. Its ability to meet and support a wide variety of concerns—fiscal, regulatory, safety, and quality—makes case management a natural selection as a complete model for delivery of care. It blends into the philosophies of accreditation agencies and addresses their requirements based on the specifics of the accreditation standards. The intrinsic value of case management is its ability to place the patient at the center of the team while supporting collaboration of the interdisciplinary healthcare team in meeting stated outcomes. This may not be the only one of its most valuable assets but also one of its most challenging to attain.

15.8. INTERDISCIPLINARY APPROACH TO PATIENT CARE

Another relationship between case management and accreditation is to examine the specific involvement of the interdisciplinary team in patient care delivery. How does the organization get individuals and/or departments to move beyond their separate spaces and to work together? The answer is to break down the barriers or silos and direct united energies into the delivery of quality, safe patient care. The healthcare organization must continuously educate each department (no matter how far removed from the actual delivery of patient care) to the overall mission. This involves commitment and dedication by the leadership team to allow and support necessary collaboration among the various professionals to achieve cohesion among the team.

Accreditation standards have driven the collapse of individual departmental requirements into patient-focused and organization functions and therefore elimination of silos and creation of cross-functional collaborations. These demands are felt by all. No longer could nursing or radiology open to an accreditation standard and measure only its individual performance. It is necessary to work with other disciplines, to know what they do, to determine how and where they overlap, and to assess the overall organizational performance. Accreditation agencies pressure healthcare organizations to refocus on their ultimate mission and to seek ways to point each department in the direction of meeting the organizational objectives.

Knowing this to be the sound, correct way for organizations to position themselves, accreditation agencies are savvy enough to know that this would require intentional and undivided efforts to achieve desired outcomes. The incentives are the same for each department or discipline, including case management—to meet the organizational mission of quality, safe, and cost-effective care. At the center of this mission lies the patient, family, and caregiver.

The introduction of quality management and performance improvement concepts have enabled healthcare organizations to educate staff and enhance their func-

tions. These also have facilitated the growth of working teams to assess, evaluate, and improve services, delivery of care, systems, and processes within the organization. What accreditation agencies have done by establishing quality assessment and improvement standards is to refocus the healthcare organization's way of thinking. They ask healthcare organizations to consider that no matter how well each separate piece of the organization performs, without communication, collaboration, and the ability to work together as teams, inefficiencies and bottlenecks may continue to occur. As a result, delivering quality services efficiently may then be hindered by duplication and miscommunication while what remains as the focus becomes the work rather than the patient.

Case management is a solution to bridging the interdisciplinary healthcare team. It provides the direction the patient needs to take to complete the course of care through an episode of illness. All team members have the opportunity to identify where and when they need to intervene to accomplish their care goals. Each team member knows who, how, and when to communicate with other team members as progression of the patient along the path takes place. Each member is also aware of the involvement of the rest of the team and has access to the specific outcomes and the associated patient responses.

The case management model facilitates a holistic approach to patient care. It recognizes the need for the many disciplines to contribute in directing the patient plan of care appropriately and efficiently. It also recognizes the need to attend to details, to deal with unexpected issues, and to allow each team member to participate in care provision and evaluation of outcomes. Case management reinforces the commitment, responsibility, and accountability of the individual disciplines and the interdisciplinary healthcare team members as a whole to efficient, safe, and timely delivery of care and treatments.

In addition, the case management model assists in educating the interdisciplinary healthcare team with regard to necessary concepts and principles for survival in today's healthcare environment. It introduces discussion of the following:

- Cost issues and treatment efficacy
- Appropriateness of resource utilization and cost containment efforts
- Standards requirements and regulatory needs
- Patient-focused care and care delivery redesign
- Care settings and appropriate levels of care
- Interdisciplinary communication and collaboration, especially across providers in different care settings

- Safety and reduction of errors or care omissions
- Quality management and performance improvement

The "teams" that previously allowed members to interact independently with the patient, family, and significant other must now interact with each other in helping the patient to journey through the maze of the healthcare system. Based on the developed case management plans, all members contribute their interventions and evaluations, allowing the next phase of care to occur and the work to flow around the patient. This approach is most necessary for providing quality, safe patient care services and keeping all healthcare providers focused on the seamless transition of the patient through the system.

The case management program provides a strong working model to accomplish many objectives efficiently. It meets patient, practitioner, team, fiscal, and accreditation agency needs with its effective and appropriate approach to delivery of quality and safe patient care services. It allows organizations to put action into theory and theory into action. Implementing a case management model puts a process in place at the level of patient care that parallels the standards of accreditation agencies. It provides a solid infrastructure to move the organization forward in its vision and attainment of delivery of quality services. It also recognizes the need to develop patient-centered systems and processes to meet patient needs and organizational objectives.

Case management provides the interdisciplinary healthcare team with ways to organize standards of care and practice into cost-effective plans that move the patient through the various healthcare settings efficiently. It positions patients and their families at the center, prepares them for transition appropriately into the community, and helps them to become ready to adopt necessary lifestyle changes and make adjustments to meet health goals. It also facilitates the existence of the healthcare team and organization around patients, supporting them through the episode of illness and assisting them in using documented data regarding practice and outcomes to shape the organization's future.

15.9. THE NATIONAL COMMITTEE FOR QUALITY ASSURANCE

The NCQA is a private, not-for-profit organization dedicated to improving healthcare quality and safety through accreditation. Since its founding in 1990, the NCQA has been driving improvement throughout the healthcare system, helping to elevate the issue of healthcare quality to the top of the national agenda. It offers accreditation in may areas including case management and health inasurance plans. Healthcare organizations must pass a comprehensive review and must annually report on their performance to achieve and maintain NCQA accreditation status (Case Manager's Tip 15.7) (NCQA, 2015a).

The NCQA has built its accreditation standards based on consensus around important healthcare quality issues and by collaborating with employers, policymakers, physicians, patients, and health insurance plans. The standards highlight what is important, how to measure it, and how to promote improvement. The NCQA's programs and services reflect continuous quality improvement, focusing on process of specific activities such as: measure, analyze, improve, and repeat. The NCQA has developed quality standards and performance measures for a broad range of healthcare organizations. These measures and standards are the tools that healthcare organizations and providers may use to identify opportunities for improvement especially when pursuing NCQA accreditation (NCQA, 2015a).

NCQA accreditation is no easy task. For example, accredited health insurance plans today face a set of more than 60 standards and must report on their performance in more than 40 areas in order to earn NCQA's accreditation. The related accreditation standards promote strategies that improve care, enhance services, and reduce costs; for example, paying healthcare providers based on performance, leveraging the Internet to share health information with patients, and disease management and provider-level measurement (NCQA, 2015a).

The range of accreditation programs NCQA offers is broad. They apply to healthcare organizations and individual healthcare professionals ranging from health insurance plans (e.g., HMOs, PPOs, and consumer-directed plans) to physician networks, medical groups, individual physicians, and programs within organizations. NCQA offers several healthcare accreditation programs including those described in Box 15.7.

 CASE MANAGER'S TIP 15.7

The National Committee for Quality Assurance Accreditation

For consumers, payers, employers, and healthcare providers, accreditation is a reliable indicator that a healthcare organization or programs are well-managed and deliver high quality, safe, and cost-conscious care and services.

Box 15.7   The National Committee for Quality Assurance Accreditation Program Offerings

For Health Insurance Plans:

- Health Plans (HP)
- Disease Management (DM)
- Case Management (CM)

For Healthcare Provider Organizations

- Accountable Care Organizations (ACO)
- Wellness and Health Promotion (HWP)

For Health Plan Contracting Organizations

- Managed Behavioral Healthcare Organizations (MBHO)
- Disease Management (DM)
- Case Management (CM)

Box 15.8   The National Committee for Quality Assurance Accreditation Standards for Health Insurance Plans (NCQA, 2015a)

Quality Management and Improvement

1. Program structure
2. Program operations
3. Health services contracting
4. Availability of practitioners
5. Accessibility of services
6. Member experience
7. Complex case management
8. Disease management
9. Practice guidelines
10. Continuity and coordination of medical care
11. Continuity and coordination between medical and behavioral healthcare
12. Marketplace network transparency and experience
13. Delegation of quality improvement activity

Utilization Management (UM)

1. UM structure
2. Clinical criteria for UM decisions
3. Communication services
4. Appropriate professionals
5. Timeliness of UM decisions
6. Clinical information
7. Denial notices
8. Policies for appeals
9. Appropriate handling of appeals
10. Evaluation of new technology
11. Experience with the UM process
12. Emergency services
13. Procedures for pharmaceutical management
14. Triage and referral for behavioral healthcare
15. Delegation of UM

Credentialing and Recredentialing of Personnel

1. Credentialing policies
2. Credentialing committee
3. Initial credentialing verification
4. Recredentialing cycle length
5. Practitioner office site quality
6. Ongoing monitoring
7. Notification to authorities and practitioner appeal rights
8. Assessment of organizational providers
9. Delegation of credentialing

The NCQA's health insurance plan accreditation is one of the oldest and most comprehensive evaluations in the healthcare industry. It is one of the few that incorporate the results of clinical performance (i.e., Healthcare Effectiveness Data and Information Set [HEDIS] measures) and consumer experience (i.e., CAHPS measures). High performing health insurance plans choose NCQA accreditation because it satisfies many stakeholders such as employers, regulators, and consumers. The USDHHS also has selected NCQA as an accrediting entity for qualified health insurance plans participating in the Health Insurance Exchange Marketplace. This is because NCQA's accreditation program focuses on the various key elements the law requires and aligns the CMS's marketplace with accreditation requirements. Box 15.8 summarizes the accreditaion standards for health insurance plans (NCQA, 2015a).

The NCQA offers health insurance plans with different accreditation status levels based on their adherence to standards and performance on the requirements including the HEDIS and CAHPS measures. Accreditation status levels include: excellent, commendable, accredited, provisional, interim, or denied. For HEDIS measures requirements, refer to Box 15.9 and for CAHPS measures refer to Chapter 11.

The NCQA's case management accreditation is a comprehensive, evidence-based program dedicated to quality improvement that can be used for case management programs in provider, payer, or community-based organizations. This accreditation program also ensures that the healthcare organization has processes implemented to enhance safe transitions of patients across care settings and providers. For organizations that are already accredited, certified, or recognized by

Box 15.8 (continued)   The National Committee for Quality Assurance Accreditation Standards for Health Insurance Plans (NCQA, 2015a)

Members' Rights and Responsibilities

1. Statement of members' rights and responsibilities
2. Policies and procedures for complaints and appeals
3. Subscriber information
4. Physician and hospital directories
5. Privacy and confidentiality
6. Marketing information
7. Delegation of members' rights and responsibilities

Member Connections

1. Health appraisals
2. Self-management tools
3. Functionality of claims processing
4. Pharmacy benefit information
5. Personalized information on health plan services
6. Innovations in member service
7. Health information line
8. Encouraging wellness and prevention
9. Delegation of member connections

Medicaid Benefits and Services

1. Medicaid benefits and services

NCQA, the case management accreditation program demonstrates a commitment to the highest degree of quality improvement and safe care delivery (Box 15.10) (NCQA, 2015b).

Case management programs according to NCQA connect people who have complex healthcare and social needs to providers and track their care over time. If successful, these programs hold the potential for reducing unnessary access to healthcare services (e.g., visits to EDs and acute care hospital admissions) by ensuring that consumers receive optimal care while in the community. Because the quality and effectiveness of case management programs varies, independent assessments of the capabilities and performance of these programs or organizations are necessary to demonstrate they deliver the highest quality care possible (NCQA, 2015b).

NCQA developed its case management accreditation program drawing on its past expertise in health insurance plans and clinician practices through the patient centered medical home (PCMH). To develop the case management accreditation program, NCQA convened a panel of experts that reviewed the latest evidence on performance of NCQA's other programs. Ultimately, the expert panel recommended the standards for case

Box 15.9   Healthcare Effectiveness Data and Information Set Measures Requirements based on the 2015 National Committee for Quality Assurance Accreditation Standards (NCQA, 2015a)

HEDIS Measures Requirements for Commercial Health Plans:

- Adult BMI assessment
- Antidepressant medication management
- Appropriate testing for children with pharyngitis
- Appropriate treatment for children with upper respiratory infection
- Medication management for people with asthma
- Avoidance of antibiotic treatment in adults with acute bronchitis
- Breast cancer screening
- Cervical cancer screening
- Childhood immunization status
- Chlamydia screening in women
- Colorectal cancer screening
- Comprehensive diabetes care
- Controlling high blood pressure
- Flu vaccinations for adults ages 18–64
- Follow-up after hospitalization for mental illness
- Follow-up for children prescribed ADHD medication
- Human papilloma virus vaccine for female adolescents
- Immunizations for adolescents
- Initiation and engagement of alcohol and other drug dependence treatment
- Medical assistance with smoking and tobacco use cessation
- Persistence of beta-blocker treatment after a heart attack
- Pharmacotherapy management of COPD exacerbation
- Prenatal and post-partum care
- Use of imaging studies for low back pain
- Weight assessment and counseling for nutrition and physical activity for children/adolescents
- Getting care quickly
- Getting needed care
- Claims processing
- Customer service
- Rating of health plan
- Rating of all healthcare services
- Rating of personal doctor
- Rating of specialist seen most often

HEDIS Measures Requirements for Medicare Health Plans

- Adult BMI assessment
- Antidepressant medication management
- Breast cancer screening
- Colorectal cancer screening
- Comprehensive diabetes care controlling high blood pressure
- Flu vaccinations for adults ages 65 and older
- Follow-up after hospitalization for mental illness
- Initiation and engagement of alcohol and other drug dependence treatment

Box 15.9 (continued)   Healthcare Effectiveness Data and Information Set Measures Requirements based on the 2015 National Committee for Quality Assurance Accreditation Standards (NCQA, 2015a)

HEDIS Measures Requirements for Medicare Health Plans (continued)

- Medical assistance with smoking and tobacco use cessation
- Osteoporosis management in women who had a fracture
- Persistence of beta-blocker treatment after a heart attack
- Pharmacotherapy management of COPD exacerbation
- Pneumococcal vaccination status for older adults
- Use of high-risk medications in the elderly
- Getting care quickly
- Getting needed care
- Rating of health plan
- Rating of all healthcare
- Rating of personal doctor
- Rating of special

HEDIS Measures Requirements for Medicaid Health Plans

- Adult BMI assessment
- Annual dental visits
- Antidepressant medication management
- Appropriate testing for children with pharyngitis
- Appropriate treatment for children with upper respiratory infection
- Medication management for people with asthma
- Avoidance of antibiotic treatment in adults with acute bronchitis
- Breast cancer screening
- Cervical cancer screening
- Childhood immunization status
- Chlamydia screening in women
- Comprehensive diabetes care standard description
- Controlling high blood pressure
- Follow-up after hospitalization for mental illness
- Follow-up for children prescribed ADHD medication
- Frequency of prenatal care
- Human papilloma virus vaccine for female adolescents
- Immunizations for adolescents
- Initiation and engagement of alcohol and other drug dependence treatment
- Medical assistance with smoking and tobacco use cessation
- Pharmacotherapy management of COPD exacerbation
- Prenatal and post-partum care
- Use of imaging studies for low back pain
- Weight assessment and counseling for nutrition and physical activity for children/adolescents
- Getting care quickly
- Getting needed care
- Customer service
- Rating of health plan
- Rating of all healthcare
- Rating of personal doctor

Box 15.10   The National Committee for Quality Assurance's Case Management Accreditation Program

NCQA's case management accreditation program has many benefits. It:

- Directly addresses how case management services are delivered, not just the healthcare organization's internal administrative processes.
- Gets right to the core of care coordination, transitions of care, and quality of care.
- Is designed for a wide variety of healthcare organizations including both providers and payers.
- Is appropriate for health insurance plans, providers, population health management organizations, and community-based case management organizations.

management programs which include the following (NCQA, 2015b):

- Identify people who are in need of case management services.
- Target the right services to people and monitor their care and needs over time.
- Develop personalized, patient-centered care plans.
- Monitor people to ensure care plan goals are reached and to make adjustments as needed.
- Manage communication among providers and share information effectively as people move between care settings, especially when there are transitions from institutional settings.
- Build in consumer protections to ensure people have access to knowledgeable, well-qualified case management staff.
- Keep personal health information safe and secure.

NCQA's case management accreditation addresses healthcare organizations' processes regarding safe transitions of patients between settings of care and providers. The standards also require case management program personnel to maintain current knowledge and competence in the latest care management techniques and to work toward continuous improvement in patient outcomes and satisfaction. The NCQA accreditation standards and guidelines for case management programs are summarized in Box 15.11. The accreditation status levels NCQA offers for these programs vary based on the program's or organization's performance against the accreditation standards. The levels include:

- *Accredited for 3 years*: awarded to organizations that demonstrate strong performance of the functions outlined in the standards for case management accreditation.

Box 15.11 The National Committee for Quality Assurance Accreditation Standards and Guidelines for Case Management—Elements by Standard (NCQA, 2015b)

Care Management

- Care management program
- Patient population
- Care management process
- Individualized care plan
- Analyzing effectiveness/identifying opportunities
- Implementing interventions and follow-up evaluation

Improving Member Satisfaction

- Assessment of member satisfaction
- Opportunities for improvement
- Improving satisfaction

Clinical Quality Improvements

- Clinical improvements

Care Transitions

- Managing transitions of care
- Supporting members (patients) through transitions
- Analyzing performance
- Identifying unplanned transitions
- Analyzing transitions of care
- Reducing transitions of care

Relationship With Contracted Facilities/Providers

- Monitoring members' health status
- Monitoring changes in members' health status
- Maintaining members' health status

Coordination of Medicare and Medicaid Coverage

- Coordination of benefits for dual-eligible members
- Administrative coordination of benefits
- Administrative coordination for chronic condition and institutional benefit packages
- Service coordination
- Network adequacy assessment

- *Accredited for 2 years*: awarded to organizations that demonstrate performance of the functions outlined in the standards for case management accreditation.
- *Denied*: awarded to organizations that are found not to meet the NCQA requirements during the accreditation survey process (NCQA, 2015b).

15.10. UTILIZATION REVIEW ACCREDITATION COMMISSION

Another case management and health insurance plan accreditation agency is URAC. As an independent leader, it promotes healthcare quality through accreditation, education, and measurement/evaluation. It also offers a wide range of quality benchmarking products that reflect the latest transformations in healthcare. URAC has developed its evidence-based measures and standards through strategic engagement with a broad range of stakeholders who are committed to improving the quality of healthcare sysytems including consumers, providers, payers, and regulators (URAC, 2015a).

In the late 1980s, and because of growing concerns over the lack of uniform and nationally recognized standards for utilization review (UR) services, URAC began to focus on improving the quality and accountability of healthcare organizations using UR programs. Today, it has expanded its services to diverse healthcare settings, including the accreditation of integrated systems such as ACOs and health insurance plans. Formally incorporated in 1990, URAC has more than 30 accreditation and certification programs (URAC, 2015a).

URAC recognizes that an accreditation organization is widely accepted by key stakeholders if it were not biased by industry interests. As a result, URAC formed as an independent organization with a governing board of directors that consisted of representatives from all affected constituencies: consumers, providers, employers, regulators, and industry experts (URAC, 2015a). It accredits many types of healthcare organizations based on their functions and provides them with a range of accreditation programs that vary from organizational review of health insurance plan standards to boosting quality within a single functional area, such as case management or credentialing of clinicans (URAC, 2015b).

Any healthcare organization that meets accreditation program standards and measures its performance can seek accreditation. This includes entities such as hospitals, HMOs, PPOs, third-party administrators (IPAs), and healthcare provider groups. The accreditation process involves a rigorous four-phase review: building the application, desktop review, on-site review, and committee review (Box 15.12). The process may take over 6 months to complete.

Health insurance plans that earn the URAC accreditation status are able to demonstrate to consumers, employers, and governmental agencies an added level of confidence in what it does. This results from the independent third-party (i.e., URAC) evaluation which requires continuous monitoring for adherence to accreditation standards of quality and customer service and engagement. URAC's health insurance plan accreditation program with measures (Box 15.13) addresses the core requirements of the Patient Protection and Affordable Care Act of 2010 (PPACA) and

---

Box 15.12   Utilization Review Accreditation Commission Accreditation process (URAC, 2015g)

- *Building the Application*: This initial phase takes several months and consists of completing the application forms and supplying supporting documentation.

- *Desktop Review*: In this phase, URAC reviewers analyze the applicant's documentation for adherence to the standards. The documentation usually consists of formal policies and procedures, organizational charts, position descriptions, contracts, sample template letters, and program descriptions and plans for departments, such as quality management and credentialing.

- *On-Site Review*: After completing the desktop review, the same accreditation review team conducts an on-site review to verify adherence to the standards. This entails an interview of management about the organization's programs, observation of staff performing their duties, audits, review of personnel and credentialing files, education, and quality management programs.

- *Committee Review*: The last phase in the process; consists of a review by the accreditation and executive committees. This review process begins with a written summary documenting the findings of the desktop and on-site reviews. The committee then renders an accreditation determination.

Box 15.13   Utilization Review Accreditation Commission's Accreditation Standards for Health Insurance Plans

Accreditation standards address key issues stated in the PPACA requirements and focus on quality improvement activities that promote patient safety across the continuum of care. Standards include the following topics:

- Wellness and health promotion
- Care coordination
- Medication safety and care compliance
- Rewarding quality
- Care delivery through a patient centered medical home network
- Mental health parity
- Health Insurance Portability and Accountability Act breach requirements
- Measures: patient centeredness, coordination of care, patient safety, health insurance plan administration
- Effectiveness of care, and health information technology integration
- Patient experience of care (CAHPS survey)

---

incorporates key market trends and health policy issues. This program aligns with the nine components for accrediting health insurance plans as outlined in the PPACA requirements for state exchanges: consumer access, utilization management, quality assurance, provider credentialing, complaints and appeals, network adequacy and access, patient information programs, measures, and the CAHPS survey (URAC, 2015b).

URAC's accountable care accreditation program focuses on population health and care coordination for improving the health of a defined segment of a population or an entire one through activities such as population needs assessment and risk stratification. Accountable care organizations considering accreditation must meet URAC's clinical integration accreditation requirements. Applicants for this accreditation program may include multispecialty physician practice groups and provider clinics, independent practice associations (IPAs) and physician-hospital organizations (PHOs). This accreditation considers the standards of clinical care integration and advanced organizational and operational capabilities in the areas of risk contracting, consumer centeredness, and quality management. It also

entails an evaluation of the provider network's ability to coordinate high-quality, efficient, and cost-effective care as demonstrated through quality and performance outcomes (URAC, 2015c).

The accountable care accreditation program ensures that providers within a network or seeking to join a network add value and assist the entire network in meeting performance and care delivery goals. It provides guidance and recognition for provider organizations committed to enhancing patients' access to high-quality services, and the delivery of cost-effective care. The accreditation standards focus on patient centeredness and engagement, health information technology, population-based risk management, quality management, and case management (URAC, 2015c). Organizations pursuing this accreditation program may demonstrate quality performance and adherence to these standards by (URAC, 2015c):

- Conducting ongoing performance monitoring using information systems designed for population management
- Promoting and enforcing the adoption of evidence-based clinical practice guidelines through the use of aligned incentives and network participation rules
- Implementing advanced population health management strategies including a plan for addressing the needs of at-risk consumers
- Managing risk through appropriate risk contracting and abiding by applicable laws and regulations

Box 15.14   Utilization Review Accreditation Commission's Case Management Accreditation Standards and Measures (URAC, 2015d)

There are seven case management standards which cover the following areas:

Case Management Program Components

- Program description
- Criteria for identification of patients eligible for case management services
- Guidelines for case management discharge
- Guidelines for case manager's caseload
- Guidelines for evidence-based care and clinical practice
- Case management care plan policy
- Guidelines for collaborative communication among stakeholders
- Access to physician consultations
- Job descriptions for consulting health professionals
- List of consulting physicians and health professionals

Consumer Education and Engagement

- Samples of health information and health education materials
- Consent for case management services and content form
- Consumer information packet
- Consumer motivation and engagement policy and procedure
- Consumer education policy and procedure
- Case management disclosure policy and process

Staff Training and Qualifications

- Case management training program and curriculum/ agenda
- Case management staff roles and responsibilities
- Case management supervisor job description
- Case manager qualifications
- Scope of practice attestation
- Verification of licensure and certifications

Case Management Assessment and Plans

- Case management assessment policy and sample tool/ template
- Medications safety
- Consumer-centered case management plan of care

Care Coordination

- Care coordination policy and procedure
- Care coordination activities—tools and templates
- Care coordination communication—tools for communication with stakeholders

Transitions of Care (with Optional Specialty Designation)

- Procedures for transitions of care
- Transitions of care planning policy
- Criteria for necessary transitions of care information
- Care transitions summary
- Transitions of care follow-up policy and procedures
- Transitions of care consumer outreach policy and procedure

Measurement Reporting to URAC

- Performance monitoring policy
- Quality committee and meeting minutes
- Information support systems policy and procedures
- List of current and planned case management information systems
- Ongoing evaluation of case management systems

Case Management Measures Which Cover the Following Domains:

- Medical readmissions to acute care
- Percentage of participants that were medically released to return to work (applies to disability management and workers' compensation programs only)
- Patient complaint and response timeliness
- Overall consumer satisfaction (excludes disability management and workers' compensation programs)
- Percentage of individuals that refused case management services
- Coleman's three-item care transitions measure
- Patient activation measure

URAC's case management accreditation program provides an essential set of standards and performance measures (Box 15.14) that address the increasing demands for excellence in coordination of care, transitions of care, improved consumer engagement, and achievement of optimal healthcare outcomes. Healthcare organizations may also pursue an optional designation for transitions of care; a specialty component of case management. This consists of comprehensive

planning and ongoing oversight of the transitions of care process, including use of guidelines by case managers when dealing with transitions involving changes in providers, care setting, or levels of care (URAC, 2015d).

URAC states that safe and effective transitions of care promote positive healthcare outcomes for consumers. Recently and because of the importance of transitions of care, it started to offer an optional designation for "transitions of care" accreditation that builds upon the fundamental principles of the case management accreditation program. This designation provides guidelines for the effective management of care transitions which involve changes in healthcare settings, levels of care, and/or providers including comprehensive planning, targeted outreach, and the timely transfer of information between parties critical to the transition. This designation recognizes those organizations that offer services for the active management of transitions of care, which is a critical component for reducing preventable readmissions and poor health outcomes.

Any organization that offers a case management program may apply for the URAC case management accreditation including hospitals, clinically integrated networks, accountable care organizations, health insurance plans, home healthcare agencies, medical management organizations, state or federal programs, behavioral health, injured workers and workers' compensation, long-term care, vocational rehabilitation, community clinics, and patient-centered medical home, provider-based practices (URAC, 2015d).

URAC offers a number of additional accreditation programs. Of special importance are the utilization management (UM) and the PCMH. The UM accreditation program entails the evaluation of the medical necessity, appropriateness, and efficiency of the use of healthcare services and procedures under the provisions of the applicable benefits of the patient's health insurance plan. It also ensures that all types of organizations conducting utilization review follow a process that is clinically sound and respects patients' and providers' rights. Generally, the standards (URAC, 2015e):

- Address the use of evidence-based guidelines
- Outline specific reviewer requirements for each level of utilization review
- Require a policy that prevents the offering of financial incentives to providers solely based on consumers' use of healthcare services
- Ensure the adequacy of utilization management programs through evaluation against broadly recognized standards and measures (URAC, 2015e)

The UM accreditation program applies to a variety of healthcare organizations and case management programs involved in the conduct of utilization review (including independent UM companies). Examples of those eligible to pursue UM accreditation are HMOs, PPOs, consumer-directed healthcare plans, hospitals, and other specialty UM organizations, such as mental health and physical medicine or rehabilitation companies (URAC, 2015e).

The PCMH accreditation program supports URAC's provider care integration and coordination of care programs. The PCMH is a quality-driven, healthcare provider-led approach to care coordination and delivery that places patients, family members, and caregivers at the center of the healthcare system, including all decisions concerning the patient's health. A PCMH provides comprehensive and individualized access to physical health, behavioral health, and supportive community and social services, ensuring patients receive the right care in the right setting at the right time and right amount (URAC, 2015f).

URAC's PCMH accreditation program consists of standards that evaluate the PCMH's ability to increase patient's access to services, support care coordination across the continuum of care, improve patient accountability through information and active or shared decision-making, and drive efficiency and effectiveness of care and services. This accreditation program uses a unique approach with a level of flexibility and customizable elements not available in other programs. On-site review allows for an interactive and consultative approach to the accreditation process and provides strong educational support. Applicants for the PCMH accreditation include healthcare providers in primary care, and may include the following:

- Primary care practices
- Pediatric practices
- Multispecialty provider groups inclusive of primary care or pediatric practitioners
- Practices in multiple types of settings such as professional healthcare offices, outpatient clinics, and academic-affiliated ambulatory care centers (URAC, 2015f).

15.11. THE JOINT COMMISSION

The TJC is an independent, not-for-profit organization that accredits and certifies tens of thousands of healthcare organizations and programs in the United States. It is the nation's oldest and largest standards-setting and accrediting agency in healthcare, founded in 1951 and has a history that is over a century old. The TJC programs are recognized both nationwide and internationally as symbols of quality that reflect commitment to widely recognized performance standards. The TJC's mission focuses on the continuous improvement of healthcare for the public and inspiring excellence in the provision of safe and effective care of the highest quality and value (TJC, 2015b).

Many types of healthcare organizations and programs within organizations are eligible for TJC accreditation or certification. These include hospitals, critical access hospitals, physician offices, nursing homes, surgery centers, behavioral health treatment facilities, providers of home care services, opioids treatment programs, and laboratory services (TJC, 2015c). Of relevance to case management is the PCMH certification which focuses on care coordination, access to care, and how effectively a primary care provider/clinician and interdisciplinary healthcare team work together and with the patient and family/caregiver (Case Manager's Tip 15.8). The TJC introduced this certification in 2011 for ambulatory care clinics which were already accredited by the TJC. It then introduced it to accredited hospitals and critical access hospitals in 2013, and to behavioral health home (BHH) in 2014 (TJC, 2015d).

The PCMH certification is consistent with federal healthcare laws, including the PPACA of 2010, and aims to improve patient care outcomes and the continuity, quality, safety, and efficiency of healthcare services. This PCMH program focuses on educating the patients and encouraging them to self-manage their health condition or illness. Patients benefit from this model of care because they have increased access to their primary care clinician and interdisciplinary

 CASE MANAGER'S TIP 15.8

The Joint Commission Accreditation Programs and Case Management

Although TJC does not offer a case management specialty accreditation or certification, except in the case of the primary care medical home practice, it reviews the case management program as part of the general hospital or other healthcare organization accreditations it offers. In this regard, accreditation of case management is subsumed under the general accreditation. For example, when a hospital or acute care facility pursues TJC accreditation, case management is reviewed under the patient care provision standard, including continuum of care, discharge and transitional planning, and interdisciplinary care planning. Therefore, an organization can improve its case management practices and program by assuring it meets TJC accreditation standards.

healthcare team; their care is tracked and coordinated with special support by the use of health information technology.

The Joint Commission's PCMH certification is based

Box 15.15   Elements of Performance of the Primary Care Medical Home Certification (TJC, 2015a)

Patient-Centered Care

- Patient-selected primary care clinician
- Primary care clinician and interdisciplinary healthcare team that works in partnership with the patient
- Consideration for the patient's culture, primary language spoken, and educational needs and preferences
- Patient involvement in establishing the treatment plan
- Support for patient self-management

Comprehensive Care

- Provision of acute, preventive, and chronic care
- Provision of continuous and comprehensive care
- Use of internal and external resources to meet patient needs
- Primary care clinician with the educational background, knowledge, and experience to handle patient needs
- Primary care clinician working collaboratively with the interdisciplinary healthcare team
- Care that addresses various phases of the patient's life span, including end-of-life
- Disease management

Coordinated Care

- Responsibility for care coordination
- Team-based approach to care

Access to Care

- Enhanced access, defined as responsiveness to patient's preferences, timely response to needs, telephonic or electronic access to care team, and use of electronic communication tools
- Availability 24 hours/day, 7 days a week
- Access for nonvisit related patient needs
- Access to patients with special communication needs

Systems-Based Approach to Quality and Safety

- Population-based care
- Use of health information technology
- Electronic prescribing
- Practice in accordance with laws and regulations including scope of practice of various clinicians
- Use of evidence-based medicine and decision support tools
- Provision of care to a panel of patients
- Patient involvement in performance monitoring and improvement efforts

on the Agency for Healthcare Research and Quality's (AHRQ) definition of a medical home, and includes five core functions and attributes (TJC, 2015d) as described below. For the elements of performance, refer to Box 15.15.

- *Patient-centered care*: Care that is relationship-based and holistic which allows an understanding and respect of each patient's needs, culture, values, and preferences.
- *Comprehensive care*: An interdisciplinary healthcare team (may include physicians, advanced practice nurses, physician assistants, nurses, pharmacists, nutritionists, mental health workers, social workers, and others) that addresses the patient's physical and mental healthcare needs, including prevention and wellness, acute care, and chronic care.
- *Coordinated care*: Care coordination occurs across the healthcare continuum, including specialty care, acute care, home care, and the provision of community and support services. This is particularly critical during transitions between sites of care or providers.
- *Access to care and services*: Access to services with shorter timeframes especially for urgent needs, around the clock telephone or electronic access to members of the healthcare team, and alternative methods of communication such as digital tools.
- *Systems-based approach to quality and safety*: The use of evidence-based guidelines and clinical decision support tools, performance measurement, and improvement methods, with special focus on the patient experience, population health management, and sharing of quality and safety data publically.

15.12. KEY POINTS

1. Case management models provide a foundation for meeting the requirements and standards of regulatory and accreditation agencies.
2. The use of case management services and plans allows the delivery of efficient, effective, safe, and quality care.
3. The use of both interdisciplinary communication and documentation tools are encouraged by the accreditation agencies including TJC, URAC, and NCQA. Case management provides a foundation for both of these.
4. Case management models embody the same principles as those outlined in the standards of accreditation agencies. One can review these

standards when developing a model/program or improving an existing one.
5. The interdisciplinary healthcare team, such as the case management team, is a focus of accreditation agencies and their standards.
6. Case management ensures that healthcare providers do the right things and do them right (i.e., enhance a safe healthcare environment that is free of errors).
7. Accreditation standards generally describe what an organization needs to do and have in place in three main areas of care delivery: patient-centered, organization-centered, and structure or function an organization must offer to both patients and healthcare professionals.
8. Accreditation standards focus on a number of aspects of an organziation including but not limited to the following: care provision systems, access to care, patient-centered care, providers' competency, knowledge and eductaional backgrounds, quality and safety, quality improvement, communication and information management, documentation and medical records, leadership and governance, ethics, risk management, transitions of care, care coordination, and utilization management.

15.13. REFERENCES

The Joint Commission. 2015a. Comprehensive accreditation manual for hospitals, 2015. Oakbrook Terrace, IL.

The Joint Commission. Accessed September 3, 2015b. About The Joint Commission. Available at www.jointcommission.org/about_us/about_the_joint_commission_main.aspx

The Joint Commission. Accessed September 3, 2015c. What is accreditation? Available at www.jointcommission.org/accreditation/accreditation_main.aspx

The Joint Commission. Accessed September 3, 2015d. Certificatiuon: Primary Care Medical Home. Available at www.jointcommission.org/certification/priamry_care_medical_home_certification.aspx

National Committee For Quality Assurance. Accessed September 3, 2015a. Health plan accreditation. Available at www.ncqa.org/Programs/Accreditation/HealthPlanHP.aspx

National Committee for Quality Assurance. Accessed September 3, 2015b. Case management accreditation. Available at www.ncqa.org/Programs/Accreditation/CaseManagementCM.aspx

URAC. Accessed September 3, 2015a. About URAC. Available at www.urac.org/about-urac/about-urac/

URAC. Accessed September 3, 2015b. Accreditation programs: Health plan programs. Available at www.urac.org/accreditation-and-measurement/accreditation-programs/health-plan-programs/

URAC. Accessed September 3, 2015c. Accreditation programs:

Accountable care organizations. Available at www.urac.org/accreditation-and-measurement/accreditation-programs/all-programs/accountable-care-accreditation/

URAC. Accessed September 3, 2015d. Accreditation programs: Case management. Available at www.urac.org/accreditation-and-measurement/accreditation-programs/all-programs/case-management/

URAC. Accessed September 3, 2015e. Accreditation programs: Utilization management. Available at www.urac.org/accredi-tation-and-measurement/accreditation-programs/all-programs/health-utilization-management/

URAC. Accessed September 3, 2015f. Accreditation programs: Patient centered medical home. Available at www.urac.org/accreditation-and-measurement/accreditation-programs/all-programs/patient-centered-medical-home/

URAC. Accessed September 3, 2015g. Accreditation programs: Accreditation process, available at www.urac.org/accreditation-and-measurement/accreditation-programs

16 Using the Internet and Digital Tools in Case Management

The public wants access to healthcare-related knowledge on the Internet at their fingertips. Healthcare providers and other agencies, including those that provide case management services, have responded with enthusiasm and have made information available in abundance. In addition, for the past decade the Internet has been increasingly used as an attractive and desirable communication tool and invaluable resource for both healthcare consumers and providers alike. It functions as an easy medium for locating, accessing, exchanging, sharing, and disseminating information. However, posting health-related information on the Internet is not limited to healthcare providers and experts; anyone can post information regardless of one's qualifications. This can make the quality, clarity, credibility, currency, and accuracy of the information questionable.

It is not a simple task for healthcare consumers to evaluate Internet-based information and resources and to make a decision whether to use them and how to guide patients and their families on the use of such health-related information. Therefore it behooves healthcare providers to guide consumers of healthcare services in selecting appropriate and reliable information and to educate them about the harms of misinformation. Because of their role in care coordination, transitions of care, patient activation, and engagement, case managers are best positioned to assume the role of guiding consumers in this area. Chapter 16 presents the case manager with a "tool kit" for effective use of the Internet as a medium for locating health-related information for, and communicating with, their patients, families, and other providers and agencies.

Searching for healthcare-related information on the Internet and the world wide web (WWW) is essential for case managers' success in the information management and communication dimension of their role. It is also important when working with patients and their families to promote:

- Patient activation
- Patient engagement
- Self-management
- Counseling about healthy lifestyle behavior
- Medications management
- Adherence to health regimen

The use of the Internet assists case managers in locating people, community support services, telephone numbers, addresses (both regular and electronic mailing addresses), patient and family education materials, and other information about community, governmental, and nongovernmental agencies and resources. This information is most helpful in care coordination, transitional planning, resource utilization, and care and outcomes management. Ultimately, the Internet serves as an information tool that is essential for both the provider and the consumer of healthcare services. However, because of the virtually limitless amount of information available on the WWW, it presents a great challenge, particularly for the consumer. No wonder patients and their families often express their frustration about the difficulty of accessing information online.

16.1. THE INTERNET

The Internet is a public, cooperative creation that operates using national and international telecommunication technologies and networks, including high-speed

455

data lines, telephone lines, satellite communications, fiberoptics, and radio networks. The history of the Internet is available on the website of the Internet Society, which can be accessed at www.internetsociety. org/internet/what-internet/history-internet. Individuals and healthcare organizations and providers connect to the Internet through a local area network (LAN) using a computer. Each computer has a unique Internet protocol (IP) address and connects to the Internet via a local server or host. The local server often connects to a larger server called a wide area network (WAN). This can result in connecting many computers and many LANs and WANs into larger networks that ultimately form the Internet and the WWW (Case Manager's Tip 16.1).

The WWW allows Internet users access to a wealth of information, materials, and documents. The amount of Internet-based information is growing by leaps and bounds every day. This information is available in many different forms, such as text, pictures, graphics, films, videos, presentations, animations, virtual reality, games (amusement and health education), and audio recordings. Compared with other modes of information (e.g., animation and virtual reality), text is the easiest to download and requires the least sophisticated type of technology. Although the Internet has many advantages, it is not free of certain challenges (Box 16.1). Case managers and other healthcare providers must be aware of these and act accordingly to ensure appropriate and safe use of this technology both by providers and consumers alike. It also is important for case managers to have some knowledge of Internet technology and computers so that they can advise consumers of healthcare on patient and family education materials and resources that are easily accessible and do not require extensive Internet and computer knowledge and skills.

 CASE MANAGER'S TIP 16.1

The Internet and Its Portability

Today, the popularity of mobile devices such as smart phones, iPads. and tablets have made the Internet portable and easily accessible by individuals while on the move, anywhere and anytime. The availability of telecommunication, photography, and teleconferencing features on computers and mobile devices have created innovative ways of communication and case management activities with the patient and family. Case managers must be knowledgable and comfortable in the use of the latest mobile devices and Internet-enhanced technologies to be able to effectively case manage their patients and meet their preferences in communciation approaches.

 CASE MANAGER'S TIP 16.2

Guide to Using the Internet

There are many websites that include tips, tools, and other Web-searching resources. Examples are as follows:

- Finding Information on the Internet: http://www.lib. berkeley.edu/TeachingLib/Guides/Internet/FindInfo. html
- Learn the Net: Knowledge When You Need It: http://www.learnthenet.com/english/index.html (also available in French and Spanish)
- Search Engine Watch: http://www.searchenginewatch. com (information and tips about searching the web)

16.1.1. Use of the Internet by Case Managers

Case managers can use the Internet (Case Manager's Tip 16.2) in many ways that benefit the provision of patient care and its related outcomes (Johnson and Tahan, 2003). These may include searching for and downloading information, communicating via individual and group electronic mail (e-mail), and engaging in online chat, support group discussions, counseling, and videoconferencing or telecommunication. Before discussing these benefits, it is important to explain the different types of IPs, also called Transmission Control Protocols (TCPs), and how Web pages are named and organized.

16.1.2. Internet Protocols

An IP/TCP is a communication language used by Web clients and servers to communicate with one another. It assembles files, documents, films, messages, and other information into smaller packets for transmission over the network/Internet. IP/TCP allows the distribution of information over the Internet and ensures that packets reach their intended destination. TCP is a higher layer than IP; TCP assembles and disassembles the information messages/packets and the IP carries the address information to assure the message is delivered and received by the intended addres or party.

There are six types of protocols used to access resources on the Internet. These are as follows:

1. The hypertext transfer protocol, known as http, provides access to the Internet by defining hypertext links to information on the WWW.
2. The file transfer protocol, known as ftp, provides for the transfer or downloading of documents, pro-

---

Box 16.1   Advantages and Disadvantages of the Internet

Some of the advantages of the Internet are as follows:

- It provides almost instantaneous access to information compared with traditional print media.
- The barriers of time and distance when attempting to access, gather, or disseminate information are resolved by using the Internet.
- Conducting timely literature or computer searches related to a particular topic; ease of access to lay information on a variety of healthcare-related topics.
- The turnaround time for making information (e.g., texts, videos, films, instructional games) available on the Internet surpasses that required by traditional publication media.
- Messages can be sent almost immediately by one Internet user to another or to a large group of users, regardless of geographical location, distance, or time.
- It provides the ability to share large size e-mail documents or files easily and efficiently.
- Communicating to a large number of people at the same time and using the same message is helpful and desirable.
- It provides the ability to navigate Web pages that address similar and related topics using hyperlinks.
- It provides the ability to use the Internet at one's own convenience and on the move with use of mobile technologies.

Some of the disadvantages of the Internet are as follows:

- Accessing the information available on the Internet relies on the availability of the server and the speed and type of the modem or wirless network.
- The benefits of face-to-face and personal contact are absent.
- Not all documents posted on the Internet are refereed/peer reviewed, which threatens their quality and credibility.
- Information available on the Internet is not thorough and does not replace traditional media and publications.
- The ease and immediacy of e-mail communication can become a source of trouble and annoyance. Expectation of immediate acknowledgement and response can be burdensome.
- The Internet is not guaranteed as a safe networking or communication medium. Sometimes computer viruses are transmitted intentionally or unintentionally, and hackers may be able to alter the information on some websites despite password protection activities.
- Downloading documents from the Internet may present some problems depending on the type of Internet-based services and availability of specific software or technologies.
- The use of e-mail as a method for distributing "junk" mail may be viewed as a nuisance.
- Maintaining privacy and confidentiality of information presents a great challenge.
- Credibility of health-related information may be questionable sometimes and the lay consumer may not be sensitive to such concern; this may result in unintended harm.

---

grams, and files from or to a file transfer server. It is also the method of sending files to and receiving files from remote computers on the Internet.

3. The Telnet, known as TELNET, allows one to log on to remote computers.

4. The simple mail transfer protocol, known as smtp, enables the sending and receiving of electronic messages.

5. The hypertext markup language, known as html, produces a hypertext document for display by a WWW browser and uses a standardized set of tags that tells the browser how to display the text and how to specify the hypertext links.

6. The user datagram protocol (UDP) is similar to TCP, however it is not affected by the size of the maximum transmission unit that is integral to the way TCP operates; it fragments the size of the message packet to manageable parts for successful transmission.

Knowledge of these protocols is not a prerequisite for accessing Internet-based resources; however, it enhances case managers' Internet navigation skills and makes them better able to educate their patients about how to access information via the Internet. If patients present their case manager with certain questions, the case manager can be prepared and ready to answer or he or she can be comfortable with how to obtain answers to these questions.

16.1.3. Web Pages

Web pages are named and organized in a specific way to help Internet users to easily locate information on the WWW. The address of a file, Web page, document, or resource available on the Internet and accessed by Web users is called the uniform resource locator (URL). URLs are unique in nature and are mutually exclusive. Most Web pages are composed applying

HTML. An example of a Web page is http://mended-hearts.org/about-us. This is the address of the home page of The Mended Hearts, Inc., which is a non-profit organization that focuses on healthcare consumers and is designed to offer help, support, and encouragement to heart disease patients and their families. Let us review the specific components of this URL as follows:

1. http:// is the prefix used to access the file; that is, the hypertext transfer protocol.
2. www.mendedhearts.org is the domain name of the server on which the file is located, in this case The Mended Hearts, Inc., main Web server.
3. www is the portion of the domain name that specifies the server. In this case, it is the Web server. Domain names do not always have a reference to the WWW.
4. mendedhearts is the subdomain of The Mended Hearts, Inc.
5. .org is a suffix that identifies an organization.
6. About-us is the directory in which the file resides. This reflects where the information resides based on the site's map.

There are more than 15 different suffixes of URLs, most commonly nused are the following:

1. *.edu* indicates a US educational institution Internet site. An example is http://www.columbia.edu, the website for Columbia University, New York.
2. *.com* indicates a commercial Internet site. An example is http://www.LWW.com, the home page of the Lippincott Williams & Wilkins publishing company.
3. *.gov* indicates a governmental Internet site. An example is http://www.ahrq.gov, the home page of the Agency for Healthcare Research and Quality.
4. *.org* indicates an organization Internet site. An example is http://www.ncsbn.org, the website of The National Council of State Boards of Nursing.
5. *.net* indicates a network-related Internet site. An example is http://www.matisse.net, a website that shares information pulled together from other sites.
6. *.mil* indicates a military website. An example is http://www.army.mil, the U.S. Army website.
7. *.info* indicates an information source. An example is http://www.afilias.info, the world's second largest company for registration of Internet domain information.
8. *.US* (or any two letters) indicates a reference to a country. An example is https://www.gov.uk/, the website of the United Kingdom's government services.

Understanding the use of different suffixes allows case managers to locate information on the WWW more expeditiously. For example, case managers must know that to locate websites of governmental agencies, they must use the suffix .gov after the acronym of the agency they are interested in locating.

16.1.4. Navigating to Knowledge

The greatest advantage of the Internet is availability and ease of access to information. Case managers and others can use the Internet to obtain any type of information, including professional and scientific literature, research outcomes, latest technologies, therapies, nonprofessional literature, patient and family education and health instructional materials, health products information, addresses and contact information of medical and consumer agencies, and commercial reports and information. So, how can one search for such information?

To locate information on the Internet, case managers can use search engines. Search engines employ specialized software to query the Internet. The software allows the search engine to constantly acquire new information, documents, files, and other resources and to update the database that makes up the search engine. When a person queries a topic, the search engine checks for matches in the database based on the key words used to search the topic. Before you search a topic, it is important to decide whether you need broad, general information or narrow, specific information because this dictates the type of search engine to be applied. Search engines are of three types: major and meta search engines (both also known as indices) and directories (Case Manager's Tip 16.3).

 CASE MANAGER'S TIP 16.3

Differentiating between Directories and Indices

Directories, also called subject catalogs, are lists of websites that have been filtered by an editor or reviewer or compiled by a person. They are limited to a fraction of the documents available on the WWW. This is because documents are added to the directory only after notification of the document author or the websiteowner. Examples of directories are Yahoo, Excite, and Medsite Navigator.

Indices are large databases of websites. The entries of an index are usually gathered automatically by search engines designed to scan the WWW for any new documents and websites on a regular basis, usually weekly or monthly, and the resulting new information is then automatically added to the database. Examples of indexes are AltaVista, Infoseek, and the Internet Sleuth.

Major search engines are comprehensive search tools that are fairly current and used for broad and general topics. The following are some popular major search engines:

AltaVista	http://www.altavista.com
Excite	http://www.excite.com
Bing	http://www.bing.com
HotBot	http://www.hotbot.com
Infoseek	http://www.infoseek.com
Lycos	http://www.lycos.com
WebCrawler	http://www.webcrawler.com
Direct Hit	http://www.directhit.com
FastSearch	http://ussc.alltheweb.com
Go	http://www.go.com
Google	http://www.google.com
GoTo	http://www.goto.com
Northern Light	http://www.northernlight.com
Snap	http://www.snap.com

Meta search engines are multiengine search sites and are used to search for specific and narrow topics. The following are some popular meta search engines:

DogPile	http://www.dogpile.com
InferenceFind	http://www.wisdomdog.com
MetaCrawler	http://www.metacrawler.com
MetaFind	http://www.metafind.com
All4One	http://www.all4one.com
ProFusion	http://www.profusion.com
SavvySearch	http://www.savvysearch.com
Highway61	http://www.highway61.com
Cyber411	http://www.cyber411.com

Directories are hierarchically organized databases and are best for locating a large amount of information on a topic. Popular Web directories include the following:

Yahoo	http://www.yahoo.com
Galaxy	http://www.galaxy.com
LookSmart	http://www.looksmart.com
OpenDirectoryProject	http://www.dmoz.com
W3 Virtual Library	http://www.virtuallibrary.com

A rule of thumb for the case manager attempting to locate information on the Internet is to use major and meta search engines because the outcomes of such searches will most likely be the information most appropriate and relevant to the keyword used in the search. For example, attempting to search for "case management" using the search engine Metafind will most possibly yield a list of references limited to the topic "case management" and not health management or disease management. Other tips on searching for information are discussed in the following section.

16.1.5. Tips on Searching for Information

Using the Internet to search a particular topic can lead to hundreds or even thousands of Web pages and documents. For example, a recent search of the topic, managed care, yielded 378 websites using the Yahoo directory; 1,979,640 sites using WebCrawler; and 20 sites using the MetaCrawler search engine. However, if you use quotation marks you can narrow down your search and make it more specific. When quotation marks were used for searching the same topic, "managed care," applying the same search engines, it yielded 297 sites in Yahoo, 31,810 sites in WebCrawler, and 20 sites in MetaCrawler. Other strategies that can be used to narrow down the search results are as follows:

- Use AND, OR, NEAR, and NOT between the keywords in the topic.
- Use a plus (+) sign in front of any word that you want included in the results.
- Use a minus (–) sign in front of any word you want excluded.
- Use an asterisk (*) to search for variations on a word.

An additional way to search a topic is by navigating the Web using the hyperlinks included in the results of an initial search. Most of the time websites related to the topic being searched include hyperlinks to other similar or related Web pages. It is not necessary to review all of the sites displayed in the results of a search. It is common that the first 20 or so sites displayed are the ones found to be the most useful and most relevant to the topic searched.

Searching the Internet is not limited to locating documents and healthcare information. It can also be used to find newsgroup postings and people. Finding newsgroups, or digital discussions and bulletin boards, can be done using search engines that are dedicated to seeking and archiving messages from these forums. Search engines such as AltaVista, InfoSeek, and Excite allow Internet users to locate newsgroups as well; however, there are other sites, such as the following, that are available specifically for the purpose of locating newsgroups:

Google Groups	http://www.groups.google.com
InReference, Inc.	http://www.inreference.com

In addition to locating newsgroups, there are special search engines available for finding people on the Internet. These engines operate through databases that gather people's electronic mailing addresses obtained from the commercial Internet access providers or through tracking the addresses of people who post messages online. If a person has an electronic mailing address but does not use it, it is unlikely for it to appear in the search or for other people to learn of its presence. Examples of these search engines are as follows:

BigYellow	http://www.bigyellow.com
World Wide Yellow Pages	http://www.yellow.com
Yahoo People Search	http://www.people.yahoo.com

16.1.6. Electronic Communication

Electronic communication is the act of transmitting information from one person to another or to a group of people using the Internet, the WWW media/network, and technology. This form of electronic communication is completed on demand. However, as with other forms of electronic communication on the Internet, information is posted by individuals or agencies at their convenience and regardless of the specific needs of or requests by others (i.e., Internet users). Examples of electronic communication are e-mail, newsgroups, bulletin boards, and listservs.

The use of e-mail is so widespread and popular today that almost everyone relies on it to conduct regular business functions. E-mail is the most common use of the Internet. It is the act of sending messages from one person to another using electronic media and telecommunication technologies. The transmission of such messages takes place via the Internet or a network. E-mail is also used as a method of communication between one individual and a group of people simultaneously; in this case it is called a listserv, bulletin board, or newsgroup (Case Manager's Tip 16.4) (Johnson & Tahan, 2003).

Listservs (also called mailing lists), bulletin boards, and newsgroups provide a forum for group discussion.

 CASE MANAGER'S TIP 16.4

Using Electronic Communication Tools with Caution

Electronic communication tools such as newsgroups, listservs, chat rooms, mailing lists, and bulletin boards are a rich source of information; however, case managers must caution patients and their families about the reliability of these tools. Patients must be advised not to blindly apply the recommendations made by participants of these forums without validating the information first with case managers or other healthcare providers. Case managers must also teach their patients how to differentiate between those that are moderated by a healthcare professional and those that are "free for all."

These methods of communication consist of a group of people with similar interests (e.g., nursing informatics, case management) or professions (e.g., case manager, social worker) who get together to share information through an e-mail–based discussion group. They are asynchronous (i.e., do not need the online presence of people engaged in the discussion at the same time) in nature and allow participants/subscribers to respond to posted messages at their own convenience. Members of these communication forums can be from around the globe; however, they use the same language in their exchange of information.

Another type of mailing list is synchronous discussion groups, or chat rooms, which provide an opportunity for real-time/concurrent conversations and discussions. Each chat room focuses on a specific topic or an area of interest. Not all chat rooms are facilitated by a moderator. Moderators function as a facilitator of the discussion and oversee the content and flow of information. They also possess the authority to disqualify subscribers who are disruptive or use obscene language from participating in a chat room discussion. Some chat rooms are oriented toward professionals such as nurses, physicians, or other healthcare providers; some others are for consumers of healthcare (patients and their families). Provider-based chat rooms focus on the discussion of topics that relate to the delivery of healthcare or the various health professions. Consumer-based chat rooms focus on topics related to health promotion, disease prevention, self-help, emotional support, and sharing personal experiences. Case managers should be knowledgeable about the advantages and disadvantages of these methods of electronic communication (Box 16.2) so that they become better able to assist healthcare consumers in selecting the most beneficial forums for communication in relation to accessing healthcare services and resources.

In response to the concerns the public has expressed regarding electronic/online communication and consultation, in October 2006, Medem, Inc., and the eRisk Working group for Healthcare, a consortium of professional liability carriers, medical societies, and representatives of state licensing boards, developed a set of guidelines for "online communication and services with patients," including e-mail and other Internet-based services. These guidelines are reviewed and updated regularly. They aim to help healthcare providers enhance the safety and reduce the risk of electronic communication and services. It is appropriate and important for case managers, especially those who use electronic communication as a case management strategy with their patients, to adopt these to the best of their ability. Medem, Inc., and the eRisk Working

---

Box 16.2   Advantages and Disadvantages of Electronic Communication (Johnson & Tahan, 2003)

Some of the advantages of electronic communication are as follows:

- The speed of transfer of information (i.e., communication).
- The ability to communicate the same message to a group of people at the same time.
- Being on mailing lists can put information and resources at providers' (e.g., case managers) fingertips.
- Easy and universal access to patients and healthcare professionals.
- The ability to transmit files electronically as e-mail attachments.
- The ability to communicate with healthcare professionals at the patients' convenience and without having to be personally present.
- Providing patients with easy access to schedule follow-up appointments or request information or advice regarding healthcare issues or treatments.
- Dissemination of health promotion and prevention information such as newsletters and patient and family education/health instruction materials.
- The tendency toward being informal in nature.
- Participation in moderated discussions with book authors, experts, and authority figures in nursing and patient care.
- Easy filing of important documents and information which makes it more accessible in future dates; for example, electronic summary of care, health instruction materials, and confirmation of follow-up care appointment with details.

Some of the disadvantages of electronic communication are as follows:

- Concern regarding the security, privacy, and confidentiality of e-mail messages.
- Dependence on availability of a electronic mail software program and an Internet server.
- The challenge to maintain compliance with the HIPPA standards.
- The presence of e-mail and Internet hackers.
- The susceptibility of communicated information for abuse or mishandling.
- Downloading attachments and files is dependent on comparable/compatible software applications.
- Similar to regular snail mail, some e-mail messages are considered "junk" mail.
- The access of advertising agencies and market researchers to e-mail account subscribers.
- Misspelling an e-mail address results in returned mail or delivery to the wrong person.
- Some subscribers of mailing lists/listservs find it easy to respond to posted messages in a flaming or obscene way because there is no face-to-face contact.
- Concerns for e-mail tone and expression of feelings; sometimes use of uppercase letters for example is misinterpreted as yelling.

Group for Healthcare cautions that these guidelines are not meant to be used as formal legal, ethical, and professional guidelines, nor as legal advice, to govern communications between the healthcare provider and patients. Healthcare providers may use them as recommendations be applied to e-mail, websites, listservs, and other methods of electronic communication (Medem, Inc. and eRisk Working Group for Healthcare, 2006). The recommendations are as follows:

- *Confidentiality*: Take reasonable steps to protect patient privacy and to guard against unauthorized access to or use of patient healthcare information. Key consideration are privacy and security and authentication.
  - *Privacy and Security*: Communicate over a secure network, with provisions for privacy and security including authentication and encryption in accordance with the Health Insurance Portability and Accountability Act (HIPAA) and other appropriate guidelines. Healthcare providers need to be aware of potential security risks, including unauthorized physical access and security of computer hardware, and guard against them with technologies such as automatic logout and password protection. Use of standard and regular e-mail does not meet HIPAA requirements.
  - *Authentication*: Take reasonable steps to authenticate the identity of correspondent(s) in an electronic communication and to ensure that recipients of information are authorized to receive it. Patient authentication, or authentication of an authorized patient proxy (i.e., authorized family member, etc.) for patient–provider online communication including the delivery of patient data is important in order to ensure patient privacy and confidentiality. Healthcare providers may establish a policy or protocol about written patient authentication and train all involved in its use; keep a written record of the patient's

authentication for online communciation; and refrain from offering to use online healthcare services where a patient's authentication is not addressed or not feasible.

■ *Unauthorized access to computers*: This can immediately compromise a patient's personal information and compromise security. Establish and follow procedures that help to guard against and mitigate this risk. The use of online communication may increase the risk of unauthorized distribution of patient information.

■ *Informed consent*: Obtain informed consent from the patient regarding the appropriate use and limitations of the methods of electronic communication.

■ *Pre-existing clinician-patient relationship*: Do not limit yourself to an online provider-patient relationship. Initiating a provider-patient relationship solely through online interaction can increase the healthcare provider's liability exposure. It is advised that online communciations be used after an in-person meeting first.

■ *Licensing jurisdiction*: Be aware of the state requirements of online communication and licensure. Communicating with patients outside the state the provider is licensed in may subject the provider to increased risk.

■ *Highly sensitive subject matter*: Advise patients of potential privacy risks associated with online communication related to highly sensitive information such as issues of mental or behavioral health.

■ *Patient eductaion and care management*: Healthcare providers are responsible for the information they share or make available online with their patients. Information provided through personal health records, automated patient education programs, or care management services must come from a credible source.

■ *Emergency subject matter*: Healthcare providers should advise their patients on the appropriate use of online communication. Patients should be advised not to use online communication in the case of emergency medical situations (e.g., chest pain, shortness of breath).

■ *Medical records*: Maintain a permanent record of the online communications pertinent to the ongoing medical care of the patient and integrate it into the patient's medical record, whether that record is paper or electronic.

■ *Authoritative information*: Make sure that the information you provide or make available via online communication, such as a website, comes either directly from you as the provider or from a recognized and credible source.

■ *Commercial information*: Avoid website-based or online communication of advertising, promotional, or marketing products because they may subject providers to increased liability, including implicit guarantees or implied warranty.

■ *Links to third party websites and other sources of information*: Post disclaimers about the links to any third party website or information that advises patients and other viewers they are leaving the provider's website and that the provider is not responsible for information conveyed via the linked website.

16.2. PATIENT AND FAMILY EDUCATION RESOURCES

Patient and family education resources are available on the Internet in abundance. Case managers are advised to employ the information searching tips presented in the previous section to locate and access these resources and to educate their patients on how to obtain healthcare-related materials online. Patients and families who are familiar with how to access and use the Internet to obtain health instruction, counseling, and support resources may feel empowered and may feel a greater sense of security. They may also feel a greater sense of control, gain more self-care and self-management skills, and assume the responsibility for their own care. Knowing that they are not alone and that other people with similar conditions are accessible via the Internet and online support discussion groups enhances their self-confidence and encourages them to adhere to their medical regimen. Case managers and healthcare consumers may access patient and family education resources through the following website types:

1. Professional societies such as the American Heart Association (http://www.americanheart.org) and the Oncology Nursing Society (http://www.ons.org)

2. Governmental agencies such as the CMS) (http://www.cms.gov) and the National Institutes of Health (http://www.nih.gov)

3. Healthcare organizations such as the Mayo Clinic (http://www.mayoclinic.org) and the Cleveland Clinic (http://www.clevelandclinic.org)

4. Commercial organizations such as WebMD (http://www.webmd.org) or Johnson and Johnson, Inc. (http://www.johnsonandjohnson.com)

5. Consumer-sponsored organizations such as The Mended Hearts, Inc. (http://mendedhearts.org) and Health Cite, Inc. (http://www.healthcite.com)

One must be able to differentiate between resources

that are developed by healthcare providers and those developed by lay people. Those sponsored by healthcare providers and agencies tend to be more reliable, current, and void of any misinformation. Case managers can assume a significant role in educating their patients/families in this area and in assisting them to locate the best health instruction materials possible. Case managers can also be an invaluable resource for streamlining and simplifying available resources for patients and their families in an effort to enhance their adherence to the medical regimen, build their self-care and self-management skills, and reduce their anxiety toward their health condition and necessary healthy lifestyle changes. Ultimately, this role enhances the achievement of desirable outcomes and may contribute to quality and safety.

16.3. OTHER USES OF THE INTERNET BY CASE MANAGERS

Case managers may rely on the Internet for the delivery, management, and evaluation of healthcare services. They can also use the Internet to access resources such as directories of healthcare providers of particular health insurance plans and managed care companies, information about healthcare benefits, governmental program information and guidelines, directories of community resources and healthcare services/agencies, and charitable organizations. Access to such information is important especially when a patient is being discharged home or transitioned to another care setting and the patient happens to be from out of state and need the arrangement of post-discharge/transition services in the state of residence. Since such transition is not a frequent occurrence for the case manager, accessing relevant resources via the Internet facilitates a timely discharge or transition. Such practice and use of Internet resources are essential for better case management services and outcomes.

Case managers may use the Internet in many ways, with the ultimate goal of enhancing the practice of case management. Some of the uses of the Internet for case managers are as follows:

- Find the latest research outcomes to implement evidence-based practice.
- Access recommendations of professional organizations and societies.
- Obtain national standards and guidelines from clearinghouses to use for improving patient care delivery and outcomes.
- Remain abreast of the latest changes in the standards of governmental and accreditation agencies.

- Share expert knowledge in specific practice areas.
- Access national benchmark databases.
- Communicate across the globe in a timely fashion.
- Receive/send announcements and newsletters electronically.
- Direct questions to authors, researchers, and experts and obtain answers expeditiously.
- Communicate among settings, levels of care, and different providers. Discuss care issues, make decisions regarding changes in the plan of care, and resolve problems in a timely fashion.
- Transmit required information electronically to other public and private agencies and organizations (e.g., utilization reviews to health insurance plans and managed care organizations, and significant events data to the state department of health and human services and/or TJC).
- Participate in continuing educational sessions online (e.g., webinars).
- Conduct research and collect data online.
- Schedule appointments for follow-up care or consults for patients.
- Communicate with patients post-discharge (e.g., post-discharge calls/contacts) and respond to patients' questions or queries regarding self-care.

16.4. ASSESSING THE QUALITY OF HEALTH INFORMATION ON THE INTERNET

The Internet is a medium of free expression. Some information is accurate, reliable, and credible; some is not and is considered harmful. Maintaining the quality of the information available on the WWW presents a great challenge considering that this medium is volatile and difficult to trace. The reason for this challenge is the fact that the provision of healthcare information on the Internet and the WWW is not regulated, except for HIPAA which pertains to privacy and confidentiality of information. Therefore it is necessary to educate patients and their families about how to examine the quality of the information posted on the Internet to prevent the application of misinformation, and when in doubt to seek the guidance of a healthcare professional. Case managers are best positioned to assume the educator role. To be effective they must be familiar with the process of assessing information available on the WWW and must apply specific criteria for this purpose.

As the Internet has become an essential tool for the provision of healthcare services, it is important that healthcare providers, including case managers, play a gatekeeper role in ensuring that consumers use only information that is considered of exceptional quality. To avoid any flaws in the process of evaluating the quality of health information available on the Internet, several authors and societies developed and recommended the use of certain necessary criteria for such evaluation. To prevent confusion about which set of criteria is more credible and best to apply, Romano, Hinegardner, and Phyillaier (2000) compared several sets and identified five common and simple-to-use criteria. Case managers may elect to use these criteria as their standard for evaluating the quality of Internet-based healthcare information. The criteria are as follows:

■ *Authority/source*: If it is an author, the website must include the author's credentials and expertise. If it is an organization, one must question its reputation and establish credibility and trustworthiness before use. The site must also include contact information.
■ *Purpose/objectivity*: The site must clearly state its purpose, its sponsor, and the intended audience.
■ *Content*: The site must disseminate accurate, useful, and relevant information to the need of the users. It must also include relevant and authoritative links to other sites.

■ *Currency*: The site must include the date of posted information and of any updates.
■ *Design*: The site must be well organized, easy to navigate, stable, and free of any clutter.

There are other sets of criteria recommended by other agencies such as the criteria set advocated for by The Health Information Technology Institute of Mitretek Systems (Box 16.3) The Institute developed its criteria by convening a Health Summit Working Group in 1996. It held another Summit in 1998 that resulted in revising the original criteria (Ambre et al., 1999). The set of criteria developed by this Summit is considered credible, is widely used, and is available all over the world. It also has been translated into several languages. The users of these criteria include policy makers, healthcare information/content developers, providers, consumers, and payers. Although these criteria are over a decade old, they continue to be applicable in today's environment.

Another source of criteria for examining the quality of health-related websites consumers may use is

---

Box 16.3 Criteria for Assessing the Quality of Health Information on the Internet

Credibility

Source

Does the site display the name and logo of the institute responsible for the information and the name and title of the author?
Does the site present the credentials and qualifications of the authors and organizations?
Does the site include any information about the sponsors or other affiliations?

Currency

Does the site display the original document posting date?
Does the site include the date(s) of revisions?

Relevance

Does the content of the documents relate to the information they purport to offer?

Site Evaluation

Does the site apply a peer review process before posting a document?
Does the site share a description of its peer review process?

Content

Accuracy

Does the site identify the data that underlie the conclusions presented?
Does the site include the clinical and/or scientific evidence that supports the position taken?

Disclaimer

Does the site display a disclaimer that describes the purpose, scope, authority, and currency of information provided?
Does the site disclose the sources of information?
Does the site share information in the context of general health information and not medical advice?

Completeness

Does the site present discussions that are comprehensive and balanced?
Does the site include pertinent facts, negative results, and a statement of any information not known about the subject addressed?

Box 16.3 (continued)   Criteria for Assessing the Quality of Health Information on the Internet

Disclosure

Purpose

Does the site display its mission or purpose clearly?

Does the information provided relate to the mission or purpose?

Profiling

Does the site make the user aware of the purpose of the information presented?

Does the site share with the user the process for collecting information and its use?

Does the site present a process for dissemination of information?

Links

Selection

Does the site include any links to other sites?

Does the site employ qualified staff for selecting appropriate and related links?

Does the site include links that are relevant to its mission and purpose?

Architecture

Does the site make it easy for the user to find his or her way backward or forward?

Does the site apply an apparent and logical structure?

Does the site use any meaningful and consistent image-based icons or textual identifiers?

Content

Does the site include links with accurate, current, credible, and relevant information?

Does the site provide information about the linked source before the user clicks to the site?

Back Linkages (Linkages From One Site to Another)

Does the site avoid any bias in the use of back linkages?

Does the site allow for back linkages?

Design

Access

Does the site include graphics and text in its layout?

Does the site allow accessibility using the lowest level available browser technology?

Does the site alert the user to the need for special technology (e.g., real player, multimedia) for access to certain information?

Navigability

Does the site focus on its purpose and target audience?

Does the site allow for simple and easy navigation?

Does the site balance between the use of graphics, text, color, and sound?

Internal Search Capability

Does the site allow for internal search capability?

Does the site provide search capability by keywords? Retrieve relevant information only?

Does the site's internal search capability apply an easy process?

Interactivity

Does the site provide the users with a feedback mechanism to communicate their comments, criticism, and corrections?

Does the site offer the users access to chat rooms or discussion groups?

Does the site employ a qualified moderator to facilitate the discussion groups?

Caveats

Does the site market products?

Does the site advertise or sell products or services?

Box 16.4   Criteria for Assessing the Quality of Health Information on the Internet—MedlinePlus Guide (United States National Library of Medicine, 2015)

Consider the source

- Responsibility for the content; may look for the "about us" information
- Transparency regarding responsibility for the site: is it governmental or a nonprofit institution, a professional organization, a health system, a commercial organization, or an individual?
- Availability of contact information; missing information raises concerns

Focus on quality

- Editorial board members: is the content peer-reviewed?
- Subject matter expertise of those involved in the site development and management
- Process of selecting or approving information made available on the website
- Information about writers, authors, or editorial policy

Be a cyber skeptic

- Claims made that seem too good to be true; deliberately obscure information; "scientific" sounding language; promise of quick, dramatic, miraculous results; only site making such claims
- Caution if the website uses a sensational writing style (e.g., excessive use of exclamation points)
- Use of simple language rather than technical jargon

Look for the evidence

- Reliance on science versus testimonials
- Available author information and credentials

Check for currency

- Date when information was posted; latest update
- Functionality of the links on the site

Beware of bias

- Financial backers of the website
- Support by public funds, donations, or by commercial advertising
- Labeling of advertisements (e.g., from our sponsor)
- Conflict of interest
- Sales versus educational purpose

Protect privacy

- Website's privacy policy; easy access to "privacy" or "privacy policy"
- Registration form for website accessibility; types of questions one must answer to gain access (e.g., personal information, social security number)

---

the MedlinePlus, which is the National Institute of Health's website for patients, their families, and consumers of health services in general. This is produced by the United States National Library of Medicine (Box 16.4), which brings to the public information about diseases, health conditions, and wellness. The website uses a language targeted to the lay person to enhance understanding. MedlinePlus offers reliable and current health information, available for free anytime and anywhere.

Another method for ensuring the credibility and reliability of health information on the Internet is adherence to the "Health on the Net (HON) Code of Conduct" for medical and health websites. Users of the Internet are able to identify if a site complies with

the HON Code of Conduct if the site has successfully achieved certification and indicates such on its home page. This is communicated by including the HON logo/seal on the main page of the website. The HON Code of Conduct is a nongovernmental, self-regulatory solution, and voluntary certification system applied to address the lack of confidence and problem of distrust in the information available on the WWW. It is the Internet's first and most widely spread ethical standard. It has been available since 1996 in more than a dozen languages, including English (Health on the Net Foundation, 2015). The HON Code of Conduct addresses one of the Internet's main healthcare information-related issues: the reliability and credibility of information made available electronically.

Applying the HON Code of Conduct means quality; that is, the website follows good standards in the presentation of healthcare information, resources, and advice, and strictly abides by the code's principles (Case Manager's Tip 16.5). The code consists of eight principles (Box 16.5): authority, complementarity, confidentiality, attribution, justifiability, transparency of authorship, transparency of sponsorship, and honesty in advertising and editorial policy.

16.5. SOCIAL MEDIA AND DIGITAL TOOLS

Social media and digital tools are computer-mediated devices and innovations which allow easy sharing of information among people in a virtual web-based environment. Information may include pictures, videos, thoughts, ideas, physiologic monitoring data, healthcare materials, and other personal stories. Social media and digital tools are a group of Internet-based applications that depend on both mobile and web-based technologies for ease of interaction and exchange of information among individuals regardless of time, space, speed, frequency, or permanence. The advent of social media technologies has drastically changed the way healthcare providers, including case managers, communicate with, and offer services to, patients and other consumers.

People use social media and digital technologies in varied ways; some use them for personal entertainment, leisure, and socialization while others use them

 CASE MANAGER'S TIP 16.5

Exercising Caution When Surfing the Internet for Health and Medical Information

Unfortunately, the use of the Health on the Net Code of Conduct does not eliminate incompetence, fraud, or communication of dishonest healthcare information. On the other hand, if a website is found not to bear the code/seal, it does not mean that it is of poor quality. Users must exercise caution when applying the information available on the Internet and judge for themselves. When in doubt, they must consult with a healthcare provider such as a case manager.

for professional purposes. Healthcare providers tend to use them to advertise their services, access profesional or technical information, or for the provision of select care activities of services to their patients. Consumers of healthcare services on the other hand may use them to communicate with their healthcare providers, seek information about a topic of interest, or to network with others and offer support. Below are some examples of how social media and digital technologies may be used in healthcare; subject matter of interest is usually healthcare-related. When using social media or digital technologies for the sharing of sensitive personal and health information or provision of certain healthcare services (e.g., counseling, consultation or advice), one must be careful not to use public networks; rather use

---

Box 16.5   Health on the Net Code of Conduct (Health on the Net Foundation, 2015)

The Health on the Net Code of Conduct consists of the following eight principles:

- *Authority*: Medical information or health advice is provided and hosted online only by medically trained and qualified professionals unless a clear statement is made that a piece of information is from a nonmedical person.
- *Complementarity*: Information provided on the website is designed to support, not replace, the relationship between a patient/user and his or her physician/healthcare provider.
- *Confidentiality*: Data related to individual patients, users, and visitors, including their identities is respected and kept confidential. The owners of the site honor or exceed the legal requirements of medical/health information privacy that apply in the country/location where the website is located.
- *Attribution*: Information included on the site is supported, when appropriate, by clear references and data sources, and dates of the last modifications are clearly stated.
- *Justifiability*: Balances claims relating to the benefits/performance of a specific treatment, commercial product, or service with appropriate evidence in the manner stated in principle four.
- *Transparency of authorship*: Designers of the website provide information in the clearest possible manner and provide contact addresses for visitors who seek further information or support. The website includes the Webmaster's e-mail address.
- *Transparency of sponsorship*: Includes information about and the identities of the sponsors of the website and the names of the commercial and noncommercial organizations that have contributed funding, services, or materials to the site.
- *Honesty in advertising and editorial policy*: Clearly states whether advertising is a source of funding to the site. If that is the case, presents a brief description of the advertising policy adopted by the site. Advertisements are presented in a manner that is easy to differentiate from original materials created by the operators of the site.

protected networks where the user must authenticate personal identity and confirm use of tools that protect privacy and confidentiality.

- *Networking*: commenting on information others have posted, creating a network of friends and families, or joining groups (e.g., support groups for specific purpose such as heart transplant receipients) created by others (e.g., fellow patients or healthcare professionals).
- *Communicating*: sharing or transmitting physicologic monitoring data to healthcare providers; for example, blood glucose levels, blood presure values, and daily weights.
- *Support groups*: creating a support group for a specific purpose (e.g., maternal grief, end stage renal disease with dialysis) or belonging to an existing support group seeking to receive or offer psychosocial support.
- *Bookmarking*: tagging websites of interest while searching through various sites. Sometimes bookmarking specific content on a website or saving such materials in one's individual user profile and specifications.
- *News*: interacting by sharing opinions, commenting on posts or articles, and voting on something; posting of articles or one's personal story such as journey with a disease or condition.
- *Photo and video sharing*: connecting with others through an exchange or sharing of videos and photos (personal and public) and commenting on others' videos and photos. Sometimes sharing health condition-related photos (e.g., picture of a wound or surgical site).

Case managers and other healthcare profesionals may use social media and digital technologies or tools (Case Manager's Tip 16.6) as a way to deliver care to patients and to remain connected with them or accessible anytime/anywhere, rergardless of whether there was a specific episode of care. Such approaches foster new and trusting relationships and may enhance adherence to health regimen, for example, through supporting the patient/family in self-management. Interactions may not always be between healthcare providers and patients; patients may use social media to connect with other patients for support and networking, especially when suffering the same health conditions or chronic illnesses.

A large percentage of patients and their families are using some form of social media applications and digital technologies today. What is interesting is the use of digital tools for health maintenance activities. For example, use of tracking devices for exercise and nutri-

---

 CASE MANAGER'S TIP 16.6

Various Forms of Social Media and Digital Tools

Case managers must be familiar with the various types of social media technologies and applications so that they are better able to advise their patients on their use and capitalize on employing such applications, as appropriate, to enhance patient's self-management abilities and safety. Some of the social media types include:

- Blogs
- Business networks
- Enterprise social networks
- Support groups
- Gaming
- Virtual worlds
- Social networks
- Professional networks
- Remote monitoring devices

---

tion/weight management allow individuals to monitor performance against established health targets. Often these targets are determined with the assistance of healthcare providers especially when they are related to the presence of a chronic health condition, rather than just wellness and risk reduction. Other types of health uses of digital and social media technologies are:

- Electronic communications about follow-up appointments (e.g., reminders, confirmations).
- Transmitting of results of physiologic monitoring to healthcare providers such as blood glucose levels for diabetics, daily weights for those suffering heart failure, and calorie count and food intake for those on weight management programs.
- Medications management (e.g., tracking of medictaions intake, use of alerts to administer a medication according to certain schedule).
- Ordering of medications and supplies online; establishing a standing schedule for the replenishment of medications and healthcare supplies with specific vendors. This practice prevents the patient from encountering a situation where medications and supplies are unavailable.
- Accessing rersults of medical tests and procedures.
- Accessing personal health records (PHRs) (Box 16.6) on the Internet and via mobile technologies. This practice allows patients to have accurate health information that is accessible anywhere, any time, without the need to physically carry health records around.
- Patient advocacy, engagement, and empowerment.

16.6. PERSONAL HEALTH RECORDS

PHRs are becoming increasingly popular especially as a result of meaningful use, certified electronic health records, patient centered medical home, transitions of care, and other programs that focus on case management services and avoidance of unnecessary or unanticipated access to healthcare services. Additionally, health insurance plans, patient advocacy groups, and employers are also promoting the use of PHRs. The use of PHRs must not be confused with a patient's medical record. Although both types may contain similar content, PHRs are meant for personal use while medical records are for use by healthcare professionals. Medical records are usually more detailed and may contain technical and medical language; PHRs are summarized and highlight salient information about a patient's health history and current state using lay language.

Considering their increasing popularity, case managers must be familiar with PHRs and engage patient's in their use while educating them about their value for enhancing health. PHRs are defined as electronic patient records containing information about an individual's health (e.g., history, medications, allergies, preferences, healthcare providers, next of kin, advanced directive, and healthcare proxy) that is stored digitally online in the virtual environment and made easily accessible anywhere, anytime, by those the patient gives the right to access. It is meant to enhance quality of care, safety, and efficiency.

The use of PHRs presents some concerns, especially regarding privacy, confidentiality, and security. eRisk Working Group for Healthcare emphasizes the need for patients to accept the use of a PHR and to grant permission in writing for such use and access by healthcare providers. It states that technology used for PHRs and other related services (e.g., electronic communication) introduce special concerns and potential risks. Therefore, Medem, Inc. and the eRisk Group advocate for the use of a special agreement between the healthcare provider and patient, family or caregiver, indicating that the patient has agreed in writing to the use of a PHR (Medem, Inc. and eRisk Group Working for Healthcare, 2006). The agreement must at a minimum cover specific aspects such as those described in Box 16.6).

Some patients use access to social media and digital communication technologies as a factor in deciding about a primary care provider and the healthcare facility to receive care when needed. This is an indication that patient and their families trust the use of these tools for the management of their healthcare needs. Despite the rising trend in the use of these technologies, case

---

Box 16.6 Personal Health Records (Medem, Inc., and the eRisk Working Group for Healthcare, 2006)

In 2006, Medem, Inc. and the eRisk Working Group for Healthcare identified several aspects of PHR use patients must agree on in writing before healthcare professionals use PHRs. They primarily focus on the patient's responsibilities and assure that there are no misunderstandings of what PHRs are and how they are used. The major points of focus are the following:

- The PHR service is provided to patients for their convenience only, and is distinct from the medical record maintained by the healthcare provider or facility. Entries in the PHR are not automatically considered as part of the medical record.
- It is the patient's responsibility to notify the healthcare provider of the presence of a PHR.
- The PHR is not a substitute for directly communicating the patient's medical or health information to the patient's primary care provider.
- It is the patient's responsibility to notify healthcare providers when new information appears in the PHR.
- There are no guarantees that the healthcare provider has seen or reviewed information available in the PHR.
- The healthcare provider should make it clear that the patient is responsible for the accuracy of the information in the PHR.
- Developing and maintaining a PHR on a healthcare provider's website requires that patients have a pre-existing relationship with that provider.
- Information available through the PHR are not a substitute for professional medical or health advice.
- Patients and caregivers should agree to contact their healthcare providers for any questions about their medical or health condition, or if they need assistance. For emergency medical services they would immediately call 911, their local emergency number, or their physician.
- Patients and caregivers should agree that their User ID and Password to access the PHR are their responsibility to maintain and protect from unauthorized access and use by third parties.

---

managers and other healthcare providers must be careful about their use in the communiciation of sensitive and private matters. Although encryption of messages is available, it does not mean transmitting sensitive information should be taken for granted (Case Manager's Tip 16.7).

Case managers currently face the challenge of maintaing adherence to ethical and legal standards when using social media and digital technologies in the pro-

CASE MANAGER'S TIP 16.7

Caution when Using Social Media and Digital Technologies in Healthcare

Often these technologies and tools are used to either store health-related information in a virtual place that is accessible anywhere, anytime, or for communication of improtant information such as physiologic monitoring data. Case managers and other healthcare providers must be careful in the use of these technologies. They must make every effort to maintain adherence to HIPAA laws and to avoid malpractice lawsuits.

A healthcare facility's culture is a key asset to prepare for patient communictaion using social media and digital technologies. Healthcare professionals in these facilities, including case managers, must be empowered to proactively engage with patients and their families and alleviate the risk for miscommunications or inapproporiate use of these tools. They also must educate the patient and family as well as other staff about the appropriate and inappropriate use of social media and digital tools.

 CASE MANAGER'S TIP 16.8

Ethical and Legal Concerns When Using Social Media and Digital Technology in Healthcare

Case managers have an obligation to provide safe and quality care to patients/families. This obligation does not preclude them for adhering to ethical and legal standards. When using social media, electronic communication, telemedicine, and digital tools in care provision, it is important for case managers to assure they are practicing within the boundaries of their practice act and the jurisdiction of the state they are licensed in.

Case managers also have the obligation to use technologies that meet ethical and legal standards. There are several organizations that established standards case managers may refer to as guides for evaluating the acceptance and appropriateness of websites state of digital tools used in healthcare. An example is Health on the Net Foundation (developed the Health on the Net Code of Conduct), the American Telemedicine Association (developed guidelines for telehealth and telemedicine), and the National Association of Boards of Pharmacy (developed a verified internet pharmacy practice sites program).

To assure adherence to ethical and legal standards at all times, case managers must be aware of them and knowledgeable about where to access them. Being proactive and regulary review changes and revisions of codes/standards or newly developed ones is necessaery for case managers to maintain adherence at all times and avoid legal and ethical risk.

vision of healthcare services. Availablility of personal health records in the virtual environment and use of electronic communications and telehealth technology allow case managers access to patients regardless of the patients' place of residence or the jurisdiction case managers are licensed and credentialed to operate in. It is easy for a case manager to provide care via the Internet to a patient without awareness that the patient resides out of the case manager's state of jurisdiction. Care in this case can be in the form of offering health advise, answering a question posed via electronic communication, reviewing physicologic monitoring data for a patient and instituting action, or coordinating services for a patient with other providers and agencies. Although the case manager's intent in these situations is to ensure patient's safety and provide care in a timely manner, he/she never intends to ignore the law (Case Manager's Tip 16.8).

Some healthcare providers offer online consultation for patients; although not as common, such practice is on the rise and case managers must be aware of the implications of online consultation especially if any of their patients are participating in online healthcare service. With the state of today's technology and the enhancements of telehealth and telemedicine, online consultations are no longer a dream. Usually an online consultation is similar to a healthcare provdier's visit and may invove the use of secure messaging. Case managers may be involved in online visits with their patients especially if they are managing patients with

multiple chronic illnesses and working on preventing avoidable admissions to acute care hospital or unplanned access to healthcare services.

Healthcare professionals have a set of obligations when engaged in online consultation activities. According to Medem, Inc. and the eRisk Working Group for health (2006), the obligations are similar to those established for online communication in addition to the following:

- *Informed consent*: Prior to initiating an online consultation, the healthcare provider should obtain the patient's informed consent to participate in the consultation, including discussing appropriate expectations, disclaimers, and service terms.
- *Fee disclosure*: Prior to an online consultation, patients should be clearly informed about any charges that might be incurred, and whether the patient's health insurance plan would reimburse for the service.

- *Identity disclosure*: Spend appropriate time at the beginning of the session on complete introductions. Review in detail any clinical information that is provided to the patient during the consultation.
- *Available information*: The healthcare provider should state and document, within the context of the consultation, that the consultation is based upon information made available by the patient during, or prior to, the online consultation (e.g., referral documents, medical record).
- *Online consultation versus online diagnosis and treatment*: Healthcare providers must distinguish between an online consultation related to a known pre-existing condition and the diagnosis and treatment of new conditions and must be mindful of patient safety.
- *Follow-up plans*: Include an explicit plan for follow-up care, as clinically indicated and clearly communicate the plan to the patient.
- *Internet pharmacies*: There are potential risks when patients are referred to online pharmacies. The National Association of Boards of Pharmacy has a Verified Internet Pharmacy Practice Sites (VIPPS) program (http://www.nabp.net/vipps/intro.asp).

16.7. PATIENT ACTIVATION, ENGAGEMENT AND USE OF TECHNOLOGY

A growing body of evidence demonstrates that patients who are more actively involved in their own healthcare experience better health outcomes and incur lower costs. Many public and private healthcare organizations are employing strategies to better engage patients, such as educating them about their conditions and involving them more fully in making decisions about their care. Patient engagement entails getting healthcare consumers to be more aware of and involved in their own care. Health information technology is integral to better patient engagement (Box 16.7). Stage two meaningful use has made patient access to one's own PHRs a critical component, mandating that at least 5% of patients electronically view, download, or transmit their personal health data. This demand is advancing patient engagement and the involvement of case managers in such.

Patient activation is a prerequiste to patient engagement. It refers to a patient's knowledge, skills, ability, and willingness to manage his or her own health and needed services. Patient engagement, on the other hand, is a broader concept that combines patient activation with specific interventions designed to increase activation and promote positive patient behavior, such as obtaining preventive care or exercising regularly. Patient engagement is also one of the strategies to

---

Box 16.7   Health Information Technology and Patient Engagement

Health technology used to enhance patient engagement may include some or all of the following features dependeing on the healthcare organization's stage of development of patient engagement programs:

- PHRs
- Patient portals
- Electronic access by patients and other healthcare providers to a summary of an episode of care and laboratory and radiologic results
- Accessing patients regardless of location (e.g., e-mail and text messaging with case managers and physicians)
- Remote monitoring (e.g., telehealth and tele-engagement) which allows patients to self-report data such as blood pressure, blood glucose levels, body weights, and use of medications
- Mobile health tools that allow patients to keep tabs on their conditions outside the hospital or doctor's office which ultimately enhance self-management and adherence
- Access to patient specific health instruction and educational videos
- Collaborative care tools that allow sharing of patient information across care settings and healthcare providers (transitions of care)
- Online support groups/community support forums

---

achieve the "triple aim" of improved health outcomes, better patient care, and lower costs.

Modern healthcare is complex, and many patients struggle to obtain, process, communicate, and understand even basic health information and services. Similar to patient activation, health literacy is another prerequisite to patient engagement. Many patients lack health literacy, or a true understanding of their medical conditions and care regimens. Some healthcare providers also fail to provide the information that patients need to make the best decisions about their own care and treatment. This further complicates the issue of patient engagement. Even when patients do receive detailed information, they can be overwhelmed or demonstrate a lack of confidence in their own choices. Those with low levels of health literacy find it difficult to follow instructions on how to care for themselves or to adhere to treatment regimens, such as taking their medicines. Case managers can assist in reducing this challenge by assessing health literacy and incorporating the finding in the patient's case management plan of care.

Recognizing these problems, the 2001 Institute of Medicine report, Crossing the Quality Chasm: A New

Health System for the 21st Century, called for reforms to achieve a "patient-centered" healthcare system. The report envisioned a system that provides care that is respectful of and responsive to individual patient preferences, needs, and values, and ensuring that patient values guide clinical decisions. Out of the recognition of the need to apply patient-centered care models, patient engagement has emerged. There are many aspects to patient engagement; commonly used are three different levels (Box 16.8).

Another important charateristic of patient engagement is shared decision making. Here patients and providers together consider the patient's condition, treatment options, the medical evidence behind the treatment options, the benefits and risks of treatment, and patients' preferences, and then arrive at and execute a treatment plan. The strategy is often used with patients who have "preference-sensitive" conditions or treatment options—that is, they may or may not choose particular treatments, or to be treated at all, depending on their own feelings about the risks versus the benefits of treatment, their ability to live well with their conditions, or other factors.

For example, although one patient with knee pain may wish to have knee replacement surgery, another may worry about the risks that the surgery may not completely relieve pain or restore mobility and may choose to forgo it in favor of managing the pain with medication and weight loss. In such cases, there are multiple, reasonable treatment options, each with their own risks and benefits, and the "correct" path forward should be guided by a patient's unique needs and circumstances.

Shared decision making involves several essential elements. First, providers and patients must recognize that a decision is required. Next, they must have at their disposal, and understand, the best available evidence. Finally, they must incorporate the patient's preferences into treatment decisions. There are various modalities through which shared decision making can be conducted. A typical process is to use decision aids such as leaflets, books, videos, health websites, and other interactive media that give patients information on the risks and benefits of various treatment options and help them make the choice that most reflects their personal values. Some organizations have developed balanced, expert-reviewed decision materials and placed them online and made them accessible to patients through electronic engagement tools (e.g., PHRs, portals, and patient-centered care technology). Using these decision aids, shared decision making can be conducted in person between providers and patients, or remotely using digital tools.

A patient's greater engagement in healthcare contributes to improved health outcomes, and information technologies can support engagement. Healthcare Information and Management Systems Society (HIMSS, 2015) equips healthcare providers to e-connect with patients and families through engagement with patient portal adoption, secure messaging, social media, and other emerging health related technologies that include, but are not limited to, the following:

- Health management technology that covers patient portals, secure messaging, Blue Button, Consumer Mediated Exchange, and patient generated health data.
- Social and behavioral tools that cover social media, texting and gaming, wearables and mobile, and the social determinants of health.
- Home health technology which covers remote monitoring and telehealth, patient education, and smart homes.
- Financial health technology which includes managing health insurance and expenses, transparency and consumerism, patient onboarding, and financial options.

Case managers are able to impact patient engagement through shared decision making, health instructions, building patient's self-management skills, healthy lifestyle behavior, follow-up, and advocacy. Patients who are engaged may exhibit behaviors such as those listed in Box 16.9.

Box 16.8   Three Levels of Patient Engagement Programs

Health technology used to enhance patient engagement may include some or all of the following features depending on the healthcare organization's stage of development of patient engagement programs:

1. Level one—patient-based: Direct patient care, in which patients get information about a condition and answer questions about their preferences for treatment. This form of engagement allows patients and providers to make decisions based on the medical evidence, patients' preferences, and clinical judgment.

2. Level two—organization-based: Organizational design and governance where healthcare organizations reach out for consumer input to ensure that they become as responsive as possible to patients' needs.

3. Level three—community-based: Policy making is where consumers are involved in the decisions that communities and society make about policies, laws, and regulations in public health and healthcare.

Box 16.9   Patient Behaviors Demonstrative of Successful Engagement

Health technology used to enhance patient engagement may result in some or all of the following behaviors dependeing on the healthcare organization's stage of development of patient engagement programs and patient activation:

- Finding safe care
- Communication and collaboration with health professionals on ongoing basis
- Paying for care
- Making good treatment decisions
- Promoting own health
- Getting preventive care
- Planning for end-of-life
- Seeking health knowledge
- Adherence to medications and treatments
- Engaging in activities that maintain functioning and reduce health declines
- Involvement in treatment and diagnostic choices
- Selecting individual providers and provider organizations based on performance, reputation, and quality
- Navigating the healthcare system easily
- Knowledge how to manage own health condition and able to self-manage symptoms and problems
- Having the skills and behavioral repertoire to manage condition
- Having the confidence to collaborate with healthcare providers, maintain functioning, and access appropriate and high quality care

16.8. CASE MANAGEMENT–RELATED WEBSITES

The following is a list of websites that are relevant to case management practice. This list is by no means exhaustive. Although the websites are placed under one topic, some relate to more than one area of focus. Case managers are advised to surf the Internet for other sites that may be more relevant to their area of practice. To do this more effectively, they are encouraged to use the tools and tips presented in Chapter 16. Please note, however, that the URL addresses in Chapter 16 are based on the information available as of early 2016. Websites are constantly being changed by their owners or Webmasters; therefore some URL addresses may no longer be correct if the website was altered in some way.

There is no limit to the amount of healthcare resources available on the WWW and the Internet. These resources are constantly changing. Information is updated daily, and in some respects, by the moment. Case managers are encouraged not to fear using the Internet as a resource. If they choose to work with their patients and families, they must do so patiently, starting with the level of knowledge and skill they are at in using the Internet or other electronic communication methods. For some healthcare consumers the Internet may work well, especially for consumers who are enrolled in disease management programs or other forms of case management services and programs.

Accreditation Agencies	
The Joint Commission	http://www.tjc.org
National Committee for Quality Assurance	http://www.ncqa.org
Commission for Accreditation of Rehabilitation Facilities	http://www.carf.org
URAC	http://www.urac.org
Case Management Organizations	
Case Management Society of America	http://www.cmsa.org
The Center for Case Management	http://www.cfcm.com
American Case Management Association	http://www.acmaweb.org
National Association of Case Management	http://www.yournacm.com/
Disease Management	
Disease Management Forum	http://www.sapien.net/dm/
National Association of Disease Management and Wellness Professionals	http://www.nadmwp.org/
Population Health Alliance	http://www.populationhealthalliance.org
Case Management Software	
Landacorp/EXL Healthcare	http://www.landacorp.com
McKesson/InterQual	http://www.mckesson.com/payers/decision-management/interqual-evidence-based-clinical-content/
Milliman Care Guidelines/Hearst Health Network	http://www.mcg.com
Athena Health	http://landing.athenahealth.com
Allscripts Care Manager	http://www.allscripts.com
Orion Healthcare technology—AccuCare	http://www.myaccucare.com
Netsmart Technologies—Care Manager	http://www.ntst.com

Certification in Case Management

Commission for Case Manager Certification	http://www.ccmcertification.org
American Nurses Association	http://www.nursingworld.org
American Institute of Outcomes Care Management	http://www.aiocm.com
National Association of Healthcare Quality	http://www.nahq.org/certify/content/exam.html
The Center for Case Management	http://www.cfcm.com
National Board for Certification in Continuity of Care	http://www.nbccc.org
Certification of Disability Management Specialists Commission	http://www.cdms.org
Rehabilitation Nursing Certification Board	http://www.rehabnurse.org
National Association of Social Workers	http://www.nasw.org
American Board of Managed Care	http://www.abmcn.org
American Board for Occupational Health Nurses	http://www.abohn.org
American Academy of Case Management	http://www.aihcp.org/cs~mgmnt.htm
National Managed Health Care Congress	http://www.nmhcc.org
American College of Managed Care Medicine	http://www.acmcm.org

Patient and Family Education Materials

New York Online Access to Health	http://www.noah.cuny.edu/
HealthFinder	http://www.healthfinder.gov
MedlinePlus—U.S National Library of Medicine	https://www.nlm.nih.gov/medlineplus/
MedWeb Consumer Health	http://www.gen.emory.edu/MEDWEB/keyword/consumer_health.html
National Health Information Resources	http://www.nhic.org

Ethics

Health on the Net Code of Conduct	http://www.hon.ch/HONcode/

Patient Rights and Safety

National Coalition of Patient Rights	http://www/tiac.net/
President's Advisory Commission on Consumer Protection	http://www.hcqualitycommission.gov
National Patient Safety Foundation	http://www.npsf.org
Institute for Safe Medication Practices	http://www.ismp.org
VHA National Center for Patient Safety	http://www.patientsafetycenter.com

Governmental Agencies

Agency for Healthcare Research and Quality	http://www.ahrq.gov
National Institutes of Health	http://www.nih.gov
Healthy People 2010	http://web.health.gov/healthypeople
National Health Information Center	http://www.nhic.org; http://www.health.gov/nhic/
Centers for Disease Control and Prevention	http://www.cdc.gov
National Institute of Safety and Health	http://www.cdc.gov/niosh/
Occupational Safety and Health Administration	http://www.osha.gov
The Department of Health and Human Services	http://www.dhhs.gov
U.S. Government Statistics	http://www.fedstats.gov
Federal Register	http://www.access.gpo.gov/
Food and Drug Administration	http://www.fda.gov/

Quality and Safety

National Committee for Quality Assurance	http://www.ncqa.org
MediQual Systems, Inc.	http://www.mediqual.com
The Quality Compass	http://www.ncqa.org/Info/QualityCompass/Index.htm
The Institute for Outcomes Research	http://www.admin@isiscor.com
Medical Outcomes Trust	http://www.outcomes-trust.org
Combined Health Information Database	http://www.chid.nih.gov
Evidence-Based Medicine Toolkit	http://www.med.ualberta.ca/ebm/
American Institute of Case Management Outcomes	http://www.aiocm.com
National Quality Forum	http://www.qualityforum.org
National Patient Safety Foundation	http://www.npsf.org

Quality and Safety (continued)

World Health Organization	http://www.who.int/patientsafety
Institute for Healthcare Improvement	http://www.ihi.org
Patient Safety Movement	http://www.patientsafetymovement.org
The Healthcare Advisory Board	http://www.advisoryboardcompany.com

Managed Care

Managed Care Information Center	http://www.themcic.com
Health Scope	http://www.healthscope.org
The HMO Page	http://www.hmopage.org
Managed Care Magazine	http://www.managedcaremag.com
American Association of Managed Care Nurses	http://www.aamcn.org
National Association of Managed Care Physicians	http://www.namcp.com
Integrated Healthcare Association	http://www.iha.org
ANA Nursing Quality Report Card	http://www.nursingworld.org
Managed Care Online	http://www.mcol.com
National Association of Boards of Pharmacy	http://www.nabp.net/vipps/intro.asp

Workers' Compensation/Occupational Health

U.S. Department of Labor, Office of Workers' Compensation	http://www.dol.gov/dol/esa/public/aboutesa/ow-cpabot.htm
Workers' Compensation Services, Inc.	http://www.workcompaudit.com
U.S. Department of Labor	http://www.dol.gov
U.S. Department of Justice, Americans With Disabilities Act	http://www.usdoj.gov/crt/ada
Employment Standards Administration	http://www.dol.gov/esa/
Occupational Safety and Health Administration	http://www.osha.gov

 16.9. KEY POINTS

1. The Internet and the WWW allow case managers immediate access to an invaluable amount of health-related information and resources that may facilitate better patient care services and outcomes.

2. Case managers must advise their patients and families not to apply any recommendations of treatments obtained from Internet resources without first consulting their primary healthcare provider or case manager.

3. Applying the tools and tips presented in Chapter 16 on how to surf the Web maximizes search results and increases the chances for obtaining information that is accurate and relevant to the topic of interest.

4. It is important for case managers to apply the criteria of evaluating the quality and safety of healthcare resources available on the Internet.

5. When they are involved in developing resources and information for use via the Internet, such as online patient and family education materials, case managers must abide by the Health on the Net Code of Conduct and Medem's guidelines.

6. There are multiple uses today for social media and digital tools in healthcare delivery and services. Case managers must be aware of these uses and educate their patients and colleagues about them as to avoid quality and safety concerns.

7. Personal health records available in the virtual environment are becoming more popular. They are not the same as medical records. Case managers must differentiate these records to their patients and must educate them about safe use of each.

8. Patient activation, shared decision making, and patient engagement are essential for improving the health of individuals and communities. Case managers play an important role in this regard.

16.10. REFERENCES

Ambre, J., Guard, R., Perveiler, F., Renner, J., & Rippen, H. (1999). Criteria for assessing the quality of health information on the Internet, Falls Church, VA. Health Summit Working Group, Mitretek Systems, (policy paper). Available online at http://www.mitretek.org/Home.nsf/Main/Publications (accessed 3/26/02).

e-Risk Working Group for Healthcare. 2001. Guidelines for online communications and consultations. Medem. Available online at http://www.medem.com/corporate/corporate_erisk_guidelines.cfm

Hancock, L. (1996). Physician's guide to the Internet, Lippincott-Raven, Philadelphia, PA.

Health Information and Management Systems Society (HIMSS). Accessed August 24, 2015. Patient Engagement. Available at http://www.himss.org/library/patient-engagement-toolkit

Health on the Net Foundation. Accessed June 12, 2015. Health on the net code of conduct. Available online at http://www.hon.ch/HONcode/Patients/Conduct.html

Johnson, T. & Tahan, H. (2003). Improving performance of clinical operations. In Montgomery K, Fitzpatrick J, Eds., Essentials of Internet use in nursing, Springer, New York, NY.

Medem, Inc., and eRisk Working Group for Healthcare. (2006). eRisk Working Group for Healthcare's Guidelines for Online Communication. Available at http://www.aao.org/SearchResults.aspx?q=erisk working group&c=1

Romano, C., Hinegardner, P., & Phyillaier, C. (2000). Some guidelines for browsing the Internet. In Fitzpatrick J, Montgomery K, Eds. Internet resources for nurses, Springer, New York, NY.

The United States National Library of Medicine, MedlinePlus. Accessed 2015. Available at http://www.nlm.nih.gov/medlineplus/healthywebsurfing.html

Appendix I— Sample Job Descriptions

This appendix presents a number of job descriptions relevant to case management practice and programs. The job descriptions are for hospital (or other type of facilities) and community case management positions.

- The job description should delineate the power and the level of independence granted in the role (i.e., case manager, discharge planner, physician advisor). It should also provide a clear description of the role, functions, and responsibilities and the minimum expected qualifications.
- Healthcare organizations, or case management employers in general, are advised to incorporate a review of the job descriptions the various personnel directly and indirectly participate in the case management program or department during the orientation or training and education programs. Goals and objectives of the role and the healthcare organization can also be shared.

The following examples of job descriptions are included here:

- Director of Case Management
- Inpatient/Acute Care Case Manager
- Social Worker
- Admitting Office Case Manager
- Emergency Department Case Manager
- Community-Based Case Manager
- Discharge Planning Specialist
- Appeals Coordinator
- Physician Advisor
- Case Management Associate

Things to Remember When Developing the Case Manager's Job Description

- Define the scope of practice and describe in general terms the role, functions, and responsibilities of the case manager.
- Delineate the specific tasks reflective of the role and responsibilities of the case manager and how these relate to the (1) roles and responsibilities of other memebrs of the interdisciplinary healthcare team (e.g., physician advisor, social worker) and (2) to the various care settings across the continuum of health and human services.
- Differentiate the case manager job description from those established for other personnel.
- Delineate the accountability, leadership, and power provided in the role.
- Define the reporting relationship, and indicate to whom the case manager is accountable.
- Define the minimum educational background required for the role.
- Specify the licensure and/or certification requirements.
- Identify the skills required for the role.
- Specify the years of experience required for the role, if any.
- Establish a job description that fits the healthcare organizations's and case management department's operations, systems, and standards of care and practice.
- Establish a job description that reflects the mission, values, beliefs, and philosophy of the institution.
- Specify if it is necessary to belong to specialty professional organizations/associations/societies (e.g.,

American Nurses Association, Case Management Society of America, National Association of Social Workers).

Things to Remember When Developing the Utilization Review Officer Job Description

- Define the scope of practice and the role functions and responsibilities of the physician advisor.
- Identify the educational background, past experience, and skills required for the role.
- Develop a job description that interfaces the physician advisor's role with the case manager's role and the role of other physicians and staff in other departments, such as medicine, surgery, social work, revenue cycle, and quality management.
- Define the interface of the physician advisor with health insurance plans, managed care organizations, managed care department within the employer's organization, board of trustees, and finance.
- Delineate the responsibilities of the physican advisor toward the utilization management plan and committee.
- Describe the responsibiities of the physican advisor in meeting regulatory standards and requirements such as discharge planning and utilization review regulation present in the Medicare Conditions of Participation.

SAMPLE JOB DESCRIPTION: DIRECTOR OF CASE MANAGEMENT

GENERAL JOB SUMMARY:

Coordinates and supervises department of case management and social work. Develops, integrates, and implements systems used in the case management process. Administratively responsible for social workers and nurse case managers, and coordinates with the manager of social work and manager of nursing case management to ensure efficient work processes which are in keeping with regulatory agency expectations. Develops effective strategies to manage denials and ensure positive financial outcomes.

REPORTS TO: Chief Medical and Chief Nursing Officers
SUPERVISES: Case Management Staff

RESPONSIBILITIES:

1. Develops, integrates, and implements systems used in the case management process. Responsible for the ongoing evolution of the case management program and its integration of inpatient and outpatient services or care settings across the continuum.

2. Ensures that positive patient and financial outcomes are achieved through the appropriate screening, discharge/transitional planning, and placement of patients in post-acute care facilities. Develops transitional strategies to address movement from inpatient to community status or across the continuum of care.

3. Refines and improves departmental processes to meet the evolving needs of patient populations, the healthcare team, and the hospital. Evaluates unit processes and staffing patterns, using employee and patient satisfaction as well as financial and operational criteria.

4. Develops, analyzes, and interprets data. Develops PI processes. Develops and communicates denial reduction strategies via education and communication with physician, staff, and payers.

5. Maintains a reliable communication channel from the department to key customers and suppliers. Considers feedback from consumers/personnel, communicates feedback to staff, and initiates corrective action as indicated.

6. Conducts criteria-based performance appraisals at regularly scheduled intervals. Counsels departmental staff appropriately demonstrating sound motivational techniques aimed at enhancing staff performance and productivity.

7. Promotes a positive work and practice environment by setting an atmosphere of open communication, transparency, and feedback. Considers and communicates feedback to and from consumers or personnel, initiates corrective action when indicated.

8. Ensures compliance of clinical and utilization review activities to meet regulatory and accreditation requirements. Plans and coordinates short- and long-term projects to continuously improve the outcomes of the case management program.

9. Develops, implements, and monitors budgets and cost controls. Collaborates with the senior leaders in the preparation of the personnel budget and in identifying and prioritizing capital budget needs.

10. Actively reviews and revises operations to reflect changes in reimbursement, regulations, accreditation, and corporate mission.

11. Establishes workflows (e.g., clinical care management, discharge and transitional planning, utilization management) that assures the provision of safe, quality, and patient-centered case management services.

12. Monitors and evaluates the performance of the case management program/department and the productivity of case managers and other personnel. Ensures that evaluation includes key core measures and value-based purchasing requirements. Prepares outcomes reports and disseminates such to key personnel.

EXPERIENCE:

- Minimum of 5 years of acute care case management experience preferred.
- Clinical background in medical-surgical preferred.
- Previous utilization management and discharge/transitional planning experience preferred.
- Working knowledge of utilization management applications such as InterQual or Milliman Care Guidelines preferred.
- Previous experience with regulatory, accreditation, and compliance requirements; previous experience in medical record audits and review.

EDUCATION:

- Current RN License
- Master's degree in nursing or related field preferred
- State certification, if appropriate
- Case management certification preferred

SKILLS:

- Excellent clinical and administrative skills and judgment.
- Strong interpersonal and communication skills, including verbal, written, and presentation skills.
- Ability to work effectively with other disciplines and departments and outside agencies.
- Computer skills essential.

Note: This job description may be modified to reflect a specific care setting or healthcare organization. Some language may be modified accordingly for appropriateness and relevance. Reporting structure may vary by healthcare organization. In some organizations, the director may report to the chief medical or chief nursing officer or both; in others the director may report to the chief financial officer, chief operations officer, or the chief clinical transformation officer.

SAMPLE JOB DESCRIPTION: INPATIENT/ACUTE CARE CASE MANAGER

JOB SUMMARY:

The case manager is responsible for facilitating the patient's hospitalization from preadmission through discharge or transition to another level of care or setting. The case manager coordinates with physicians, nurses, social workers, and other interdisciplinary healthcare team members to expedite appropriate cost effective and safe, quality care. The case manager applies clinical expertise and medical appropriateness criteria to resource utilization and discharge/transitional planning. Will advise the healthcare team and provide leadership as needed.

REPORTS TO: Director of Case Management
SUPERVISES: Case Management Support Staff

RESPONSIBILITIES

1. Utilization Management
   a. Using established criteria, reviews appropriateness of patient's admission, need for continued hospital stay, and discharge criteria.
   b. Discusses with attending physician and/or advisor the appropriateness of medical necessity, estimated length of stay, resource utilization, consultation, treatment, and discharge plans.
   c. Obtains from third party payer timely and accurate certification for medical necessity, status, level of care, and any information required for discharge.
   d. Responds in a timely manner to third party requests for concurrent and continued stay reviews and sharing of clinical information.
   e. Issues letters of denial and reinstatement within regulatory timeframe.
   f. Responds timely to denials, concurrent or retrospective.

2. Discharge/Transitional Planning
   a. Initiates discharge or transitional planning by assessing the patient's and family's needs and documenting the assessment on the interdisciplinary plan of care.
   b. Provides timely discharge/transitional planning for patients and coordinates home care services and durable medical equipment needs.
   c. Within 24 hours of admission, identifies patients and families who have complex psychosocial, financial, and legal discharge planning needs and refers those patients to social work.
   d. Collaborates with social workers to assure complex patients receive appropriate and timely discharge planning and counseling as needed.
   e. Collaborates (and delegates to) with case management support staff in the coordination of transportation services, ordering of durable medical equipment, and arranging follow-up care appointments for patients.
   f. Completes the Patient Review Instrument in a timely manner.

3. Care Coordination
   a. Ensures that the interdisciplinary care plan and discharge/transition plan are consistent with patient's clinical care course, continuing care needs, and covered services.
   b. Identifies, screens, and assesses in a timely manner those patients and families/significant others who require a social work referral and intervention such as counseling, crisis management, and Medicaid application.
   c. Actively participates in interdisciplinary patient care management rounds.
   d. Participates in patient flow communication and follow up on improvement strategies.
   e. Discusses estimated length of stay, treatment, and discharge plan with the attending physician, as indicated.
   f. Coordinates discharge teaching and health instructions. Ensures that teaching is completed by members of the interdisciplinary team.

g. Consults with physician advisors, nursing staff, and staff in ancillary departments and coordinates the elimination of barriers to efficient delivery of care in the appropriate setting.

h. Resolves and eliminates conflicts in the patient treatment plan.

4. Integrates case management plan into overall interdisciplinary patient care plan through interdisciplinary collaboration and communication.

5. Documents patient care plan, interventions, progress, and outcomes promptly and completely in medical record.

6. Identifies service gaps (e.g., care delays and variances) and participates in other hospital and departmental programs to address and improve quality of care. Collaborates with social workers to identify, track, and resolve avoidable delay days and saved days through hospital stay.

7. Collects data on core measures and variances from quality screening criteria approved by the quality assurance committee. Forwards these data to the quality management department for continued support of the clinical departments.

8. Communicates to risk management all incidents that are potentially compensable events or present risk for malpractice litigation.

9. Follows regulations from payers, government, and state; adheres to standards of accreditation agencies.

EXPERIENCE:

- 1–3 years of acute care case management experience preferred.
- Clinical background in assigned unit/service line preferred.
- Previous utilization management and discharge planning experience preferred.
- Working knowledge of InterQual or Milliman Care Guidelines preferred; previous experience with regulatory and compliance requirements; previous experience in chart review.

EDUCATION:

- Current RN License
- Bachelor's degree in nursing required; master's degree preferred
- State certification, if appropriate
- Case management certification preferred

SKILLS:

- Excellent clinical and administrative skills and judgment.
- Strong interpersonal and communication skills, including verbal, written, and presentation skills.
- Ability to work effectively with other disciplines and departments and outside agencies.
- Computer skills essential.

Note: This job description may be modified to reflect a specific care setting, clinical specialty, patient population, or healthcare organization. Some language may be modified accordingly for appropriateness and relevance. Reporting structure may vary by healthcare organization. In some organizations, the inpatient case manager may report to the director of case management; in some others, and depending on the size of the organization, the inpatient case manager may report to a manager of case managers within the case management department.

SAMPLE JOB DESCRIPTION: SOCIAL WORKER

JOB SUMMARY:

The social worker coordinates and facilitates discharge and transitional planning activities in collaboration with the case manager and the interdisciplinary healthcare team. Complex discharge planning should be referred to the social worker, who will evaluate the patient and/or family needs, and make recommendations based on the assessment findings.

REPORTS TO: Director of Case Management
SUPERVISES: Case Management Support Staff

RESPONSIBILITIES:

1. Identifies, screens, and assesses in a timely manner those patients and families/significant others who require social work service consults.

2. Integrates social work plan of care into the case management plan and the overall interdisciplinary plan of care and through interdisciplinary collaboration.

3. Provides professional social work services in the areas of comprehensive case management, discharge planning, continuing care services, advocacy, clinical social work services (e.g., crisis intervention, counseling, and appropriate education to patients and families/significant others utilizing appropriate modalities).

4. Understands and uses hospital and community based resources and government funding. Refers patients, families/significant others, and hospital staff to appropriate services to ensure continuity and quality, safe care. Develops and uses specialized knowledge of resources related to the needs of specific patient populations. Facilitates Business Department's efforts to obtain insurance coverage for hospital and community based services.

5. Documents the patient care plan, interventions, and outcomes promptly and completely in the patient's medical record. Completes statistical reports as required by the department and other programs.

6. May provide field instruction to social work students. Under supervision, as directed by state social work act, may professionally direct activities of social work assistants, other department assistants, or volunteers. May teach professionals or nonprofessionals within or outside the hospital.

7. Identifies service gaps and participates in other hospital and departmental programs to address and improve quality of care. Collaborates with case managers to identify, track, and resolve avoidable delay days and saved days through hospital stay.

8. Participates in and may assume leadership of hospital and departmental committees.

9. Collaborates with case managers to assure complex patients receive appropriate and timely discharge planning services.

10. Coordinates charity care and services for patients in need.

EXPERIENCE:

- 1–3 years as an acute care social worker experience preferred.
- Experience preferably in clinical area of requested position.
- Experience in case management preferred.

EDUCATION:

- Master's degree in social work from accredited school of social work
- State certified as a professional social worker
- Case management certification preferred

SKILLS:

- Excellent social work, clinical and administrative skills, and judgment.
- Strong interpersonal and communication skills, including verbal, written, and presentation skills.
- Ability to effectively work with other disciplines and departments and outside agencies.
- Computer skills essential.

Note: This job description may be modified to reflect a specific care setting, clinical specialty, patient population, or healthcare organization. Some language may be modified accordingly for appropriateness and relevance. Reporting structure may vary by healthcare organization. In some organizations, the social worker may report to the director of case management; in some others, and depending on size of the organization, the social worker may report to a social work manager within the case management department.

SAMPLE JOB DESCRIPTION: ADMITTING OFFICE CASE MANAGER

JOB SUMMARY:

The admitting office case manager carefully reviews scheduled admissions, transfers, and other patients to determine if established criteria for admission to inpatient or ambulatory care setting are met. The case manager works closely with patient access and registration, attending physicians, and third party payers to facilitate the appropriate setting for care. The position serves as resource to the patient/family regarding issues that may impact the admission, length of stay, or patient discharge.

REPORTS TO: Director of Case Management
SUPERVISES: Case Management Support Staff

RESPONSIBILITIES:

1. Using established utilization management criteria, reviews medical necessity and appropriateness of level of care of patient's admission.
2. Determines clinical appropriateness of observation, outpatient, and other designated patients expected to stay overnight (<48 hours).
3. Discusses with attending physician and/or physician advisor the appropriateness of medical necessity and compliance with any federal or state regulations.
4. Responds timely to third party payer requests for concurrent clinical information.
5. Facilitates use of alternative care settings when appropriate to patient's presenting needs.
6. Reviews all same-day admissions before the scheduled day of surgery or admission to ensure that health insurance plan authorization has been appropriately obtained and to determine the need for appropriateness of setting or any discharge planning needs.
7. Reviews all requests for transfers from other facilities to ensure that the patient's condition necessitates the transfer and provides feedback to the sending facilities regarding determination.
8. Refers patients/families to discharge/transitional planning or other appropriate services or community resources.
9. Notifies inpatient case manager of issues related to health insurance plan coverage, benefits, special patient/family circumstances, or other situations that may impede ongoing care or discharge.
10. Responds timely to denials, concurrent or retrospective.
11. Participates in patient flow activities and improvement strategies.
12. May participate in or lead multidisciplinary teams.

EXPERIENCE:

- 1–3 years of acute care case management experience preferred.
- Clinical background in assigned unit/service line, specialty, or patient population is preferred.
- Previous utilization management experience preferred.
- Working knowledge of coding procedures, InterQual and Milliman Care Guidelines preferred.
- Previous experience with regulatory, accreditation, and compliance requirements.
- Previous experience in chart audits and reviews.

EDUCATION:

- Current RN License
- Bachelor's degree in nursing required, master's degree preferred
- State certification, if appropriate
- Case management certification preferred

SKILLS:

- Excellent clinical and administrative skills and judgment.
- Strong interpersonal and communication skills, including verbal, written, and presentation skills.
- Ability to effectively work with other disciplines and departments and outside agencies.
- Computer skills essential.

Note: This job description may be modified to reflect a specific care setting, clinical specialty, patient population, or healthcare organization. Some language may be modified accordingly for appropriateness and relevance. Reporting structure may vary by healthcare organization. In some organizations, the admitting office case manager may report to the director of case management; in some others, and depending on size of the organization, the admitting office case manager may report to a manager of case managers within the case management department.

SAMPLE JOB DESCRIPTION: EMERGENCY DEPARTMENT CASE MANAGER

JOB SUMMARY:

The emergency department (ED) case manager carefully reviews patients who are being admitted or placed on observation status by the ED physicians. The case manager works closely with ED physicians, the ED social worker, nursing, and any other ancillary service providers in that department. The case manager serves as a resource to both ED physicians and admitting physicians in determination of medical necessity status and level of care. There are times when the ED case manager may contact third party payers to facilitate authorization for the appropriate care setting for the patient. The position serves as a resource to the patient/family and fellow healthcare professionals regarding issues that may impact the admission, length of stay, or patient discharge.

REPORTS TO: Director of Case Management
SUPERVISES: Case Management Support Staff

RESPONSIBILITIES:

1. Utilization Management
   a. Using established criteria, reviews appropriateness of patient's admission, including both status and level of care.
   b. Discusses with both ED and attending physicians and/or physician advisor the appropriateness of medical necessity and compliance with any federal or state regulations and accreditation standards.
   c. Responds timely to third party payer requests for concurrent clinical information, should the patient be held in the ED awaiting an inpatient bed or transfer to another facility.
   d. Identifies issues of clinical resource utilization and/or delays in service/care (based on service standards) with the emergency department staff and refers these issues to the appropriate department head/vice president for resolution.

2. Discharge/Transitional Planning
   a. Facilitates use of alternative settings and services when appropriate to patient's presenting needs.
   b. Refers patients/families to discharge planning or other appropriate services or community resource.
   c. Refers patient to and arranges for home care services.
   d. Arranges for the patient follow-up care appointment and communicates with patient's primary care provider about the discharge from the ED and coordinated services if any.
   e. Assures adherence to EMTALA law.

3. Care Coordination
   a. Facilitates the initiation of diagnostic services, treatment planning, and therapeutic treatment while patient is present in the ED of admitted patients.
   b. Collaborates with the social worker as patient's need arises and facilitates and expedites discharge of patients to alternate care settings.
   c. Facilitates diagnostic testing, treatment planning, and therapeutic care for the ED patient.
   d. Notifies inpatient case manager of issues related to health insurance plan coverage, benefits, special patient/family circumstances, or other situations that may impede ongoing care, discharge to home, or transition to another level of care/facility.
   e. Participates in patient flow activities and improvement strategies, including ED turnaround time for tests, treatment and release, and admission.
   f. May initiate assessment on inpatient or observation service patients who are held in the ED.
   g. Identifies patients with multiple chronic conditions or other complex issues, especially those who frequently access the ED for care, and develops appropriate patient care management and discharge plans for them.

4. Resource Management
   a. Participates in strategies to decrease patients with frequent ED utilization.
   b. Prevents need to admit patients who do not meet medical necessity criteria and coordinates other services for these.

5. May participate in or lead interdisciplinary team rounds and handoff communication.

EXPERIENCE:

- 1–3 years of acute care case management experience preferred.
- Clinical background in assigned unit/service line, patient population preferred.
- Previous utilization management experience preferred.
- Working knowledge of InterQual and Milliman Care Guidelines preferred.
- Previous experience with regulatory, accreditation, and compliance requirements.
- Previous experience in chart audits and reviews.

EDUCATION:

- Current RN License
- Bachelor's degree in nursing required; master's degree in nursing preferred
- State certification, if appropriate
- Case management certification preferred

SKILLS:

- Excellent clinical and administrative skills and judgment.
- Strong interpersonal and communication skills, including verbal, written, and presentation skills.
- Ability to effectively work with other disciplines and departments and outside agencies.
- Computer skills essential.

Note: This job description may be modified to reflect a specific care setting, clinical specialty, patient population, or healthcare organization. Some language may be modified accordingly for appropriateness and relevance. Reporting structure may vary by healthcare organization. In some organizations, the ED case manager may report to the director of case management; in some others and depending on size of the organization may report to a manager of case managers within the case management department.

SAMPLE JOB DESCRIPTION: COMMUNITY-BASED CASE MANAGER

JOB SUMMARY:

The case manager is responsible for facilitating the patient's care process in the outpatient setting. The case manager coordinates with physicians, nurses, social workers, and other health team members to expedite medically appropriate cost-effective care. The case manager applies clinical expertise and medical appropriateness criteria to resource utilization, referrals to outside agencies, and use of services across the continuum. Will advise the health-care team and provide leadership as needed.

REPORTS TO: Director of Case Management
SUPERVISES: Case Management Support Staff

RESPONSIBILITIES:

1. Uses high-risk screening criteria to assess patients' level of care needs. Completes this on admission to the outpatient setting and every 3 months thereafter, or more often as needed.
2. Completes a comprehensive physical, psychosocial, and financial assessment of the patient/family to determine priorities in developing a case management plan of care.
3. Coordinates the plan of care with all members of the interdisciplinary team.
4. Identifies patients and families who have complex psychosocial, financial, and/or legal needs and refers those patients to social work.
5. Interacts with patients and families on an as-needed basis to modify and update the plan of care based on the assessment.
6. Obtains from third-party payer certification for use of services across the continuum (e.g., home care services); responds to third-party payer requests for concurrent clinical information.
7. Updates and modifies the interdisciplinary plan of care as needed based on an assessment of the patient's achievement of expected outcomes of care.
8. Collaborates with patients/families to coordinate community services and appropriate resources that meet the patient's/family's needs and goals including self-management and health literacy.
9. Discusses with primary care providers and/or physician advisors the appropriateness of resource utilization, consultations, and treatment plan.
10. Collects data on variances identified in the outpatient care setting. Consults with physician advisors, nursing staff, and staff in ancillary departments and coordinates the elimination of barriers to efficient delivery of care in the appropriate setting.
11. Communicates to risk management all incidents that present potential risk for malpractice and litigation.
12. Ensures that medical record documentation supports the level of care provided.
13. Conducts interdisciplinary case conferences (e.g., nursing, medicine, social work, community health) as needed to ensure the following:
    a. Completion and reporting of diagnostic testing and results/test reports
    b. Completion of treatment appropriate to the episode of illness
    c. Modification of the plan to meet the continuing needs of the patient
    d. Communication of relevant issues and third-party payer information to the team
14. Discusses estimated length of treatment, frequency of outpatient visits, or other care modalities with the attending physician, as indicated.
15. Ensures that all critical elements of the plan of care are communicated to the patient and family and are documented on the interdisciplinary plan of care.
16. Collaborates in developing, implementing, and evaluating teaching/learning strategies for the patient/family in the community.

17. Performs ongoing evaluation of the plan of care to ensure that current and potential complications are identified and to evaluate the effectiveness of interventions.

18. Ensures that patient appointments are made for follow-up visits. Addresses no-shows as necessary.

19. Communicates with other case managers along the continuum, including acute care, home care, managed care, and long-term care.

20. Uses appropriate resources and methods to resolve conflict with others.

21. Demonstrates active collaboration with other members of the health team to achieve the case management programmatic goals.

22. Maintains clinical competency and current knowledge of regulatory, accreditation, and payer requirements.

EXPERIENCE:

- 1–3 years of acute care case management experience preferred.
- Clinical background in assigned unit/service line (ambulatory care), specialty, or patient population is preferred.
- Previous case management, chronic care management experience preferred.
- Working knowledge of InterQual and Milliman Care Guidelines preferred.
- Previous experience with regulatory, accreditation, and compliance requirements.

EDUCATION:

- Current RN License
- Bachelor's degree in nursing required, master's degree preferred
- State certification, if appropriate
- Case Management certification preferred

SKILLS:

- Excellent clinical and administrative skills and judgment.
- Strong interpersonal and communication skills, including verbal, written, and presentation skills.
- Ability to effectively work with other disciplines and departments and outside agencies.
- Computer skills essential.

Note: This job description may be modified to reflect a specific care setting, clinical specialty, patient population, or healthcare organization. Some language may be modified accordingly for appropriateness and relevance. Reporting structure may vary by healthcare organization. In some organizations, the community-based case manager may report to the director of case management; in some others and depending on size of the organization the community-based case manager may report to a manager of case managers within the case management department.

SAMPLE JOB DESCRIPTION: DISCHARGE PLANNING SPECIALIST

JOB SUMMARY:

The discharge planning specialist serves as a resource to case managers and/or social workers working with patients who present with complex discharge planning needs. The discharge planning specialist also carries a case load of complex patients, identified by either day, dollar, or time intensity outlier. Analyzing data to understand the reason for referrals for complex discharge planning is also a part of this role.

REPORTS TO: Director of Case Management
SUPERVISES: Case Management Support Staff

RESPONSIBILITIES

1. Coordinates the discharge/transition plans for patients with complex discharge needs, including those with greater psychosocial acuity, having time intensive needs, those who require legal guardianship procedures, or have unusual needs (e.g., discharge to another country).
2. Serves as a resource to any social worker or case manager who has a complex patient requiring extensive discharge planning services.
3. Serves as a resource for city, state, national, and international discharge planning challenges.
4. Collects and analyzes data regarding referrals and complex cases.
5. Follows job description of staff social worker.
6. Follows regulations from payers, government, state, and accrediting agencies.
7. May participate in or lead interdisciplinary patient care management teams.
8. Participates in quality, outcomes, and value-based purchasing activities including gathering of data on core measures.
9. Report concerns that may present potential for malpractice and litigation to risk management.
10. Coordinates guardianship procedures; communicates with crisis intervention teams and protective services; facilitates transitions to other complex long-term care settings.

EXPERIENCE:

- 3–5 years as an acute care social worker.
- Experience in complex case management and discharge planning.
- Experience in clinical specialty preferred.

EDUCATION:

- Master's degree in social work
- State certification, if appropriate
- Case management certification preferred

SKILLS:

- Excellent clinical and administrative skills and judgment.
- Strong interpersonal and communication skills, including verbal, written, and presentation skills.
- Ability to effectively work with other disciplines and departments and outside agencies.
- Computer skills essential.
- Ability to manage difficult and complex situations with calmness and organization.
- Knowledge of guardianship procedures and familiarity with working with medical attaches in consulates

Note: This job description may be modified to reflect a specific care setting, clinical specialty, patient population, or healthcare organization. Some language may be modified accordingly for appropriateness and relevance. Reporting structure may vary by healthcare organization. In some organizations, the discharge planning specialist may report to the director of case management; in some others and depending on size of the organization the discharge planning specialist may report to a social work manager within the case management department.

SAMPLE JOB DESCRIPTION: APPEALS COORDINATOR

JOB SUMMARY:

The appeals coordinator serves as a resource to case managers and/or social workers working with patients who present with complex needs and who encounter service denials from the health insurance plan. The appeals coordinator reviews denials and prepares the appeals paperwork in collaboration with other case managers and physician advisors. The appeals coordinator analyzes data to understand the reason for denials, the financial impact, and to identify opportunities for improvement.

REPORTS TO: Director of Case Management
SUPERVISES: Case Management Support Staff

RESPONSIBILITIES:

1. Acts as a resource to case managers relative to concurrent and retrospective denials of payment and serves as a consultant to the case managers relative to the appeal process.
2. Acts as a liaison between payers and the case managers in response to specific payer issues.
3. Maintains and updates, within 24 hours of receipt, the payer database and facilitates distribution of same to appropriate members of the case management team.
4. Attends appeal hearing, as appropriate, to represent the institution.
5. Analyzes denials and appeals for financial impact, patterns, and trends.
6. Provides information to the director of case management regarding patterns or trends (practitioners, diagnosis, patient location, physician of record, and types of denials) associated with appeals.
7. Participates with the managed case department in reviewing payer contracts to assess the feasibility of the clinical reviews being requested and utilization management procedures.
8. Extracts from the medical record clinically pertinent information to respond to resource demands and develop concise corrective action steps.
9. Develops, reviews and revises case management policies and procedures in conjunction with the case managers.
10. Serves as the on-site appeals coordinator and a resource to the case managers in interpreting payer information requests.
11. Responds to retrospective denials.
12. Uses appropriate resources and methods to resolve conflicts with others.
13. Meets assigned deadlines and quality standards without a reminder from supervisors or others.
14. Maintains adherence to policies and practices regarding confidentiality and patient's rights.
15. Maintains clinical competency and current knowledge of regulatory, accreditation, and payer requirements to perform job responsibilities.
16. Collaborates with other departments, such as business office, admitting, managed care and revenue cycle, finance, in regard to appeals and denials.
17. Participates as a member of utilization review and management committees.

EXPERIENCE:

- 1–3 years of acute care case management experience preferred.
- Clinical background in nursing.
- Previous utilization management experience including denials and appeals preferred.
- Working knowledge of InterQual and Milliman Care Guidelines preferred.
- Previous experience with regulatory, accreditation, and compliance requirements.
- Previous experience in chart audits and reviews.

EDUCATION:

- Current RN license
- Bachelor's degree in nursing required; master's degree in nursing preferred
- State certification, if appropriate
- Case management certification preferred

SKILLS:

- Excellent clinical and administrative skills and judgment.
- Strong interpersonal and communication skills, including verbal, written, and presentation skills.
- Ability to effectively work with other disciplines and departments and outside agencies.
- Computer skills essential.

Note: This job description may be modified to reflect a specific care setting, clinical specialty, patient population, or healthcare organization. Some language may be modified accordingly for appropriateness and relevance. Reporting structure may vary by healthcare organization. In some organizations, the appeals coordinator may report to the director of case management; in some others and depending on size of the organization, the appeals coordinator may report to a manager of case managers within the case management department, or director of revenue cycle/management.

SAMPLE JOB DESCRIPTION: PHYSICIAN ADVISOR

JOB SUMMARY:

The physician advisor serves as an advocate and expert for medical necessity with hospital physicians. This position is responsible for reviewing all concurrent and retrospective denials escalated by the case management staff. This physician reviews cases for medical necessity against established criteria and collaborates with physicians to provide appropriate documentation to demonstrate medical necessity. Additionally this position provides education to hospital physicians regarding medical necessity and appropriate documentation.

REPORTS TO: Chief Medical Officer and Director of Case Management
SUPERVISES: Appeals Coordinator or none

RESPONSIBILITIES

1. Supports clinical review function of the case management program in area of medical necessity of patients for admission to acute care.
2. Meets with case management and healthcare team members to discuss selected cases.
3. Works with hospital and clinical committees to develop processes and guidelines to improve documentation for medical necessity and appropriateness of care.
4. Participates in Utilization Management/Review Committee. Acts as the chair of this committee.
5. Acts as liaison between managed care companies, government auditing bodies, and the hospital to assure optimal payment when appropriate.
6. Reviews all potential or actual denials (whether concurrent or retrospective) that are referred by the case managers for medical necessity or appeals coordinator.
7. Reviews cases that present level of care concerns or are considered inappropriate for acute care admission.
8. Acts as a resource to attending and consulting physicians regarding their decisions about appropriateness of hospitalization, procedures and/or surgeries, continued stay, and use of resources.
9. Acts as resource to attending and consulting physicians regarding federal and state utilization and quality regulations.
10. Assures timely response on issues presented by the case management staff, including:
    a. Those concurrent cases felt to be medically justified, despite lacking adherence to standardized criteria, will be pursued using the concurrent appeal process.
    b. Those retrospective cases felt to be medically justified, despite lacking adherence to standardized criteria, and will be pursued by preparing a clinical justification appeal letter to be included in the appeal packet sent to the payer.
    c. Retrospective denials that are prioritized for completion based on the date by which the appeal must be submitted to the payer.
    d. For concurrent cases not fitting into any of the above categories, the case is pursued with the attending physician of record to obtain clinical information about the patient that may not be apparent from a review of the medical record but that may be sufficient to justify an acute care stay and ensure that the patient is in the most appropriate setting or the level of care needed.
11. Prepares a monthly activity report of appealed cases and the outcomes of those appeals. The report includes trends of escalation and denials and an action plan to address those trends.
12. Participates in physician education programs regarding reimbursement, clinical criteria, and documentation as needed.
13. Serves as a liaison between the physician staff and the case management staff.
14. Maintains positive, working relationships with the Medical Directors of the third parties.

EXPERIENCE:

- 5 years medical staff experience.
- Previous utilization management experience preferred.
- Working knowledge of InterQual and Milliman Care Guidelines preferred.
- Respect of peers is essential.
- Previous experience with regulatory, accreditation, and compliance requirements.

EDUCATION:

- Licensed medical doctor with specialty board certification (if required by other medical staff physicians)
- Utilization management certification preferred

SKILLS:

- Excellent clinical and administrative skills and judgment.
- Strong interpersonal and communication skills, including verbal, written, and presentation skills.
- Ability to effectively work with other disciplines and departments and outside agencies.
- Computer skills essential.

Note: This job description may be modified to reflect a specific care setting, clinical specialty, patient population, or healthcare organization. Some language may be modified accordingly for appropriateness and relevance. Reporting structure may vary by healthcare organization. In some organizations, the physician advisor may report to the chief medical officer, director of case management, or revenue cycle/management (i.e., finance).

SAMPLE JOB DESCRIPTION: CASE MANAGEMENT ASSOCIATE

JOB SUMMARY:

The case management associate works under the direction of a department leadership team member to provide administrative support for case management processes. The associate can perform tasks identified by the case management team for discharge planning, utilization management, and care coordination support. The position does not provide any support that requires professional intervention.

REPORTS TO: Director of Case Management
SUPERVISES: None

RESPONSIBILITIES:

1. Completes tasks related to transfer of patients to post-acute care facilities including:
   a. Communication with facility related to bed availability, including use of case management electronic discharge system
   b. Sharing of internal referral information electronically or via fax
   c. Assuring transfer of documentation/medical record complete
   d. Arranging transportation, confirmation of arrangements, and communication with families regarding transfer arrangements
   e. Maintaining and managing awareness of post-acute settings, such as skilled nursing facilities, home care agencies, infusion services, durable medical equipment services, hospice, acute rehab, and long term acute care facilities
   f. Demonstrating independence and proactive initiation of duties related to transfer of patients described above
2. Provides patient and/or family with second important message letters, as directed by case management staff.
3. Secures requested information for the healthcare team, patient, and/or family. This could include prescription availability, insurance requirements, and community resources.
4. Uses case management electronic system to support case management utilization management and discharge planning processes, as directed.
5. Supports the case management staff in tasks related to care coordination, discharge planning, and/or utilization management.
6. Assists with data collection.
7. Keeps team members updated with progress of assigned tasks. Escalates issues to case manager, social worker, or leadership staff in a timely manner.
8. Maintains and adjusts schedule to enhance the performance of the department.
9. Arranges for follow-up care appointments for patients and transmits summary of care documents to primary care providers.
10. Documents accurately and thoroughly all transactions during the shift, according to department policy.

EXPERIENCE:

- One year of related work in a healthcare environment preferred.
- Sound knowledge of basic medical terminology preferred.
- One year in a position involving experience in similar or related duties.
- Demonstrates positive and interpersonal relations in dealing with all members of the team.

EDUCATION:

- High school graduate required
- Associate Degree preferred, or two years' experience commensurate with job

SKILLS:

- Computer and data entry knowledge essential.
- Strong interpersonal and communication skills.
- Excellent organizational skills.
- Ability to effectively work with a healthcare team.

Note: This job description may be modified to reflect a specific care setting, clinical specialty, patient population, or healthcare organization. Some language may be modified accordingly for appropriateness and relevance. Reporting structure may vary by healthcare organization. In some organizations, the case manager associate may report to the director of case management; in some others and depending on size of the organization may report to a manager or supervisor of case managers or social workers.

Appendix II: Sample Performance Appraisals/ Review

This appendix presents an example of a competency-based performance appraisal. This example can be used as a guide to develop perfromance appraisls and review documents for personnel in the case management department. This example can also be applied in case management programs of any healthcare organization across the continuum of care whether payer, provider, or employer based.

- The competency-based performance appraisal should reflect the various domains assumed in a particular role (i.e., case manager, discharge planner, physician advisor, case manager associate). It should also provide a clear description of how perfromance is evaluated to reflect productivity and effectiveness in the role.

- The competency-based performance appraisal should always be criteria based. Evaluating performance is important for determining the effectiveness of those who partake in the case management program or department. Each domain should have specific allocated weight dependent on the amount of time one spends on average on such domain and the improtance or risk associated with the domain.

- Healthcare organizations or case management employers in general are advised to incorporate reviewing the process of evaluating performance in the training and education of those involved in the case management department, especially at the time they assume their roles and on an ongoing basis. Goals and objectives of the role and the healthcare organization can also be shared.

Things to Remember When Developing Performance Appraisals for Those Involved in the Case Management Department

The tips provided below are for the case manager's role; however they also are applicable to any role within the case management program (e.g., social worker, discharge planner, physician advisor, or case manager associate). A similar process or concept can be used to develop performance appraisals for the other roles.

- Develop a performance appraisal that is competency-based and reflective of the job description and the role dimensions of the case manager.
- Clearly define the rating system used in the performance appraisal.
- Specify the minimum acceptable rating (performance) or the performance threshold.
- Make expectations clear and well known.
- Include the skills, knowledge, abilities, and competencies required for the job in the performance appraisal.
- Delineate the frequency of evaluating performance and whether formal or informal.
- Identify the competencies related to the role.
- State the competencies in a measurable and practical way.
- Determine the criteria for merit increases or bonuses and make those known.
- Communicate the percentage of time the case manager is expected to spend in each of the role dimensions to the degree possible or appropriate. Remember that the percentage for each dimension may vary according to the practice area or

specialty (e.g., acute inpatient care setting versus emergency department) or the person assuming the role (e.g., nurse case manager or social worker case manager).

■ Today, there are many vendors who offer electronic human resource information systems for use in the performance review and appraisal of personnel in an organization. These systems usually mimic the traditional paper/manual procedures and documents. These systems include the following:

—Demographic and background information about the healthcare professional (e.g., case manager) which communicate the person's name, credentials, and qualifications (e.g., educational degrees and certifications), date of hire, performance appraisal period, and place of work (e.g., specialty, care setting, patient population if appropriate).

—Core values section that the organization may have implemented and expect each healthcare professional to demonstrate adherence to (e.g., customer service, teamwork, respect, innovation, and patient-centered care).

—Role functions and specific areas of responsibilities which describe the technical knowledge and skills the person must exhibit when taking care of patients. These relate directly to the role; for example, case manager's roles and fucntions.

—Opportunities for continued development and growth. This section sometimes reflect deficiencies or advancement. It identifies the deficient or suboptimal areas of performance with a plan for improvement and further development. Sometimes this section may articulate new or expanded responsibilities in an effort for advancement in one's role and ultimately a promotion to another level.

—Signatures and comments section confirming that the performance review has been completed and the involved parties are clear on its content and plan for near future activities.

■ The performance review is not a once a year type activity. Often it happens informally (i.e., may not always be documented) throughout the year and on a regular basis and once per year it is formally documented and includes advancement decisions and incentive planning and confirmation. It is important to for the case management leader to provide feedback to the case management team members on an ongoing basis and not just annually. The feedback must also reflect what is going well as well as areas for improvement.

Guide for a Case Manager's Competency-Based Performance Appraisal

Role Dimension	Relative Weight[1]	Key Performance Area[2]	Performance Expectations[3]	Performance Level Achieved[4]	Comments
Clinical/Client Care Management	30% 0.3	1. Appraises the need for case management services through gathering and evaluation of relevant assessment data. 2. 3. 4.	• Assess client's condition to identify suitability for case management services. • Evaluates the client based on the selection criteria for case management. • Seeks the client's consent for the services to be provided and discusses goals of care.	Level: 3 Subscore: ___ 3 x 0.3 = 0.9	
Managerial and Leadership	10% 0.1	1. Advocates for clients through effective partnership with clients, their families, payer representatives, and healthcare team members. 2. 3.	• Establishes an effective relationship with client, family, care giver, and healthcare team. • Communicates with providers and payers important information in a timely manner; obtains authorizations for care. • Facilitates and maintains client's autonomy in decision making.	Level: 2 Subscore: ___ 2 x 0.10 = 0.2	
Discharge and Transitional Planning	20% 0.2	1. Assesses client for readmission risk using the readmission risk assessment upon admission and before discharge. 2. 3. 4.	• Completes timely assessment of client for post-discharge needs and transfer or discharge to most appropriate care setting. • Coordinates post-discharge needs and services with external vendors and service agents. • Prepares client and family for discharge assuring appropriate self-management skills and health knowledge.	Level: 3 Subscore: ___ 3 x 0.2 = 0.6	
Utilization Management and Financial or Business	20% 0.2	1. Applies medical necessity criteria in the evaluation and designation of level of care. 2. 3. 4.	• Prevents duplication or fragmentation of services or use of unnecessary resources. • Seeks authorizations for specific services and prevents service denials. • Procures, coordinates, and facilitates appropriate allocation of resources based on client's needs.	Level: 2 Subscore: ___ 2 x 0.2 = 0.4	
Information Management and Communication	15% 0.15	1. Integrates the quality, safety, efficiency, and cost-effectiveness principles into outcomes management. 2. 3.	• Establishes measureable clinical, financial, and quality of care goals and outcomes. • Identifies and manages variances and care delays. • Maintains open communication with the client/family and members of the interdisciplinary healthcare team. • Collects value-based purchasing related data; prepares core measure reports; disseminates reports to key personnel.	Level: 3 Subscore: ___ 3 x 0.15 = 0.45	
Professional Development and Advancement	5% 0.05	1. Maintains a competitive professional status and involves self in professional activities including specialty certification. 2. 3.	• Maintains membership in professional organizations. • Participates in regional or national taskforce in areas of professional practice and health policy. • Applies appropriate research evidence in practice. • Participates as a speaker at regional or national conferences. • Writes and publishes to contribute to knowledge for practice.	Level: 2 Subscore: ___ 2 x 0.05 = 0.1	

Total Score = 2.75 (275)
Maximum Score = 3 (300)

[1] The total relative weight per dimension and must be distributed among the key performance areas appropriate to each dimension.
[2] These are only examples. Other more detailed expectations must be developed depending on the job description and the practice setting.
[3] These are only examples. Others may be added depending on the job description. For example, if there are four performance areas in the clinical/client care management dimension, the total relative weight for the four areas must equal 0.4.
[4] Performance level achieved applies the same scale the healthcare organization uses for all personnel. In this example a three-point scale is used.

1 = does not meet expectations; 2 = meets expectations; 3 = exceeds expectations. To calculate the subscore per domain, multiply the level rating given for the domain by the relative weight assigned to the domain. To determine the overall rating, add the performance levels achieved for each domain: this should not always range between one and three since the rating scale consists of three points, three being the maximum while one is the minimum.

Index

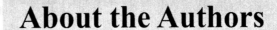

About the Authors

Toni Cesta

Toni G. Cesta, Ph.D., RN, FAAN is Partner and Health Care Consultant in Case Management Concepts, LLC, a consulting company which assists institutions in designing, implementing and evaluating acute care and community case management models, new documentation systems, and other strategies for improving care and reducing cost.

The author of nine books, and a frequently sought after speaker, lecturer and consultant, Dr. Cesta is considered one of the primary thought leaders in the field of case management.

Dr. Cesta writes a monthly column called *Case Management Insider* in the Hospital Case Management journal in which she shares insights and information on current issues and trends in case management.

Prior to her current work as a case management consultant, Dr. Cesta was Senior Vice President—Operational Efficiency and Capacity Management at Lutheran Medical Center in Brooklyn, New York. She was responsible for case management, social work, discharge planning, utilization management, denial management, bed management, the patient navigator program, the clinical documentation improvement program and systems process improvement. Prior to her position as Senior Vice President at Lutheran Medical Center, Dr. Cesta has held positions as Corporate Vice President for Patient Flow Optimization at the North Shore—Long Island Jewish Health System and Director of Case Management, Saint Vincents Catholic Medical Centers of New York, in New York City and also designed and implemented a Master's of Nursing in Case Management Program and Post-Master's Certificate Program in Case Management at Pace University in Pleasantville, New York. Dr. Cesta completed seven years as a Commissioner for the Commission for Case Manager Certification.

Dr. Cesta has been active in the research and development of case management for over 25 years. Her research in case management has included two funded studies measuring the effects of a case management model on congestive heart failure and fractured hip patient populations, with measures of patient satisfaction, quality of life, and short and long term clinical perceptions and outcomes.

Dr. Cesta has presented topics on case management at national and international conferences and workshops. Her books include *Nursing Case Management: From Essentials to Advanced Practice Applications*, *The Case Manager's Survival Guide: Winning Strategies for Clinical Practice*, *Survival Strategies for Nurses in Managed Care* and *Core Skills for Hospital Case Managers*.

Dr. Cesta is Consulting Editor of "Hospital Case Management Journal" and "Discharge Planning Advisor". In addition, she serves as editorial advisory board member of several case management journals and publications including *Strategies for Healthcare Excellence* and *The Journal of Care Management*.

Dr. Cesta has a BS in Biology from Wagner College, a BS in Nursing from Adelphi University, an MA in Nursing Administration from New York University, and a Ph.D. in Nursing Research and Theory Development from New York University.

Dr. Cesta is a Fellow of the American Academy of Nursing. Among her awards are included the "Nursing Service Administration Award" from the New York State Nurses Association, the Jessie M. Scott Award for excellence in research, practice and education from the American Nurses Association, and three "Book of the Year" awards from the *American Journal of Nursing*. In 2010, she was awarded the Brooklyn Leaders Award from the Arthritis Foundation.

Hussein M. Tahan, PhD, RN

Hussein M. Tahan, PhD, RN, is the system vice president for nursing professional development and workforce planning for MedStar Health. He is responsible for developing a strategic vision and action plan for the professional development of nursing associates across the organization, and implementing a workforce planning model that allows leaders to forecast the organization's need for nursing talent. Tahan works collaboratively with MedStar's senior vice president and chief nursing officer, and entity chief nursing officers to drive innovation in these areas of responsibility. He serves as an executive liaison to the MedStar Nursing Professional Development Council and offers nursing input for system initiatives.

Hussein has more than 25 years of experience in acute-care nursing, having worked in a variety of settings and healthcare systems. Prior to joining MedStar in December 2014, he was corporate director of Nursing Research and Education at New York-Presbyterian Hospital, New York, where he led a team of professionals engaged in the training and education of more than 6,000 nurses, implemented the use of innovative learning technologies, developed an evidence-based practice (EBP) framework for practical application by the clinical nurse at the bedside, and oversaw the work of collaborative governance councils in the areas of nursing education and EBP/Research. Additionally, Hussein led the implementation of workforce measures and reporting for Nursing across the hospital. He also chaired the executive committee on care management program redesign with special focus on care transformation. While at the New York-Presbyterian Hospital, Hussein held a number of leadership roles including director of Nursing, Cardiovascular Services, Care Coordination, and executive director of International Health Services.

Hussein holds a Doctor of Philosophy in nursing from Columbia University, a Master of Science in nursing administration from the College of Mount St. Vincent, both in New York, and a Bachelor of Science in nursing from the American University of Beirut in Lebanon. His scholarly activities include a strong publication, presentation and research record in the area of case management, care coordination and transitions of care. He co-authored four textbooks, two of which received the *American Journal of Nursing* Book of the Year Award.

Hussein has served on various national panels pertaining to nursing/patient care and quality, including the National Quality Forum Care Coordination Technical Advisory Panel, the GE Healthcare/Monitoring Solutions Consumer Advisory Board, the Agency for Healthcare Research and Quality peer review panel on Comparative Effectiveness of Case Management for Adults with Medical Illness and Complex Care Needs, and the Center for Medicare and Medicaid Innovation Bundled Payment Demonstration Projects peer review committee. Hussein serves currently on the editorial advisory board of the *Professional Case Management* and *CMSA Today* journals, as knowledge editor of the *Case Management Body of Knowledge Peer-Reviewed Web Portal* sponsored by the Commission for Case Manager Certification, and is a peer reviewer for the *Lippincott Williams and Wilkins, Journal of Nursing Administration*, and *Nursing Outlook*. In 2013, Nursing Outlook recognized Tahan with a "Certificate of Excellence in Reviewing."

Tahan is a member of the American Organization of Nurse Executives, American Nurses Association, Case Management Society of America, the National Transitions of Care Coalition, The Association for Nursing Professional Development, and elected fellow of the New York Academy of Medicine.